PCR *in situ* Hybridization
Protocols and Applications

Third Edition

PCR *in situ* Hybridization
Protocols and Applications

Third Edition

Gerard J. Nuovo, M.D.
Director, MGN Medical Research Laboratories
Setauket, New York

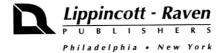
Lippincott - Raven
PUBLISHERS
Philadelphia • New York

Printed in the United States of America

9 8 7 6 5 4 3 2 1

Library of Congress Cataloging-in-Publication Data
Nuovo, Gerard J.
   PCR *in situ* hybridization: protocols and applications/Gerard J. Nuovo.
   p. cm.
   Includes bibliographical references and index.
   ISBN   0–397–58749–X
   1. Polymerase chain reaction.   2. In situ hybridization.   3. Cytodiagnosis.
   4. Papillomavirus infections—Cytodiagnosis.   5. HIV infections—Cytodiagnosis.
   I. Title.
RB43.8.P64N86   1996
616.07'582—dc20

                                                                    96-25449
                                                                        CIP

Contents

Preface

Interactions between the surgical pathologist and the molecular biologist have been somewhat limited for several reasons. Training in molecular biology for the pathologist may be limited to a few lectures in medical school. Few molecular biologists have the occasion to study in-depth microscopic analyses of tissues. Furthermore, some of the frequently used procedures of molecular biology, such as Southern blot hybridization and the polymerase chain reaction (PCR), do not allow for the direct correlation of the molecular analysis with the cytopathology and histopathology of the sample. *In situ* hybridization has helped to bridge this gap, but its relatively low sensitivity when compared to other methodologies, especially PCR, has somewhat limited its usefulness.

The methodology for detecting amplified DNA and cDNA in intact cells has now been available for over five years. I strongly believe that the technique is much easier to perform now than 2 to 3 years ago. Many groups have published protocols for *in situ* PCR. This has allowed for direct comparisons of different techniques, which helps one determine which variables are essential for successful PCR within an intact cell. Perhaps most important, we now understand a great deal more about the chemistry of PCR as it occurs within an intact cell. Such data form the basis of Chapters 3, 6, and 7. Although much of this understanding involves optimizing target-specific amplification, the wealth of information that now exists on the nonspecific pathways of PCR, both in solution phase and *in situ*, has made it possible for us to manipulate the conditions for our benefit during *in situ* PCR, as stressed in Chapters 3 and 6. Finally, the instrumentation is now becoming as sophisticated as the technology. Several companies now market machines for *in situ* PCR. The machine from Perkin-Elmer Corporation will allow one to do at least 10 slides at a time and eliminate the need for mineral oil.

One feature of PCR *in situ* hybridization that I have found very exciting over the last five years is the concomitant increased interaction between the surgical pathologist and the molecular biologist, as each need the other's specific expertise to do the methodology and interpret the results. I sincerely believe that such interactions will greatly enhance the study of many areas, such as oncogenesis and the dynamics of infectious diseases, that are now extensively studied by PCR.

A most fascinating and exciting aspect of *in situ* PCR is the realization that one is synthesizing DNA inside a cell. A given tissue section may contain over 100,000 cells. Thus, one could argue that the most incredible accomplishment of *in situ* PCR is the ability to perform tens of thousands of separate PCR reactions in an area less that 1 μm in size!

There are some important differences between PCR in a 50 μl volume in a GeneAmp tube and PCR in a cell of 4 to 20 μm in diameter, which has less than 1,000th of the volume. There are two obvious physical differences. First, there is the marked difference in the surface-to-volume ratio. In a 0.5 μl tube, the ratio of the surface area to volume is about 1:2. With *in situ* PCR, assuming one uses a coverslip of 10 mm and a volume of 10 μl, the surface-to-volume ratio is over 20 times greater. The second difference is that the contents of the amplifying solution in solution phase PCR is mostly water, with relatively scanty amounts of DNA and even less amounts of proteins. With *in situ* PCR, the nucleus of a fixed cell is a relatively dense matrix of DNA, RNA, and proteins that, if the fixative is formalin, will be extensively cross-linked to form a complex, three-dimensional labyrinth. This nuclear skeleton is sometimes referred to as the *nuclear matrix*. The cytoplasm of the cell also consists of a complex, three-dimensional matrix that is composed of its skeleton, made primarily of the intermediate filaments, and a wide variety of other proteins and RNA. The cytoplasm also contains an interconnecting array of proteins, called the *endoplasmic reticulum,* that is involved in RNA and protein trafficking. The important concept is that the relatively dense and complex protein–nucleic acid matrix found in the cytoplasm and nucleus will require some critical differences in technique for successful *in situ* PCR versus solution phase PCR. However, it can also be exploited to serve as an anchor for the amplicon during *in situ* PCR to prevent its migration out of the cell. Finally, it will cause some important differences in the various DNA synthesis pathways that can be operative with *in situ* PCR versus solution phase PCR. The important ramifications of these differences are discussed at length in this book.

The purposes of this book are:

1. To provide the necessary theoretical framework of molecular biology and histology to understand the basics of *in situ* PCR
2. To provide an in-depth discussion of the different DNA synthesis pathways operating during *in situ* PCR
3. To provide in-depth protocols for standard *in situ* hybridization, solution phase PCR, PCR *in situ* hybridization (for DNA), and reverse transcriptase (RT) *in situ* PCR (for RNA)
4. To provide a simplified start-up protocol for *in situ* PCR
5. To provide an in-depth discussion of the applications of *in situ* hybridization, PCR *in situ* hybridization, and RT *in situ* PCR
6. To present an alternative to the aluminum boat method, specifically, the Perkin-Elmer *in situ* PCR thermal cycler 1000

It is my sincere hope that the accomplishment of these goals will allow anyone, despite the strengths and weaknesses of prior training, to master logically and relatively rapidly the *in situ* PCR technique, to experience the excitement of seeing a DNA or RNA sequence amplified within a cell easily recognized on morphologic grounds, and to realize that, in many cases, there may not be any other way to localize the target to that specific cell type.

I would like to end this preface by briefly expanding on point 5, specifically with regard to the application of HIV-1 detection. Not long ago, it was being argued that HIV-1 was the cause of AIDS due, in part, to the difficulty in detecting HIV-1 DNA in the target CD4 cell prior to the onset of AIDS. It is now considered a basic tenet of HIV-1 pathogenesis that HIV-1 infects billions of CD4 cells even prior to the development of AIDS. This key concept is the foundation for the marked shift in antiretroviral therapy to early and aggressive (multidrug) treatment. It is important to remember that the initial description of the massive, primarily latent infection of HIV-1 prior to the development of AIDS was made by PCR *in situ* hybridization in combination with RT *in situ* PCR. Indeed, Chapter 9 demonstrates the power of *in situ* PCR in the understanding of the sexual transmission of the virus, and the various serious manifestations of the infection, including lymph node infection and AIDS dementia.

Acknowledgments

Although every book represents the input and assistance of many people, it is particularly true of this work. The group at Cetus Corporation, now Roche Molecular Systems, especially Drs. John Sninsky, Will Bloch, and Michele Manos, provided essential early technical, theoretical, and material assistance. Dr. Bloch played a major role in the theory and testing of the PCR hot start technique, which is the focus of Chapter 4 and was a major breakthrough for the PCR *in situ* technique. This Third Edition reflects many discussions and experiments conducted with the superior assistance of John Atwood at Perkin-Elmer Corporation. I would also like to acknowledge the material and financial assistance of the Perkin-Elmer Corporation, which has also been very important for the work described in the book. Much of the *in situ* hybridization material is a direct offshoot of the superior work done by Drs. Susan Bromley and Dennis Groff of Oncor Corporation. Dr. Brian Holaway of Boehringer Mannheim was instrumental in helping with the direct labeling of amplified nucleotides, which is discussed at length in this book. I am especially indebted to Ms. Phyllis MacConnell. I have had the great pleasure to know and work with Ms. MacConnell from day one of my work with *in situ* PCR. Her expert technical assistance, which was instrumental in developing and testing the technique, is perhaps overshadowed only by her expert editorial assistance in all three editions of this book. Ms. Angella Forde, Frances Gallery, and Kim Rhatigan provided important technical expertise. I am much indebted to Dr. Naji Abumrad for his support of my work at SUNY/Stony Brook. I gratefully acknowledge the help of Dr. Roger Pomerantz with the studies on HIV-1. I will always be indebted to Drs. Christopher Crum and Saul Silverstein for assistance with my initial foray into molecular biology. I owe a very special thanks to two people who have been instrumental in the Third Edition of the book. Carl Odhner is responsible for upgrading many of the computer-generated graphics. Ms. Sandra Sue Otera is responsible for upgrading many of the photomicrographs. Both of these people are consummate professionals, and most of the improvements in the quality of the Third Edition are due to them. I also wish to thank my parents, Mr. James and Mrs. Mary Nuovo, for their support and my good, life-long friend, Mr. Bruce Parizo, whose support and personal example, during the good times and bad, have always meant a great deal to me. I would like to thank the kind people at the Finishing Touch for their professional and expert help with the color photographs, and Peter and Ron Morrell at Morrell Instruments for their technical expertise. Finally, perhaps the person most responsible for the research that led to this book, is Mr. Salim B. Lewis, president of the Lewis Foundation, whose financial support and personal example were and continue to be major motivating factors in my work.

PCR *in situ* Hybridization
Protocols and Applications

Third Edition

1

Introduction

Perhaps no technique has had a greater impact than the polymerase chain reaction (PCR) on the practice of molecular biology in the research laboratory, in diagnostics, and in forensic medicine. For example, a virus or a rearranged gene can be rapidly detected with this technique when only a few cells in a tissue sample contain the DNA sequence of interest (1–6). Furthermore, one can detect a few copies of mRNA, rapidly synthesize, clone, and sequence virtually any segment of DNA, or determine if a minute sample came from a particular criminal suspect.

Despite the incredible power of the PCR there has been one major limitation since its discovery in 1985. It was not possible to correlate PCR results with the pathological features of tissue, because preparation for the PCR required that the DNA or RNA be extracted from the sample. In many cases it would be extremely useful to be able to identify the particular cell containing the DNA or cDNA sequence being amplified. For example, when human immunodeficiency virus type 1 (HIV-1) DNA is detected by PCR before the AIDS disease is apparent, what cell type is serving as the reservoir of latent infection, and what percentage of the target cells are harboring the virus (7–12)? Despite much interest in developing techniques, it has been difficult to answer these simple, yet very important questions. Only one to a few copies of HIV-1 DNA may be present in a cell, and this small number would likely escape detection by standard *in situ* hybridization methodology. Although quantitative PCR could provide some information about the amount of HIV-1 DNA

present in a person infected by the virus prior to the development of AIDS, it cannot reveal the specific cells that are infected and may not be accurate when analyzing relatively infrequent targets.

It is interesting to remember that just a few years ago there was a strong controversy about whether HIV-1 was the cause of AIDS. This controversy was centered on data provided by standard *in situ* hybridization and quantitative PCR that suggested that only about 1 in 10,000 of the target CD4 cells was infected in the asymptomatic period of infection. It was difficult to understand how such an apparent low infection rate was consistent with the hypothesis that HIV-1 actually was the cause of AIDS. *In situ* PCR was to demonstrate that, during the asymptomatic period of infection, on average about *1 in 3* of the CD4 cells in the lymph node was infected by HIV-1 and that the infection was primarily latent. About 1 in 20 of these HIV-1 proviral-containing cells was productively infected, which corresponds to *1 to 2 billion* actively infected cells in the asymptomatic individual. Clearly, this number supports the theory that AIDS is primarily a viral disease and underscores the need to direct therapy against viral replication; this is discussed in detail in Chapter 9.

Another example of the utility of *in situ* PCR can be seen when the HIV-1 virus and the Epstein-Barr virus (EBV) are both detected by PCR in an AIDS patient with lymphoma. Can these viruses be present in the same cell (13–16)? One can detect EBV with *in situ* hybridization by taking advantage of its ample synthesis of certain messages while in the latent state. However, regions of the EBV DNA frequently chosen as the target for *in situ* hybridization are usually present in 10 to 15 copies per infected cell and may be missed by standard *in situ* analysis. As noted above, the copy number of HIV-1 DNA per cell is usually too low to be detected by *in situ* hybridization. Using the PCR *in situ* hybridization technique, my colleague Joanne Becker and I have shown that EBV and HIV-1 infect different cell types in the tissues of people with AIDS lymphoma (17). It was also demonstrated that HIV-1 was absent in the lymphoma cells, whereas the detection rate of EBV in lymphoma cells varied considerably from case to case. Again, it can be argued that these observations could not have been made with any other methodology.

Of course, there are many other instances besides HIV-1 where the low copy number of the target may preclude its direct detection by standard *in situ* hybridization. Common examples include point mutations, latent or subclinical viral infection, and, in many instances, mRNAs as well as RNA viruses. One reason that RNA targets may be in copy numbers below the threshold of standard *in situ* hybridization is the amplification inherent in the synthesis of proteins from a given RNA. It will be demonstrated in this book that, by using reverse transcriptase (RT) *in situ* PCR, one can readily and reproducibly detect even low copy RNA targets.

Due to the extreme sensitivity of solution phase PCR there have been problems with sample contamination. If human papillomavirus (HPV) is detected in a cervical swab by PCR but not by a less sensitive test such as Southern blot hybridization, how can one be sure that the positive result does not represent contamination from another woman's sample or from viral DNA present in the laboratory (18–21)? The serious nature of this potential problem is underscored by the fact that cervical HPV-related infection is a sexually transmitted disease, and thus a positive diagnosis can have severe emotional implications for the patient. In spite of the employment of careful laboratory practices and the availability of several excellent PCR-related methods to limit contamination

(22–25), those who use this technique know that the problem may occur now and then, usually at the most inopportune times.

An important strength of the *in situ* PCR is its natural resistance to sample contamination. This methodology offers a built-in check for contamination based on an expected localization of the target within specific cell types or cell components and an apparent inherent prevention of contamination within the reaction due to a migration barrier effect. Under precisely defined conditions, including the use of a cross-linking fixative and optimal protease digestion time, there is striking limitation of migration of the PCR product. This containment of product can be seen in the distinct variety of cytoplasmic patterns for different human and viral RNAs detected by RT *in situ* PCR and in the exclusively nuclear-based signal for a DNA target of *in situ* PCR (Fig. 1-1). Although the biochemical basis for this migration barrier is presently unclear, "inhibition of migration" of the *in situ* PCR product appears to be effective in reverse, that is, from the amplifying solution into the cell. We added microgram amounts of labeled DNA to the amplifying solution, performed *in situ* PCR, and, after a high stringency wash, did not observe this labeled DNA to be present in the cells that lacked the corresponding target. This phenomenon is discussed at length later in the book. For now, suffice it to say that, under the proper conditions, one will not get a false-positive signal with *in situ* PCR due to influx of labeled PCR product from the amplifying solution to the cell.

The technique whereby the extreme sensitivity of PCR is combined with the cell-localizing ability of *in situ* hybridization is described. Why did it take 5 years to develop the technique to amplify DNA and cDNA in the nucleus or in the cytoplasm of intact cells after the initial discovery of PCR? *In situ* detection of amplified DNA in paraffin-embedded fixed cells and tissue has been problematic for several reasons. A method had to be developed to make target DNA available to the amplifying solution without destroying cell morphology. Optimal concentrations of the various amplifying reagents such as the primers, magnesium, and the DNA polymerase needed to be determined and, as is stressed throughout this book, may differ markedly with the optimal conditions for solution phase PCR. Perhaps the greatest operational difference between solution phase PCR and *in situ* PCR is that, although each may suffer from nonspecific pathways of DNA synthesis, primer oligomerization can greatly influence the specificity and sensitivity of solution phase PCR, whereas nonspecific DNA synthesis secondary to primer-independent pathways may predominate during *in situ* PCR. An anticipated problem that hindered the development of the *in situ* PCR was the belief that the amplified DNA would be poorly retained in the cell nucleus. Although this may be true in certain circumstances, such as when cells or tissues have been fixed in acetone or ethanol, migration of the PCR product can be made negligible during *in situ* PCR by the use of cross-linking type fixatives under well-defined conditions. In addition, if the reaction is to be carried out directly on glass slides, which has been a major goal of ours as this would allow the analysis of archival specimens, loss of tissue adherence and tissue drying must be circumvented (26–29).

The marriage of PCR and *in situ* hybridization has produced strange bedfellows. Many scientists expert at PCR view tissue as useful only after it is ground up and its nucleic acids extracted; microscopic examination is usually not on their list of research tools. On the other hand, many good histopathologists who have used *in situ* hybridization as an extension of their histologic analyses have at most dabbled in PCR and are not nearly as comfortable with primer oligomerization and mispriming as they are with nuclear atypia and squamous metaplasia. Assuming that the reader knows little about either PCR or *in situ* hybridization and cellular morphology, I would like to begin with a discussion of the basics of molecular biology with a focus on *in situ* hybridization. A new feature of the third edition is in Chapter 2, which is a brief review of the basics of histology for the nonpathologist to assist the basic researcher in the interpretation of *in situ*

hybridization analysis. The basics of PCR are presented for the nonmolecular biologist, assuming little prior knowledge of the subject. Although there are sections that may seem too basic for some readers, depending on their experiences, I hope that this approach will help to facilitate the collaboration of the basic researcher and the morphologist. Of course, those readers expert in a specific area such as PCR might wish to skim the basics of the molecular biology chapter and would probably be best served by focusing their attention on the theory and practice of *in situ* hybridization and *in situ* PCR. Nonetheless, I strongly believe that it is essential to stress both the basic biochemistry of PCR and the practical aspects of the histologic analysis of tissues for the scientist to get the maximum benefit from the use of *in situ* PCR. I hope that this goal will be achieved by including enough basic information about each topic.

After PCR *in situ* hybridization and RT *in situ* PCR techniques are described in detail, several chapters are devoted to a description of the application of these methodologies. The discussion of application focuses on the HPV virus and the HIV-1 virus, because they lend themselves well to a combination of molecular and cytological/histological analyses.

There are several other changes from the second edition of this book. A major addition is the protocol for one-step RT *in situ* PCR. This one-step procedure, based on the enzyme rTth, greatly simplifies the detection of RNA targets in cells. The second edition included much detail with regard to the theory of PCR *in situ* hybridization and RT *in situ* PCR. The third edition continues with a detailed and expanded discussion about the biochemistry of the DNA synthesis as it occurs within the nucleus or cytoplasm of a cell. I strongly believe that an in-depth description of the data and resultant hypotheses will assist readers, especially those with a basic science background, to understanding the rationale for the protocols presented in this book as well as in planning their own experiments to test some of the theories presented here. No doubt the reader will also gain a greater understanding of what

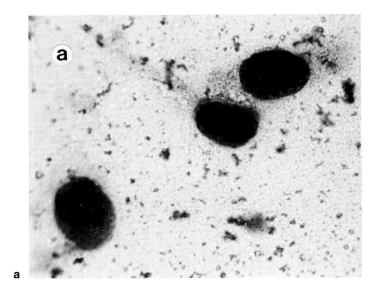

a

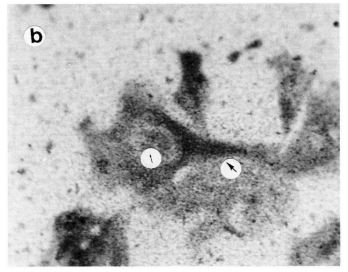

b

Figure 1-1. *Marked subcellular localization of the amplicon with RT* in situ *PCR after formalin fixation and optimal protease digestion.* The signal with *in situ* PCR for a DNA target (in this case, matrix metalloprotease-92 [(**MMP-9**)]) localizes to the nucleus with no apparent crossover to the cytoplasm (**a**). These are HT 1080 cells, derived from a sarcoma, which have ample, stellate cytoplasm that is not evident with the nuclear fast red counterstain. After DNase digestion and RT *in situ* PCR using primers specific for MMP-9, an intense cytoplasmic signal (*large arrow*) is evident (**b**); note the loss of the nuclear-based signal (*small arrow*). There are a variety of localizing patterns for different viral RNAs as evident after RT *in situ* PCR. For example, hepatitis C RNA localizes to part of the nuclear membrane (**c**). HIV-1 RNA is seen in the nucleus of scattered cells in this section of brain from a person who had AIDS dementia (**d**).

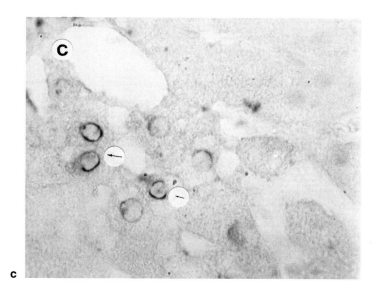

c

d

Figure 1-1. *Continued.*

is occurring at a molecular level in the cell during the PCR part of the process. The third edition describes several attempts to circumvent problems due to DNA repair, such as using labeled primers and different approaches to interfering with the primer-independent pathway, to allow for target-specific direct incorporation of the reporter system with *in situ* PCR. New data on other potential causes of background, or a false-positive signal, are presented in this third edition with recommendations on how to recognize and avoid these problems. To this end, the third edition now includes a section that discusses the most common problems I have seen with *in situ* PCR with recommendations on how to avoid them. I sincerely thank the many people who called and wrote me to share their *in situ* PCR problems, as this was instrumental in organizing this section on troubleshooting. I have also tried to streamline and simplify the techniques. The new data presented on primer oligomerization and oligoprobes versus full-length probes provides the theoretical basis, it is hoped, to demonstrate to the reader that these probes, which are much easier to use due to their much greater signal-to-background ratio, are the probes of choice for PCR *in situ* hybridization. Another addition to the appendix is a glossary. The part of the appendix that describes the various commercially available reagents and materials needed for PCR *in situ* hybridization has been expanded and includes the catalogue numbers of the products. Also new to the third edition are protocols and data for detection of bacterial nucleic acids by *in situ* PCR.

Many hands-on workshops since the second edition has further convinced me that there is a strong need to describe an *in situ* PCR start-up protocol for the beginner. For those with little actual experience using *in situ* PCR, I strongly suggest beginning with the start-up protocol. Although the signal generated with this protocol is nonspecific, its successful completion will demonstrate that the investigator is able to synthesize DNA inside the nucleus and detect the product. It has been my repeated experience that when this is mastered, target-specific detection by *in situ* PCR usually follows shortly thereafter.

Several of the chapters share some overlap of material. For example, the start-up protocol has many features in common with RT *in situ* PCR. I have included similar discussions of key topics in these chapters. This was done with the belief that it would be more convenient and less distracting for the reader to have key information available in each section without having to page through looking for a referenced figure or discussion.

Although the focus of this book is the process of *in situ* PCR including necessary fixation, reagents, and post-PCR conditions for successful PCR *in situ* hybridization and RT *in situ* PCR, another essential component of the methodology, especially with regard to its large-scale application, is the technology of the thermal cycling machine. To this end, Chapter 11 describes the thermal properties and performance characteristics of some innovative machinery developed by Perkin-Elmer Corporation for PCR *in situ* hybridization. In my opinion, the major advantage of the Perkin-Elmer *in situ* PCR thermal cycler 1000 is that it is much more user friendly than my aluminum boat method, which is described in Chapter 5. Workshops have demonstrated to me that initial success with *in situ* PCR, especially for the person with little experience with tissue sections or glass slides, occurs more quickly with the *in situ* PCR thermal cycler 1000. Early problems with bubbles, which created nonamplifying zones, have been solved.

It has been with a mixture of amazement and excitement that we have seen the further emergence of *in situ* PCR as a mainstream technique. To this end, I have included a list of publications using *in situ* PCR that have been published since the second edition. The list is growing rapidly and I apologize to any group whose paper I inadvertently omitted. The size of the list attests to the increasing use of this important tool in the research and diagnostic laboratory (30–85).

To conclude this introductory section, the objectives of the third edition are as follows:

1. To provide the necessary theoretical framework of molecular biology and histology to understand the basics of *in situ* PCR
2. To provide an in-depth discussion of the different DNA synthesis pathways operative during *in situ* PCR
3. To provide in-depth protocols for standard *in situ* hybridization, solution phase PCR, PCR *in situ* hybridization (for DNA) and RT *in situ* PCR (for RNA)
4. To provide a simplified start-up protocol for those beginning *in situ* PCR
5. To provide an in-depth discussion of the applications of *in situ* hybridization, PCR *in situ* hybridization, and RT *in situ* PCR, focusing on human papillomavirus, hepatitis C, human immunodeficiency virus type 1, and cytokine expression
6. To present an alternative to the aluminum boat method, specifically, the Perkin-Elmer *in situ* PCR thermal cycler 1000
7. To present a glossary, troubleshooting section, and list of reagents in the appendix

REFERENCES

1. Saiki RK, Gelfand DH, Stoffel S, et al. Primer-directed enzymatic amplification of DNA with a thermostable DNA polymerase. *Science* 1988;239:487–491.
2. Nuovo GJ: Human papillomavirus DNA in genital tract lesions histologically negative for condylomata: analysis by *in situ*, Southern blot hybridization and the polymerase chain reaction. *Am J Surg Pathol* 1990;14:643–651.
3. Lawyer FC, Stoffel S, Saiki RK, Myambo KB, Drummond R, Gelfand DH. Isolation, characterization, and expression in E. coli of the DNA polymerase gene from the extreme thermophile, Thermus aquaticus. *J Biol Chem* 1989;264:6427–6437.
4. Faloona F, Weiss S, Ferre F, Mullis K. Direct detection of HIV sequences in blood: high gain polymerase chain reaction. 6th Int Conf AIDS, San Francisco, CA (Abstract 1019).
5. Nuovo GJ, Darfler MM, Impraim CC, Bromley SE. Occurrence of multiple types of human papillomavirus in genital tract lesions: analysis by *in situ* hybridization and the polymerase chain reaction. *Am J Pathol* 1991;58:518–523.
6. Shibata DK, Arnheim N, Martin WJ. Detection of human papilloma virus in paraffin-embedded tissue using the polymerase chain reaction. *J Exp Med* 1988;167:225–230.
7. Chadwick EG, Yogev R, Kwok S, Sninsky JJ, Kellogg DE, Wolinsky SM. Enzymatic amplification of the human immunodeficiency virus in peripheral blood mononuclear cells from pediatric patients. *J Infect Dis* 1989;160:954–959.
8. Escaich S, Wallon M, Baginski I, et al. Comparison of HIV detection by virus isolation in lymphocyte cultures and molecular amplification of HIV DNA and RNA by PCR in offspring of seropositive mothers. *J AIDS* 1991;4:130–135.
9. Horsburgh CR, Ou C, Jason J, et al. Concordance of polymerase chain reaction with human immunodeficiency virus antibody detection. *J Infect Dis* 1990;162:542–545.
10. Genesca J, Wang RYH, Alter HJ, Shih JWK. Clinical correlation and genetic polymorphism of the immunodeficiency virus proviral DNA obtained after polymerase chain reaction amplification. *J Infect Dis* 1990;162:1025–1030.
11. Sninsky JJ, Kwok S. Detection of human immunodeficiency viruses by the polymerase chain reaction. *Arch Pathol Lab Med* 1990;114:259–262.
12. Ou CY, Kwok S, Mitchell SW, et al. DNA amplification for direct detection of HIV-1 in DNA of peripheral blood mononuclear cells. *Science* 1988;239:295–297.
13. Lusso P, DeMaria A, Malnati M, et al. Induction of CD4 and susceptibility to HIV-1 infection in human CD8+ T lymphocytes by human herpesvirus 6. *Nature* 1991;349:533–535.
14. Said JW. Lymphoreticular system. In: Nash G, Said JW, eds. *Pathology of AIDS and HIV infection.* Philadelphia: WB Saunders;35–60.
15. Knowles DM, Inghirami G, Ubriaco A. Molecular genetic analysis of three AIDS-associated neoplasms of uncertain lineage demonstrates their B-cell derivation and the possible pathogenetic role of the Epstein-Barr virus. *Blood* 1989;73:792–799.
16. Borisch-Chappuis B, Nezelof C, Muller H. Different Epstein-Barr virus expression in lymphomas from immunocompromised and immunocompetent patients. *Am J Pathol* 1990;136:751–758.
17. Becker J, Nuovo GJ. *In situ* detection of PCR-amplified EBV and HIV-1 nucleic acids in hyperplastic lymph nodes and lymphomas. *J Histochem Cytochem* 1996 *[in press].*
18. Bauer HM, Ting Y, Greer CE, et al. Genital human papillomavirus infection in female university students as determined by a PCR-based method. *JAMA* 1991;265:472–477.
19. Lorincz AT. Human papillomavirus testing. *Diagn Clin Test* 1989;27:28–37.
20. Tidy JA, Parry GCN, Ward P, et al. High rate of human papillomavirus type 16 infection in cytologically normal cervices. *Lancet* 1989;i:434.
21. Tidy J, Farrell PF. Retraction: Human papillomavirus subtype 16b. *Lancet* 1989;ii:1535.
22. Melchers WJG, Schift R, Stolz E, Lindeman J, Quint WGV. Human papillomavirus detection in urine samples from male patients by the polymerase chain reaction. *J Clin Microbiol* 1989;27:1711–1714.
23. van den Brule AJC, Meijer CJL, Bakels V, Kenemans P, Walboomers JMM. Rapid detection of human papillomavirus in cervical scrapes by combined general primer-mediated and type-specific polymerase chain reaction. *J Clin Microbiol* 1990;28:2739–2743.
24. Wright PA, Wynford-Thomas D. The polymerase chain reaction: miracle or mirage? *J Pathol* 1990;162:99–117.
25. Higuchi R, Kwok S. Avoiding false positives with PCR. *Nature* 1989;339:237–238.

26. Nuovo GJ, MacConnell P, Forde A, Delvenne P. Detection of human papillomavirus DNA in formalin fixed tissues by *in situ* hybridization after amplification by the polymerase chain reaction. *Am J Pathol* 1991;139:847–854.

27. Nuovo GJ, Gallery F, MacConnell P, Becker J, Bloch W. An improved technique for the detection of DNA by *in situ* hybridization after PCR-amplification. *Am J Pathol* 1991;139:1239–1244.

28. Nuovo GJ, Becker J, MacConnell P, Margiotta M, Comite S, Hochman H. Histological distribution of PCR-amplified HPV 6 and 11 DNA in penile lesions. *Am J Surg Pathol* 1992;16:269–275.

29. Haase AT, Retzel EF, Staskus KA. Amplification and detection of lentiviral DNA inside cells. *Proc Natl Acad Sci USA* 1990;87:4971–4975.

30. Nuovo GJ, Gorgone G, MacConnell P, Goravic P. *In situ* localization of human and viral cDNAs after PCR-amplification. *PCR Method Appl* 1992;2:117–123.

31. Nuovo GJ, Gallery F, MacConnell P. Analysis of the distribution pattern of PCR-amplified HPV 6 DNA in vulvar warts by *in situ* hybridization. *Mod Pathol* 1992;5:444–448.

32. Nuovo MA, Nuovo GJ, MacConnell P, Steiner G. Analysis of Paget's disease of bone for the measles virus using the reverse transcriptase *in situ* polymerase chain reaction technique. *Diagn Mol Pathol* 1993;1:256–265.

33. Nuovo GJ, Lidonocci K, MacConnell P, Lane B. Intracellular localization of PCR-amplified hepatitis C cDNA. *Am J Pathol* 1993;17:683–690.

34. Nuovo GJ, Gallery F, Hom R, MacConnell P, Bloch W. Importance of different variables for optimizing *in situ* detection of PCR-amplified DNA. *PCR Method Appl* 1993;2:305–312.

35. Chumas J, Nuovo GJ. Detection of human papillomavirus RNA in unusual variants of adenocarcinoma of the cervix. *J Histotech [in press]*.

36. Seidman R, Peress N, Nuovo GJ. *In situ* detection of PCR-amplified HIV-1 nucleic acids in skeletal muscle in patients with myopathy. *Mod Pathol* 1994;7:369–375.

37. Kelleher MB, Duggan TD, Galutira D, Nuovo GJ, Haegert D. Progressive multifocal leukoencephalopathy in a patient with Alzheimer's dementia. *Diagn Mol Pathol* 1994;3:105–113.

38. Nuovo GJ, Becker J, Simsir A, Margiotta M, Shevchuck M. *In situ* localization of PCR-amplified HIV-1 nucleic acids in the male genital tract. *Am J Pathol* 1994;144:1142–1148.

39. Lidonnici K, Lane B, Nuovo GJ. A comparison of serologic analysis and *in situ* localization of PCR-amplified cDNA for the diagnosis of hepatitis C infection. *Diagn Mol Pathol* 1995;4:98–107.

40. Bagasra O, Hauptman SP, Lischer HW, Sachs M, Pomerantz RJ. Detection of human immunodeficiency virus type 1 provirus in mononuclear cells by *in situ* polymerase chain reaction. *N Engl J Med* 1992;326:1385–1391.

41. Nuovo GJ, Margiotta M, MacConnell P, Becker J. Rapid *in situ* detection of PCR-amplified HIV-1 DNA. *Diagn Mol Pathol* 1992;1:98–102.

42. Nuovo GJ, Forde A, MacConnell P, Fahrenwald R. *In situ* detection of PCR-amplified HIV-1 nucleic acids and tumor necrosis factor cDNA in cervical tissues. *Am J Pathol* 1993;143:40–48.

43. Patterson BK, Till M, Otto P, et al. Detection of HIV-1 DNA and messenger RNA in individual cells by PCR-driven *in situ* hybridization and flow cytometry. *Science* 1993;260:976–979.

44. Embretson J, Zupancic M, Ribas JL, Racz P, Tenner-Racz T, Haase AT. Massive covert infection of helper T lymphocytes and macrophages by HIV during the incubation period of AIDS. *Nature* 1993;362:359–362.

45. Embretson J, Zupancic M, Beneke J, Ribas JL, Burke A, Haase AT. Analysis of human immunodeficiency virus infected tissues by amplification and *in situ* hybridization reveals latent and permissive infections at single cell resolution. *Proc Natl Acad Sci USA* 1993;90:357–361.

46. Nuovo GJ, Gallery F, MacConnell P, Braun A. *In situ* detection of PCR-amplified HIV-1 nucleic acids and tumor necrosis factor RNA in the central nervous system. *Am J Pathol* 1994;144:659–666.

47. Chiu KP, Cohen SH, Morris DW, Jordan GW. Intracellular amplification of proviral DNA in tissue sections using the polymerase chain reaction. *J Histochem Cytochem* 1992;40:333–341.

48. Nuovo GJ, Becker J, Margiotta M, Burke M, Fuhrer J, Steigbigel R. *In situ* detection of PCR-amplified HIV-1 nucleic acids in lymph nodes and peripheral blood in asymptomatic infection and advanced stage AIDS. *J AIDS* 1994;7:916–923.

49. Long AA, Komminoth P, Lee E, Wolfe HJ. Comparison of indirect and direct in-situ polymerase chain reaction in cell preparations and tissue sections. Detection of viral DNA, gene rearrangements and chromosomal translocations. *Histochemistry* 1993;99:151–162.

50. Embelton M, Gorochov J, Jones PT, Winter G. In cell mRNA: amplifying and linking rearranged immunoglobulin heavy and light chain V-genes within single cells. *Nucleic Acids Res* 1992;20:3831–3834.

51. Nuovo GJ, Gallery F, MacConnell P. Analysis of non-specific DNA synthesis during solution phase and *in situ* PCR. *PCR Method Appl* 1994;4:342–349.

52. Cheng J, Nuovo GJ. The utility of RT *in situ* PCR in the diagnosis of viral infections. *J Histotech* 1994;17:247–251.

53. Nuovo GJ. *The utility of PCR in situ hybridization for the detection of HIV-1 DNA and RNA.* New York:Plenum Press;1995;268–279.

54. Chow LH, Bubramanian S, Nuovo GJ, Miller F, Nord EP. Endothelial receptor expression in the renal medulla identified by *in situ* RT PCR. *Am J Physiol* 1995;269:449–457.

55. Nuovo GJ, MacConnell P, Valea F, French DL. Correlation of the *in situ* detection of PCR-amplified metalloprotease cDNAs and their inhibitors with prognosis in cervical carcinoma. *Cancer Res* 1995;55:267–275.

56. Gruber BL, Sorbi D, French DL, Marchese MJ, Nuovo GJ, Arbeit LA. Elevated circulating MMP-9 (gelatinase B) in rheumatoid arthritis. *Arthritis Rheum [in press]*.

57. Dubrovsky L, Ulrich P, Nuovo GJ, Manogue KR, Cerami A, Burkinsky M. Nuclear localization signal of HIV-1 as a novel target for therapeutic intervention. *Mol Med* 1995;1:217–230.

58. Brandwein M, Biller H, Nuovo GJ. Histologic distribution of EBV DNA in hairy leukoplakia: a study by *in situ* PCR. *Mod Pathol* 1996;9:298–303.

59. Nuovo GJ, Preissner M, Bronson R. Vitronectin expression in the male genital tract. *Mol Hum Reprod* 1995;10:2187–2191.

60. Yoo BJ, Selby MJ, Choe J, et. al. Transfection of a differentiated human hepatoma cell line (Huh7) with in vitro transcribed hepatitis C Virus (HCV) RNA and establishment of a long term culture persistently infected with HCV. *J Virol* 1995;69:32–38.

61. Nuovo GJ, Forde A. An improved system for reverse transcriptase *in situ* PCR. *J Histotech* 1995;18:295–299.

62. Galanakis D, Nuovo GJ, Spitzer S, Kaplan C. Demonstration of fibrinogen mRNA in human trophoblasts by reverse transcriptase PCR *in situ*. *Thrombosis Res* 1996;81:263–269.

63. Nuovo GJ, Simsir A, Steigbigel R, Kuschner M. Rapid detection of hantavirus infection in tissue sections by reverse transcriptase *in situ* PCR. *Am J Pathol* 1996;148:685–692.

64. Schmidtmayerova H, Notte HS, Nuovo GJ, et al. HIV-1 infection alters chemokine β peptide expression in human monocytes: implications for recruitment of leukocytes into brain and lymph nodes. *Proc Natl Acad Sci USA [in press]*.

65. McHugh RW, Hazen P, Eliezri Y, Nuovo GJ. Human papillomavirus type 35 DNA in a periungual squamous cell carcinoma and axillary lymph node metastases. *Arch Dermatol [in press]*.

66. Nuovo GJ. Current concepts in pathologic diagnoses: viral diseases. *J Histotech* 1995;18(Spec. Iss.):475–483.

67. Nuovo GJ. PCR *in situ* hybridization. In: Wiedbrauk DL, Farkas DH, eds. *Molecular Methods for Viral Detection*. San Diego: Academic Press; 1995:237–259.

68. Simsir S, Nuovo GJ. PCR and RT PCR *in situ* hybridization: applications in viral detection. *Trends Biotechnol* 1995;11:13–23.

69. Nuovo GJ. The theoretical framework of *in situ* PCR. In: Nuovo GJ, Leursen K, eds. *Methods: companion to methods in enzymology. [in press]*.

70. Kransnokvtsky S, Khan A, Nuovo GJ. The utility of *in situ* PCR for the study of human papillomavirus-related diseases. In: Nuovo GJ and Leursen K, eds. *Methods: companion to methods in enzymology: [in press]*.

71. Steigbigel R, Nuovo GJ. New insights into HIV-1 pathogenesis as determined by *in situ* PCR. In: Nuovo GJ and Leursen K, eds. *Methods: companion to methods in enzymology [in press]*.

72. Bagasra O, Pomerantz RJ. HIV-1 provirus is demonstrated in peripheral blood monocytes in vivo: a study utilizing *in situ* PCR. *AIDS Res Hum Retroviruses* 1993;9:69–76.

73. Bagasra O, Sheshamma T, Pomeranz R. Polymerase chain reaction *in situ*: intracellular amplification and detection of HIV-1 proviral DNA and other specific genes. *J Immunol Methods* 1993;158:131–145.

74. Chen RH, Fuggle SV. *In situ* cDNA polymerase chain reaction. A novel technique for detecting mRNA expression. *Am J Pathol* 1993;143:1527–1534.

75. Gosden J, Hanratty D. PCR *in situ*: A rapid alternative to *in situ* hybridization for mapping short, low copy number sequences without isotopes. *Biotechniques* 1993;15:78–80.

76. Heniford BW. Variation in cellular EGF receptor mRNA expression demonstrated by *in situ* RT polymerase chain reaction. *Nucleic Acids Res* 1993;3159–3166.

77. Komminoth P, Long AA. Evaluation of methods for hepatitis C virus detection in liver biopsies: comparisons of histology, immunohistochemistry, *in situ* hybridization, and *in situ* PCR. *Pathol Res Pract* 1994;190:1017–1025.

78. Martinez A, Cuttitta F. Non radioactive localization of nucleic acids by *in situ* PCR and *in situ* RT PCR in paraffin embedded sections. *J Histochem Cytochem* 1995;43:739–747.

79. Metha A. Detection of herpes simplex virus sequences in the trigeminal ganglia of latently infected mice by and *in situ* PCR method. *Cell Vision* 1994;1:110–115.

80. O'Leary JJ. Importance of fixation procedures on DNA template and its suitability for solution phase PCR and PCR *in situ* hybridization. *Histochem J* 1994;26:337–346.

81. Patel V, Heniford B, Weiman T, Hendler F. Detection of epidermal growth factor receptor mRNA in tissue sections from biopsy specimens using *in situ* PCR. *Am J Pathol* 1994;144:7–14.

82. Pestaner C, Bibbo M, Seshamma T, Bagasra O. Potential of the *in situ* PCR reaction in diagnostic cytology. *Acta Cytol* 1994;38:676–680.

83. Sallstrom J, Alemi M, Wilander E. Pitfalls of *in situ* PCR using direct incorporation of labeled nucleotides. *Anticancer Res* 1993;13:1153–1155.

84. Teo IA, Shaunak S. PCR *in situ*: an appraisal of an emerging technique. *Histochem J* 1995;27:647–659.

85. Ueki K, Richardson EP, Louis DN. *In situ* PCR demonstration of JC virus in progressive multifocal leukoencephalopathy, including an index case. *Annals Neurol* 1994;36:670–673.

2

The Basics of Molecular Biology and Histologic Analysis

MOLECULAR BIOLOGY

Terminology

Any specialty has its own jargon, and molecular biology is no different. It is essential to understand terms such as *probe*, *hybridization*, *homology*, and *stringency* if one wants to perform or critically analyze studies based on molecular biology. The first part of this chapter introduces such terms and describes the different tests based on the principles of molecular biology. As noted in the Introduction, the material is presented at a basic level, assuming no or minimal prior knowledge of the topic. Thus, this part of the chapter may be of more interest to the anatomic pathologist; the PhD or the person with a solid background in molecular biology may wish to skim or simply skip this section. A more advanced discussion of PCR and the various nonspecific pathways that can compete with target-specific amplification is provided in Chapter 3. The second part of this chapter is for the nonpathologist and provides the basics of how to distinguish the different cell types that may be present in a given tissue section.

Nucleic Acid Sequence

The central foci of molecular biology are the *nucleic acids* RNA and DNA. Each is composed of four separate building blocks called *nucleotides*. The bases that give the nucleotides their specificity for RNA include adenine, guanine, cytosine, and uracil; for DNA, uracil is re-placed by thymine. The nucleotides consist of the base and a triphosphate group each attached to a 5-carbon sugar (see Fig.2-2b); the ribose sugar lacks the 2′ OH group in DNA, hence the term *deoxynucleic acid*. The nucleotides are connected to each other to form a chain-like arrangement that comprises its *sequence* (Fig. 2-1). The linkage between any two nucleotides is formed by the complexing of a phosphate group on carbon 5 with the OH group on carbon 3 via a phosphodiester bond, yielding pyrophosphate. Dideoxynucleotides, which are discussed later in the book, can terminate DNA synthesis, as they lack the OH group on carbon 3. That is, although the phosphate group on carbon 5 of a dideoxynucleotide can form a phosphodiester bond with the OH group on carbon 3 of the last nucleotide that was added to the growing DNA chain, the absence of an OH group on its carbon 3 prevents the formation of a phosphodiester linkage with another free nucleotide.

RNA is composed of a single strand, whereas DNA is composed of two paired strands. For the paired strands to match up, they must face each other in the opposite or complementary direction. The complementary strands of DNA are kept together primarily by the *hydrogen bonds* that form between the bases adenine (A) and thymine (T) (two bonds) and cytosine (C) and guanine (G) (three bonds) (Fig. 2-2a and b). It is this specific hydrogen bonding between the *matched base pairs* A and T (or, for RNA hybridization as it occurs in laboratory assays, A and U) and C and G that is the foundation of all molecular biological tests. Indeed, it can be

Nucleotide

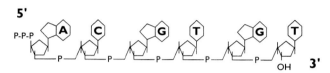

Sequence

Figure 2-1. *The sequence of single-stranded DNA.* The building block of DNA and RNA is the nucleotide, which consists of a 5-carbon sugar attached to a triphosphate group (on carbon 5), an OH group (on carbon 3), and a base (on carbon 1). RNA has an OH group on carbon 2 that DNA lacks (hence, deoxyNTP). The single-stranded DNA molecule is composed of four different nucleotides that differ by the base attached to carbon 1. The nucleotides are linked via a phosphodiester bond. Note that the triphosphate group is located at the 5' end of the strand whereas the free OH group is at the 3' end.

argued that the base pair matching between two complementary nucleic acid strands is the *most* important concept in the entire field of molecular biology. Although a single *base pair* match of A–T or C–G would separate easily, there is strength in numbers. The more base pair matches there are, the greater the number of hydrogen bonds that will form between the two DNA strands and the less likely the strands will separate. Note that the figures represent the two ends of each DNA strand as having a triphosphate group (on carbon 5) and a hydroxyl group (on carbon 3), respectively, as discussed above. These groups define the 5′ and 3′ ends of DNA. This arrangement is the basis of DNA synthesis in general and PCR in particular as the triphosphate group of a single nucleotide will invariably be linked with the 3′ OH group of the growing chain via the phosphodiester bond. The OH group at carbon 3 of the single nucleotide *cannot* form a phosphodiester bond with the one triphosphate group at the 5′ end of the single-stranded DNA molecule, as is discussed later in this chapter.

Hybridization of Nucleic Acid Strands

When two DNA strands meet, they orient each other in opposite or antiparallel directions to allow base pair matching to occur. If there are no base pair matches, the strands will not join together. However, if there are sufficient base pair matches the strands will join together or *hybridize.* The specific term used to describe the degree of base pair matching that determines whether the strands stay together is *homology.* How much homology is needed for two strands to stay together? Although it is true that "the more, the better," another important variable is how close the base pair matches are to one other. Adjacent base pair matches in a sequence will hold together more strongly than the same number of base pair matches widely dispersed over the DNA sequence (Fig. 2-3). Adjacent base pair matches are common between related DNA sequences such as the myoglobin gene of humans and chimpanzees. They rarely occur as a random event between two dissimilar DNA sequences. This selectivity con-

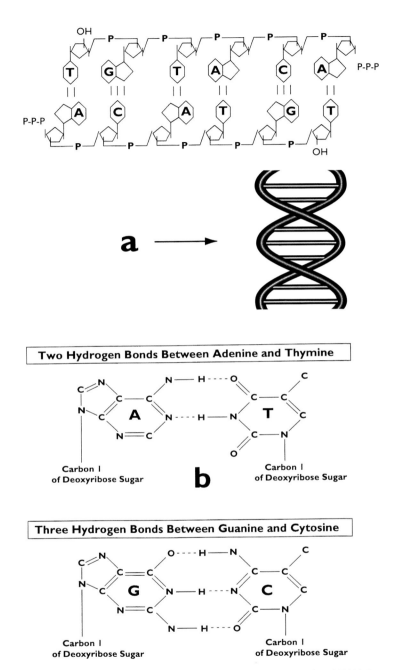

Figure 2-2. *The formation of double-stranded DNA.* **a:** Two single strands of DNA in opposite orientations are linked by the hydrogen bonds that form between the complementary base pairs GC and AT. This leads to the helical structure of the double-stranded molecule. **b:** Two hydrogen bonds form between A and T compared with three hydrogen bonds that form between G and C. The increased strength of the GC base pair match can facilitate nonspecific binding of single-stranded DNA to itself or to other single-stranded molecules. This may be one mechanism of nonspecific binding during filter hybridization or, more importantly, PCR, as discussed in Chapter 3.

tributes greatly to the high specificity of the molecular-based tests. This is especially important when one considers that in a given hybridization reaction between homologous DNA sequences there will be hundreds of base pairs available for hybridization. For example, human papillomavirus (HPV) DNA contains about 8,000 base pairs, and one can easily construct labeled HPV DNA that comprises the entire 8,000 base pair region. It is amazing to realize that the probability would be 1 in 65,536 that even eight sequential base pairs in a nonhomologous (e.g., human) DNA sequence would be homologous to an eight base pair stretch in the HPV DNA. An eight base pair region of homology would not be adequate to keep the DNA complex hybridized at room temperature, and this would only have 1:1,000 the degree of base pair matching of the homologous HPV DNA probe–target hybridized complex! As discussed later, the completely homologous HPV hybridized complex would easily remain hybridized at temperatures over 70°C, whereas the rarer, more dispersed HPV–human hybridized complexes would dissociate at this temperature, assuring us target-specific detection of HPV. To continue with this example, this is not to say that HPV–human DNA hybrids cannot potentially cause false-positive results due to persistent hybridization under certain conditions. The important point is that these conditions can be controlled to favor highly homologous DNA hybrids and to disfavor poorly homologous hybrids.

There will be times, especially during PCR, when much smaller DNA hybrids, usually around 20 base pairs, will be generated. Under these conditions, a few base pair mismatches may make the difference between hybridization and separation. Hydrogen bonds are the glue that keeps two hybridized strands together, and many chemicals and other conditions can effect hydrogen bonding. The term *stringency* describes hybridization reaction conditions that relatively favor or disfavor hydrogen bonding. Because this is a key term, let us illustrate it with an example. Let us assume that three DNA molecules, each 10 base pairs long, share variable homology—one base pair match, five base pair matches, and, finally, complete homology of ten base pair matches (Figs. 2-4 to 2-6). The

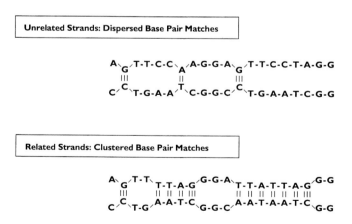

Figure 2-3. *Variable base pair matching between related and unrelated hybridized DNA strands.* Base pair matches, the primary force that keeps hybridized DNA together, are more effective as such if they are clustered close to one another. In closely related DNA molecules, such as the same gene from two closely related species, the base pair matches are typically closely grouped. Conversely, the base pair matches between unrelated DNA strands, such as HPV 6 and a comparably sized strand of human DNA, tend to be more widely dispersed. This facilitates the detection of the related sequences, because they are more likely to remain hybridized during the detection process compared with the random, more dispersed grouping shown at the top of this figure.

small number of base pairs is being used for illustrative purposes to show that the important concept is the relative percentage of base pair matching. Under low stringency conditions the strands with 10% homology will separate (Fig. 2-4). The hybridized strands with 50% and 100% homology remain together at low stringency (Figs. 2-5, 2-6). These three figures show the effects of different homologies on hybridized DNA complexes with varying stringencies. Note how increased stringency will disrupt the hydrogen bonds between some base pair matches. If enough base pair matches stay intact, then the complex remains hybridized; otherwise, it denatures. Note that some base pairs are disrupted as one goes to low stringency conditions (e.g., from room temperature to 45°C). Sufficient base pair matches remain to keep the hybridized strands with 50% and 100% homology together. However, if one adds a chemical such as formamide that may further disrupt the hydrogen bonds, there may not be sufficient remaining bonds to keep the strands with 50% homology together though sufficient hydrogen

bonding persists in the strands with complete homology to keep them hybridized (Figs. 2-5, 2-6). This change in conditions that disfavors hydrogen bonds and thus demands more homology for nucleic acid strands to remain hybridized is referred to as increasing the *stringency* of the reaction or, more commonly, as *high stringency.*

Another term that reflects hydrogen bonding is referred to as the *melting temperature* or (*Tm*). If paired strands of DNA that share homology are hybridized, at any given time some of the strands will remain hybridized whereas others will have separated. This separation is referred to as *denaturation*. The *Tm* or melting temperature is defined as that temperature under the specific reaction conditions where one-half of the hybridized strands are still hybridized and the other half are denatured (Fig. 2-7). The ratio of hybridized to denatured DNA strands will vary depending on the degree of homology, as well as on any condition that may affect hydrogen bonding such as formamide concentration or temperature. The concentration of salt will

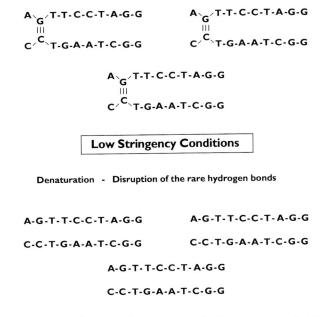

Figures 2-4 to 2-6. *The effects of varying homology and stringency on hybridized DNA complexes.* **Figure 2-4.** The 10% homology between the two strands is not sufficient to support hybridization even under low stringency conditions.

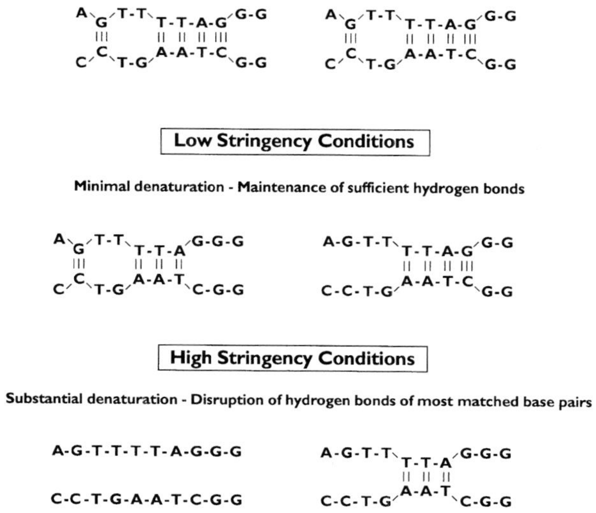

A‑G‑T‑T ‑T‑T‑A‑G ‑G‑G
C‑C‑T‑G ‑A‑A‑T‑C ‑G‑G

A‑G‑T‑T ‑T‑T‑A‑G ‑G‑G
C‑C‑T‑G ‑A‑A‑T‑C ‑G‑G

Low Stringency Conditions

Minimal denaturation - Maintenance of sufficient hydrogen bonds

A‑G‑T‑T ‑T‑T‑A ‑G‑G‑G
C‑C‑T‑G ‑A‑A‑T ‑C‑G‑G

A‑G‑T‑T ‑T‑T‑A‑G ‑G‑G
C‑C‑T‑G ‑A‑A‑T‑C ‑G‑G

High Stringency Conditions

Substantial denaturation - Disruption of hydrogen bonds of most matched base pairs

A‑G‑T‑T‑T‑T‑A‑G‑G‑G
C‑C‑T‑G‑A‑A‑T‑C‑G‑G

A‑G‑T‑T ‑T‑T‑A ‑G‑G‑G
C‑C‑T‑G ‑A‑A‑T ‑C‑G‑G

Figure 2-5. There is 50% homology. Sufficient hydrogen bonding between the nondisrupted base pair matches remains at low stringency for hybridization of most of the complexes. Further disruption of remaining hydrogen bonds at high stringency, however, leads to denaturation of most of the DNA complexes.

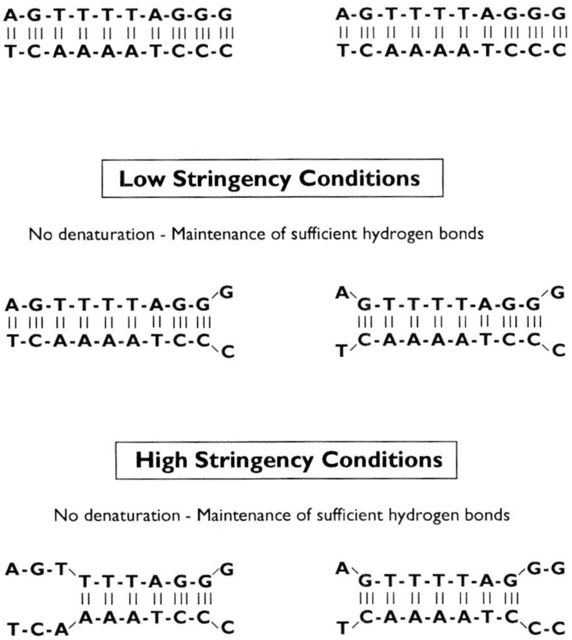

A‑G‑T‑T‑T‑T‑A‑G‑G‑G
T‑C‑A‑A‑A‑A‑T‑C‑C‑C

A‑G‑T‑T‑T‑T‑A‑G‑G‑G
T‑C‑A‑A‑A‑A‑T‑C‑C‑C

Low Stringency Conditions

No denaturation - Maintenance of sufficient hydrogen bonds

A‑G‑T‑T‑T‑T‑A‑G‑G ‑G
T‑C‑A‑A‑A‑A‑T‑C‑C ‑C

A‑G‑T‑T‑T‑T‑A‑G‑G ‑G
T‑C‑A‑A‑A‑A‑T‑C‑C ‑C

High Stringency Conditions

No denaturation - Maintenance of sufficient hydrogen bonds

A‑G‑T ‑T‑T‑T‑A‑G‑G ‑G
T‑C‑A ‑A‑A‑A‑T‑C‑C ‑C

A‑G‑T‑T‑T‑T‑A‑G ‑G‑G
T‑C‑A‑A‑A‑A‑T‑C ‑C‑C

Figure 2-6. The complete homology between the two strands allows hybridization to remain at high stringency despite the disruption of the hydrogen bonds of some of the base pair matches.

also affect the degree of hybridization, because the positively charged sodium ion can interact with the negatively charged triphosphate group on the terminal carbon 5 and, in this way, reduce the ionic repulsion between adjoining nucleic acid strands. Thus, increasing salt concentrations increases the relative percentage of complementary homologous DNA strands that are hybridized. Figure 2-7 illustrates how the Tm will shift to lower temperatures if some conditions are adjusted to disfavor hydrogen bonding. A common and simple way to disfavor hydrogen bonding is to add formamide, as is evident from the formula used to calculate the Tm; also note from the formula how increasing the salt concentration increases the Tm and thus makes DNA hybrids more stable:

$$Tm = 81.5°C + 16.6 \log [Na^+] \text{ (as molarity)}$$

$$+ 0.41 \text{ (% G + C content)} - 0.61$$

$$\text{(% formamide)} - \text{(500/# base pairs in the}$$

$$\text{DNA–DNA hybrid [1,2])}$$

For practical purposes, when one is dealing with completely homologous relatively long (>500 base pair) DNA strands under standard conditions (25% formamide and 100 mM Na^+ with a GC content of 50%), the Tm will be 69.9°C. Thus, one must bring the temperature substantially above 70°C in order to denature most of the DNA. This explains why denaturing is usually done at about 100°C and the temperature then brought to about 40°C. At 40°C, the probe and target (see below) will hybridize and remain attached since they share strong homology. However, the probe will dissociate from unwanted segments of DNA at 40°C because the temperature will be much above the Tm for such complexes. Specifically, assuming 10 of 500 base pair matches between probe and nontarget DNA, 25% formamide, 100 mM Na^+, and a GC content of 50%, the Tm would be 19.9°C. The adjustment of conditions to favor probe-to-target DNA hybridization while denaturing probe–nontarget hybrids is the basis

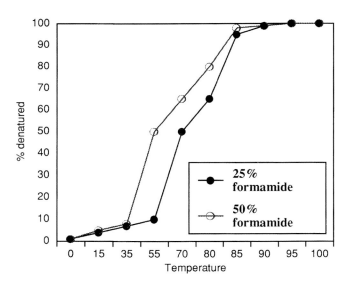

Figure 2-7. *Graphic representation of the melting curve of hybridized DNA.* Hybridized DNA complexes will denature with increasing temperatures according to the "S-shaped" pattern depicted. Increasing the formamide concentration twofold will "shift the curve to the left," which means that, at most temperatures, a greater percentage of the DNA complexes will have separated. With 25% formamide, the temperature at which one-half of the DNA hybrids are denatured (i.e., the melting temperature or Tm) is at 70°C, whereas at 50% formamide a temperature of 55°C will denature one-half of the DNA complexes under the conditions depicted. A similar decrease of 15°C in the Tm is affected by decreasing the sodium concentration tenfold.

of the superior specificity of molecular hybridization based analyses.

For example, to illustrate these important points, let us assume that the probe is HPV 31 and the tissue contains both HPV 31 and HPV 52. HPV 52 shares weak homology with HPV 31. Under low stringency conditions both HPVs would be detected, but at high stringency one would no longer see any evidence of the hybridization between HPV 31 and 52 (Figs. 2-8, 2-9). Note that more HPV 52 is present than HPV 31. This illustrates a simple but important point—the actual number of hybridized molecules between the probe (see below) and

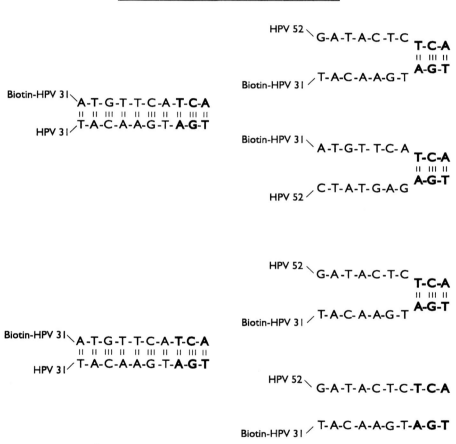

Low Stringency Conditions

Figure 2-8. *Graphic representation of dual infection, low stringency conditions.* The area of homology between HPVs 31 and 52 are represented by the boldface **T–C–A** and **A–G–T**. The HPV 31 probe is labeled with biotin. Under low stringency conditions, there is sufficient hybridized HPV 31 probe and HPV 52 target for detection of the HPV 52. At low stringencies, the HPV 31 probe–HPV 52 complexes (*right*) may produce a more intense hybridization signal than that generated from the HPV 31–31 complexes (*left*) due to the greater amount of HPV 52 present in the sample. However, under high stringency conditions, the HPV 31–HPV 52 complexes would dissociate owing to disruption of the remaining hydrogen bonds. Thus, the HPV 52 would no longer be detectable. However, the HPV 31 in the sample would still be detected due to the complete homology between the probe and target (See also Fig. 2-9).

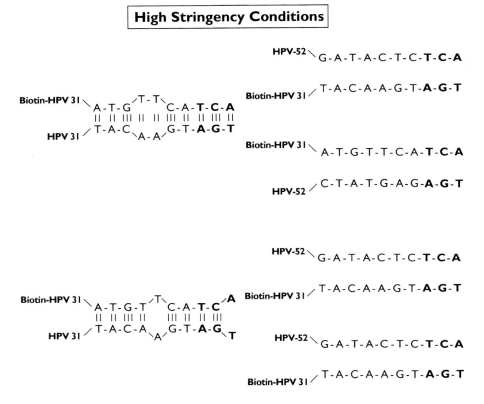

Figure 2-9. *Graphic representation of dual infection, high stringency conditions.*

two different strands will be a function of the degree of homology *and* the relative number of the two distinct strands. At low stringency, the absolute number of hybridized HPV 31=HPV 52 may be greater than HPV 31= HPV 31 because of the greater number of HPV 52 molecules.

Cloning

Cloning refers to the process of purifying large amounts of a specific DNA fragment or *insert*. This can be accomplished by various methods. A common technique is to attach the specific strand of DNA that one wishes to clone to a known carrier segment of DNA. The carrier segment is usually a *plasmid* that is a circular double-stranded DNA molecule capable of self-replicating. A key factor is that

the plasmid DNA must offer a selective advantage to the bacteria it will be introduced into. The most common advantage is resistance to an antibiotic, such as ampicillin. The bacterium used in the cloning technique, usually a strain of *Escherichia coli*, is incapable of producing ampicillinase (ß-lactamase) and thus will not survive in a growth medium that contains the ampicillin antibiotic. However, if the bacterium is exposed to the plasmid and some of it incorporates the plasmid DNA in a process called *transformation*, this bacterium will grow and produce colonies (Fig. 2-10). The colonies, recognized on the agar growth medium plates as whitish aggregates of about 2 to 5 mm in size, represent millions of bacteria that were all derived from the same parent bacterium that incorporated the plasmid. These bacteria should all contain the copy of the plasmid DNA. It is essential for cloning that the DNA sequence to be purified be attached to the plasmid. This selection can be done in a process termed *ligation*, which involves the attaching of complementary regions of linear DNA. Of course, this is similar to what occurs in hybridization. However, whereas in hybridization the complementary DNA strands attach and may separate if the strin-

gency conditions are varied, in ligation they attach and then are covalently bonded to each other via the phosphodiester bond. The enzyme that has this capability is termed *DNA ligase*.

Another part of the process of cloning and DNA ligation is the generation of the complementary strands of DNA on the plasmid and the DNA segment chosen for cloning. These com-

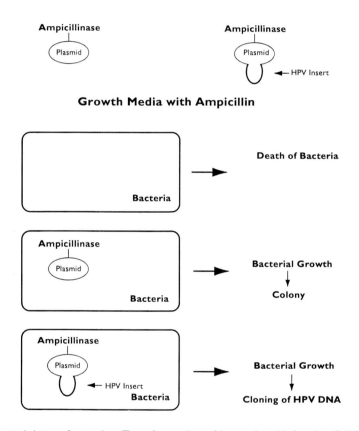

Figure 2-10. *Bacterial transformation.* Transformation of bacteria with foreign DNA is a commonly used method of cloning. A bacterium, often a strain of *E. coli*, is chosen that is sensitive to an antibiotic, usually ampicillin. Thus, the bacteria would not grow in a media that contained ampicillin (*top*). To transform the bacteria, one can use a circular, self-replicating segment of DNA called a plasmid. By placing the gene that dictates the synthesis of ampicillinase on the plasmid, its entry into the bacteria will allow for the selective growth of the microbe and the production of a colony (*middle*). The plasmid can be attached to any segment of DNA (called the insert) by using a restriction endonuclease that digests each segment followed by linkage at the cut site by the enzyme DNA ligase (*bottom*) (see Fig. 2-11). If the plasmid does not recircularize, it is much less efficient at bacterial transformation, which makes transformation by linearized plasmid that lack the insert very unlikely. Grown in large quantities the transformed bacteria allows one to mass produce or clone the insert after extracting and purifying the plasmid–insert ligand.

plementary regions are made by the action of a large family of enzymes that cut or digest DNA at highly specific sites within a given sequence. Since these enzymes cut DNA segments internal to the 5′ and 3′ ends, they are referred to as *endonucleases* or, more common, *restriction endonucleases*. An example of the action of a common endonuclease called *Bam*HI is pre-

sented in Fig. 2-11. Note what may happen if this endonuclease encounters only one of its target sequences (GGATCC) in the plasmid. If only one site (or two sites separated by a few base pairs) is encountered, then the circular plasmid will become a linear molecule. This is easily recognized on an agarose gel, as the linear band migrates at a slower rate than the tightly coiled

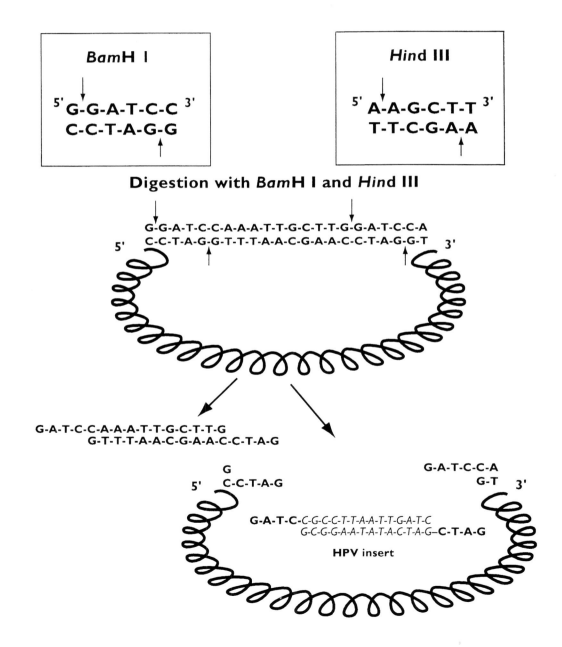

circular band of the plasmid (Fig. 2-12). However, if many GGATCC sites are available in the plasmid DNA, it will be divided into many small linear strands that will migrate on the gel according to their sizes (Fig. 2-12). This digestion will likely disrupt the gene that confers the ampicillinase activity of the plasmid. However, this gene, which is essential for transformation, will remain intact if only one or few digestion site(s) for *Bam*HI is available, assuming there is no such site on the ampicillase gene region, which indeed is the case.

It is important to realize that the plasmid that has been linearized by an endonuclease that cuts it at one site loses most of its ability to transform a bacterium. The plasmid must be recircularized to regain this ability. This can be done in one of two ways. First, DNA ligase could be added and the two ends reattached. Although this procedure can be used as a measure of the activity of DNA ligase, it would not be useful with regard to cloning, as one must attach the insert of interest. The second method would involve using DNA ligase with the plasmid and the DNA sequence that one wished to clone that has also been digested by the same endonuclease. In this mat-

ter, they would have complementary ends and, thus, would hybridize (Fig. 2-11). Once this was achieved, DNA ligase could form the covalent phosphodiester bond (see Fig. 2-21), and the plasmid with its insert could then readily transform a bacterium.

Two other points should be made regarding cloning. First, some restriction endonucleases will cleave DNA without producing the four base "overhang" illustrated in Fig. 2-11. Such blunt-end DNA segments can be cloned by DNA ligase, although with much less efficiency than when there are fragments with "sticky" overhanging ends. This is because the DNA segments with blunt ends cannot hybridize. Second, in a given ligation reaction one cannot differentiate which bacteria contain the recircularized plasmid from those that contain the plasmid and insert, as both will show resistance to ampicillin. There are two ways to demonstrate that a given bacteria colony contains the plasmid and ligated insert of interest:

1. Perform filter hybridization. This can be achieved by transferring the bacteria colonies growing on the agar plate to a filter, denatur-

Figure 2-11. *Restriction endonucleases.* A large series of enzymes have the ability to break the phosphodiester bond linking any given two nucleotides in the double-stranded DNA molecule. These enzymes digest the phosphodiester bond between the 5' and 3' ends of the molecule and are thus called DNA endonucleases or, more commonly, restriction endonucleases. There are several important implications to having a large strand of DNA digested at only one or two sites by a given endonuclease: (i) If the DNA strand was circular, it will now be linear and migrate differently on an agarose gel (see Fig. 2-12). (ii) If the DNA strand was linear, digestion can be demonstrated by a shift from one band to several smaller bands on an agarose or acrylamide gel. (iii) Most importantly, if the endonuclease digests the DNA asymmetrically, which is common, the 5' and 3' ends at the site of digestion can easily be ligated to any other segment of DNA digested by the same endonuclease.

In this example, two commonly used restriction endonuclease are depicted: *Bam*HI and *Hin*dIII (*top*). The DNA strand is circular and 2,600 base pairs in size. Note how the strand does not have the 5'A–A–G–C–T–T 3' sequence that is digested by *Hin*dIII. However, it has two sites digested by *Bam*HI. Thus, after digestion one obtains two linear strands, one 15 base pairs in size and the other 2,585 base pairs (*middle*). After *Bam*HI digestion, one could ligate another DNA molecule also digested with *Bam*HI. In this example, a small fragment of HPV that resulted after *Bam*HI digestion has the complementary 5' overhang regions (bold face, *bottom*) needed to hybridize and then be ligated to the plasmid.

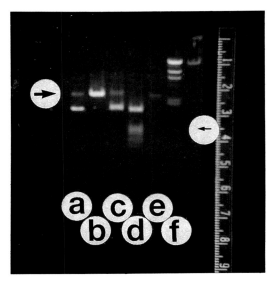

Figure 2-12. *Digestion of the plasmid pUC19 by various restriction endonucleases.* pUC 19 is a commonly used plasmid in cloning; it contains the ampicillinase gene (see Fig. 2-10). *Lane a* is the uncut plasmid. The multiple bands represent the open or "nicked" circle (*top*), the linear (*middle, large arrow*), or the tightly coiled form (*bottom*) that the plasmid can assume. Although each form is 2,600 base pairs, they migrate differently due to their different configurations. Compare this to *lane b*, where only the linear form is seen after digestion with *Bam*HI. Thus, this enzyme cuts the plasmid at one site. *Lane c* shows the pattern for an enzyme that does not digest pUC19 (*Eco*RV), whereas *lane d* shows multiple small bands indicative of an enzyme (*Hin*f) that digests the plasmid at many sites. *Lane e* also indicates a "one cut" endonuclease (*Eco*RI). *Lane f* is the marker lane, which consists of the lambda phage digested with *Hind*III. The bands correspond to approximately 23,000, 9,000, 6,000, 2,300, 2,100, and 500 (*small arrow*) base pairs.

ing the DNA, and then hybridizing with a probe specific for the clone (Fig. 2-13).

2. Isolate the bacteria colony, grow it overnight in growth media that contains ampicillin, then lyse the microbes, extract the DNA, and digest it with the endonuclease used initially to produce the ends that were bonded by DNA ligase. This can only be done with the endonuclease(s) that produced the overhangs. If the insert is present, one will see it on the agarose gel as a distinct band of the expected size. For those endonucleases that produce blunt ends, one must digest with two different endonucleases that cut the plasmid at one site on either side of the inserted cloned fragment. Usually one can find two such endonucleases with ease because most plasmids have many sites linked together that are digested only once by a restriction endonuclease. These polylink-

ers greatly facilitate the cloning process by offering a variety of endonucleases that can be used, assuming they also cut the insert one wishes to clone at just one site.

Hybridization Assays

Molecular biology methodologies are based on the use of a known nucleic acid sequence to hybridize with and thus identify a specific nucleic acid strand in the sample being tested. The known strand is usually labeled and is called the *probe.* The unlabeled strand in the sample being analyzed that is homologous to the probe is called the *target.* Standard probe labeling techniques include radioactively modifying nucleotides with isotopes such as ^{3}H, ^{35}S, and ^{32}P or ^{33}P and using nonisotopic nucleotide tags that can be detected by a variety of methods including, to name a few, fluorescence and colorimetric changes. The most common colorimetric reaction is based on biotin-labeled nucleotides, which avidly bind streptavidin that, in turn, is conjugated to alkaline phosphatase, which can then catalyze the precipitation of a substrate visible with light microscopy (Fig. 2-14). However, endogenous biotin may be present in certain tissues, such as kidney and liver, producing nonspecific reactions and increased background when using the biotin system for *in situ* hybridization. Another commonly used system employs digoxigenin-tagged nucleotides, often as digoxigenin dUTP. Digox-

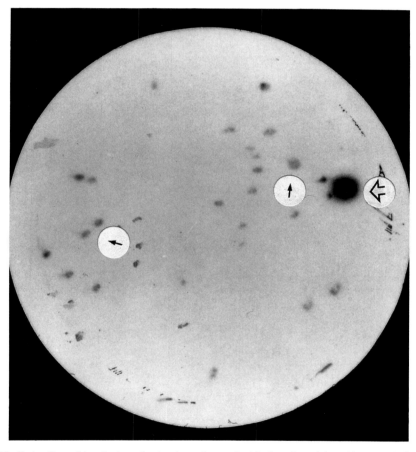

Figure 2-13. *Detection of bacteria colonies transformed with the plasmid and insert.* pUC19 and HPV 51 DNA were each digested with the enzyme *Hind*III. This enzyme digests the plasmid once and HPV 51 twice (7,900 base pairs and about 100 base pairs). Ampicillin-sensitive *E. coli* bacteria were transformed by the DNA present after ligating the pUC19 and HPV 51 fragments. To differentiate those colonies that contain only pUC19 from those that contained the plasmid ligated to HPV 51, the colonies were transferred to a filter, and the DNA denatured (see text) and then hybridized to a ^{32}P-labeled HPV 16 probe; this shares sufficient homology with HPV 51 to yield a hybridization signal. The colonies with a signal (*closed arrows*) were shown to contain the 7,900 base pair HPV 51 insert after isolating a large amount of the plasmid DNA and detecting the 7,900 and 2,600 base pair bands after digesting it with *Hind*III. The *open arrow* depicts 100 pg of purified HPV 16 DNA, which serves as a positive control for the hybridization step.

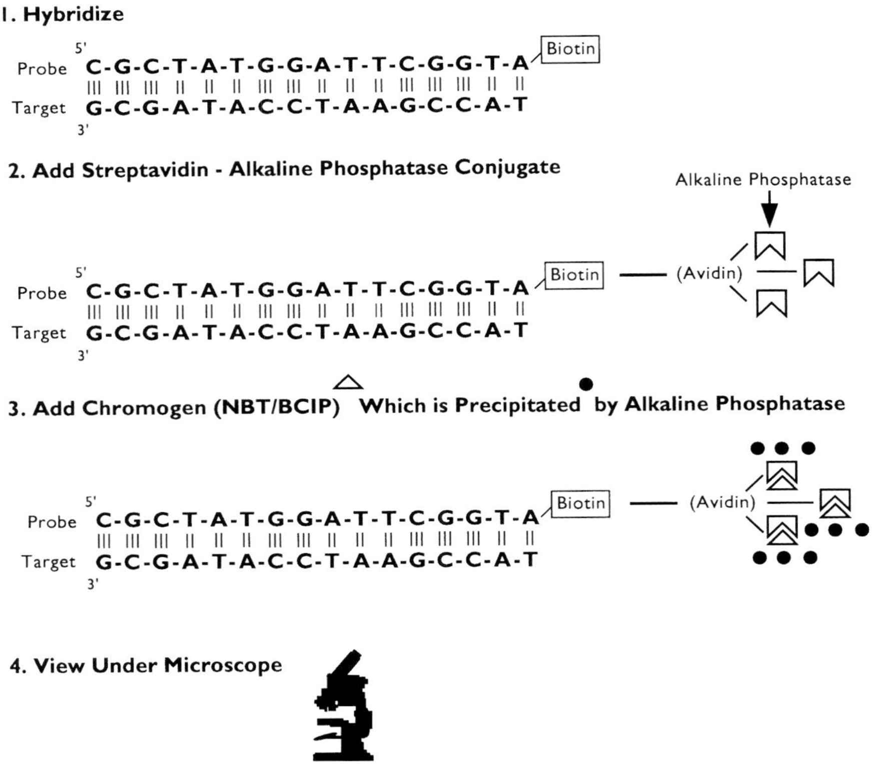

1. Hybridize

```
        5'
Probe   C-G-C-T-A-T-G-G-A-T-T-C-G-G-T-A┐Biotin
        ||| ||| ||| || || || || ||| ||| || ||
Target  G-C-G-A-T-A-C-C-T-A-A-G-C-C-A-T
        3'
```

2. Add Streptavidin - Alkaline Phosphatase Conjugate

Alkaline Phosphatase

```
        5'
Probe   C-G-C-T-A-T-G-G-A-T-T-C-G-G-T-A┐Biotin ——— (Avidin)
        ||| ||| ||| || || || || ||| ||| || ||
Target  G-C-G-A-T-A-C-C-T-A-A-G-C-C-A-T
        3'
```

3. Add Chromogen (NBT/BCIP) Which is Precipitated by Alkaline Phosphatase

```
        5'
Probe   C-G-C-T-A-T-G-G-A-T-T-C-G-G-T-A┐Biotin ——— (Avidin)
        ||| ||| ||| || || || || ||| ||| ||| ||| ||| || ||
Target  G-C-G-A-T-A-C-C-T-A-A-G-C-C-A-T
        3'
```

4. View Under Microscope

Figure 2-14. *Detection of a biotin-labeled probe–target complex.* Biotin-labeled nucleotides incorporated into the probe, which has hybridized to the target, avidly bind streptavidin. This, in turn, is conjugated to alkaline phosphatase. The enzyme will precipitate a variety of chromogens, including NBT/BCIP which can be visualized by light microscopy.

igenin is not found in mammalian tissues (it is derived from the foxglove plant), and, thus, nonspecific reactions due to endogenous products are reduced.

Let us examine some examples of detection of probe–target complexes and use these to illustrate some of the points described above. Figure 2-15 shows the localization of HPV 11 in a low-grade cervical squamous intraepithelial lesion (SIL). The signal is a blue precipitate and marks the presence of alkaline phosphatase conjugated to streptavidin, which, in turn, is bound to the biotin on the probe that is hybridized to the target. The other panel in Fig. 2-15 shows the detection of a serial section with a ^{35}S-labeled probe of HPV 11. Note

that the virus is most abundant toward the surface of the lesion as might be expected given that HPV is transmitted by sexual contact. Also note that the two different detection systems give similar results. Needless to say, the biotin system is safer and much faster to work with than the isotopic label. Biotin-based hybridization assays can be completed in 1 day rather than the 3 to 14 days needed for [35]S. Nonisotopic labeling requires fewer steps and, of course, does not necessitate the disposal of hazardous waste, as is true for ^{35}S and other radioactive isotopes.

Figure 2-16 shows an infection by multiple types of HPV in one case of a cervical SIL. This multiple infection is a rare event, occur-

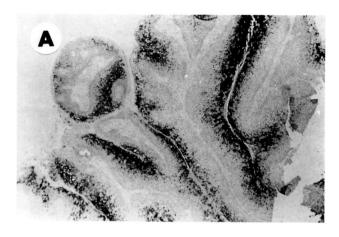

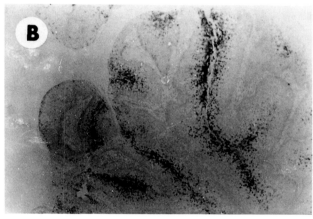

Figure 2-15. *Detection of the probe–target complex by* in situ *hybridization:* ^{35}S *-and biotin-based systems.* The detection of hybridized DNA complexes is usually achieved by labeling a known DNA strand called the probe with nucleotides to which are attached radioactive isotopes or molecules that can be detected enzymatically. Two common schemes involve ^{35}S and biotin labeling, respectively. The tissue is a vulvar condyloma that contains HPV 6 DNA. Viral DNA was detected using either a biotin-labeled probe (**A**) or ^{35}S (**B**); note that the intensity of the hybridization signals is similar. The biotin-based signal reflects precipitation of NBT/BCIP by the enzyme alkaline phosphatase (see Fig. 2-14). The ^{35}S-based signal reflects exposure of the photosensitive emulsion that is placed on the slide after hybridization by the decay of the radioisotope, producing small black grains. Higher magnifications of the NBT/BCIP precipitate (**C**) and the black grains (**D**) are provided. An advantage of the radioactive system is that the number of grains can be correlated with copy number or, for RT *in situ* PCR, the intensity of the positive control versus the cDNA-specific signal (see Chapter 7).

ring in only about 2% of cases as determined by *in situ* and filter hybridization (3). Note that different groups of cells are infected by different HPV types. Compare this pattern with an example of cross-hybridization between two distinct HPV types where the cells

in the same region of the tissue are positive (Fig. 2-17). Note the weak cross-hybridization between HPV 31 and HPV 52 (Fig. 2-16). The weak signal evident between these two viruses at low stringency is eradicated at high stringency. These results exemplify some

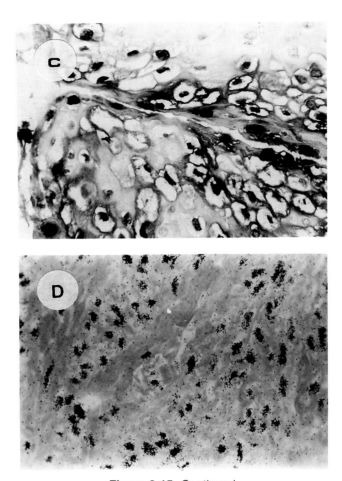

Figure 2-15. *Continued.*

important influences on the hybridization signal. The presence and intensity of a hybridization signal will be a function of the *degree of homology* between the target and probe, the *amount* of target, and the conditions of *stringency*. If there had been less HPV 31 in the tissue sample, there would not have been a signal detected between it and HPV 52 under conditions of low stringency. Figure 2-16 illustrates the points graphically depicted in Figures 2-8 and 2-9.

Figure 2-17 shows a striking example of the importance to the hybridization signal of the degree of homology between the target and probe. The target is HPV 6. Note that a signal is evident at low stringency if a genomic HPV 11 probe is used (Fig. 2-17a,b). A signal was also seen at high stringency (not shown). A genomic (or full-length) probe means that the entire HPV 11 genome, which, as noted above, is about 8,000 base pairs, was labeled. HPVs 6 and 11 share over 80% homology in parts of their genome (4). However, some parts will show poor homology. If subgenomic probes are made from regions where the degree of homology is poor, a signal will be present when the HPV 6 subgenomic probe is used but not when the HPV 11 subgenomic probe is used (Fig. 2-17c,d).

Several techniques have evolved based on the ability of a labeled probe to bind to and

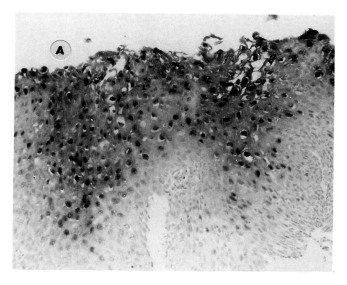

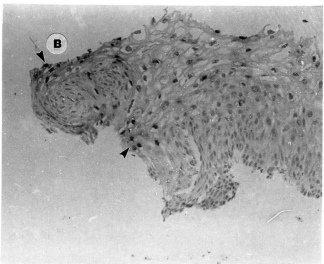

Figure 2-16. *Infection by multiple HPVs in a cervical squamous intraepithelial lesion.* HPV DNA was detected by an HPV 31 probe (**A**) and an HPV 52 probe (**B**) in two different groups of cells in this cervical SIL, indicative of a dual infection. A weak hybridization signal was seen in the area that contained HPV 31 when the HPV 52 probe was used (**C**, *arrowheads*), reflecting cross-hybridization at low stringency. Note how this cross-hybridization signal is lost under high stringency conditions (**D**, *arrowheads*). This SIL actually contained another type, HPV 56, as is evident in (**E**, *arrowheads*), where the group of cells positive with this probe is distinct from the group positive for HPV 52 (**B**, *arrowheads*).

thus permit the detection of the target nucleic acid sequence of interest. One approach is to extract the DNA, both target and nontarget, from a sample and bind it to a filter where it can then be hybridized with the labeled probe. This is called *filter hybridization*. Often the sample DNA is directly placed on the filter with the aid of a vacuum manifold, which has a slot-like space for each sample, hence the term *slot blot* (or dot blot) hybridization. Al-

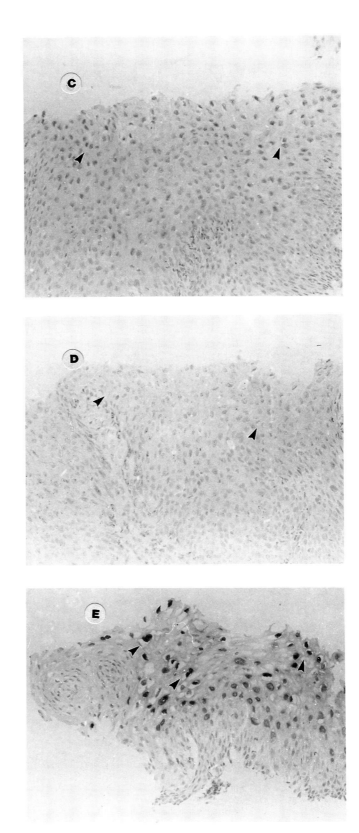

Figure 2-16. *Continued.*

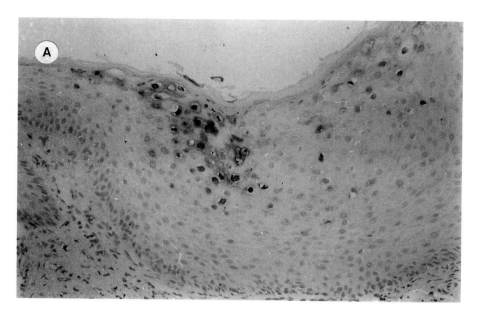

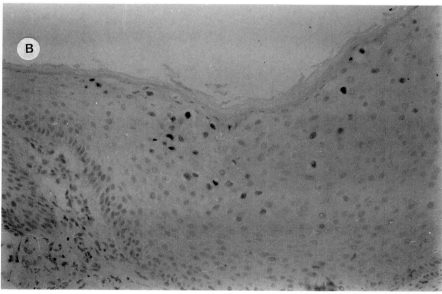

Figure 2-17. *Cross-hybridization between HPVs 6 and 11.* This low-grade penile SIL contained HPV 6 as demonstrated by PCR using type-specific primers. A hybridization signal is evident at low stringency when genomic HPV 6 (**A**) and HPV 11 (**B**) probes are used; the latter signal reflects the areas of strong homology shared between these two HPV types. However, if subgenomic probes are made that are chosen from regions where there is poor homology between these two HPV types, a signal is evident at low stringency with the HPV 6 probe (**C**) but *not* the HPV 11 probe (**D**). The subgenomic probes are from ONCOR (Gaithersburg, MD).

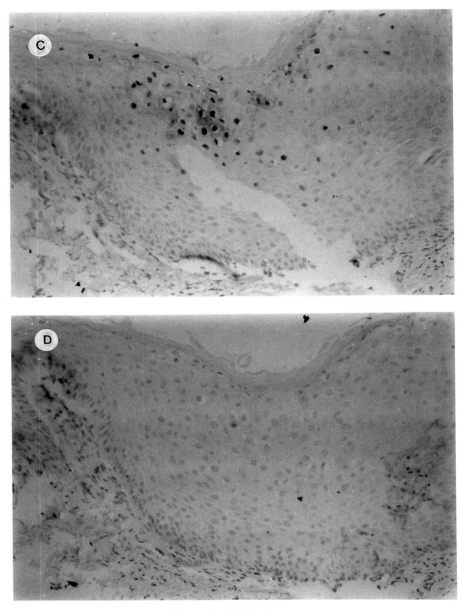

Figure 2-17. *Continued.*

ternatively, the sample DNA may first be separated according to size and configuration by electrophoresis on a gel and then transferred to a filter. This procedure is termed *Southern blot* hybridization (Fig. 2-18). The preparatory process for both of these techniques re-

quires that the DNA be extracted from the tissue, which precludes direct histologic correlation of the test results. In a third technique based on hybridization of a target and the probe, the target DNA is not extracted but rather left in the intact cell where it may bind

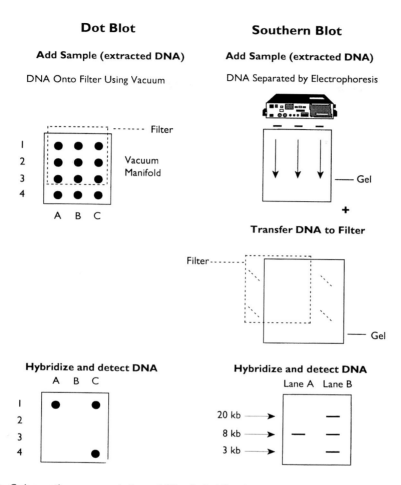

Figure 2-18. *Schematic representation of filter hybridization analysis.* In filter hybridization, DNA is extracted from fresh cells or tissue and then either directly applied to a filter (slot blot) or transferred from a gel to a filter after electrophoretic separation (Southern blot). The drawings illustrate the information about the size of the DNA target evident by Southern blot hybridization that is not provided by slot blot analysis.

to the probe. This, of course, is *in situ* hybridization. The final assay based on molecular biological principles is the polymerase chain reaction (PCR), which is discussed later in this chapter.

A brief comparison of filter hybridization and *in situ* hybridization is in order so that the reader may better appreciate the advantages and limitations of the different methodologies. As depicted in Table 2-1, an important difference between filter and *in situ* hybridization is their detection threshold. Detection of a DNA sequence by *in situ* hybridization implies a selective increase in its numbers due to, for example, active viral proliferation common in early HPV infections (see Fig. 2-15). On the other hand, only one virus need be present per every 100 cells for detection by the Southern blot, though at this low copy number the *in situ* test would be scored as negative (Fig. 2-19). Why is there such a disparity in detection thresholds? There are probably several reasons.

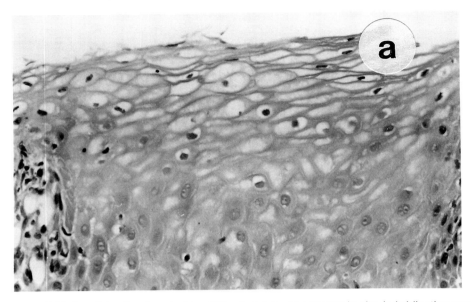

Figure 2-19. *Differing detection thresholds of filter hybridization versus* in situ *hybridization analyses.* HPV DNA was detected by Southern blot hybridization in this cervical biopsy specimen (**b**, *lane a, lane b* is a molecular weight marker, HPV16 digested with PST1.) that lacked the histological features of a SIL (**a**). However, as is true for most of these "nondiagnostic" tissues, the virus was not detected by *in situ* analysis (**c**). This implies that the number of viral genomes per infected cell is less than ten. This should be contrasted to cervical tissues that show the cellular crowding and nuclear atypia diagnostic of a SIL, which are often intensely positive for HPV by standard *in situ* hybridization (see Fig. 2-16 and 2-17).

The probe may find it more difficult to find the target if it has to transverse the labyrinth of nuclear proteins and nucleic acids during the *in situ* analysis rather than the easier route to the more "naked" DNA that has been attached to a filter in slot blot or Southern blot hybridization. A second explanation may be that the extraction and purification of DNA characteristic of filter hybridization lead to a concentrating effect of rare nucleic acid sequences.

Protocols for *in situ* hybridization are presented in Chapter 4. A protocol for filter hybridization analyses is discussed in the next section.

Table 2-1. *Selected features of the three major molecular hybridization assays*

	In situ	Southern blot	Slot blot
Detection threshold	10–20 Copies/cell	1 Copy/100 cells	1 Copy/200 cells
Samples	Fresh or fixed	Fresh	Fresh
Background	Low	Low	Low–high
Time	≤ Day	2–7 Days	1–5 Days
Cell localization	Yes	No	No
Specialized equipment	None	Transfer unit gel cast/ electrophoresis unit	Vacuum manifold
Samples/run	≤25	≤15	≤75
Detection latent infection	No	Yes	Yes

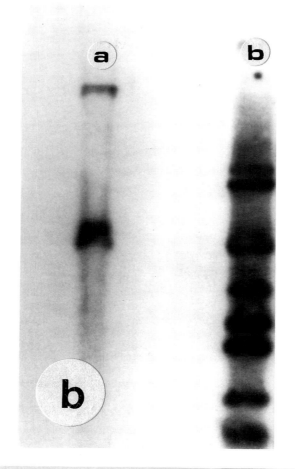

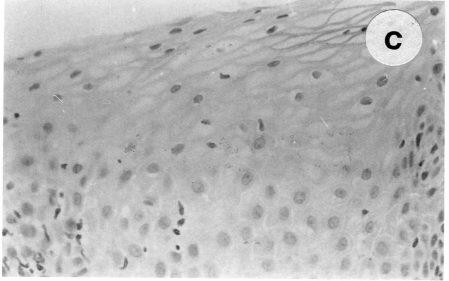

Figure 2-19 . *Continued.*

PROTOCOLS FOR SLOT BLOT AND SOUTHERN BLOT HYBRIDIZATION

DNA Extraction

Description

The DNA that can be extracted from fixed, paraffin-embedded tissue can be used for slot blot or Southern blot hybridization analyses. However, the extraction process reduces the yield of the DNA such that one may not detect a target that had been present, especially if the copy number in the tissue was low. For example, the detection rate of HPV DNA by Southern blot hybridization has been shown to be 100% in frozen, unfixed vulvar warts (which are invariably HPV positive), but was only 27% in DNA extracted from a part of the same tissue that was fixed and then embedded in paraffin (5). This decreased detection rate likely reflects sequestration of the DNA on cellular proteins that may be counteracted by extended protease digestion times or other chemical treatments that tend to solubilize DNA. Nonetheless, it is recommended that one perform filter hybridization analyses on unfixed tissues. During the process of extracting the DNA from tissue samples, it is useful to dissociate it from cellular proteins by digesting with a proteinase. The proteins can then be removed by extraction in phenol, which, in turn, can be removed from the fluid phase by extraction in a chloroform-containing solution. DNA precipitation can then be achieved using ethanol and salt.

Protocol 2-1: DNA Extraction and Purification

1. Place a 3-mm to 7-mm tissue section, preferably unfixed, into a sterile 1.5 ml tube. Add 190 μl of a solution that contains 0.1 M Tris HCl (pH 7.5) and 1% SDS. To this solution add 10 μl of a solution of proteinase K (10 mg/ml stock solution). The tissue may be macerated by adding some sterile "sea sand" to the tube and grinding it with a plastic or glass rod.
2. Incubate the tissue from 3 hours to overnight at 55°C.
3. Add 200 μl of phenol; vortex well.
4. Add 200 μl of chloroform:isoamyl alcohol solution (24:1 ratio), vortex, and centrifuge for 1 minute.
5. Add to supernatant 200 μl of the chloroform:isoamyl alcohol solution, vortex, and centrifuge for 1 minute.
6. Add to supernatant 25 μl of a 3 M sodium acetate solution, 900 μl of 100% ethanol stored at −20°C, and vortex well.
7. Incubate at −70°C for 30 minutes (or −20°C for 2 hours to overnight), centrifuge at 15,000 rpm for 15 minutes, decant solution, and dry pellet.
8. Resuspend pellet in 25 μl of water.

The usual yield from the extraction process is about 25 μg of total cellular DNA. Hence, one would anticipate a concentration of approximately 1 μg/ml, which can be analyzed with a spectrophotometer at 260-nm wavelength. If one measures 2 μl of the resuspended pellet in a volume of 300 μl in the spectrophotometer, an optical density (OD) of 0.13 would correspond to a concentration of 1 μg/ml in the resuspended pellet.

DNA Analysis

Description

The DNA sample is applied directly to the filter for slot blot analysis. This can be done by placing 1 to 2 μg of the DNA sample onto the filter and letting it dry. However, it is more advantageous to put 1 to 2 μg of the sample into a separate tube, increase the volume to 50 μl, and then add the sample to the filter using a vacuum manifold and bench top vacuum source. It is a simple matter to denature the DNA in slot blot hybridization. The filter is treated in a solution that contains 0.5 M NaOH and 1.5 M NaCl for 5 minutes followed by two separate washes in a solution that contains 1.0 M Tris HCl (pH 7.5) and 1 M NaCl for 10 minutes each.

For Southern blot analysis, one needs to prepare a 1% agarose gel. Then 5 to 10 μg of the DNA sample are added to each slot in the gel followed by electrophoresis. Note that a smaller amount of DNA is suggested for slot blot hybridization to reduce excessive background. The problem of background experienced with the slot blot technique is much less of an issue with Southern blot analysis due to the purifying effect of the electrophoresis step. After electrophoresis, the DNA must be transferred to a filter. This is done after treating the gel with an alkaline solution to denature the DNA, then inactivating the NaOH. Although the transfer of the DNA from gel to filter can be done by capillary action using an overnight transfer with absorbent paper, a vacuum-mediated transfer is recommended. Vacuum mechanisms are now available from several commercial sources (e.g., ONCOR Corporation, Stragene) that allow for efficient transfer in 30 minutes. The filter is then heated at 80°C for 1 to 2 hours to bind the single-stranded DNA irreversibly to the filter after which the hybridization procedure is carried out. The following is the protocol for placing the DNA onto the filter.

Protocol 2-2: DNA Analysis

1. For slot blot analysis, add 1 μg of DNA per slot using a vacuum manifold. It is important to include 1 μg of a negative control and a set of dilutions from 1 to 1 ng of the positive control. Denature the DNA using a wash in 0.5 M NaOH and 1.5 M NaCl (5 minutes) followed by two washes in 1.0 M Tris/1.0 M NaCl (10 minutes each).
2. For Southern blot analysis, prepare a 1% agarose gel by adding 1 gm of agarose to 100 ml of Tris acetate buffer (ONCOR Corp.). The agarose can be placed into solution by heating to boil in a microwave oven. The edges of the Lucite gel mold can be sealed with a small amount of the agarose solution. As the solution cools to about 50°C, 10 μl of an ethidium bromide solution can be added to the agarose solution, which can then be added to the Lucite mold. The agarose should be poured immediately after adding the ethidium, which is carcinogenic. This part of the procedure should be done in a vacuum hood. After the gel hardens, remove the Lucite ends and gel comb and to each lane add 10 to 15 μg of sample. Each allotment of sample should

include 2 μl of a bromophenol blue solution. This combination simplifies addition of the sample to the gel as well as providing for a molecular weight marker.

The negative lead (black) should be placed at the top of the Lucite box and the positive lead (red) at the bottom. The electrophoresis should be performed at 60 to 80 V, and the current should be about 30 to 50 mAmp. It is important to run a molecular weight marker with the sample; many are available from a variety of commercial sources (see Appendix).

Allow the sample to run about one-half to two-thirds down the gel; then photograph the gel using a UV box. Do successive washes in

a. 0.2 N HCl for 15 minutes on a shaker (depurinate DNA to allow for more efficient transfer by breaking up larger sized fragments); rinse with water
b. 0.2 M NaOH for 15 minutes (denature DNA); rinse with water
c. 20 × SSC:1 M Tris HCl (pH 7.5) (at 10:1 ratio) for 30 minutes; water rinse
d. Repeat step c to neutralize the NaOH solution
e. Transfer DNA from the gel to a Nytran filter using a 10 × SSC solution and either capillary action or a vacuum-driven apparatus
f. Wash filter in 2 × SSC solution
3. For either slot blot or Southern blot hybridization, bake filter at 80°C for 1 to 2 hours; place in sealable plastic bag.

DNA Hybridization

The protocol that follows is based on the use of ^{32}P-labeled probes. At this stage nonisotopic systems do also perform well, routinely detecting 1 pg in a sample, especially if one uses the chemiluminescent–alkaline phosphatase-based systems. Still, my own experience is that of obtaining consistently lower backgrounds with intense signals with the ^{32}P-based system.

Before discussing the protocol for detection of a specific target with a labeled probe by filter hybridization analysis, it is important to review the different types of probes that can be used. The size of the probe is an important factor. As is discussed in detail in Chapter 4, the typical probes used for *in situ* hybridization and for filter hybridization techniques is at times referred to as a *full-length probe,* so named because they are derived from a full length-clone inserted into a plasmid vector. To distinguish it from the plasmid vector, as described above, the DNA that is cloned in the plasmid is called the *insert.* The insert DNA is usually greater than 250 base pairs in size. For example, the full-length inserts of HPV 16 and HIV-1 that are readily available as clones in plasmids are about 8,000 and 12,000 base pairs, respectively. Alternatively, much smaller segments of DNA may be synthesized. When labeled, these smaller segments are referred as *oligoprobes* and are usually from 18 to 40 base pairs in size.

Later in this chapter is a discussion of the different methods available to synthesize a labeled probe. The important point at this stage is that the labeling of genomic probes of 250 base pairs or larger produces a large series of probes that will be around 100 to 200 base pairs. The labeling of an oligomer does not much affect the size of the DNA probe available for hybridization, which, as noted above, is usually about 20 base pairs. Thus, a labeled oligoprobe is usually only about one-tenth the size of the labeled full-length probe. As discussed above, the strength of the hybridization is related to the number of base pair matches between target and probe. This is reflected in the formula for Tm provided above. Assuming that all other conditions are equal (Na^+ = 0.1 M, GC content = 50%, and formamide concentration = 50%), it follows that *the Tm for the 250 base pair full length probe will be*

$$Tm = 81.5°C - 16.6 + 20 - 30 - (500/250)$$

$$= 54.9 - 2 = 52.9°C$$

and *the Tm for the 25 base pair oligoprobe will be*

$$Tm = 81.5°C - 16.6 + 20 - 30 - (500/25)$$

$$= 54.9 - 20 = 34.9°C$$

The results of these calculations show that if one does the hybridization at a temperature of 50°C under the conditions of salt and formamide defined above, the signal for the full-length probe will be retained whereas the hybridization signal for the oligoprobe will be greatly diminished and possibly lost. Although one might consider doing a hybridization at a temperature of 25°C for either the oligoprobe or the full-length probe, this would result in too much background for the full-length probe. It is preferable to use different hybridization conditions for the full-length probe than for the oligoprobe. The following are the recommended conditions for each type of probe.

Hybridization Conditions for Full-Length Probes

Formamide (50%)	2.0 ml
20 × SSC	0.8 ml
25% Dextran sulfate	0.9 ml
Sonicated salmon sperm	0.1 ml
Probe (100Ng/nl)	0.2 ml
Total	4.0 ml

Hybridization Conditions for Oligoprobes

Formamide (10%)	0.4 ml
20 × SSC	0.8 ml
25% Dextran sulfate	0.9 ml
Water	1.6 ml
Sonicated salmon sperm	0.1 ml
Probe (100Ng/nl)	0.2 ml
Total	4.0 ml

Similarly, the conditions of the posthybridization wash must be adjusted differently for the oligoprobe and for the full-length probe:

Posthybridization Wash Conditions for Full-Length Probes

Temperature	57°C, 15 min
20 × SSC	1 ml
2% SDS	1 ml
Water	98 ml

The calculation for Tm under these conditions is

$$Tm = 81.5°C - 32.2 + 20 - (500/250) = 67.3°C$$

Thus, the wash conditions are 10°C below the Tm, often referred to as Tm−10.

Posthybridization Wash Conditions
for Oligoprobes

Temperature	54°C, 10 min
20 × SSC	10 ml
2% SDS	0.5 ml
Water	84.5 ml

The calculation for Tm under these conditions is

$$Tm = 81.5°C − 16.6 + 20 − (500/25) = 64.2°C$$

Thus, the wash conditions are at Tm−10.

Note that the posthybridization washes for the oligoprobe and the full-length probe are both at Tm − 10. This is a high stringency wash, designed to remove background while retaining a high percentage of probe and target in a hybridized complex. However, note that we had to use a much higher concentration (10 times greater) of salt in the wash with the oligoprobe to compensate for the tenfold decrease in the size of the probe/target complex. If the concentration of salt (10 mM or 0.01 M) in the wash for the full-length probe is used for the oligoprobe wash, there would be a change in the Tm for the oligoprobe.

The calculation for Tm under these conditions with the oligoprobe is

$$Tm = 81.5°C − 33.2 + 20 − (500/25) = 48.3°C$$

Thus, the wash conditions are at Tm+6.

Because the temperature of the wash under these conditions would be greater than the Tm, much of the signal would be lost, and one would risk obtaining a false-negative result. Of course, the temperature of the wash could be decreased to 43°C to maintain Tm−5. The important point is that the same hybridization or wash conditions cannot be used for the full-length probes and for the oligoprobes.

The reference list includes several reviews and discussions of molecular biology in general, comparative studies of filter hybridization, *in situ* hybridization, and PCR analyses and some studies highlighting the clinical or pathological utility of filter hybridization analyses (5–60). The last three (58–60) are general molecular biology references for the reader who wishes to review in more detail topics such as the biochemistry of nucleic acids. Finally, Fig. 2-20 shows an example of HPV 16 DNA detected by slot blot hybridization and Southern blot hybridization analyses.

THE BASICS OF PCR

Terminology

Before we begin our discussion of how PCR works, certain terms need to be defined. Essential components of PCR are short segments of DNA called *oligonucleotides* (usually about 20 base pairs long). Because these short DNA sequences will serve as the primers or initiation points of DNA amplification in PCR, they are commonly referred to as *primers.* The synthesis of oligonucleotides is a simple matter, and several commercial laboratories perform this service for a fee of about $50 to $200 per 20 base pair sequence. To choose an oligonucleotide to detect a given DNA strand, one must know at least part of the sequence of that molecule. There is extensive literature detailing the partial and in many cases complete sequences of oncogenes, viruses, and so forth. (61–73). Indeed, an ambitious project, if carried to completion, will map out the entire sequence of the human genome.

Another important topic involves the orientation of the native, double-stranded DNA molecule. Each of the building blocks of DNA, the nucleotides, has two ends that participate in their joining. Although mentioned above, let us review this information, which is central to understanding the PCR. Attached to the carbon 5 of the ribose sugar is the triphosphate group. This end is referred to as the *5 prime (5′)* end of the nucleotide. The other important reference point of the nucleotide is the OH group on carbon 3 of the ribose sugar, which is referred to as the *3 prime (3′)* end. When two nucleotides are joined together, the 5′ triphosphate group of one joins with the 3′ OH group of the other nu-

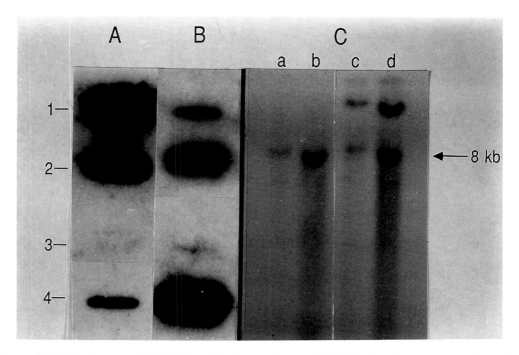

Figure 2-20. *Southern and slot blot hybridization analyses of HPV infection in squamous cell carcinoma of the finger.* In **A**, *slots 1* and *2* represent DNA extracted from two different squamous cell cancers of the finger, *slot 3* is the DNA from normal skin of the finger, and *slot 4* is 200 pg of HPV 16 DNA. Note that a hybridization signal is evident using a ^{32}P-labeled probe of HPV 16 in the samples in *A1* and *A2*. In **B**, *slots 1* and *2* represent the DNA from slots *A1* and *A2* analyzed for HPV 16 at low stringency, whereas *slots 3* and *4* are the DNA from *slots 1* and *2* analyzed for HPV 16 at high stringency (0.2 × SSC at 60°C for 10 minutes). Note that the signal for case *A2* is maintained at high stringency, whereas it is lost for case *A1* under these conditions. This strongly suggests that case *A2* is HPV 16 and case *A1* contains an HPV type related to but distinct from HPV 16. To corroborate this conclusion, Southern blot hybridization was done. In **C**, *lane a* is the pattern seen after sample *A2* was digested with *Bam*HI; *lane b* is purified HPV 16 DNA. Note that in each case a band at 8 kb is evident after hybridization with the HPV 16 probe at a high stringency wash; this is the expected result for HPV 16. *Lanes c* and *d* are undigested DNA from case *A2* and purified HPV 16 DNA, respectively. The sample from *A1* was shown by Southern blot hybridization analysis with digestion using various endonucleases to contain HPV 33.

cleotide, and pyrophosphate is released (Fig. 2-21). The result is a dinucleotide that has a free 3′ OH group on one side and a free 5′ triphosphate group on the other side. The enzyme that catalyzes the synthesis of DNA, called *DNA polymerase*, can join only the free 5′ triphosphate group of the single nucleotide to the 3′ OH group of the larger growing chain (Fig. 2-22). Because DNA polymerase can function only on the 3′ OH group of the growing chain with the 5′ triphosphate unavailable, DNA synthesis occurs in a *5′ to 3′ direction* (Fig. 2-22). The goal of PCR is to synthesize a large amount of a given region in a DNA sequence. The fact that DNA polymerase can function only in a 5′ to 3′ direction allows, by the use of one primer that is complementary to the lower or 3′ DNA strand and another primer that is complementary to the upper or 5′ strand and chosen downstream (i.e., toward the right) of the first primer, the synthesis of the double-stranded sequence of interest. The size of this sequence will be defined by the distance between the two primers. A new term has been introduced: *downstream*. This term refers to the position of a particular sequence on the double-stranded hybridized complex. By con-

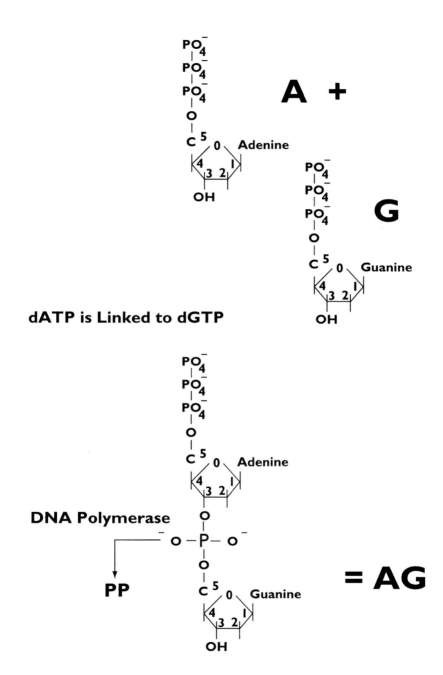

Figure 2-21. *Linkage of two nucleotides.* Each of the two nucleotides (dATP and dGTP) have an OH group attached to carbon 3 and a triphosphate group attached to carbon 5. When the two nucleotides are linked by the action of DNA polymerase, a phosphodiester bond is formed as the carbon 5 phosphate group of the dGTP links to the carbon 3 OH group of the dATP, releasing pyrophosphate (PP).

vention, the 5′ end of the strand is always written in the upper left of the hybridized complex (Fig. 2-23). Thus, the 3′ end of the DNA molecule is at the left side of the lower strand and the right side of the upper strand. To describe a particular DNA sequence in the larger DNA molecule as being downstream of another DNA sequence means that it is closer to the 3′ end of the upper strand (Fig. 2-23).

An illustration of the relationship of sequences in complementary strands of DNA is shown in Fig. 2-23. The native DNA molecule with its two complementary strands are oriented in opposite directions to allow base pair

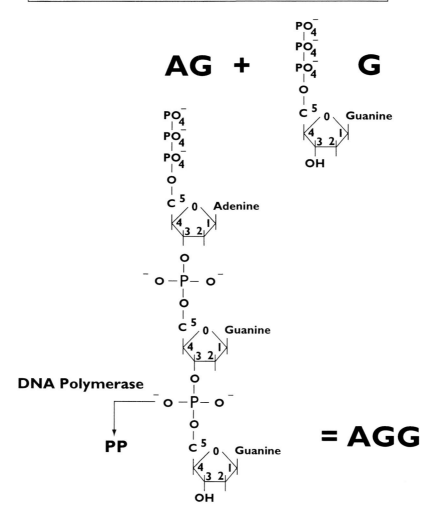

Figure 2-22. *The 5′ to 3′ direction of the growing DNA chain.* As more nucleotides are added to the growing DNA strand, the carbon 5 phosphate group of the mononucleotide is always linked to the carbon 3 OH group of the larger molecule. Because the 5′ triphosphate group at the end of the growing chain is not involved in further DNA synthesis, whereas each new nucleotide is added to the 3′ OH group of the growing DNA segment, DNA synthesis is said to occur in the 5′ to 3′ direction.

matching to occur. Note the standard 5′ to 3′ orientation of the upper strand of DNA. If primer A is chosen complementary to the lower strand and primer B complementary to the upper strand, *and* if primer B is downstream of primer A, then DNA synthesis *must* occur from one primer toward the other primer (Fig. 2-23).

The final item to discuss is the DNA polymerase itself. For DNA polymerase to bring about the addition of a nucleotide to the 3′ OH group of the growing chain, it must locate an area of transition from single-stranded to double-stranded DNA. The enzyme will "fill in the gap," and DNA will be synthesized using the single strand as its template (Fig. 2-23). In PCR this is achieved when the primer hybridizes or *anneals* to the much larger denatured DNA molecule. It is important to realize that this process of DNA synthesis will occur in *any* area of DNA where the double-stranded sequence has been denatured and part, but not all, has rehybridized. Aided by proteins that can denature specific regions of the DNA molecule, partial denaturation and reannealing occur in nature as essential events in DNA and RNA synthesis. Clearly, the synthesis and expression of a given DNA sequence can occur at a specific moment in time. This natural process is essential in embryogenesis and is perturbed in oncogenesis. During the preparation of tissue sections, one inadvertently causes gaps in the DNA sequence when heating the cells and their DNA. These single-stranded gaps may also serve as a template for DNA synthesis by DNA polymerase; in effect, one creates a very long "primer" (see Fig. 3-5).

PCR Theory

The essential reagents needed for PCR include the DNA (double-stranded) sample, the primers,

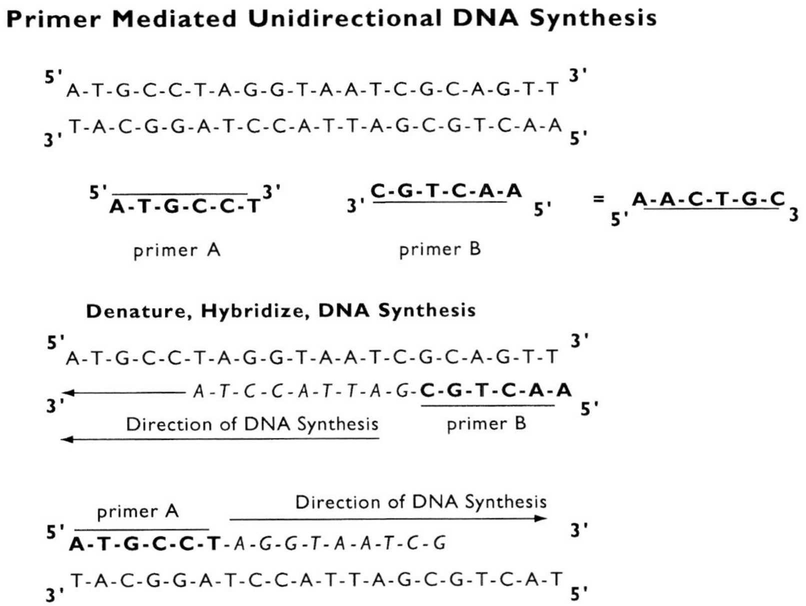

Primer Mediated Unidirectional DNA Synthesis

Figure 2-23. *"Inward" primer-mediated DNA synthesis.* To amplify a specific region during PCR, it is essential that DNA extension from one primer be directed toward the DNA synthesis being mediated by the other primer. This is easily accomplished by choosing the two primers in the following manner: *primer A* has the same sequence as part of the upper strand; *primer B* has the same sequence as part of the lower strand *but* is made in reverse order (i.e., 5′ to 3′); and *primer B* is downstream of *primer A*. Thus, *primer A* will anneal with the lower strand and *primer B* will anneal with the upper strand, and DNA synthesis will be toward the "center".

the DNA polymerase with its essential cation magnesium, a buffer (the exact composition is discussed later), and the four nucleotide building blocks dATP, dCTP, dGTP, and dTTP, which I collectively refer to as the *dNTPs*. Recall that DNA polymerase cannot synthesize new DNA using a double-stranded DNA. Thus, the first step is to denature the DNA. This can be done by increasing the temperature of the sample to 95°C. Even though there is typically no formamide in the reaction mixture, most of the DNA will denature, because 95°C is sufficiently greater than the Tm of native double-stranded DNA unless an excessive amount of salt is present in the sample. A problem becomes immediately apparent. How will the DNA polymerase withstand this high temperature? Most enzymes would be destroyed if exposed to such temperatures even for a very brief time. A major advance in PCR methodology was the isolation of DNA polymerases that could withstand the high temperatures needed for denaturation. One source of this DNA polymerase is a bacterium that lives in hot springs called *Thermus aquaticus* (74–76)—hence, the term *Taq* (DNA) polymerase (AmpliTaq, Perkin-Elmer Cetus, Norwalk, CT). This is not to say that *Taq* polymerase is invulnerable at high temperatures. The thermal stability of *Taq* polymerase is 20 minutes at 97.5°C. Thus, the enzyme can withstand the 94°C for the 5 minutes needed to denature the sample DNA and the repeated 94°C cycles used throughout the amplification process.

In solution phase PCR, the *Taq* polymerase is added to a total amplifying solution volume of 50 to 100 μl in a 0.5 ml plastic tube. In contrast, the volume of the amplifying solution for PCR *in situ* hybridization is usually 10 μl, which is placed under a coverslip of about 1 cm in size. It is readily apparent that the surface area-to-volume ratio for PCR *in situ* hybridization is much greater than the ratio for solution phase PCR. This difference has important implications for the stability of the *Taq* polymerase. A much greater surface area may lead to a shorter half-life of the enzyme during PCR *in situ* hybridization. Although this does not preclude performing PCR *in situ* hybridization, it does underscore the importance of strict regulation of the denaturing tempera-

ture and time when using this technique. As is discussed in more detail in Chapter 5, the initial denaturing time and *actual* temperature should not exceed 3 minutes and 94°C, respectively, for PCR *in situ* hybridization rather than the 5 minutes and 94° to 97°C recommended for solution phase PCR.

After the DNA is denatured, one more event must occur before DNA synthesis can be catalyzed by the enzyme. As mentioned earlier, for DNA polymerase to begin DNA synthesis, it must find an area of transition from double-stranded to single-stranded DNA. If the temperature remains at 95°C, most of the DNA will remain single stranded. However, if the reaction is brought to room temperature, much of the template DNA will renature, preventing the DNA polymerase from functioning. Clearly, it would be advantageous to reach an intermediate temperature at which the competition between native DNA and primer DNA for the target favors the latter to allow the primers to hybridize to the desired DNA sequence. At the proper temperature, which is typically around 55°C, sufficient primer–target DNA hybridization will occur to create an initiation point for DNA synthesis by *Taq* polymerase (Fig. 2-24). The primers will seek out regions with similar homology, and, if a 20 base pair primer finds a region that is completely complementary, it will likely hybridize to it and remain hybridized at 55°C. On the other hand, if a primer hybridizes to a region where only two of the base pairs match, the hydrogen bonding will be so weak that at 55°C this complex would most probably denature (see Fig. 2-4). That is to say, when such weak bonding occurs, the Tm of the reaction will be much below 55°C. But, what if an intermediate situation occurs where 15 of 20 base pairs are complementary. Will this complex remain hybridized? Such intermediate hybridization complexes, although lacking 100% homology, *may* indeed stay annealed at these elevated temperatures. Whether they remain annealed or denatured depends on factors such as the temperature, the salt concentration, and, as discussed earlier, the arrangement of the homologous base pairs (i.e., are they directly adjacent to or dispersed throughout the sequence, the former giving a

Step 1. Choosing the Primers

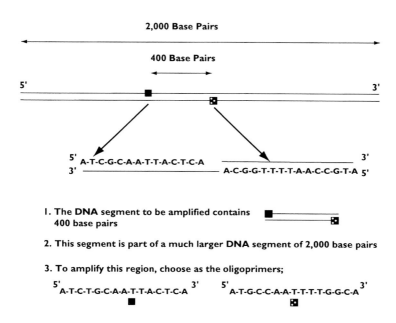

1. The **DNA** segment to be amplified contains 400 base pairs

2. This segment is part of a much larger **DNA** segment of 2,000 base pairs

3. To amplify this region, choose as the oligoprimers;

Figure 2-24. *The polymerase chain reaction.* The various parts of PCR are presented in four parts: choosing the primers; the denaturation step, synthesis of the actual PCR templates, and amplification.

Step 1: choosing the primers. In this example, a 400 base pair region of a gene 2,000 base pairs long will be amplified. The DNA sequence is written with the upper strand in the 5' to 3' orientation, by convention. In ordering primers to amplify this region, one would select a sequence identical to a region of the upper strand (5' A–T–C–T–G–C–A–A–T–T–A–C–T–C–A) and another sequence identical to a sequence in the dowstream region of the lower strand written in the "reverse" or 5' to 3' direction (5' A–T–G–C–C–A–A–T–T–T–T–G–G–C–A). This second primer is, thus, complementary to a downstream region of the upper strand.

Step 2: denaturation. For the primers to anneal to the target, one must first denature the DNA by heating to 94°C. The temperature is then decreased to 55°C to allow for the primers to anneal to their complementary region of the target.

Step 3: synthesis of the DNA template. After the primers anneal, *Taq* polymerase rapidly extends the primer by adding thousands of base pairs in a matter of minutes. Note that the DNA synthesized after this first PCR cycle has two important features: (i) it is very long (>1,000 base pairs in this example); (ii) it has at its 5' end a primer; and (iii) it includes a region that is *complementary* to the other primer. The DNA synthesized in cycle 1 serves as the template in cycle 2.

Step 4: amplification of the 400 base pair target. The two templates synthesized in cycle 2 lead to the synthesis of DNA fragments that have a primer at their 5' end and a region complementary to their primer at their 3' end. These serve as the actual templates for PCR amplification. With successive denaturing and annealing/extension cycles, one exponentially synthesizes the DNA segment between primers 1 and 2.

Step 2. Denaturing the Template DNA

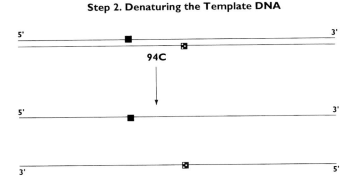

Figure 2-24. *Continued*, Step 2.

Step 3. Synthesis of the PCR Template

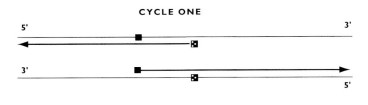

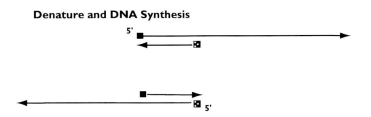

Figure 2-24. *Continued*, Step 3.

more strongly bound complex; see Fig. 2-3) plus the amount of primer and nontarget DNA.

Hybridization of the primer and nontarget DNA is referred to as *mispriming* and can lead to the synthesis of nonspecific DNA during PCR. It is apparent that this mispriming is analogous to background described above in filter hybridization or *in situ* hybridization. That is, it reflects unwanted binding of the primer (or probe) with a segment of DNA with which it shares some, but not complete, homology. It is essential to appreciate that whether these nonspecif-

ic complexes remain hybridized is to a large extent a function of the reaction conditions during PCR or the hybridization and wash conditions for filter and *in situ* hybridization analyses. The subject of mispriming as a potential pathway of nonspecific DNA synthesis in PCR and its control by the hot start maneuver as an essential step for successful PCR *in situ* hybridization is discussed in detail in Chapter 3.

Let us assume that the primer has found a single-stranded region of the DNA and hybridized to it. DNA polymerase will find this region and

Step 4. Amplification of the 400 Base Pair Segment

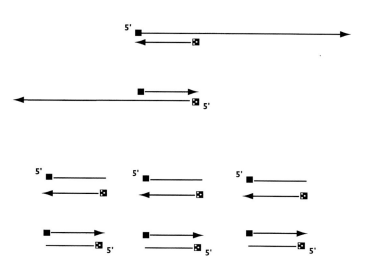

Figure 2-24. *Continued,* Step 4.

DNA will be rapidly synthesized, and thus, the primer will be extended in a 5' to 3' direction (Fig. 2-24, step 3). Of these two events of primer annealing and primer extension, the primer annealing is the rate-limiting step. The *Taq* polymerase is very efficient and may add thousands of nucleotides in a complementary fashion to the template in a matter of a few minutes. In most PCR reactions, the final product is less than 500 base pairs in size. This is the basis for the statement that an extension step is usually *not* needed with PCR or *in situ* PCR.

The next step is to separate the newly synthesized DNA from the template. This is easily accomplished by raising the temperature to 94°C for 1 minute. Note that there will be two newly synthesized segments of DNA, each having one of the two primers at its 5' point of origin (Fig. 2-24, step 4). Also note that DNA synthesis in the two strands is *toward* the other primer; indeed, in the first cycle of PCR the DNA that is synthesized always includes an area complementary to the other primer. If this process continued, we would get an arithmetic increase in the amount of these DNA segments. After 25 cycles, assuming only one DNA sequence that hybridized to the primers was avail-

able, we might be able to synthesize about 50 copies of the molecule. That is poor production and would be below the detection levels of conventional assays, such as Southern blot hybridization, typically used to detect the newly synthesized DNA. Furthermore, the newly synthesized fragment could include nontarget sequences distal to the region of interest. An example of this would be integrated HIV-1 DNA; even if the synthesis begins with the HIV-1-specific primers, the DNA polymerase may synthesize adjoining human DNA if allowed to proceed. What is needed is an exponential accumulation of the target DNA sequence. This has been accomplished by choosing the primers as illustrated in Fig. 2-24, step 1.

As illustrated in the cartoon presented in Fig. 2-24, step 3, denaturation, followed by annealing after the first cycle allows primer 1 to hybridize with the newly synthesized DNA strand that has primer 2 at its 5' end; similarly, primer 2 will hybridize to the new DNA strand that has primer 1 at its 5' end. It is clear that the large strands made in the first cycle of PCR are important intermediary templates. In the second cycle, much smaller DNA strands are made. They will have a primer on their 5′ end and they will *terminate* at their 3′ end at a region complementary to the other primer. These shorter fragments, whose size is determined by the distance of primer 1 to primer 2 (in this case, 400 base pairs), are the actual template for PCR. This is illustrated in Fig. 2-24, step 4.

Each denaturing and annealing sequence is referred to as a *cycle*. The maximum of target-specific product that can be produced is 2^n, where n is the number of cycles. Most of those who have used the PCR for experimental studies or sample testing have found 20 to 30 cycles to be sufficient. Thus, at 30 cycles one could theoretically produce 2^{30} or 1,073,741,824 copies of just one DNA molecule! Although this number in itself is mind-boggling, the degree of amplification may appear even more impressive if one considers a typical PCR reaction that seeks to detect a virus in a human cell. Say, for example, that one analyzes 100,000 cervical cells (a small-sized biopsy specimen) for HPV. We will assume that only 100 viral particles are present in the entire tissue. Therefore, at the initiation of PCR there is roughly 1 viral segment of DNA for every 1 billion similarly sized fragments of human DNA. However, after about 3 hours and 40 cycles the amount of viral DNA may be greater than the amount of human DNA in the sample. Although the reaction does not work with 100% efficiency, it is routine to amplify as little as 0.01 pg of DNA to 100 ng (10^7-fold- amplification), which may then be visualized on an agarose or acylamide gel stained with ethidium chloride (Fig. 2-25).

PCR Methodology

Now that the theory behind PCR has been discussed, let us elaborate on the actual bench top protocol. Many protocols have been published, and the reader is referred to several papers in this regard (69–91). This section will outline the procedure our laboratory uses with special reference to pitfalls and "helpful hints."

An abbreviated form of the protocol is given in Protocol 2-3. A more detailed description of the various steps follows Protocol 2-3.

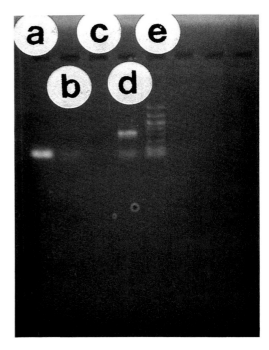

Figure 2-25. *Visualization of amplified DNA on an agarose gel. Lanes a,*(CSF), *b,*(PBMC), and *c* *(PBMC)* are clinical samples that were analyzed for CMV (*a*) and HSV (*b* and *c*) by PCR. No bands of the expected size (CMV, 260; HSV, 105) are evident. To demonstrate the integrity of the DNA in the PBMCs, PCR with *bcl-2*-specific primers was done. As evident in *lane d,* an intense band of the expected size (250 base pairs) is evident. *Lane e* is a 100 base pair ladder starting at 50 to 100 base pairs. The prominent band in *lane a* represents, most likely, primer oligomerization at the expected size of <50 bp.

Protocol 2-3: PCR Protocol

Tissue preparation

1. Cut one 4- to 10-μm paraffin-embedded section
2. Xylene 1 minute, vortex, centrifuge 5 minutes
3. 95% ETOH 1 minute, centrifuge 5 minutes
4. Dry, suspend in 180 μl water
5. Add 20 μl of protease K (10 mg/ml), store 4 to 15 hours at 55°C
6. Inactivate protease at 95°C for 10 minutes, store at 4°C

PCR reaction mixture (to each tube add)

1. 5 μl PCR buffer (as per the GeneAmp kit [Perkin-Elmer])
2. 3 μl MgCl$_2$ (25 μM stock)
3. 6 ml dNTPs (stock, add 25 μl each of 10 mM of dATP, dCTP, dGTP, and dTTP to 100 μl of water)
4. 5 μl sample
5. 1 + 1 μl of primer 1 and primer 2 (20 μM stock)
6. 26.7 μl water
7. 0.3 μl *Taq* polymerase to 2 μl of water in *separate tube on ice*

We have noted increased success of amplification if the DNA in the sample is precipitated in sodium acetate and ethanol prior to amplification and then resuspended in 200 μl water.

Cycling protocol

1. Heating block to 82°C; at 55°C, add the *Taq* polymerase solution, abort file, to 94°C for 3 minutes (manual hot start), overlay with 100 μl heated mineral oil (82°C); switch to 94°C for 3 minutes (manual hot start)
2. Cycling begins; 55°C for 2 minutes and 94°C for 1 minute
3. 25 to 35 cycles; 4°C until ready to process sample

Detection

1. Electrophorese 25 μl of reaction mixture
2. Southern blot hybridization analysis

DNA Extraction

The first step involves the extraction of the DNA from the test sample. If the sample will be taken from paraffin-embedded tissue, the type of fixative used in the processing should be determined. Fixatives such as 10% neutral buffered formalin and 95% ethanol work well (80,82). However, fixatives that contain either picric acid (e.g., Bouin's solution) or heavy metals such as mercury (e.g., Zenker's) will have altered the DNA such that it may no longer be amplified (80,82). For tissues fixed in the de-

sired manner, we recommend using a disposable blade to reduce the possibility of contamination from one sample to another. One 4- to 10-μm tissue section is cut into an Eppendorf tube. To remove the paraffin, resuspend the tissue in 400 μl of xylene, vortex briefly, and then centrifuge for 5 minutes at 15,000 rpm. The xylene is then decanted and residual xylene removed by adding 400 μl of 95% ethanol, vortexing, and centrifuging at 15,000 rpm for 5 minutes. Decant the ethanol, and allow the tissue to dry. The tissue, now free of paraffin, is then suspended in 190 μl of sterile water.

Before continuing the description of the protocol, additional mention should be made of how to limit the problem of contamination during the PCR procedure. The extreme sensitivity of this technique can be its own worst enemy, as contamination of a few target molecules into the sample may lead to a false-positive result. The reader is referred to some of the large amount of literature describing ways to limit contamination. Some of the recommendations include establishing a work area dedicated only to PCR, using cotton-plugged pipette tips, and using various chemical and other sterilization techniques that attempt to render the PCR product nonamplifiable in subsequent reactions (17,33,39). One such chemical-mediated method to reduce the risk of contamination during PCR utilizes the enzyme uracil *N*-glycosylase in conjunction with dUTP. This enzyme has the ability to degrade DNA that contains dUTP nucleotides. However, the enzyme is not functional at the high temperatures used in PCR. Thus, during PCR one can amplify DNA that contains dUTP even if uracil *N*-glycosylase is included in the reaction mixture. However, if some of the amplified product inadvertently carries over to another tube during a subsequent PCR reaction, the uracil *N*-glycosylase will destroy it. The ability of this interesting enzyme to function as a chemical hot start during *in situ* PCR is discussed in Chapter 3.

Our laboratory experience has taught us the utility of "dedicated" pipettemen, a separate laboratory work area restricted to PCR, and the practice of never working out of stock solutions. After making these changes, an initial rate of contamination in our laboratory of about 20% has been reduced to about 1%. However, we have not noted any utility in doing PCR in ventilation hoods or using cotton-plugged pipette tips. The preceding comments are not presented as the final word on PCR contamination, but rather are the results of our experience. Other laboratories may find utility in these latter procedural steps, depending on their particular circumstances.

To return to the protocol, fixatives such as buffered formalin work by cross-linking native proteins with nucleic acids (5,34–36). In this form it may be difficult for the primers to hybridize to their homologous sequences due to the formation of cross-links with native proteins. This problem may be resolved by pretreatment of the deparaffinized tissue with a protease. Our best and most reproducible results have been obtained with the use of proteinase K (1 mg/ml at 55°C for 3 to 15 hours). After the digestion is completed, one must inactivate the proteinase K, which can destroy *Taq* polymerase. Proteinase inactivation is easily accomplished by heating at 95°C for 10 minutes.

Although one can use the DNA from formalin-fixed tissues for successful solution phase PCR, it should be appreciated that, even after adequate protease digestion to release the DNA target from protein–DNA cross-links, there may be other problems. For example, prolonged storage of the formalin-fixed, paraffin-embedded tissue blocks, that is, for several years, has been associated with a decreased ability to amplify DNA sequences. This is especially true if the target size is over 500 base pairs (21). For this reason, when using paraffin-embedded tissue sections that have been stored for 3 years or more, it would be advantageous to use a primer pair that dictates the synthesis of a PCR product from 100 to 200 base pairs in length. The explanation for this apparent degradation over time of formalin-fixed DNA awaits further study. It should be appreciated, however, that PCR products (sometimes referred to as *amplicons*) greater than 200 base pairs can be amplified from the DNA extracted from paraffin-embedded tis-

sues; indeed, PCR products have been obtained from ancient DNA extracted from mummies. Furthermore, we have experienced good results using RT *in situ* PCR to detect RNA in tissues embedded for several years. The point, however, is that the probability of success in obtaining a desired amplicon may be increased for some tissues and for some targets by decreasing the size of the amplicon when dealing with paraffin-embedded tissues.

Summary of the DNA Extraction Steps

1. Use fresh or fixed cells or tissue; do not use fixatives that contain heavy metals or picric acid.
2. For paraffin-embedded tissue sections, cut one or two sections each about 5 μm in size with disposable blade and place in sterile 1.5-ml tube.
3. Add 400 μl of xylene, vortex briefly, and centrifuge at 15,000 rpm for 5 minutes.
4. Decant, add 400 μl of 95% ethanol, vortex briefly, and centrifuge at 15,000 rpm for 5 minutes.
5. Decant, either air dry or dry with a speed-vacuum, and resuspend in 190 μl of sterile water.
6. Add 10 μl of proteinase K (10 mg/ml stock solution).
7. Digest at 55°C for 4 to 15 hours.
8. Heat inactivate the protease at 95°C for 10 minutes; store at 4°C.
9. Precipitate DNA with .3M sodium acetate and 100% ethanol; resuspend in 200 μl water.

PCR Step

The next step is the preparation of the reaction mixture. Because the extracted DNA sample may contain inhibitors of PCR such as blood, magnesium chelators, or excess magnesium, and because PCR is very sensitive, it is better to use "a little" and not "a lot" of sample. A good rule of thumb is a 1:10 to 1:20 dilution of sample to the final reaction mixture volume. The other reagents are listed in Protocol 2-3. The concentrations listed in Protocol

2-3 are effective across a wide range of primer pairs and targets. However, the optimal concentration of magnesium and primers may vary with some targets. It may be useful to use a known positive sample at the recommended concentrations and, for example, ± 1 mM for magnesium and ± 0.5 μM for the primers. Variables such as the commercial source of the DNA polymerase that one is using and the presence of magnesium chelaters may alter the optimal concentration of magnesium for a given sample. The GC content of primers may influence the optimal primer concentration, requiring lower concentrations to reduce the risk of primer oligomerization. It should be stressed that it may be highly advantageous to adjust the concentration of the $MgCl_2$ over a range of 1.0 to 5.0 mM. Over this range, we have noted that the amplification of some target–primer pairs may vary more than 100-fold. Optimal amplification for some primers was 1.0 mM $MgCl_2$, whereas for others the optimal $MgCl_2$ was 4.5 mM (G.J. Nuovo, *unpublished observations, 1994*). On a practical level, I find that variations in the magnesium are the most likely to lead to changes in the yield of amplification. Higher concentrations tend to give more product, although aberrant or extra bands are more likely with the higher magnesium. Clearly, if one is getting poor amplification with a given target, it may be useful to try the PCR reaction at the range of magnesium concentrations noted above. Interestingly, the concentration of $MgCl_2$ during PCR *in situ* hybridization is much less variable and appears to be optimal at 4.5 mM for a wide variety of targets and primer pairs. This is discussed in detail in Chapter 5.

Although the protocol listed in Protocol 2-3 is based on the DNA polymerase *Taq* polymerase, other enzymes are available that may be preferable under certain conditions. For example, targets with high GC-rich areas can present problems because of their high propensity to form internal loops, driven by the three hydrogen bonds that form between every GC pair. Areas rich in AT pairs are much less likely to form such loops, as they only generate two hydrogen bonds per match. When attempting to amplify targets that have in excess of 80%

GC content, we have found that it is preferable to use higher denaturing (97°C) and annealing (65° to 72°C) temperatures. Although *Taq* polymerase and the other thermostable DNA polymerases that are commercially available can function at these temperatures, they have a half-life at 97.5°C that is usually around 10 minutes. The Stoffel fragment of *Taq* polymerase, which lacks the 289 N-terminal amino portion of the enzyme, has an increased thermal stability (20 minute half-life at 97.5°C) that allows the use of higher temperatures with a greater probability that sufficient enzyme will still be functional during the critical last cycles of PCR. The enzyme also has a broader range of optimal magnesium concentrations. Finally, it lacks the 5′ to 3′ exonuclease activity of *Taq* polymerase, which is useful in studying the effects of this activity during PCR. These studies have aided in the analysis of the nonspecific pathways during *in situ* PCR, as is discussed in Chapter 3.

A wide variety of cycling protocols have been published (5,20–36). All, of course, begin with a denaturing step, followed in most cases by an annealing step, an extension step, and the denaturing step. Standard protocols would indicate 37° to 55°C for 1 to 2 minutes for annealing, 55° to 72°C for 1 to 2 minutes for extension (i.e., primer extension secondary to DNA synthesis), and 94°C for denaturing for 1 to 2 minutes for 20 to 40 cycles. However, as noted earlier, the rate-limiting step is primer annealing and not extension of the primer by *Taq* polymerase (Dr. Will Bloch, Applied Biosystems Incorporated, *personal communication*, 1992). Other rate-limiting variables with PCR include the concentration of the primer and *Taq* polymerase. If the latter two are very high, as is the case with the amplifying solution protocol presented in this chapter, then primer extension will present a very small fraction of the total time needed for successful amplification. Thus, we have eliminated the extension step, which not only saves time but also extends the reaction life of the *Taq* polymerase.

Heat sensitivity is another important issue with regard to the *Taq* polymerase. Although it is highly resistant to elevated temperatures, it is by no means indestructible, and the elevated temperatures (usually ≥55°C, especially, of course, the denaturing temperatures) encountered in PCR slowly degrade the enzyme. Thus, insufficient functional *Taq* polymerase may remain toward the end of the cyclings, which, given the exponential progression of PCR, is the critical time in terms of synthesizing large amounts of product. These considerations lead to an important question. Is the actual temperature during the procedure or the time spent at a given elevated temperature more deleterious to *Taq* polymerase? Or, to say it in another way, is more *Taq* polymerase rendered inoperable at 97°C for 3 minutes or at 94°C for 6 minutes? It has been found that the latter is more deleterious (Dr. Will Bloch, *personal communication,* 1992). For this reason, we prefer to limit the initial denaturing step to 3 minutes at 94°C and 1 minute for subsequent denaturations. These times will be dependent, in part, on the actual thermocycler one is using. The Perkin-Elmer 9600 and 480, which change temperatures quickly, allow for a rapid transfer of heat, especially with the thin-walled tubes, and thus, one can use 94°C for shorter times (the initial denaturing step to 3 minutes at 94°C and 1 minute for subsequent denaturations). Because the Perkin-Elmer TC-1 and similar machines from other companies require longer times to reach 94°C, 5 minutes for the initial denaturation and 1.5 minutes for subsequent denaturations are suggested.

It is also important to note that the annealing temperature is better kept toward the higher end of the range to help limit the potential for primer oligomerization and mispriming. The Tm for these nonspecific pathways may be calculated from either the Tm formula presented earlier in this chapter or from computer-generated programs. Although these calculations may be useful as a general rule, annealing temperatures of 55° to 60°C will usually inhibit the nonspecific pathways, which, if unimpeded, could overwhelm the target-specific pathway. Of course, these elevated temperatures work best when used in association with the hot start maneuver. Withholding the DNA polymerase until the reaction temperature reaches 55°C is

an essential step to inhibit nonspecific pathways, as they are most likely to predominate at around room temperature. Experimental data that demonstrate the need for the hot start modification to PCR is presented in Chapter 4.

Many other protocols for PCR have been published (37–62). It may be appreciated that the protocol listed above has fewer steps and may be easier to follow than others. With some experience, readers will be able to determine which modifications to the standard protocols are best suited for their particular laboratories.

Summary of the Amplifying Step of PCR

1. Add to a 0.5-ml tube the following reagents:
    5 μl of PCR buffer II (GeneAmp kit)
    3 μl of MgCl$_2$ (25 mM stock solution)
    6 μl of the dNTP solution (25 μl of dATP [10 mM stock solution], 25 μl of dCTP [10 mM stock solution], 25 μl of dGTP [10 mM stock solution], 25 μl of dTTP [10 mM stock solution], 100 μl of sterile water)
    1 μl of primer 1 (20 μM stock solution)
    1 μl of primer 2 (20 μM stock solution)
    5 μl of sample DNA (extracted as per protocol listed above)
    27 μl of sterile water
    ± 0.5 μl of digoxigenin dUTP (1 μM stock solution)
2. For each reaction tube, place 2 μl of sterile water in a separate tube.
3. Begin with file of 82°C (soak file); at onset of this file, add 0.3 μl of *Taq* polymerase for each reaction to the tube with the second water that should be kept on ice (this is the so-called manual hot start maneuver).
4. When temperature reaches 60°C, add 2.0 μl of the *Taq*-containing solution per tube, then 100 μl of preheated sterile mineral oil. The oil can be preheated on a separate dry bath or in a separate 0.5-μl tube in the thermal cycler.
5. When the temperature reaches 82°C, abort file, then heat to 94°C for 3 minutes.
6. Cycle at 55°C for 2 minutes, then 94°C for 1 minute for 25 to 35 cycles.
7. Cool to 4°C until tubes are removed.

Detecting the Amplified Product

This section deals with the detection of the newly synthesized DNA. Some (hopefully most) of this amplified DNA will be the target of interest, but, under standard conditions, nonspecific synthesis from mispriming and primer oligomerization will also occur. It should be stressed, however, that although the hot start maneuver increases the specificity and sensitivity of PCR, some nonspecific DNA may be synthesized (as discussed in Chapter 3). Thus, one still needs to prove the specificity of the PCR product, even when using the hot start maneuver.

Several methods are available for detecting DNA. They can be divided into methods that detect any synthesized DNA and methods that detect only the amplified target. The simplest way to detect amplified DNA is nonspecific and uses electrophoresis with a gel made with agarose or, for smaller fragments, acylamide. In this way, one can separate the DNA according to its size and configuration. Electrophoresis is well suited to PCR, because one attempts to generate large numbers of DNA fragments of the same size. A common way to visualize the DNA directly on the gel is to use intercalating agents such as ethidium bromide, which fluoresce with ultraviolet light (Fig. 2-25). The ethidium bromide solution should always be handled with gloves, as it is carcinogenic. Known size standards can be used to determine whether the size of the amplified fragment is as expected from the known distance between the primers. In my experience, it is highly unlikely to see nonspecific DNA synthesis produce bands when the hot start maneuver is used and when the PCR product is from 75 to 250 base pairs in size. Another point to consider is that amplification may occur with less than optimal efficiency, and the final amount of synthesized DNA may be below the detection threshold for direct visualization with ethidium bromide (about 100 ng of DNA). For this reason, more sensitive techniques are often employed.

Another nonspecific method for detection of the PCR product utilizes a reporter molecule in the amplification solution. The formula for direct incorporation of digoxigenin dUTP

was given in Protocol 2-3. With direct incorporation of biotin or digoxigenin dUTP, one only needs to transfer the PCR-synthesized DNA to a filter and then detect the biotin or digoxigenin by the use of alkaline phosphate-conjugated complexes of streptavidin or antidigoxigenin, respectively. Pathologists especially favor this procedure, because detection of alkaline phosphatase-linked complexes is an everyday procedure in the immunohistochemistry laboratory. One may employ colorimetric detection by the use of chromogens such as NBT and BCIP, which yield a blue precipitate, to cite just one commonly used detection method (Fig. 2-26) (24). Many other reporter molecules, including, but not limited to, biotin and ^{32}P may be employed. The advantage of ^{32}P is that the DNA is simply transferred to a filter and then developed by autoradiography. The obvious disadvantage is the need to dispose of the large amount of ^{32}P-contaminated material generated from the procedure. I recommend using digoxigenin or some other nonisotopic system because such sys-

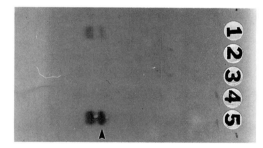

Figure 2-26. *Detection of the PCR product: digoxigenin incorporation.* During PCR, one can incorporate the reporter molecule directly into the PCR product. In this case, PCR was done for HPV from a variety of cancers. After transferring the DNA after electrophoresis from the agarose gel to a filter, one needs only to detect the digoxigenin. Note the bands evident in *lanes 1* and *5*; the *arrow* marks 450 base pairs, which is the expected size of the amplicon. The presence of multiple bands usually indicates a magnesium concentration that is slightly too high. This method is much quicker than that shown in Fig. 2-27, as it eliminates the need for a hybridization step. However, it is essential that one inhibits the nonspecific pathways. This can be done with the hot start maneuver, as discussed in Chapter 3.

tems now offer detection thresholds of 0.1 pg of DNA. This level of detection is similar to what can be obtained with ^{32}P. Many companies sell digoxigenin-and biotin-labeled molecular weight markers, which greatly assist in determining the size of the amplified product. The 0.1-pg detection threshold offers a 10^6-fold increase over ethidium staining.

As discussed above, there are two commonly used techniques that can be used to detect DNA—slot blot and Southern blot hybridization analyses. When using either technique to detect the amplified product after PCR, it is important to choose as the probe a labeled segment internal to the primers that will detect the amplified product but not other DNA synthesized as the result of mispriming or primer oligomerization. I strongly recommend that one use Southern blot hybridization rather than slot blot because it gives one the added assurance of a hybridization signal with the size of the amplified DNA (Fig. 2-27). Slot blot hybridization is much more prone to producing false-positive results, because there may be so much DNA concentrated on the filter that a signal is evident even though the DNA could be derived from nonspecific amplification and share relatively poor homology with the probe (63). The recommended protocols for dot blot and Southern blot hybridization are listed above, and protocols used by other investigators are listed in the bibliography (20,24,64–90). Commercially available kits for both techniques that are easy to use are readily available (e.g., Southern blot kit from ONCOR).

Because the oligoprobes that are used to detect the amplified product are small, often from 18 to 45 base pairs, the labeling methods of nick translation and random primers, discussed at length in Chapter 4, will not work well, as they require DNA templates of at least 200 base pairs for optimal activity. A more efficient method involves the enzyme terminal transferase, which can place labeled nucleotides on the 3′ end of the oligonucleotide. Through the generosity of Dr. Brian Holaway at Boehringer Mannheim, I was able to compare two such terminal transferase-based systems for the labeling of oligoprobes. One system places one dideoxydigoxigenin dUTP molecule on the 3′

end, whereas the other links a variable number, often 5 to 20, of dATPs and digoxigenin dUTPs on the 3′ end of the probe. Although the latter 3′ tailing method produces more background, in our experience it has a much greater sensitivity due to the larger number of digoxigenin molecules present on a given probe. Similarly, one can make oligoprobes with much higher specific activity using the tailing method with ^{32}P. I strongly recommend the 3′ tailing method for oligoprobe synthesis in detection of the amplified product in both PCR and PCR *in situ* hybridization. This topic is discussed at length, with demonstration of some of the experimen-

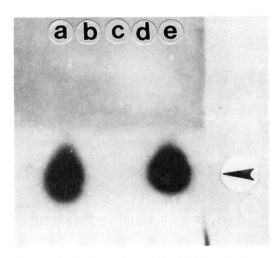

Figure 2-27. *Detection of the PCR product: hybridization with an oligoprobe.* PCR was done using primers specific for the Epstein-Barr virus (EBV) in several lymphomas from AIDS patients. No bands were evident in the agarose gel after ethidium staining (not shown). The DNA was transferred to a filter that was hybridized to a ^{32}P-labeled probe made by labeling the EBV DNA segment internal to the two primers. The band in *lane a* is the expected size of the amplified EBV fragment. *Lanes b* and *c* are other lymphoma samples, *lane d* the negative control (water), and *lane e* the positive control, which was DNA extracted from an EBV-containing Burkitt's lymphoma cell line. It is important to stress that the stringency conditions used in these experiments (1× SSC and 50°C for 10 minutes) were much less than those used for the Southern blot depicted in Fig. 2-20, where a full-length HPV 16 probe was used. Increasing the stringency of the wash to 0.2 × SSC and 60°C for 10 minutes as used in the HPV 16 assay would have abolished the signal in this blot.

tal data, in Chapter 5. Recall that it is important to use much different hybridization and wash conditions for oligoprobes and for full-length probes in filter hybridization. This important topic is discussed again in Chapter 5 in the context of PCR *in situ* hybridization.

BASICS OF HISTOLOGY

Introduction

This final section is provided for the investigator with little experience in examining tissue sections. It provides a brief overview of the organization of different tissue types and the specific features of different cell types to assist the reader in identifying what cell type contains the target of interest.

Tissue Processing

After a tissue section is removed, it is placed in a fixative. The most common fixative in the surgical pathology laboratory is 10% buffered formalin. The tissue is placed into a plastic mold and then into an automatic processor. The tissue processor is programmed to fix the tissue for an additional 4 hours, dehydrate it through ethanol and xylene, and then embed it into paraffin. To achieve paraffin embedding, the tissue must be heated at 65°C for 4 hours. The wax is then cooled, the tissue is placed in a plastic block which is then placed on a microtome. This is a machine that allows one to cut 4-μm "ribbons" of tissue that are floated on a water bath. The technician then puts a glass slide in the water bath and "scoops" the ribbon up and in this way places the tissue on the slide. The slide is then baked for 15 to 60 minutes at 60°C to remove any remaining water. The tissue can be stored this way for years. When ready for use, the paraffin is removed by washing the slide for 3 to 5 minutes in xylene and then 100% ethanol. It can then be stained or analyzed by other assays, such as *in situ* hybridization.

Different Cell Types

There are three different categories of cells that one may see in a tissue section. These are epithelial, stromal, and inflammatory cells. Each is discussed in turn. First, a brief discussion of the organization of the cell is in order.

The Components of a Cell

A cell is composed of a *nucleus* and the *cytoplasm*. In epithelial and stromal cells (described below), the cytoplasm is ample. In one type of inflammatory cell, the lymphocyte, only a scant amount of cytoplasm is evident, whereas the other types of inflammatory cells have ample cytoplasm. In most cells, the size of the nucleus is from 4 to 10 μm in diameter. The *nucleus* contains *chromatin*, which is a complicated matrix of DNA and associated proteins, notably the histones. In active cells, a prominent area of the nucleus is the *nucleolus*, which contains ample ribosomal RNA and associated proteins. The routine stain for histologists is hematoxylin and eosin. Hematoxylin binds to nucleic acids and produces a blue color (see Color Plate 15 following p. 242). The nucleus, thus, will have a blue color. Eosin binds to proteins and produces a pink color. Thus, the cytoplasm usually stains a light pink. Important exceptions are cell types that contain a large amount of, usually, a specialized protein. Common examples include squamous cells, which may contain a large amount of keratin, and skeletal muscle cells, which contain abundant myosin and actin. The abundant amount of protein yields an intense pink color to the cytoplasm of these cells (see Color Plate 1 following p. 242). However, nucleoli sometimes stain pink due to, at times, large amounts of rRNA-related proteins.

The *cytoplasm* contains *organelles* involved in RNA and protein trafficking (*endoplasmic reticulum, ribosomes*, and *Golgi complex*), energy production and usage (*mitochondria*), processing of native and foreign proteins (*lysosomes* and *vacuoles*), and variable amounts of lipids and storage carbohydrates, notably glycogen. The nucleus, nucleoli, and some of these organelles are evident in the electron microscopic photographs shown in Fig. 2-28.

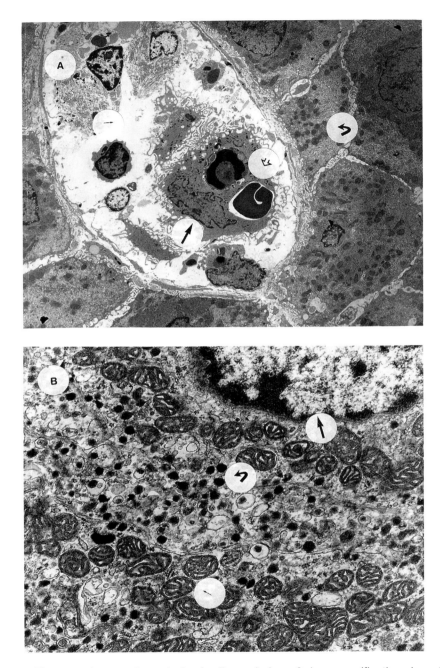

Figure 2-28. *Electron microscopic analysis of cell morphology.* **A:** low magnification view of the liver. Note the sinusoidal space that contains leukocytes (*small arrow*). The nucleus of a leukocyte is also shown (*large arrow*); note the ingested red blood cells (*open arrow*). The hepatocytes are much larger and show many tubular structures (*curved arrow*), which are mitochondria. ×2,000. **B:** The mitochondria are shown at higher magnification in another cell type from the anterior pituitary gland. Note their convoluted membrane-based structure (*small arrow*) and part of the nucleus (*large arrow*). The many small, black, and round structures are neurosecretory granules (*curved arrow*), which contain hormones such as growth hormone.

Epithelium

Epithelial cells are found on the surface of most tissues. By invaginations, they also form simple to complex structures known as *glands*. There are three types of epithelial cells: squa- mous cells, glandular cells, and transitional cells.

Squamous epithelium is *stratified*, and the cells, as they approach the surface, are *large and flat*. Squamous cells synthesize *keratin*. On the skin, this is evident as a layer of pink either dense

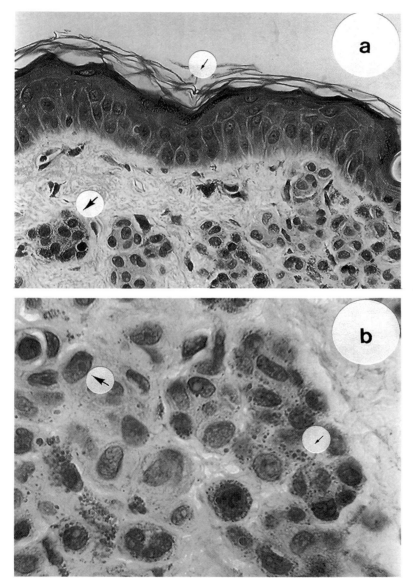

Figure 2-29. *Histologic features of keratinized squamous epithelium: the skin.* The stratified squamous epithelium shows at its surface a "basket weave" type of keratin (*small arrow*), which is typical of the epidermis of skin. Note the nests of cells (*large arrow*) in the stroma (called the dermis) (**a**). These rep- resent a benign proliferation of cells called melanocytes, which contain the pigment melanin in their cy- toplasm (**b**, *small arrow*). The prominent nucleoli typical of these cells are also indicated (*large arrow*).

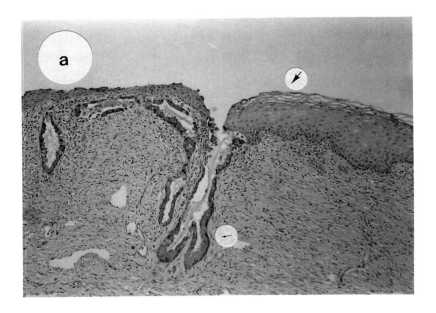

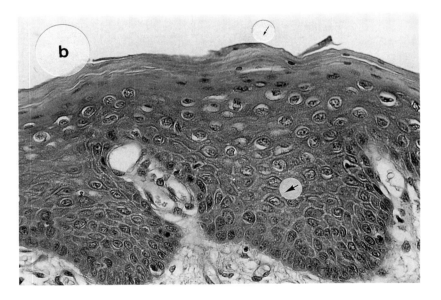

Figure 2-30. *Histologic features of nonkeratinized squamous epithelium: the cervix.* This section of the cervix shows the nonkeratinized stratified squamous epithelium typical of mucosal sites (*large arrow*); note the simple tubular or branching glands that are also evident (**a**, *small arrow*). In another section at higher magnification, the stratified squamous epithelium is inflamed and is showing minimal keratinization at its surface (**b**, *small arrow*), which serves a protective function. Also evident in this section is another feature of inflammation: The squamous cells at the base are separated from one another by small spaces (this is called spongiosis; *large arrow*). In the cervix and other sites where squamous and glandular epithelia meet, it is common to see squamous metaplasia, where the glandular cells (*small arrow*) are being replaced by immature squamous epithelium (*large arrow*). A capillary is also shown (**c**, *open arrow*) (see Fig. 2-34).

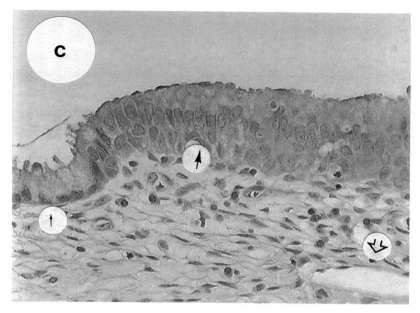

Figure 2-30. *Continued.*

or more open "basket weave" material without nuclei; this forms a waterproof barrier for the skin (Fig. 2-29). Also note the melanocytes, which synthesize the dark pigment melanin, giving the skin its color, that are forming a benign tumor in this skin biopsy material. The keratin is usually not evident on the nonskin (mucosal) surfaces lined by squamous epithelium (Fig. 2-30). Such sites include the cervix, anorectal junction, oral cavity, and esophagus. Note in Fig. 2-30a that the squamous epithelium is associated with a branching, tubular structure; these are glands. The fact that the squamous epithelium is, in areas, overlying the glands is due to a process called *squamous metaplasia* (Figure 2-30c). *Metaplasia* refers to the process whereby one cell type (usually epithelium) is replaced by another cell type; in this case, glandular epithelium is replaced by squamous epithelium.

Glandular cells are usually a *single layer thick* (called *simple*), and the cells have *basal arranged nuclei* with prominent secretions or other specialized cell processes, such as cilia or microvilli (Fig. 2-31). The secretions may contain mucus, especially in the gastrointestinal tract and the cervix (Fig. 2-31), which is notorious for nonspecifically sticking to probes during *in situ* hybridization and, thus, causing background. Glandular cells line the gastrointestinal tract from the lower esophagus, stomach, small and large intestines to the anorectal junction, respiratory tract, gallbladder, uterus, fallopian tubes, salivary and sweat glands, breast, prostate, and seminal vesicles. Glandular epithelium also comprises much of the liver, pancreas, and kidneys.

Transitional epithelium lines the bladder and the structures that both enter and exit the bladder. It consists of *stratified epithelium* in which the surface cells have typical *dome* or *umbrella shapes*. Keratin production is not evident (Fig. 2-32).

Stromal (Mesenchymal) Cells

Underneath the epithelium is a dense fibrous network that provides much of the support of the body. The primary cell of this region is the **fibroblast**, which synthesizes the major protein of the body, *collagen*. The fibroblast is a *long, tapered* cell with a *spindle-shaped nu-*

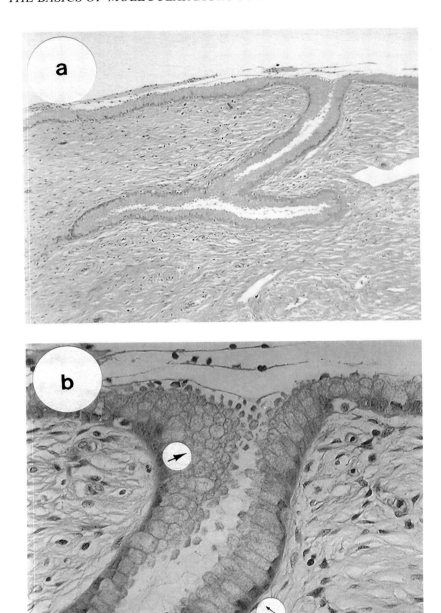

Figure 2-31. *Histologic features of glandular epithelium.* This section of the cervix shows the simple branched glands typical of the distal region of the cervix (**a**). At higher magnification (**b**), note the single layer of cells that have basal arranged nuclei (*small arrow*) and ample cytoplasm. The cytoplasm has vacuoles that are the mucus made by these cells (*large arrow*).

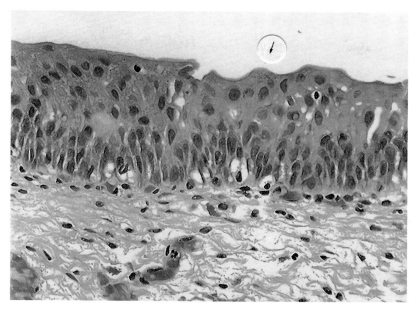

Figure 2-32. *Histologic features of transitional epithelium.* This section of the bladder shows stratified epithelium that is lined by nonkeratinizing cells that are flattened and have a cap-like surface (*arrow*), typical of urothelium.

cleus. It is typically encased in the dark pink collagen fibrils (Fig. 2-33). A common consequence of tissue damage is a *scar,* which consists in large part of collagen synthesized by fibroblasts. Figure 2-33 shows a scar that formed in the heart after a myocardial infarction; note the entrapped, partly degenerated muscle fiber. The nutrients of the body are provided by the blood vessels that are found in the stroma. The **arterioles** (which carry blood from the heart), **venules** (which carry blood back to the heart), and **lymphatics** (which carry lymph to the heart) are usually found in groups of three. The arterioles have relatively thick walls, whereas the venules and lymphatics are thin walled (Fig. 2-34). These vessels are found deep in the stroma. Nearer the surface, **capillaries** are found. The four different vessel types are lined by *flattened, spindle-shaped* cells called **endothelial** cells (Fig. 2-35). Capillaries contain red blood cells and are the actual sites of oxygen exchange. Depending on the site, smooth muscle cells and adipocytes (fat cells) are often encountered in the stroma. The **smooth muscle cells** often run in linear groups called *fascicles*; these cells have *long, tapered, pink cytoplasm* and *spindle-shaped nuclei* with abruptly tapered or *cigar-shaped* ends (Fig. 2-35); they also comprise the walls of arteries. On cross section, a small halo is often seen around the nuclei of the smooth muscle cells. **Adipocytes** are unique in having a very large cytoplasm that consists primarily of a *large droplet of fat* (Fig. 2-36).This fat is removed during the xylene, ethanol washes in the tissue processing and appears as a clear space. The nucleus has a crescent shape, as it is compressed by the fat droplet.

Other specialized mesenchymal cells include **chondrocytes**, which form cartilage, **skeletal muscle cells**, **Schwann cells**, and **osteocytes**, which form bone. Chondocytes are enclosed in a clear space, called *lacuna*, and are surrounded by a *dense bluish material* that consists of mucopolysaccharides (Fig. 2-36). Cartilage does not contain blood vessels. Skeletal muscle cells are among the largest cells in the body and have a very large amount of dark pink cy-

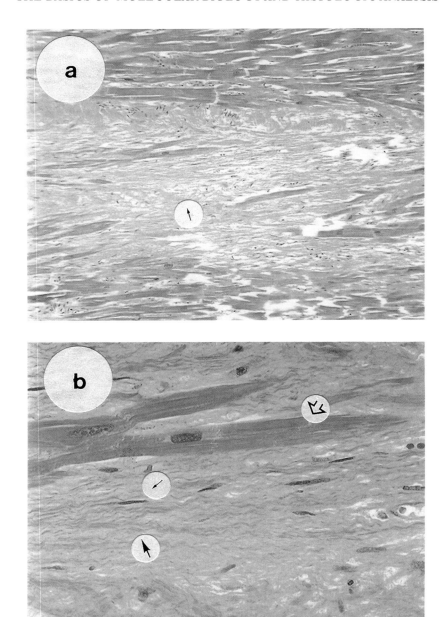

Figure 2-33. *Cells of the stroma: fibroblasts and scar tissue.* **a:** This section of the heart about 3 months after a myocardial infarction shows a large region where only a few muscle cells are evident. This is scar tissue. **b:** At higher magnification, the scar consists of many wavy fibrils—collagen (*large arrow*)—that are made by fibroblasts, which are the cells that have long, tapered cytoplasm and spindle-shaped nuclei (*small arrow*). Note the trapped skeletal muscle cell with its enormous cytoplasm (*open arrow*) that contains discrete fibrils, which correspond to actin and myosin.

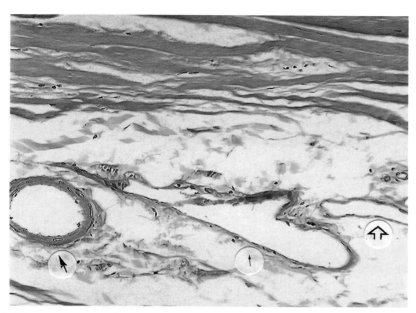

Figure 2-34. *The arrangement of arterioles, venules, and lymphatics in tissue.* Three different vessels are evident in this section: a large, thin-walled vessel (*small arrow*), which is the venule; a smaller, thick-walled vessel (*large arrow*), which is the arteriole; and a small, thin-walled vessel (*open arrow*), which is the lymphatic. These three vessels usually are seen in close proximity deep in the tissue; toward the surface the small, thin-walled capillaries are evident (see Fig. 2-30).

toplasm that contains the contractile proteins *actin* and *myosin* (Fig. 2-33). These form characteristic *cross-striations*. The nuclei are displaced toward the periphery, except for cardiac muscle, where they are centrally located (Fig. 2-33). Schwann cells surround nerve fibers; they make myelin, which is the insulation of the nerves. The Schwann cells have spindle-shaped nuclei that are often *comma shaped* (Fig. 2-36). Osteocytes are the central cells of bone in which the collagen matrix is complexed with minerals such as calcium and phosphate (Fig. 2-36); note the mixture of cells and fat that comprises the bone marrow. The bone marrow is the site of synthesis of red blood cells, neutrophils, eosinophils, and the multinucleated megakaryocytes (which synthesize platelets, which are involved in clotting).

Inflammatory Cells

Inflammatory cells (see Color Plate 2 following p. 242) include the **neutrophils**, in-volved in acute inflammation, **eosinophils, lymphocytes, plasma cells**, and **macrophages**, involved in chronic inflammation. Neutrophils have *multiple lobed nuclei* and *granules* in the cytoplasm, which contain many lysosomes. Eosinophils, involved in allergic responses, have *cytoplasmic granules* and *bilobed nuclei*. Lymphocytes, found in lymph nodes, stroma, and occasionally the epithelium, are *small round cells* with *dark blue nuclei* and *inconspicuous cytoplasm*. When activated in response to a foreign antigen, their nuclei enlarge and their chromatin becomes less dense; nucleoli are prominent due to intense RNA synthesis. Plasma cells make antibodies. They have *eccentric nuclei* with a characteristic *clock-face chromatin* and ample cytoplasm with a *perinuclear clearing* corresponding to a prominent Golgi complex system. Macrophages have *crescent-shaped nuclei* with a characteristic *central groove*. The cytoplasm is *ample* and often contains many *small vacuoles*. Macrophages often become *multinucleate* in response to chronic inflammation.

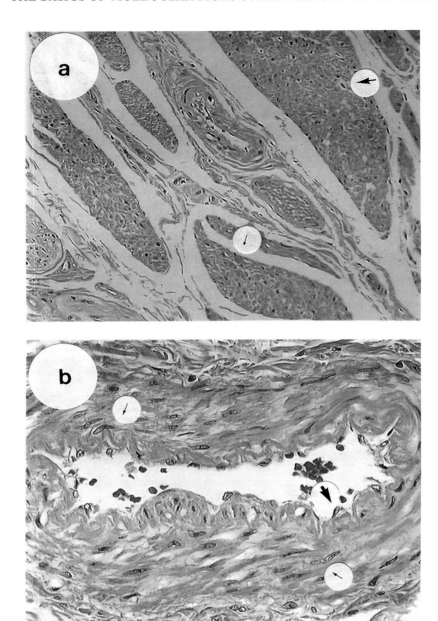

Figure 2-35. *Histologic features of smooth muscle cells.* **a:** Smooth muscle cells, found in contractile organs such as the stomach, small intestine, and colon, as well as the endometrium and bladder, usually run in interlacing groups called fascicles (*small arrow*). In the fascicles cut at cross sections, the clearing around the nuclei of smooth muscle cells, which is typical of this tissue, is evident (*large arrow*). **b:** At higher magnification, smooth muscle cells are seen to have spindled, sometimes wavy nuclei (*small arrow*); the area is the media (muscle wall) of an artery. Note the flattened endothelial cells lining the vessel wall (*large arrow*).

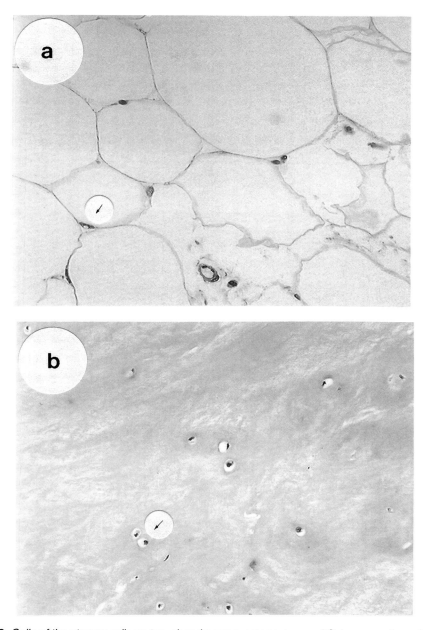

Figure 2-36. *Cells of the stroma: adipocytes, chondrocytes, osteocytes, and Schwann cells.* **a:** Adipocytes have enormous single droplets of fat in their cytoplasm, which compresses the nucleus to a round or crescent shape (*arrow*). **b:** Chrondrocytes are encased in small clear areas called lacuna (*arrow*) and are surrounded by a dense matrix that gives the tissue its strength. **c:** Bone contains osteocytes (*small arrow*); note the dense collagenous matrix that is mineralized for additional strength. Bone marrow is also indicated (*large arrow*). **d:** Section of nerve (*small arrow*). The Schwann cell, which makes myelin, has a spindle-shaped nucleus that may be comma shaped (*large arrow*).

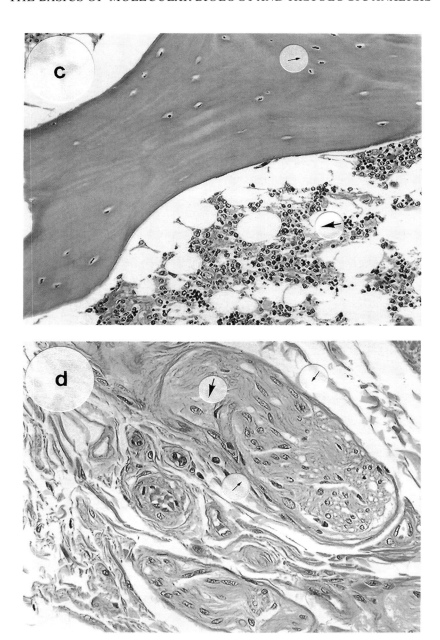

Figure 2-36. *Continued.*

Cancer Cells

Cancer cells have as their characteristic feature *uncontrolled, disorganized proliferation.* This corresponds to certain typical histological features including *variable cell density* (disorganized cell growth) and *nuclear atypia* (variability in nuclear size, shape, and color) (Fig. 2-37). In comparison, benign tumors have an *organized growth pattern* and *minimal nuclear atypia*, as well as a *capsule. Invasion* and *metastases* are other features of malignant tumors; the invasion is often associated with an *intense fibroblast reaction* with *collagen formation* (Fig. 2-37). This gives cancers their hard consistency and is referred to as *desmoplasia.*

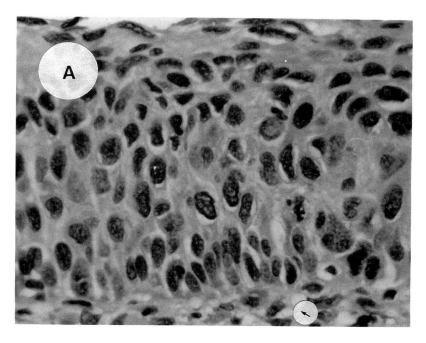

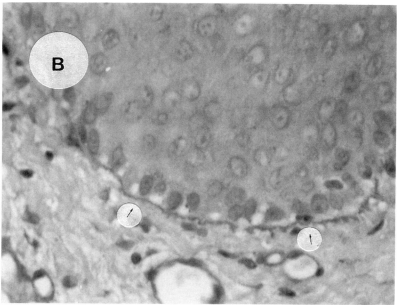

Figure 2-37. *Histologic features of cancer cells.* **A:** Note the crowded, disorganized appearance of this section of carcinoma *in situ*; the variable cell density and nuclear atypia (including the very dark, hyperchromatic nuclei) are characteristic of this early, noninvasive form of neoplasia. **B:** Note the intact basement membrane as seen with the PAS stain (*arrow*). **C:** A squamous cell cancer where nest of cells (*arrow*) are invading blood vessels.

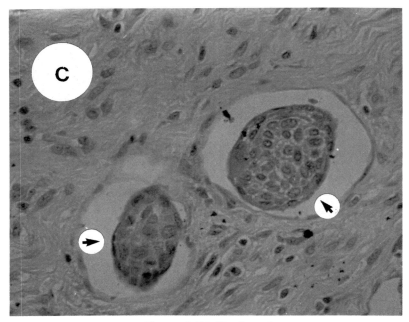

Figure 2-37. *Continued.*

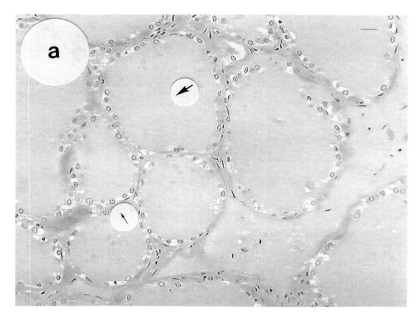

Figure 2-38. *Histologic features of different tissues: thyroid, testes, and liver.* **a:** The thyroid consists of groups of epithelium (*small arrow*) that secrete a large amount of protein called thyroglobulin (*large arrow*). **b:** The testes contains modified stromal cells called Leydig cells (*small arrow*) that make testosterone. Also note the tubules, which contain the germ cells that evolve into spermatids (*large arrow*). **c:** The liver consists of single cell "plates" of epithelium—the hepatocytes (*small arrow*). **d:** Note the groups of vessels and collagen in the portal tract (*large arrow*).

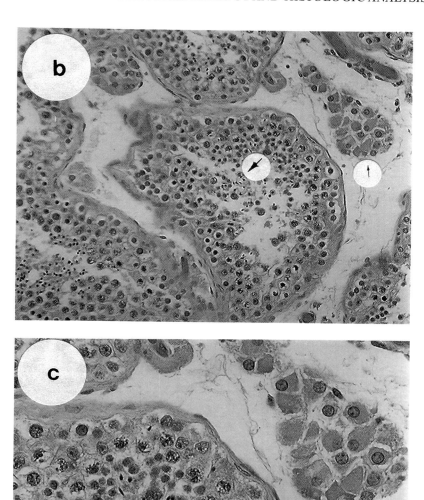

Figure 2-38. *Continued.*

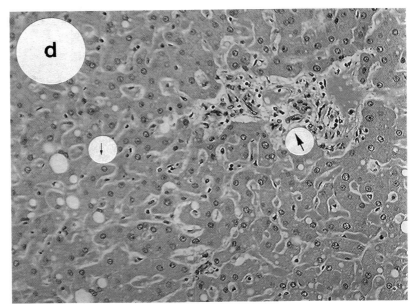

Figure 2-38. *Continued.*

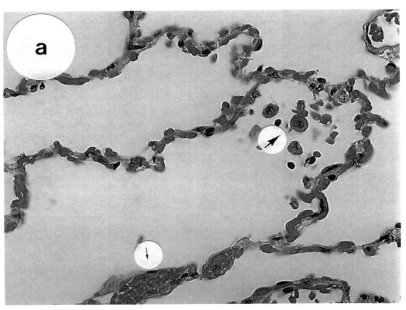

Figure 2-39. *Histologic features of different tissues: lung, pancreas, and kidney.* **a:** The lung consists of large air sacs (the alveoli) that are lined by capillaries (*small arrow*): Note the macrophages in the alveoli (*large arrow*). **b:** The pancreas contains a large amount of epithelium that secretes many enzymes needed for digestion (*small arrow*). The pancreas also contains groups of endocrine cells (which secrete directly into blood vessels) that make, among other hormones, insulin; these are called the islets of Langerhans (*large arrow*). **c:** The cortex, or outer part, of the kidney contains large numbers of glands called proximal convoluted tubules (*small arrow*) that reabsorb much of the electrolytes and water lost via the glomerulus (*large arrow*). **d:** Higher magnification views of proximal convoluted tubules. Note that the glomerulus consists of a group of capillaries (*small arrow*) overlaid by highly specialized epithelial cells (the podocytes; *large arrows*) and stromal cells (the mesangial cells;*open arrow*).

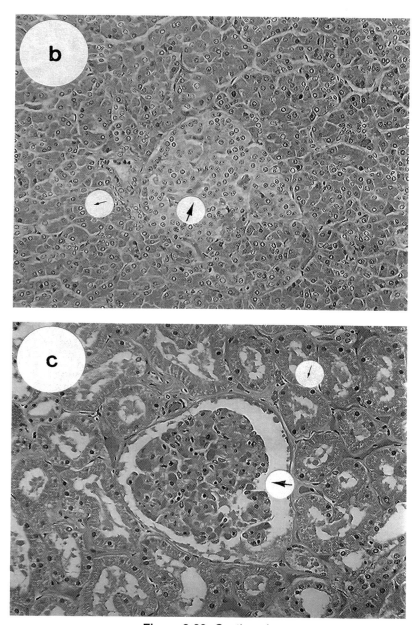

Figure 2-39. *Continued.*

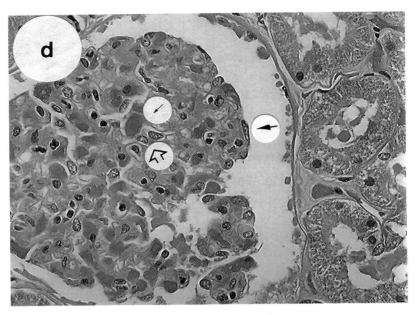

Figure 2-39. *Continued.*

Histology of Different Tissues

It is truly amazing to consider how variable different tissues can look, given that they are usually composed of different mixtures of stromal, epithelial, and inflammatory cells. Figures 2-38 and 2-39 show a brief overview of surgical pathology to illustrate this point; thyroid, testes, liver, lung, pancreas, and kidney are shown. It is hoped that this brief review will assist the nonpathologist in interpreting his or her *in situ* PCR data with tissue sections. Also, certain tissue types, such as in the central nervous system, the female genital tract, and lymph nodes, are discussed in detail in the chapters on HIV-1 and HPV. The reader is referred to several excellent textbooks on normal and abnormal tissue histology for further details (91,92).

REFERENCES

1. Gloss B, Bernard HU. The E6/E7 promoter of human papillomavirus type 16 is activated in the absence of E2 proteins by a sequence aberrant Sp1 distal element. *J Virol* 1990;64:5577–5584.

2. Dartmann K, Schwartz E, Gissmann L, zur Hausen H. The nucleotide sequence and genomic organization of human papilloma virus type 11. *Virology* 1986;151:124–130.

3. Dollard SC, Chow LT, Kreider JW, Broker TR, Lill NL, Howett MK. Characterization of an HPV type 11 isolate propagated in human foreskin implants in nude mice. *Virology* 1989;171:294–297.

4. Durst M, Croce CM, Gissmann L, Schwarz E, Huebbner K. Papillomavirus sequences integrate near cellular oncogenes in some cervical carcinomas. *Proc Natl Acad Sci USA* 1987;84:1070–1074.

5. Nuovo GJ, Silverstein SJ. Comparison of formalin, buffered formalin, and Bouin's fixation on the detection of human papillomavirus DNA from genital lesions. *Lab Invest* 1988;59:720–724.

6. ElAwady MK, Kaplan JB, O'Brien SJ, Burk RD. Molecular analysis of integrated human papillomavirus 16 sequences in the cervical cancer line SiHa. *Virology* 1987;159:389–398.

7. Goldsborough MD, DiSilvestre D, Temple GF, Lorincz AT. Nucleotide sequence of human papillomavirus type 31: a cervical neoplasia-associated virus. *Virology* 1989;171:306–311.

8. Horwitz BH, Weinstat DL, DiMaio D. Transforming activity of a 16-amino-acid segment of the bovine papillomavirus E5 protein linked to random sequences of hydrophobic amino acids. *J Virol* 1989;63:4515–4519.

9. Hrisomalos TF, Boggs DL, Fife KH. Human papillomavirus type 6 long control region and human cellular DNA contain related sequences. *J Virol* 1990;64:5188–5191.

10. Kirii Y, Iwamotot S, Matsukura T. Human papillomavirus type 58 DNA sequence. *J Gen Virol* 1991;38:424–428.

11. Rosen M, Auborn K. Duplication of the upstream regulatory sequences increases the transformation potential of human papillomavirus type 11. *J Gen Virol* 1991;38:484–487.
12. Rozenblatt S, Eizenberg O, Ben-Levy R, Lavie V, Bellini WJ. Sequence homology within the morbilliviruses. *J Virol* 1985;53:684–690.
13. Volpers C, Streeck RE. Genome organization and nucleotide sequence of human papillomavirus type 39. *Virology* 1991;181:419–423.
14. Yogo Y, Kitamura T, Sugimoto C, et al. Isolation of a possible archetypal JC virus DNA sequence from non-immunocompromised individuals. *J Virol* 1990;64:3139–3143.
15. Lawyer FC, Stoffel S, Saiki RK, Myambo KB, Drummond R, Gelfand DH. Isolation, characterization, and expression in E. coli of the DNA polymerase gene from the extreme thermophile, Thermus aquaticus. *J Biol Chem* 1989;264:6427–6437.
16. Saiki RK, Gelfand DH, Stoffel S, et al. Primer-directed enzymatic amplification of DNA with a thermostable DNA polymerase. *Science* 1988;239: 487–491.
17. Innis MA, Gelfand DH, Sninsky JJ, White TJ. *PCR protocols; A guide to methods and applications.* San Diego: Academic Press;1990.
18. Nuovo GJ, MacConnell P, Forde A, Delvenne P. Detection of human papillomavirus DNA in formalin fixed tissues by *in situ* hybridization after amplification by the polymerase chain reaction. *Am J Pathol* 1991;139: 847–854.
19. Nuovo GJ, Gallery F, MacConnell P, Becker J, Bloch W. An improved technique for the detection of DNA by *in situ* hybridization after PCR-amplification. *Am J Pathol* 1991;139:1239–1244.
20. Schiffman MH, Bauer HM, Lorincz AT, et al. A comparison of Southern blot hybridization and polymerase chain reaction methods for the detection of human papillomavirus DNA. *J Clin Microbiol* 1991;29:573–579.
21. Greer CE, Peterson SL, Kiviat NB, Manos MM. PCR amplification from paraffin-embedded tissues: effects of fixative and fixative times. *Am J Clin Pathol* 1991;95: 117–124.
22. Bauer HM, Ting Y, Greer CE, et al. Genital human papillomavirus infection in female university students as determined by a PCR-based method. *JAMA* 1991; 265:472–477.
23. Greer CE, Lund JK, Manos MM. PCR amplification from paraffin-embedded tissues: recommendations on fixatives for long-term storage and prospective studies. *PCR Method Appl* 1992;95:117–124.
24. Nuovo GJ, Darfler MM, Impraim CC, Bromley SE. Occurrence of multiple types of human papillomavirus in genital tract lesions: analysis by *in situ* hybridization and the polymerase chain reaction. *Am J Pathol* 1991;58:518–523.
25. Shibata DK, Arnheim N, Martin WJ. Detection of human papilloma virus in paraffin-embedded tissue using the polymerase chain reaction. *J Exp Med* 1988;167: 225–230.
26. Brandsma JL, Lewis AJ, Abramson A, Manos MM. Detection and typing of papillomavirus DNA in formaldehyde-fixed paraffin-embedded tissue. *Arch Otolaryngol Head Neck Surg* 1990;116:844–848.
27. Lorincz AT. Human papillomavirus testing. *Diagn Clin Test* 1989;27:28–37.
28. Melchers WJG, Schift R, Stolz E, Lindeman J, Quint WGV. Human papillomavirus detection in urine samples from male patients by the polymerase chain reaction. *J Clin Microbiol* 1989;27:1711–1714.
29. Telenti A, Aksamit AJ, Proper J, Smith TF. Detection of JC virus DNA by polymerase chain reaction in patients with progressive multifocal leukoencephalopathy. *J Infect Dis* 1990;162:858–861.
30. van den Brule A, Claas E, du Maine M, et al. Application of anticontamination primers in the polymerase chain reaction for the detection of human papilloma virus genotypes in cervical scrapes and biopsies. *J Med Virol* 1989;97:203–209.
31. Van den Brule AJC, Meijer CJL, Bakels V, Kenemans P, Walboomers JMM. Rapid detection of human papillomavirus in cervical scrapes by combined general primer-mediated and type-specific polymerase chain reaction. *J Clin Microbiol* 1990;28:2739–2743.
32. Wright PA, Wynford-Thomas D. The polymerase chain reaction: miracle or mirage? *J Pathol* 1990;162:99–117.
33. Higuchi R, Kwok S. Avoiding false positives with PCR. *Nature* 1989;339:237–238.
34. Nuovo GJ. Buffered formalin is the superior fixative for the detection of human papillomavirus DNA by *in situ* hybridization analysis. *Am J Pathol* 1989;134:837–842.
35. Dubeau L, Chandler LA, Gralow JR, Nichols PW, Jones PA. Southern blot analysis of DNA extracted from formalin fixed pathology specimens. *Cancer Res* 1986; 46:2964–2970.
36. Moench TR, Gendelman HE, Clements JE, Narayan O, Griffin DE. Efficiency of *in situ* hybridization as a function of probe size and fixation technique. *J Virol Methods* 1985;11:119–130.
37. Bedell MA, Hudson JB, Golub TR, et al. Amplification of human papillomavirus genomes in vitro is dependent on epithelial differentiation. *J Virol* 1991;65:2254–2260.
38. Erlich HA, Gelfand D, Sninsky JJ. Recent advances in the polymerase chain reaction. *Science* 1991;252: 1643–1650.
39. Griffen NR, Bevan IS, Lewis FA, Wells M, Young LS. Demonstration of multiple HPV types in normal cervix and in cervical squamous cell carcinoma using the polymerase chain reaction on paraffin wax embedded material. *J Clin Pathol* 1990;43:52–56.
40. Haase AT, Retzel EF, Staskus KA. Amplification and detection of lentiviral DNA inside cells. *Proc Natl Acad Sci USA* 1990;87:4971–4975.
41. Kawashima M, Favre M, Obalek S, Jablonska S, Orth G. Premalignant lesions and cancers of the skin in the general population: evaluation of the role of human papillomavirus. *J Invest Dermatol* 1990;95:537–542.
42. Lauer SA, Malter JS, Meier JR. Human papillomavirus type 18 in conjunctival intraepithelial neoplasia. *Am J Ophthamol* 1990;110:23–27.
43. Lynas C, Cook SD, Laycock KA, Bradfield JWB, Maitland NJ. Detection of latent virus mRNA in tissues using the polymerase chain reaction. *J Pathol* 1989;157: 285–289.
44. Mariette X, Gozlan J, Clerc D, Bisson M, Morinet F. Detection of Epstein-Barr virus DNA by *in situ* hybridization and polymerase chain reaction in salivary gland biopsy specimens from patients with Sjogren's syndrome. *Am J Med* 1991;90:286–294.
45. McDonnell JM, Mayr AJ, Martin WJ. DNA of human papillomavirus type 16 in dysplastic and malignant le-

sions of the conjunctiva and cornea. *N Engl J Med* 1989; 320:1442–1446.

46. Park JS, Jones RW, McLean MR, Currie JL, Woodruff JD, Shah KV. Possible etiologic heterogeneity of vulvar intraepithelial neoplasia. *Cancer* 1991;67:1599–1607.
47. Riou G, Favre M, Jeannel D, Bourhis J, LeDoussal V, Orth G. Association between poor prognosis in early stage invasive cervical carcinomas and non-detection of HPV DNA. *Lancet* 1990;1171–1174.
48. Shibata D, Fu YS, Gupta JW, Shah KV, Arnheim N, Martin WJ. Detection of human papillomavirus in normal and dysplastic tissue by the polymerase chain reaction. *Lab Invest* 1988;59:555–559.
49. Stetler-Stevenson M, Crush-Stanton S, Cossman J. Involvement of the bcl-2 gene in Hodgkin's disease. *J Natl Cancer Inst* 1990;82:855–858.
50. Syrjanen S, Saastamoinen J, Chang F, Ji H, Syrjanen K. Colposcopy, punch biopsy, *in situ* DNA hybridization, and the polymerase chain reaction in searching for genital human papillomavirus infections in women with normal pap smears. *J Med Virol* 1990;31:259–266.
51. Tidy JA, Parry GCN, Ward P, et al. High rate of human papillomavirus type 16 infection in cytologically normal cervices. *Lancet* 1989;i:434.
52. Young LS, Bevan IS, Johnson MA, et al. The polymerase chain reaction: a new epidemiological tool for investigating cervical human papillomavirus infection. *Br J Med* 1989;298:14–17.
53. Kiyabu MT, Shibata D, Arnheim N, Martin WJ, Fitzgibbons PL. Detection of human papillomavirus in formalin-fixed, invasive squamous carcinomas using the polymerase chain reaction. *Am J Surg Pathol* 1989;13: 221–224.
54. Johnson MA, Blomfield PI, Bevan IS, Woodman CBJ, Young LS. Analysis of human papillomavirus type 16 E6–E7 transcription in cervical carcinomas and normal cervical epithelium using the polymerase chain reaction. *J Gen Virol* 1990;71:1473–1479.
55. Cristiano K, DiBisceglie AM, Hoofnagle JH, Feinstone SM. Hepatitis C viral RNA in serum of patients with chronic non-A, non-B hepatitis: detection by the polymerase chain reaction using multiple primer sets. *Hepatology* 1991;14:51–55.
56. Persing DH. Polymerase chain reaction: trenches to benches. *J Clin Microbiol* 1991;29:1281–1285.
57. Telenti A, Marshall WF, Smith TF. Detection of Epstein-Barr virus by polymerase chain reaction. *J Clin Microbiol* 1990;28:2187–2190.
58. Nuovo GJ. Human papillomavirus DNA in genital tract lesions histologically negative for condylomata: analysis by *in situ*, Southern blot hybridization and the polymerase chain reaction. *Am J Surg Pathol* 1990;14: 643–651.
59. Nuovo GJ, Hochman H, Eliezri YD, Comite S, Lastarria D, Silvers DN. Detection of human papillomavirus DNA in penile lesions histologically negative for condylomata: analysis by *in situ* hybridization and the polymerase chain reaction. *Am J Surg Pathol* 1990;14: 829–836.
60. Nuovo GJ, Lastarria D, Smith S, Lerner J, Comite SL, Eliezri YD. Human papillomavirus segregation patterns in genital and non-genital warts in prepubertal children and adults. *Am J Clin Pathol* 1991;95:467–472.

61. Koulos J, Symmans F, Nuovo GJ. Human papillomavirus detection in adenocarcinoma of the anus. *Mod Pathol* 1991;4:58–61.
62. Delvenne P, Engellenner W, Ma SF, Mann WJ, Chalas E, Nuovo GJ. Detection of human papillomavirus DNA in biopsy proven cervical intraepithelial lesions in pregnant women. *J Repro Med* 1992; 37: 829–833.
63. Eliezri YD, Silverstein SJ, Levine RU, Nuovo GJ. Occurrence of human papillomavirus DNA in cutaneous squamous and basal cell neoplasms. *J Am Acad Dermatol* 1990;23:836–842.
64. Maniatis M. *Principles of molecular biology*. New York: Cold Spring Harbor; 1990.
65. Southern EM. Detection of specific sequences among DNA fragments separated by gel electrophoresis. *J Mol Biol* 1975;98:503–517.
66. Bergeron C, Shah K, Daniel R, Ferenczy A. Search for human papillomavirus in normal, hyperplastic and neoplastic endometria. *Obstet Gynecol* 1988;72:383–387.
67. Burk RD, Kadish AS, Calderin S, Romney SL. Human papillomavirus infection of the cervix detected by cervicovaginal lavage and molecular hybridization: correlation with biopsy results and Papanicolaou smear. *Am J Obstet Gynecol* 1986;154:982–989.
68. Gal D, Friedman M, Mitrani-Rosenbaum S. Transmissibility and treatment failures of different types of human papillomavirus. *Obstet Gynecol* 1989;73:308–311.
69. Garuti G, Boselli F, Genazzani AR, Silvestri S, Ratti G. Detection and typing of human papillomavirus in histologic specimens by *in situ* hybridization with biotinylated probes. *Am J Clin Pathol* 1989;92:604–612.
70. Maitland NJ, Cox MF, Lynas C, Prime SS, Meanwell CA, Scully C. Detection of human papillomavirus DNA in biopsies of human oral tissue. *Br J Cancer* 1987;56: 245–250.
71. McNichol PJ, Dodd JG. Detection of papillomavirus DNA in human prostatic tissue by Southern blot analysis. *Can J Microbiol* 1990;36:359–3622.
72. Palmer JG, Scholefield JH, Coates PJ, et al. Anal cancer and human papillomavirus. *Dis Colon Rectum* 1989; 32:1016–1022.
73. Pater MM, Dunne J, Hogan G, Ghatage P, Pater A. Human papillomavirus types 16 and 18 sequences in early cervical neoplasia. *Virology* 1986;155:13–18.
74. Scully C, Maitland NJ, Cox MF, Prime SS. Human papillomavirus DNA and oral mucosa. *Lancet* 1987;i:336.
75. Steinberg BM, Topp WC, Schneider PS, Abramson AL. Laryngeal papillomavirus infection during clinical remission. *N Engl J Med* 1983;308:1261–1264.
76. Wilczynski SP, Bergen S, Walker J, Lia SY, Pearlman LF. Human papillomaviruses and cervical cancer: analysis of histopathologic features associated with different viral types. *Hum Pathol* 1988;19:697–704.
77. Vermund SH, Schiffman MH, Goldberg GL, Ritter DB, Weltman A, Burk RD. Molecular diagnosis of genital human papillomavirus infection: comparison of two methods used to collect exfoliated cervical cells. *Am J Obstet Gynecol* 1989;160:304–308.
78. Willett GD, Kurman RJ, Reid R, Greenberg M, Jenson AB, Lorincz AT. Correlation of the histologic appearance of intraepithelial neoplasia of the cervix with human papillomavirus types. *Int J Gynecol Pathol* 1989;8:18–25.
79. Caussy D, Orr W, Daya D, Roth P, Reeves W, Rawls W. Evaluation of methods for detecting human papillo-

mavirus deoxyribonucleotide sequences in clinical specimens. *J Clin Microbiol* 1988;26:236–243.

80. Villa LL, Franco ELL. Epidemiologic correlates of cervical neoplasia and risk of human papillomavirus infection in asymptomatic women in Brazil. *J Natl Cancer Inst* 1989;81:337–340.

81. Nuovo GJ. A comparison of slot blot, Southern blot and *in situ* hybridization analyses for human papillomavirus DNA in genital tract lesions. *Obstet Gynecol* 1989; 74:673–677.

82. Faloona F, Weiss S, Ferre F, Mullis K. Direct detection of HIV sequences in blood: high gain polymerase chain reaction. In: *Proceedings of the sixth international conference on AIDS*. Abstract 1019. San Francisco: Humana Press; 1988.

83. Nuovo GJ. *In situ* hybridization protocols. In: Choo KHA, ed. *Methods in molecular biology.* San Diego: Humana Press; 1993.

84. Nuovo GJ. PCR *in situ* hybridization. *Clin Immunol Newslett* 1992;12:106–112.

85. Nuovo GJ. *In situ* detection of DNA after polymerase chain reaction amplification. In: Celis JE, ed. *Cell biology: a laboratory handbook.* Orlando: Academic Press; 1993;477–487.

86. Nuovo GJ. The clinical utility of detection of human papillomavirus DNA in the lower genital tract. *Infect Medicine* 1995;11:172–183.

87. Nuovo GJ. *In situ* hybridization. In: Damjanov I, Linder J, eds. *Anderson's textbook of pathology.* 10th ed. San Diego: Academic Press; 1995.

88. MacConnell P, Nuovo GJ. RT *in situ* PCR for the detection of viral RNA and mRNAs. In: Siebert PD, Larrick JW, eds. *Reverse transcriptase PCR.* San Diego: Academic Press;1994:402–419.

89. Nuovo GJ. PCR *in situ* hybridization. In: Wiedbrauk DL, Farkas DH, eds. *Molecular methods for viral detection.* San Diego: Academic Press; 1994:237–259.

90. Simsir S, Nuovo GJ. PCR and RT PCR *in situ* hybridization: applications in viral detection. *Trends Biotechnol* 1994;18:102–115.

91. Sternberg SS, ed. *Histology for pathologists.* New York: Raven Press; 1992.

92. Silverberg SS, ed. *Principles and practice of surgical pathology.* 2nd ed. New York: Churchill Livingstone; 1990.

3

Nonspecific Pathways of PCR

In the previous chapter we focused on the principles and actual methodology of molecular biology, including PCR. In essence, PCR represents the primer-dictated synthesis of DNA by *Taq* polymerase at the two 5′ boundaries of the target. Mention was made of the fact that the primers do not only bind to the target but may anneal to nontarget DNA or to themselves. The latter two alternative pathways may induce the *Taq* polymerase to synthesize unwanted DNA. The purpose of this chapter is to discuss these nonspecific pathways at length and to reveal ways in which the reaction conditions may increase the probability that the primers bind only to the target of interest.

THE FOUR PATHWAYS FOR *TAQ* POLYMERASE

DNA synthesis via a nonspecific pathway may interfere with the amount of target-specific DNA that is amplified and thus compromise the sensitivity of the PCR assay. However, it should be recognized that DNA synthesis via the nonspecific pathways can provide useful information. For example, detection of DNA synthesized via mispriming or primer oligomerization indicates that an adequate hot start maneuver was not employed. Furthermore, detection of unwanted DNA indicates that the absence of a target-specific signal is probably not due to inadequate *Taq* polymerase activity. Much more importantly, the DNA synthesized during DNA repair and mispriming can be used as a model system, albeit nonspe-

cific, to become acquainted with the process of *in situ* PCR. It has been my experience that, when teaching people who have little or no experience with *in situ* hybridization, immunohistochemistry, or *in situ* PCR, successful completion of *in situ* PCR using paraffin-embedded tissue sections, where DNA repair is invariably operative, leads to a much greater likelihood of successful detection of target-specific DNA or cDNA in cells. Indeed, a signal with the positive control for RT *in situ* PCR (no DNase) is *mandatory* for success with this technique, as it demonstrates that the protease and fixation times will allow the DNase digestion to render all genomic DNA nonamplifiable. This is essential if one is to be able to incorporate a reporter molecule during PCR into the cDNA target of interest that was generated during the RT step.

A key concept in the discussion of nonspecific DNA amplification during PCR is that *Taq* polymerase is very efficient at synthesizing DNA once the primers have provided a starting point for synthesis (1–21). The site where *Taq* polymerase will begin DNA synthesis is a function of where the single-stranded primer anneals with another single-stranded DNA molecule. The annealing of primers, depending on their concentration and on the concentration of the *Taq* polymerase, are the rate-limiting factors in PCR, rather than the activity of *Taq* polymerase once primer annealing occurs. What choices do the primers have in their sites of binding? Three of the choices are detailed in Figs. 3-1 to 3-3. The first option is for the primer to hybridize with the com-

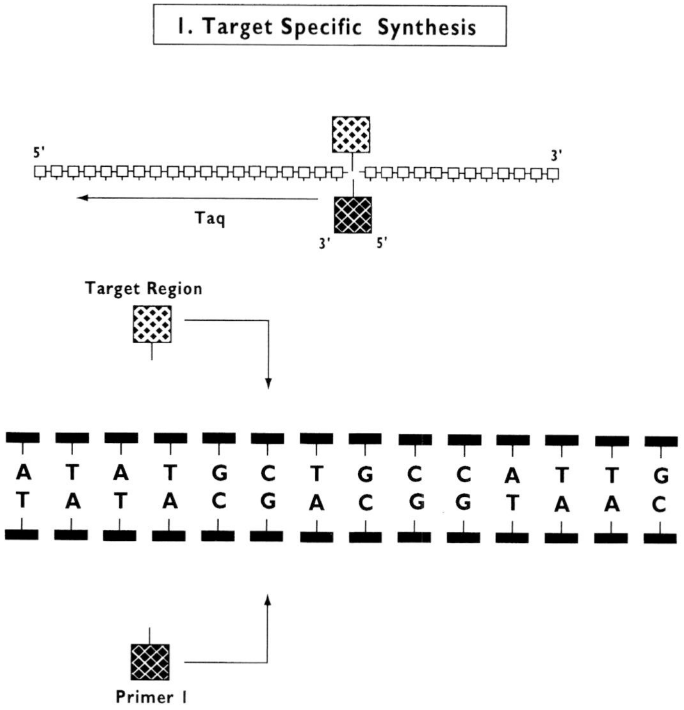

Figure 3-1. *The three primer-dependent pathways in PCR: target-specific amplification.* The primer may bind to the corresponding region of the target DNA and thus initiate DNA synthesis. Complete homology would be expected between the primer and the target.

plementary region of the target where one would expect complete homology (Fig. 3-1). The second option is for the primer to bind to nontarget areas where there is some but, most likely, not complete homology (Fig. 3-2). Finally, the primers may bind to each other, with the intervening gap serving as the initiation point of DNA synthesis (Fig. 3-3).

It should also be emphasized that target-specific amplification is not the only process in PCR where the amplified DNA produces a distinct band when analyzed by ethidium staining or Southern blot transfer. Although the size of the product from primer oligomerization and mispriming is often less than 100 base pairs, it is possible for these nonspecific products to be larger than 100 base pairs and thus

produce a band that may be confused with the amplified target. One such possible mechanism is depicted in Fig. 3-4. Clearly, caution must be exercised when determining whether the DNA from PCR is target-specific based only on the size of the product. This is especially true for products that are from 75 to 150 base pairs in size. As is stressed later in this chapter, the hot start maneuver greatly increases the likelihood that a band visible after PCR will be target-specific.

The most important difference between pathway 1 (target-specific) and the other two pathways (mispriming and primer oligomerization) is in the degree of homology. There is 100% homology in the target-specific pathway and less than 100% homology in the other two

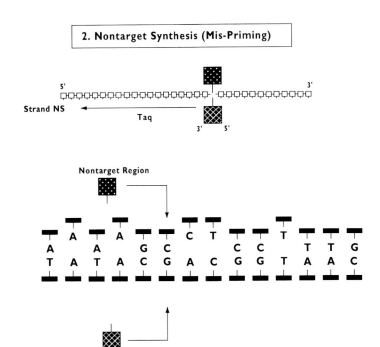

Figure 3-2. *The three primer-dependent pathways in PCR: nontarget DNA synthesis (mispriming).* The primer may bind to a region distinct from the target DNA. Although there would have to be some complementarity between the primer and the nontarget region, complete homology would not be expected. However, sufficient homology to facilitate binding and a base pair match at the 3′ end could initiate DNA synthesis and result in strand NS.

primer-mediated DNA synthesis pathways in PCR. Because of the lesser homologies that occur in mispriming and primer oligomerization, their respective Tms must be lower than for the target-specific pathway. For example, if the primer is 25 base pairs and the greatest number of base pair matches is 20 for mispriming and 10 for primer oligomerization, the calculated Tms (see Chapter 2 for calculation of Tm) for each pathway are

1. Primer-specific pathway, 62°C
2. Mispriming, 42°C
3. Primer oligomerization, 22°C

Note that the 20/25 and 10/25 base pair match for mispriming and primer oligomerization, respectively, is higher than probably occurs with these two pathways under experimental conditions. These numbers are used to illustrate how, even under these conditions, the Tm is much less than for complete homology.

It follows that if one can control the reaction conditions of PCR such that the *Taq* polymerase is not operative until a temperature of, for example, 50°C is reached, then the mispriming and primer oligomerization pathways should be inhibited without substantial suppression of the target-specific pathway. This simple example illustrates the importance of the hot start modification to PCR.

It is important to stress that primer-mediated DNA amplification is not the only mechanism whereby *Taq* polymerase may synthesize new DNA during PCR. DNA synthesis may

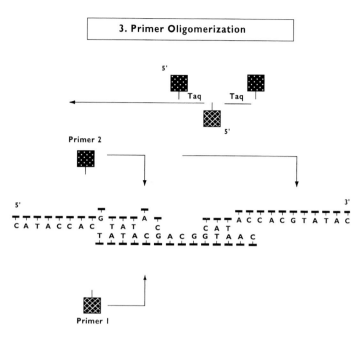

Figure 3-3. *The three primer-dependent pathways in PCR: primer oligomerization.* Primer 1 may bind to complementary regions of primer 2. If there is a 3′ match this could lead to DNA synthesis, as *Taq* polymerase fills in the single-stranded regions. Fragments larger than 20 to 40 base pairs may be synthesized by this process, which may reflect exonuclease activity of *Taq* polymerase and/or relatively rapid annealing and denaturing of the primer oligomers.

occur without the presence of primers. For example, DNA may have "loops" whereby the double-stranded molecule abruptly changes to a single-stranded sequence. These loops are more likely to occur in GC-rich areas, because more hydrogen bonds arise with this base pair complexing than with A and T matches (3 versus 2). Utilizing its nuclease activity, *Taq* polymerase could theoretically cut and extend the DNA in the region. Second, DNA may have nicks whereby a variety of chemical insults can ultimately induce the breakage of phosphodiester bonds. As illustrated in Fig. 3-5, such sites can serve as initiation points for DNA synthesis. Figure 3-6 represents another possible example of the DNA nick mechanism. The one base pair "nick" can be sufficient to initiate DNA synthesis during PCR, although this would probably require relatively high temperatures to disrupt the base pair matches that are on either side of the nick. However, gaps of many base pairs in size could induce DNA synthesis by *Taq* polymerase, even without any denaturation of the template DNA (Fig. 3-5). This chapter examines the primer-dependent and primer-independent pathways that may be operative during both solution phase PCR and *in situ* PCR. It is important to realize that, although each mechanism may be operative when PCR is performed within a 0.5-ml tube or within a nucleus, different nonspecific pathways occur more commonly in solution phase PCR than in *in situ* PCR. Before a generalized discussion of the topic, a specific example is given to demonstrate the importance of nonspecific DNA synthesis to the specificity and sensitivity of PCR.

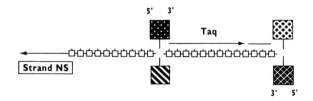

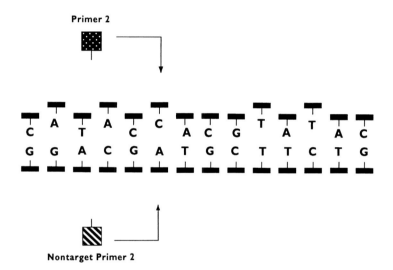

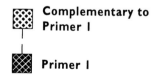

Figure 3-4. *Geometric amplification of nontarget DNA synthesis during PCR.* After denaturation, strand NS, which has primer 1 at its 5′ end, would be available for primer annealing. If primer 2 found a region on strand NS with sufficient complementarity and a base pair match at the 3′ end, then this could dictate the synthesis of a fragment with primer 2 at the 5′ end and the region complementary to primer 1 at the 3′ end. This could in subsequent cycles lead to the exponential amplification of this nontarget sequence evident as a distinct band whose size would be the sum of the number of base pairs in the two primers plus the intervening sequence. Although such events are unlikely, the much greater concentration of nontarget DNA relative to target DNA increases the possibility of this occurring.

In Next Cycle, Primer 1 hybridizes to complementary region

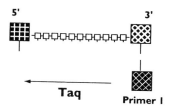

Extension by Taq polymerase produces a 3' end complementary to Primer 2

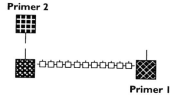

In Next Cycle, Taq synthesizes a DNA segment that has Primer 2 at the 5' End and the region complementary to Primer 1 at the 3' end

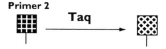

Continued synthesis leads to amplification of DNA whose size is distance of Primer 1 to Primer 2

Figure 3-4. *Continued.*

THE CONTRIBUTIONS OF THE SPECIFIC AND NONSPECIFIC PATHWAYS IN PCR DURING THE AMPLIFICATION OF HPV DNA IN SiHa CELLS

SiHa cells are a cell line derived from a carcinoma of the uterine cervix. As would be expected (see Chapter 8), the cells contain human papillomavirus (HPV) DNA. Specifically, each cell contains one copy of HPV 16 DNA. The SiHa cells were fixed in 10% buffered formalin for 15 hours, embedded in paraffin, and several 4 μm sections placed in 1.5-ml tubes. The paraffin was removed and the total DNA extracted using protease digestion followed by phenol/chloroform extraction and ethanol precipitation (see protocol 2-1 in Chapter 2). PCR was performed on 1 μg of the total cellular DNA with HPV-16-specific primers that correspond to the E7 region of the viral genome (22).

At the onset of PCR, the temperature is increased from room temperature to 94°C at the rate of about 1° per second. At the end of the initial denaturing step most of the sample DNA will be single stranded and thus incapable of hybridizing with other single-stranded DNA molecules such as the primers. However, it is important to realize that as the temperature increases to 94°C there will be some single-stranded DNA available for primer annealing even at much lower temperatures. As illustrated in Fig. 3-7, if one assumes the Tm is 65°C for the sample DNA, then about 10% will be single-stranded at room temperature (20°C). This leads us to a consideration of the Tm for the hybridization kinetics of the primers and the three primer-dependent annealing options available for it. As noted in the calculations above, the Tm of the HPV 16 primer–human DNA annealing and HPV 16 primer oligomerization pathway is approximately 42°C and 22°C, respectively. At the lower temperatures (i.e., near room temperature) the mispriming and primer oligomerization pathways may be operative, since the temperature is below their Tm. This also applies to the target-specific primer annealing pathway. However, the much larger amount of nontarget (human) DNA and primers relative to the target increases the likelihood for nonspecific DNA synthesis at these lower temperatures.

Mispriming generates a nonspecific DNA segment that has at its 5' end a primer. If the other primer found a region in this segment of sufficient homology, then one would generate two DNA fragments that have at their respective 5' ends a primer and at their 3' ends a region complementary to the other primer. Clearly, this is equivalent to what occurs during the second cycle of PCR for the target and, thus, would allow nonspecific geometric am-

plification (Fig. 3-4). Although such events are rare, the fact that in most reactions the amount of nontarget DNA is often 10^7 greater than the amount of target DNA would increase its likelihood.

A key element of these experiments with the SiHa cells was the use of the labeled nucleotide digoxigenin dUTP (Boehringer Mannheim, Indianapolis, IN). By using this label, any DNA synthesis, be it target specific or from mispriming, primer oligomerization, or DNA repair, may be detected. Figure 3-8 shows the results after PCR was performed on 1 μg of total cellular DNA extracted from SiHa cells and the product transferred to a filter after electrophoretic separation. Under standard conditions (all reagents, including the *Taq* polymerase, added at room temperature) using either a single primer pair or multiple primer pairs (the rationale for multiple primer pairs is discussed at length in Chapter 5), only a smear is evident after the colorimetric detection of incorporated digoxigenin (Fig. 3-8a, lanes A and C). The digoxigenin is detected by the use of an alkaline phosphatase antidigoxigenin antibody conjugate. The expected band at 450 base pairs (arrow) was not evident. Southern blot hybridization was performed using a ^{32}P-labeled HPV 16 probe. Under these conditions, only the nucleotides incorporated into HPV-16-specific DNA will be detected. Note that no signal is evident in lanes A and C after Southern blot hybridization, which corresponds to "cold start" conditions (Fig. 3-8b). One concludes that most, if not all, of the DNA detected in this reaction is due to DNA synthesis that originated in the primers either binding to human sequences or to themselves or, perhaps, DNA repair. DNA repair can be easily addressed by omitting the primers from the amplification solution. When this is done, no DNA synthesis is recorded, because the extensive protease digestion that is obligatory during the extraction of the DNA from the tissue eliminates the DNA repair mechanism. It can be concluded that the DNA synthesized in the above-mentioned experiment with SiHa cells reflects either mispriming or primer

DNA cross linked with proteins (formalin fixation) gaps with 5' overhangs

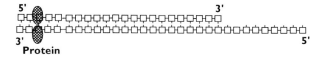

Denature

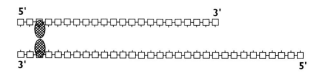

Re-anneal, extension by Taq with incorporation of digoxigenin dUTP

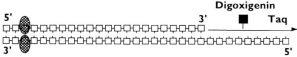

Figure 3-5. *Primer-independent DNA synthesis during PCR: repair of large gaps.* During the processing of DNA, single-stranded gaps may develop. If a cross-linking fixative is used, the protein–DNA cross-links will prevent the DNA strands from completely separating at 94°C. This would allow for the repair of the gap during the annealing step of the PCR reaction.

oligomerization. The intensity of the colorimetric reaction evident in Fig. 3-8 reflects the large amount of DNA that may be synthesized in these unwanted pathways. These experiments were repeated with one modification: the *Taq* DNA polymerase was not added until the temperature of the thermal cycler block reached 55°C. Note that, based on the detection of a single band of the expected size, all detectable DNA synthesis was shifted to HPV-16-specific amplification using a single primer pair when this *hot start modification* to PCR was employed (Fig.3-8a, lane B). This band does indeed demonstrate an intense signal when Southern blot hybridization is performed

using the ³²P-labeled HPV 16 probe, demonstrating that it does represent target-specific amplification (Fig. 3-8b, lane B).

It was suggested above (Fig. 3-7) that the ratio of target to nontarget DNA may play a role in determining which annealing pathway the primers will follow. If so, could one shift some DNA synthesis to the target-specific pathway if more target DNA was added to the sample even under "cold start" conditions? Let us return to the above experiment for the answer. Since each SiHa cell contains one copy of HPV 16 DNA, 1 μg of total cellular DNA will contain about 3 pg of HPV 16 DNA. The conditions were identical in the next series of

DNA cross linked with proteins
Small DNA nicks

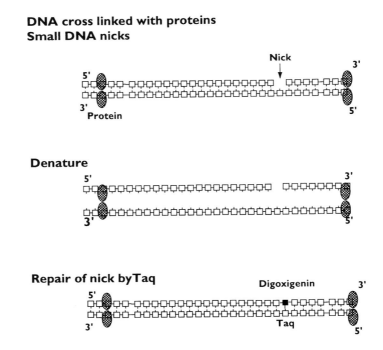

Figure 3-6. *Primer-independent DNA synthesis during PCR: repair of small nicks.* The mechanism of *Taq* polymerase-mediated nick repair during PCR is similar to that described above for gap repair (Fig. 3-5). The important difference is that the nick is much smaller. If this mechanism was the predominant mechanism of DNA repair, one would anticipate that it might be repaired by T4 DNA ligase, which is not the case. Furthermore, one could hypothesize that repair of DNA nicks during PCR by *Taq* polymerase would produce a much weaker signal than repair of large gaps due to the much lesser amount of incorporation of the reporter molecule.

experiments except that 10 pg of purified HPV 16 was added to the initial test sample that contained 1 μg of total cellular DNA. The results are shown in Fig. 3-9. Note that although a smear, which is less intense than in the initial experiment, is evident under standard conditions (i.e., "cold start"), a well-defined band of the expected size for HPV 16 is also noted (Fig. 3-9, lanes A and C). Southern blot hybridization using the ^{32}P-labeled HPV 16 probe confirmed the specificity of the amplification. The conclusion that can be made from this and other similar experiments is that targets of low copy number might not be detected using standard PCR presumably because the primers are preferentially initiating the synthesis of un-

wanted DNA. If one could eliminate or greatly reduce these undesirable pathways, primer-mediated synthesis of target-specific sequences might follow for these low copy sequences. The hot start method for PCR does increase both the detection threshold to 1 to 10 copies per sample (from 1,000 to 5,000 copies) (Fig. 3-9) (23–28).

Before concluding this section, additional mention should be made of the detection threshold of PCR, which was alluded to in the above experiments. Many articles quote a detection threshold of 1 to 10 copies of the target DNA in PCR (29–51). This may be accurate when only the target DNA is present in the reaction mixture. However, as indicated by the experi-

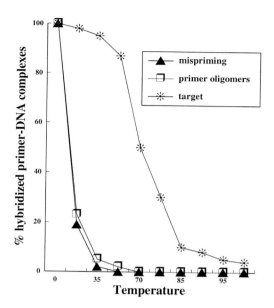

Figure 3-7. *Relative differences in the Tms for the three different primer-binding pathways.* The Tms of mispriming and primer oligomerization are much below that of target-specific binding. At low temperature (<25°C), these unwanted pathways have a selective advantage over target-specific amplification for two reasons: (i) the concentrations of the primers and nontarget DNA are much greater relative to the target DNA, and (ii) for large targets, such as on human DNA, the target may not be available for hybridizing under conditions in which primer oligomers can form.

ments above, this is highly inaccurate if additional DNA is included in the sample, which, of course, is typically the case in solution phase PCR. Under these conditions, it has been demonstrated by a variety of investigators that the detection threshold of solution phase PCR is from 1,000 to 5,000 copies. If one is analyzing a biopsy that contains 100,000 cells, then this would correspond to one copy per 20 to 100 cells. This is similar to the detection threshold for filter hybridization analysis, as discussed in Chapter 2. However, if the hot start modification is employed in solution phase PCR, then the detection threshold is from 1 to 10 copies in the background of 1 μg of nontarget DNA.

The next section examines some nonspecific pathways in both solution phase PCR and *in situ* PCR. Although on a theoretical basis many different nonspecific pathways may be operative during PCR and *in situ* PCR, we will focus on the pathways mentioned above and illustrated at the beginning of this chapter:

1. Target-specific amplification
2. Mispriming
3. Primer oligomerization
4. DNA repair

PRIMER-INDEPENDENT DNA SYNTHESIS DURING PCR

Note that mechanisms 1, 2, and 3 are each primer dependent, whereas pathway 4 is primer-independent. Thus, it is simple to test the relative contribution of the DNA repair pathway in both *in situ* PCR and solution phase PCR by omitting the primers when doing the assay. For simplicity's sake we will first discuss the data obtained from *in situ* PCR, then from solution phase PCR. It is hoped that through this discussion the similarities and differences in the various nonspecific pathways that may be operative during PCR will come to light.

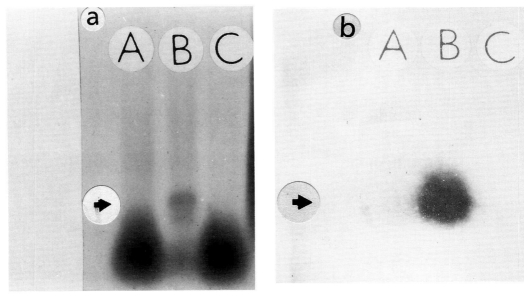

Figure 3-8. *Differential amplification of DNA in hot start and standard solution phase PCR.* An attempt was made to amplify the type-specific E7 region of HPV 16 using 1 µg of cellular DNA extracted from SiHa cells, which contain one copy of the virus per cell. **a:** Southern blot hybridization visualized nonisotopically after digoxigenin incorporation. **b:** autoradiography using a ^{32}P-labeled HPV 16 probe. In each panel, *lane A* reports on standard PCR with a single primer pair; *lane B* on hot start PCR with a single primer pair; and *lane C* on standard PCR with multiple primer pairs. The arrow represents the expected size for amplified HPV 16 DNA (450 base pairs). Note how only nonspecific amplification is evident under standard conditions when either single (*lane A*) or multiple primer pairs (*lane C*) are used. However, amplification of HPV 16 DNA is seen with a single primer pair and the hot start modification (*lane B*) either with **a:** direct incorporation of the digoxigenin dUTP or **b:** after hybridization with a ^{32}P-labeled probe.

In Situ PCR

The primer-independent pathway of DNA synthesis may occur during *in situ* PCR; however, it is highly dependent on several reaction conditions. More specifically, it depends on whether cytospin preparations (which are typically not heated during their preparation) or paraffin-embedded tissues are used. An example of the disparity of the primer-independent pathway during *in situ* PCR in cytospins and paraffin-embedded tissue is provided in Fig. 3-10. Note the intensity of the signal obtained from *in situ* PCR regardless of whether nonspecific primers (by *nonspecific* is meant that the primers have no corresponding target in the cells in the tissue) are included or no primers are present in the paraffin-embedded tissue sections. This nonspecific signal is evident even if the hot start method is used. However, no signal is evident if the primers are omitted in the cytospin preparation. Clearly, a primer-independent pathway is operative in the paraffin-embedded tissue section and responsible for much of the signal. It would seem paradoxical, however, that this pathway does not seem to be operative during *in situ* PCR in the cytospin preparation. How do cytospin samples differ from paraffin-embedded tissue sections? Cytospin slides are prepared in a very different manner from tissue sections. The cells are fixed in 10% buffered formalin for 4 to 15 hours, then placed on the silane slide by using a cytospin centrifuge. Alternatively, although tissues are also fixed in formalin for typically 4 to 15 hours, they are then subjected to treatments with xy-

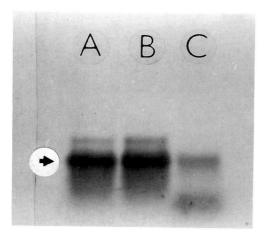

Figure 3-9. *The effect of the target DNA concentration on the specificity of the DNA synthesized in standard and hot start PCR. This experiment differed from the one depicted in Fig. 3-8 only by the addition of 10 pg of HPV 16 DNA to the 1 μg of SiHa total cellular DNA, which contains about 3 pg of HPV 16. As noted in Fig. 3-8, the panel shows Southern blot hybridization visualized nonisotopically after digoxigenin incorporation. Lane A reports on standard PCR with a single primer pair; lane B on hot start PCR with a single primer pair; and lane C on standard PCR with multiple primer pairs. The arrow represents the expected size for amplified HPV 16 DNA (450 base pairs). The appropriately fourfold increase in the HPV 16 concentration shifted the DNA synthesis in PCR under "cold start" conditions to HPV-16 specific as evidenced by a band at the expected size using either a single primer pair (lane A) or multiple primer pairs (lane C), although residual primer oligomerization is evident in lane C, which probably reflects the fourfold increase in primer concentration, relative to lanes A and B.*

lene and graded ethanols. Each of these washes typically lasts from 1 to 3 hours. Finally, the tissue is infiltrated with heated paraffin at 65°C for 4 hours. The tissue is then embedded in paraffin using a plastic mold and sectioned.

Concerning the differences in processing tissue and cytospin samples, we speculated that the heating step for tissue may be most likely to be deleterious to the DNA , thus explaining the difference noted in the primer-independent signal between paraffin-embedded tissue sections and cytospins. To examine this, tissue biopsies were frozen, and 4-μm sections were placed on silane slides by use of a cryostat machine. For the nonpathologist, a cryostat machine contains a blade and block kept at about –20°C. In this fashion, one may embed unfixed tissue in a gel-like material, freeze it, put it in the block, and then cut 4-μm sections. After sectioning, the tissue was fixed from 4 to 15 hours by placing the silane-coated slide in 10% buffered formalin. Thus, the heating step as well as the xylene and ethanol washes were avoided. The primer-independent signal was not evident in the tissue sections under these conditions (Fig. 3-11). However, it could be generated by heating the slide for 4 hours at 65°C after fixation of the frozen tissues, as is discussed shortly. Similarly, if a cytospin preparation of peripheral blood mononuclear cells (PBMC) is exposed to 4 hours at 65°C after 15 hours of fixation in 10% buffered formalin, a signal will be evident after pepsin digestion and *in situ* PCR in the absence of primers (Fig. 3-12). It is important to stress that this is "dry" heat in the absence of any aqueous solution. If the heating step is done and, at the same time, the tissue or cells are covered with an aqueous solution, the primer-independent signal is not seen. This must be the case because frozen, fixed, unheated tissue does not yield a primer-independent signal during *in situ* PCR, even though the amplifying solution is routinely being heated to 94°C for 1 minute for many cycles.

In summary, the primer-independent signal requires heating of the cells and tissue after formalin fixation. It is presumed that the primer-independent signal represents repair of single-stranded nicks and gaps in the double-stranded DNA molecule. These gaps are either being generated by the heating step or are "exposed" by the 4-hour treatment at 65°C through denaturing of regions that have breakage in the phosphodiester bonds. This model is graphically depicted in Fig. 3-5. If this model is correct, the primer-independent signal should be eliminated by pretreating the tissues with a solution containing a dideoxynucleotide, which would not allow for further extension of any given gap (Fig. 3-13).

To test this hypothesis, we studied the effect on the primer-independent signal of pretreat-

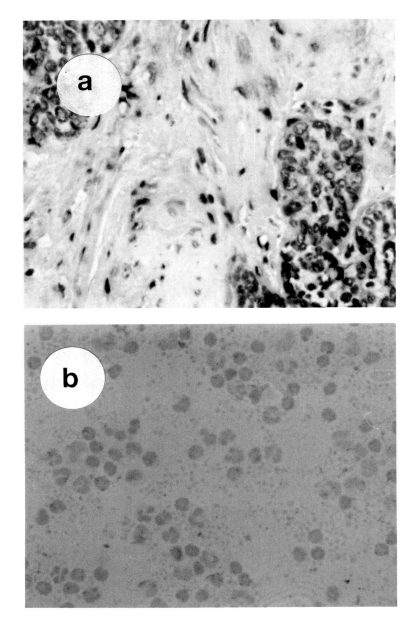

Figure 3-10. *The primer-independent signal during* in situ *PCR.* **a:** An intense signal is evident in over one-half of the cells in this paraffin-embedded cervical biopsy tissue with *in situ* PCR if the primers are omitted from the amplifying solution. **b:** This primer-independent signal is not evident in this cytospin preparation of lymphocytes if the cells are not heated during their processing (compare with Fig. 3-12).

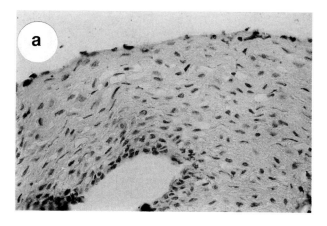

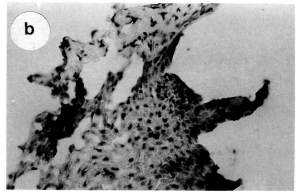

Figure 3-11. *The dependency of the primer-independent signal during* in situ *PCR on heating of the sample: tissue sections.* **a:** No primer-independent signal is evident in this skin section if the tissue is frozen, sectioned in a cryostat, placed on a silane slide, and then fixed in 10% buffered formalin. **b:** However, the primer-independent signal can be generated if the tissue is heated to 65°C for 1 hour after formalin fixation.

ing paraffin-embedded tissue sections with a dideoxynucleotide-containing solution before *in situ* PCR. In these experiments, the tissue sections were proteased and one or more of the three sections on the glass slide were treated with the following **dideoxy blocking solution:**

3 μl of GeneAmp buffer
5.6 μl of MgCl₂ (4.5 mM final concentration)
4.6 μl of dNTP solution (200 μM final concentration of each nucleotide)
3 μl of a 10 mM ddTTP solution (1,000 μM final concentration)
1 μl of a 2% bovine serum albumin solution
11.8 μl of sterile water
1 μl of *Taq* DNA polymerase

The section(s) were incubated in this solution for 30 minutes at 55°C, followed by *in situ* PCR with direct incorporation of digoxigenin dUTP. The results of these experiments are provided in Table 3-1. Varying protease times were used in these experiments to emphasize how critical this variable is to the results with *in situ* PCR in general and dideoxy blockage in particular. Note the following points:

1. When the primer-independent signal in tissue that is not blocked is optimal (defined as a 3+ signal), no signal is noted after the dideoxy blockage.
2. When the signal in nonblocked tissue is suboptimal due to inadequate (i.e., too little) pro-

Table 3-1. *The effect of protease digestion time on the primer-independent signal with* in situ *PCR with and without pretreatment in dTTP*

Fixation time (hr)	Protease digestion time (min)				
	15	30	45	60	90
8					
No treatment	1+[a]	3+	2+	2+	—
Dideoxy treatment	2+	0	1+	2+	—
16					
No treatment	0	1+	2+	3+	2+
Dideoxy treatment	2+	2+	1+	0	1+

[a]% of cells positive (1–25%=1+, 26–50%=2+, >50%=3+).

tease digestion, a signal is present after the dideoxy blockage that is usually stronger than the signal in the unblocked tissue.

3. A signal is evident after dideoxy blockage, when the protease digestion time exceeds the optimal time defined above.

The first observation demonstrates that the primer-independent signal can be blocked by dideoxy treatment. This provides further evidence that the primer-independent signal reflects repair of single-stranded DNA gaps (Fig. 3-13). The second and third observations demonstrate how dependent the dideoxy results are on protease digestion. Interestingly, when the protease time is too short, not only is a signal evident in the dideoxy blocked tissue, but it is often stronger than that seen in the serial section not treated with the dideoxy nucleotide on the same glass slide. One may speculate that

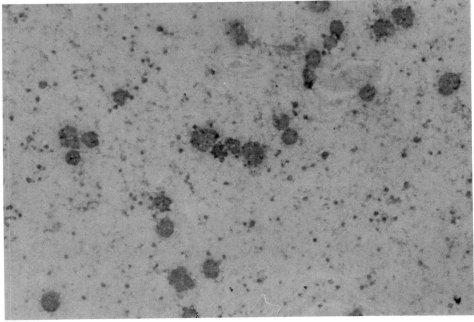

Figure 3-12. *The dependency of the primer-independent signal during* in situ *PCR on heating of the sample: cytospin preparations.* A primer-independent signal was evident in the cytospin preparation of the PBMC (see Fig. 3-10) if the cells were heated at 65°C for 3 hours after fixation.

DNA cross linked with proteins (formalin fixation)
Gaps with 5' overhang

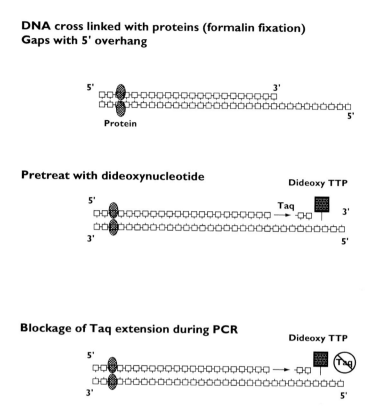

Figure 3-13. *Elimination of the primer-independent signal evident during* in situ *PCR with blockage by a dideoxynucleotide.* If the primer-independent signal represents repair of single-stranded gaps in the DNA (see Fig. 3-5), then one can hypothesize that this pathway could be blocked by pretreating the sections in a solution that contains a dideoxynucleotide and a DNA polymerase.

the suboptimal signal seen with the inadequately blocked tissue and suboptimal protease digestion is due to the relative inability of the *Taq* polymerase to repair the DNA nicks due to the adjacent protein–nucleic acid cross-links. That is, the persistent protein–DNA cross-links may not allow the "repair" of most gaps with a ddTTP molecule. However, one may further speculate that under these conditions the exonuclease activity of *Taq* polymerase may be operative during the dideoxy pretreatment, thus exposing additional nicks during the PCR process, resulting in an enhanced signal relative to the section that was not pretreated with the *Taq* polymerase and ddTTP. This could result in the enhanced signal shown in Table 3-1 (Figs. 3-14, 3-15). Although this topic is discussed in more detail in Chapter 7, the important point with regard to this section is twofold:

1. The primer-independent signal is intense after *in situ* PCR of formalin-fixed, paraffin-embedded tissues, assuming optimal protease digestion.
2. The mechanism of the primer-independent signal is likely repair of single-stranded DNA nicks and gaps.

We theorized that when protease digestion is suboptimal the exonuclease activity of *Taq* polymerase during the dideoxy blockage may be responsible for enhanced signal during *in situ* PCR. To test this theory, we substituted for *Taq* polymerase the Stoeffel fragment of the enzyme, which lacks the exonuclease function.

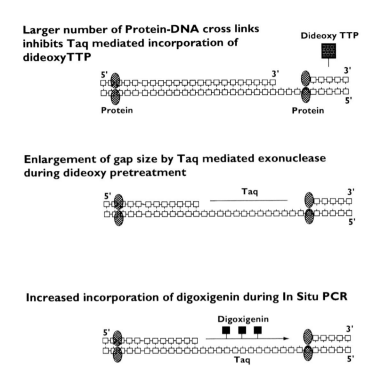

Figure 3-14. *Enhancement of the signal during* in situ *PCR by pretreatment with* Taq *polymerase and a dideoxynucleotide under suboptimal protease digestion conditions.* The primer-independent signal can be blocked after optimal protease digestion with a dideoxynucleotide. However, if the protease digestion time is suboptimal, one can obtain a signal that is more intense than the serial section on the same glass slide not pretreated with the *Taq* polymerase and the dideoxy solution (see Table 3-1). It is theorized that this enhancement may relate to the enlargement of the gaps via the exonuclease activity of *Taq* polymerase during the pretreatment DNA synthesis. Consistent with this statement is the loss of this enhancement if the Stoeffel fragment, which lacks the exonuclease function, is used in the pretreatment step and a similar enhancement with DNase digestion and suboptimal protease digestion. See Chapter 6 for a more detailed discussion of this topic.

This substitution eliminated the enhanced signal seen with dideoxy blockage after suboptimal protease (42).

Another interesting result from experiments with dideoxy blockage was the presence of a signal when protease digestion times were above optimal (3+) for the nonblocked tissue. One possible explanation is that during the blockage step the DNase activity of *Taq* polymerase is being enhanced by the increased disruption of protein–DNA cross links. According to this hypothesis, the dideoxy blockage step may be viewed as a competition between the polymerase activity of *Taq*, which adds the ddTTP and thus blocks further DNA synthesis at that site, and the exonuclease activity of the *Taq* during the 30-minute pretreatment in the dideoxy solution, which exposes other damaged sites to nonspecific DNA synthesis during the PCR part of the procedure. If this is true, one would anticipate that increased incubation time (from 30 to 60 minutes) in the dideoxy block solution for tissues that have been proteased above the optimal time may inhibit the signal. However, this was not observed (52). Furthermore, the enhanced signal with the dideoxy blockage and *Taq* polymerase beyond optimal protease digestion was not elim-

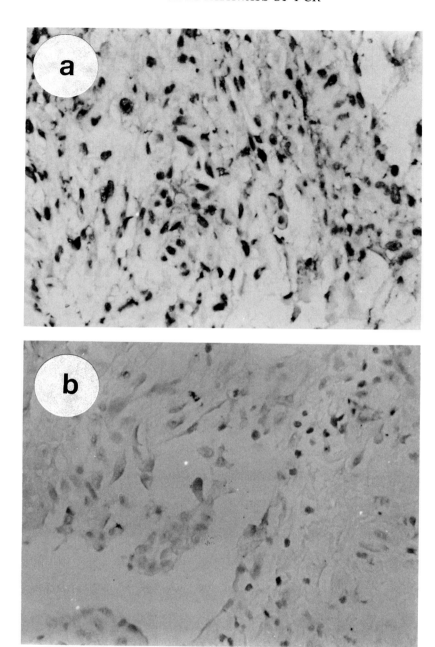

Figure 3-15. *Effect of pretreatment with a dideoxynucleotide on the primer-independent signal during* in situ *PCR.* **a:** An intense signal was seen in most cells in this liver biopsy specimen fixed in formalin for 8 hours with *in situ* PCR after 30 minutes of protease digestion. **b:** The signal was not evident if the protease digestion time was decreased to 10 minutes. **c:** The signal evident after 30 minutes of protease digestion was eliminated by pretreatment in a solution that contained ddTTP. **d:** However-er, a strong signal was seen after 10 minutes digestion if the *in situ* PCR was preceded by the dideoxy pretreatment.

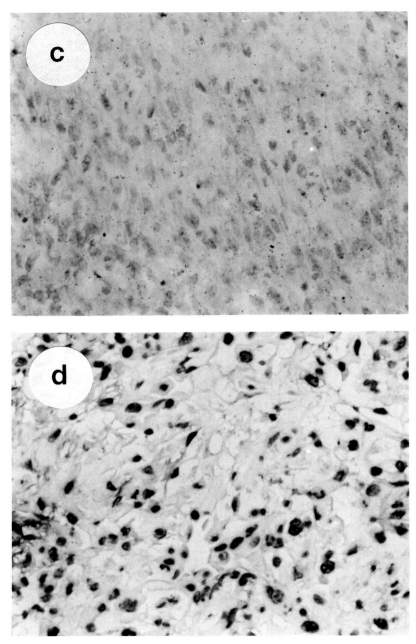

Figure 3-15. *Continued.*

inated when the *Taq* was substituted with the Stoeffel fragment during the dideoxy blockage, suggesting that this observation is not exonuclease dependent.

The previous paragraphs discussed observations that suggest that the primer-indepen-

dent pathway during *in situ* PCR results from the 5′ extension of single-stranded gaps by *Taq* polymerase that can be blocked by incorporation of a dideoxy nucleotide. A critical point with regard to DNA repair in tissue sections undergoing *in situ* PCR is that the resultant signal is *highly* dependent on fixation times in buffered formalin and on protease digestion times. To demonstrate this point, we took fresh 3- to 10-mm lung and vulvar tissue samples and fixed them in buffered formalin for 4 hours, 6 hours, 8 hours, 15 hours, 48 hours, and 1 week. The sections were embedded in paraffin after fixation, and three serial levels were placed on each silane slide to allow for direct comparisons of the results after *in situ* PCR where no primers were used. For the nonpathologist, serial sections or levels are the slices of the same tissue that are separated by only 4 μm; since most cells are over 4 μm in size, this allows direct comparisons between the same cells or adjacent cells. The digestion reagent was pepsin (2 mg/ml at room temperature). Digestion time ranged from 0 to 90 minutes. Representative examples of these experiments are shown in Figs. 3-16 and 3-17, and the results are compiled in Tables 3-2 and 3-3. Note that tissues fixed for 4 to 6 hours showed a maximum signal with *in situ* PCR after 15 minutes of pepsin digestion. However, no signal was seen after 15 minutes protease digestion when tissues were fixed for either 48 hours or 1 week (Tables 3-1 and 3-2). Tissues fixed for longer times need much longer protease digestion times, from 75 to 90 minutes, in order to get an optimal result with *in situ* PCR as defined by the presence of an intense, albeit nonspecific, signal in over 50% of the cells.

Another important factor with regard to the effects of prolonged (>15 hour) fixation on the *in situ* PCR signal is the digestion reagent used (Table 3-3). Proteinase K has greater specific activity at 1 mg/ml when compared with pepsin at 2 mg/ml. Proteinase K digestion and pepsin digestion were used on tissues fixed for either 48 hours or 1 week in order to determine if the nonspecific signal would be enhanced. As shown in Table 3-3, when the tissue was fixed for 1 week an improved signal was achieved with a 90-minute proteinase K digestion; an optimal signal was not obtainable under these conditions using pepsin digestion (Fig. 3-18). However, 90-minute digestion with proteinase K destroyed the morphology when the tissue was fixed for 48 hours (Fig. 3-18). These data demonstrate one of the reasons that I prefer pepsin digestion; one tends to obtain better morphologic detail. Stated another way, overdigestion is, in my experience, much more common when proteinase K is used than when pepsin is used. However, proteinase K is an acceptable reagent for *in situ* PCR, and, indeed, for tissues fixed for 1 week or longer, such as those obtained from autopsies, it may at times be the protease of choice. Nonetheless, I still recommend that one start with pepsin and go up to 120 minutes of protease digestion. In my experience, this will allow for successful *in situ* PCR in most cases.

The data presented in Tables 3-2 and 3-3 lead to an obvious question. Why would DNA repair be so dependent on the time of fixation and protease digestion? Two possible models

Table 3-2. *The effect of protease digestion time on the primer-independent signal with in situ PCR as a function of the time of fixation in 10% buffered formalin*

Fixation time (hr)	Protease digestion time (min)			
	0	5	10	15
4	0[a]	0.5+	0.5+	3+
6	0	0.5+	1+	3+
8	0	0	0	0
16	0	0	0	0

[a]The signal was graded as 0, 1+ (5–25% of the cells with a weak to moderate signal), 2+ (26–50% of the cells with a moderate to strong signal), or 3+ (>50% of the cells with a moderate to strong signal); 0.5+ means that only a few cells showed a weak signal.

Table 3-3. *The effect of protease digestion time on the primer-independent signal with* in situ *PCR as a function of the time of fixation in 10% buffered formalin*

Fixation time	Protease digestion time (min)				
	30	45	60	75	90
4–6 hours	Overdigested[a]				
8 hours	1+	2+	—	—	—
16 hours	0	1+	1+	2+	3+
48 hours	0	0.5+	1+	2+	3+[b]
1 week	0	0	1+	1+	2+–3+[c]

[a]Overdigested refers to loss of tissue morphology; there is a concomitant loss of the *in situ* PCR signal.
[b]The signal was 2+ when proteinase K (1 mg/ml) was substituted for the pepsin; the tissue morphology was preserved with the pepsin digestion but not with the proteinase K digestion.
[c]The 2+ signal was with pepsin, and the 3+ signal was with proteinase K digestion; tissue morphology was preserved with both proteases.

are presented in Figs. 3-19 and 3-20. In model 1, *Taq* entry is the rate-limiting step. In model 2, "exposure" of the single-stranded DNA gaps such that it can be acted upon by *Taq* polymerase is the rate-limiting event that is related to protease digestion time and the length of formalin fixation. Although we cannot determine unequivocally which of these nonmutually exclusive hypothetical models may be more important, several observations suggest that the second model may, at least in part, explain the data presented in Tables 3-3 and 3-4. First, consider the relationship of the length of formalin fixation and protease digestion time on the signal evident after standard *in situ* hybridization. These data, although discussed in detail in Chapter 4, are presented here for the purposes of discussion.

A comparison of the data in Tables 3-3 and 3-4 with those in Tables 3-2 and 3-3 clearly demonstrates that the optimal signal with standard *in situ* hybridization is similar for tissues fixed over a very large range of times. Importantly, the protease digestion time needed to obtain an optimal signal with standard *in situ* hybridization is much less for *in situ* PCR with longer fixation times. Specifically, for tissues fixed for 15 hours, the optimal protease time for *in situ* hybridization is 30 minutes, whereas it is 90 minutes for *in situ* PCR. It is important to realize that *Taq* polymerase, the largest molecule used in PCR, is equivalent in size (about 60 Å) to a 100 base pair single-stranded probe (about 75 Å), which is the standard for *in situ* hybridization. If *Taq* entry were the key parameter for DNA repair with *in situ* PCR,

TABLE 3-4. *The effect of protease digestion time on the signal with standard* in situ *PCR as a function of the time of fixation in 10% buffered formalin*[a]

Fixation time	Protease digestion time (min)				
	0	5	10	15	30
4 hours	0[b]	1+	3+	3+	Overdigested
6 hours	0	1+	2+	3+	—
8 hours	0	0	1+	3+	3+
15 hours	0	0	1+	2+	3+
24 hours	0	0	1+	2+	3+
48 hours	0	0	1+	2+	3+
1 week	0	0	0	1+	3+

[a]Pepsin was used at 2 mg/ml at 37°C. The probe was the biotin-labeled representative alu sequence.
[b]The signal was graded as 0, 1+ (5–25% of the cells with a weak to moderate signal), 2+ (26–50% of the cells with a moderate to strong signal), or 3+ (>50% of the cells with a moderate to strong signal).

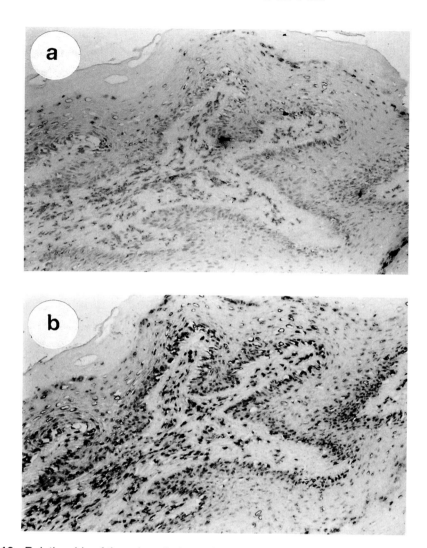

Figure 3-16. *Relationship of the primer-independent signal to the times of formalin fixation and protease digestion: short fixation time.* Skin tissue was fixed for 6 hours in 10% buffered formalin. **a:** A few cells showed a weak primer-independent signal during *in situ* PCR after 4 minutes of pepsin digestion. **b:** Many more cells showed an intense signal after 13 minutes of digestion in pepsin at 2 mg/ml.

one would anticipate similar optimal protease times for *in situ* hybridization and *in situ* PCR. This supports the second model of DNA repair, presented in Fig. 3-20, where the longer protease digestion time with longer fixation time reflects the need to unmask the many regions of DNA repair such that the *Taq* polymerase, which has diffused to the area, can access these

regions. Stated another way, with either standard *in situ* hybridization or PCR *in situ* hybridization for a specific DNA target, one has to expose just the target; for *in situ* hybridization this is a minimum of 20 copies, and for PCR *in situ* hybridization this needs only be one copy. With the primer-independent signal during *in situ* PCR (with labeling of the am-

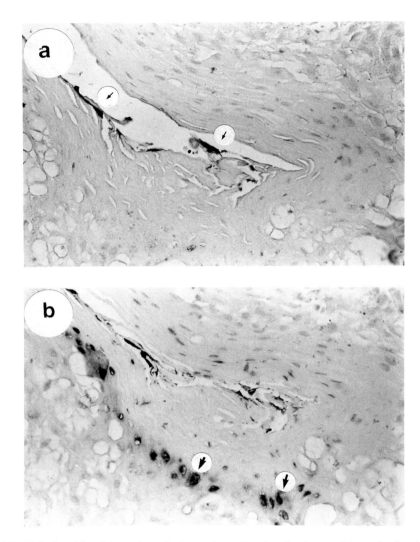

Figure 3-17. *Relationship of the primer-independent signal to the times of formalin fixation and protease digestion: intermediate fixation time.* Skin tissue was fixed for 48 hours in 10% buffered formalin. **a:** No primer-independent signal was evident after 15 minutes of protease digestion (the *black lines* on the surface are ink used to mark the boundaries of the tissue; *small arrrows*). **b:** A weak signal was evident during *in situ* PCR if the digestion time in pepsin at 2 mg/ml was increased to 50 minutes (*arrows*). **c:** The signal became optimal after 90 minutes of protease digestion (*arrow*).

plicon), one has to expose, most likely, thousands of similar-sized "targets" (i.e., gaps), to get the maximum signal; hence, increased protease digestion time reflects the need for a more complete "unmasking" of the DNA.

Another observation that supports the second model to explain the relationship of the signal with DNA repair during *in situ* PCR and protease and formalin fixation times comes from experiments with the Stoeffel fragment of *Taq* polymerase. This fragment is much smaller than *Taq*, as it lacks the N-terminal 289 amino acid portion of the parent *Taq* enzyme. We have shown that the primer-inde-

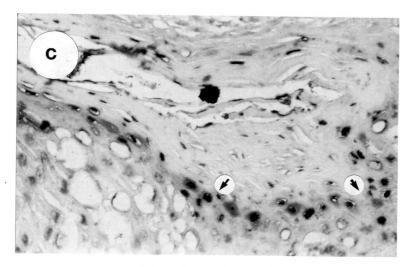

Figure 3-17. *Continued.*

pendent signal after *in situ* PCR is equally strong with *Taq* polymerase or with the Stoeffel fragment when protease digestion times are optimal (Fig. 3-21) and actually stronger for *Taq* polymerase if protease digestion times are suboptimal (Fig. 3-15). If model 1 is correct, one would anticipate a stronger signal with the Stoeffel fragment with suboptimal protease times given its smaller size. This statement must be tempered by the realization that one would have to demonstrate that the Stoeffel fragment diffused more readily through the nucleic acid–protein cross-links in the nucleus. Clearly, further study is needed to explain these interesting observations and to test the model presented in Fig. 3-20.

"Prolonged" denaturation may be a method to inhibit the DNA repair mechanism. It has been theorized that either treatment with a NaOH solution or with microwave "retrieval" before *in situ* PCR might inhibit the DNA repair pathway during the PCR step by forcing the DNA strands to remain separated, perhaps by breakage of their protein cross-links. (For the nonpathologist, microwave retrieval pretreatment consists of immersing the slide in a buffer and subjecting it to two rounds of boiling in a microwave at 5 minutes each.) If true, this would be an important observation, as it could permit target-specific incorporation of the reporter nucleotide for DNA targets in paraffin-embedded tissue, which is discussed at length in Chapter 5. We tested both the NaOH and microwave retrieval pretreatment steps on the strength of the primer-independent signal in paraffin-embedded tissue. There was no discernible effect on the primer-independent signal, which was still intense after optimal protease digestion. The one difference was that these pretreatments decreased the optimal protease digestion times. Not surprisingly, these pretreatments also increased the likelihood of loss of morphology.

The repair of DNA gap model for the primer-independent signal with *in situ* PCR clearly would predict that adequate DNase digestion would eliminate the signal. We have been able to prevent DNA repair by DNase digestion prior to the *in situ* PCR step. This observation is the cornerstone of RT *in situ* PCR, as discussed in Chapter 7. However, as is true for the nonspecific DNA repair signal itself, the results one obtains with DNase digestion are strongly dependent on both the length of time the tissue has been fixed in 10% buffered formalin and the protease digestion time. These data are presented in Table 3-5. It should be stressed that the DNase digestion was done

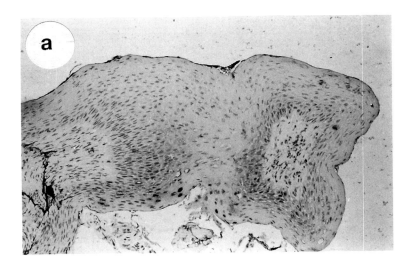

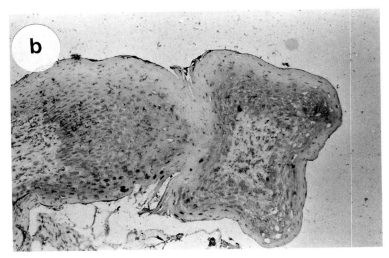

Figure 3-18. *Relationship of the primer-independent signal to the times of formalin fixation and protease digestion: prolonged fixation time.* Skin tissue was fixed for 1 week in 10% buffered formalin. Minimal signals are evident after digestion in pepsin at 2 mg/ml at either 15 minutes (**a**) or 60 minutes (**b**; an equivalent signal was seen after 90 minutes of digestion). The signal became optimal after 90 minutes of digestion in proteinase K at 1 mg/ml (**c**).

overnight. Considering the enormous amount of DNA present in the nucleus that could participate in one of the nonspecific pathways, it is not surprising that such extended periods of digestion with the DNase are needed, as discussed with the model presented in Fig. 3-20. Note the following points from the data in Table 3-5:

1. When the signal with the non-DNased tissue is optimal, the primer-independent signal is eradicated with DNase digestion.
2. When the signal with the non-DNased tissue is suboptimal due to inadequate protease digestion, the primer-independent signal for the DNase-treated tissue is enhanced compared with the serial section

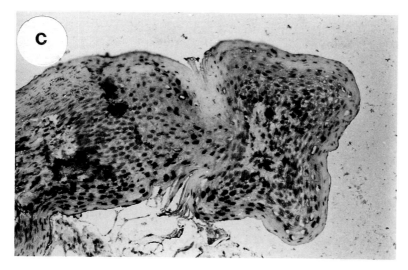

Figure 3-18. *Continued.*

on the same glass slide that was not digested with DNase.

The first observation demonstrates that DNase digestion was adequate in rendering the native DNA nonamplifiable. This serves as the negative control for RT *in situ* PCR, as, if one is to use direct incorporation of the reporter molecule after the RT step, it is critical to be assured that any resulting signal must be derived from the cDNA and that the native DNA has been rendered inoperative (Fig. 3-22).

The second observation can be considered a "paradoxical" enhancement of the primer-independent signal with DNase digestion in the setting of inadequate protease digestion. Clearly, this is similar to what was observed with dideoxy blockage and *Taq* polymerase for tissues that were not adequately proteased. Recall that this "dideoxy-pretreatment enhanced signal" with suboptimal protease was not seen if the Stoeffel fragment was used in the dideoxy step, suggesting that the exo"DNase" activity of *Taq* polymerase was responsible. Possible explanations for these observations are explored in Chapter 7 (see Fig. 7-8). Suffice it to say at this stage that the DNase digestion data again lend support to the second model to explain the relationship of DNA repair with protease digestion and formalin fix-

Table 3-5. *The effect of protease digestion time on the primer-independent signal with* in situ *PCR with and without overnight digestion in RNase-free DNase*

Fixation time (hr)	Protease digestion time (min)			
	15	30	45	60
8				
No digestion	1+[a]	3+	2+	—
DNase digestion	2+	0	0	—
16				
No digestion	0	1+	1+	3+
DNase digestion	2+	1+	0	0

[a]See Table 3-1 for definition of signal intensity.

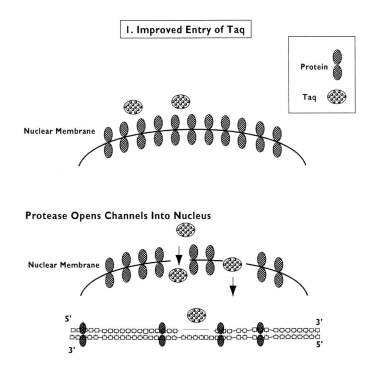

Figure 3-19. *A proposed model for the relationship of the primer-independent signal with the protease digestion time and formalin fixation time:* Taq *entry.* One possible reason for the strong relationship between the times of formalin fixation and protease digestion for *in situ* PCR is presented. Increasing fixation times in formalin may inhibit entry of *Taq* polymerase into the nucleus during PCR by decreasing pore size in the nuclear membrane. Protease digestion is required for *Taq* entry. Consistent with this hypothesis is the similar relationship between the signal evident with standard *in situ* hybridization and the protease digestion time (see Chapter 4 for a more detailed description of this subject). However, another mechanism must be operative during *in situ* PCR, as a signal is evident with standard *in situ* hybridization at protease times much less than for *in situ* PCR.

ation times. That is, with inadequate protease digestion, the DNase, although it has diffused to the nucleus, cannot access the regions of DNA repair to render them nonamplifiable. However, under these conditions it may be able to extend or create some of these putative gaps, thus enhancing the signal relative to the section that was not treated with the DNase. With adequate protease digestion, the DNase can now degrade the entire genome to the point that the single-stranded gaps no longer could support extension by *Taq* polymerase. For the purposes of this discussion of the primer-independent signal, there are three important points to emphasize:

1. Under optimal protease conditions, the primer-independent signal should be present in over 50% of the cells in a tissue section.
2. Under the same protease conditions, this signal can be completely eliminated with overnight DNase digestion.
3. These two observations define the critical positive and negative controls for RT *in situ* PCR and guide the start-up protocol described in Chapter 6.

Before leaving the topic of DNase digestion elimination of the nonspecific signal, mention should be made of a common misinterpreta-

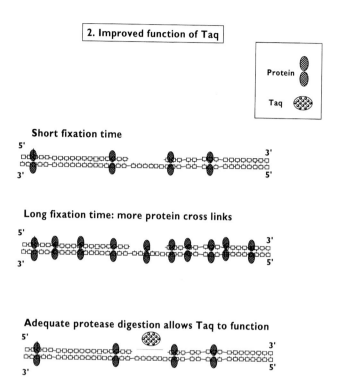

Figure 3-20. *A proposed model for the relationship of the primer-independent signal with the protease digestion time and formalin fixation time:* Taq *activity.* It is hypothesized that additional protease digestion is needed after *Taq* entry for *in situ* PCR, because remaining protein–DNA cross-links interfere with the ability of the *Taq* polymerase to repair the single-stranded gaps.

tion. Specifically, many people have reported to me that they obtained a signal in the negative control (DNase digested overnight) and assume it represents a too low DNase concentration. Assuming one is using 10 U of RNase-free DNase per section, the persistence of a signal in the negative control represents a protease digestion time that is *too short* rather than an inadequate amount of DNase (Fig. 3-23). Increasing the concentration 5× of the DNase will usually *not* eliminate the nonspecific signal under these conditions. However, increasing the protease digestion time using the guide presented in Tables 3-2 and 3-3 followed by DNase digestion will result in the elimination of the signal (Fig. 3-23). Another misconception is that DNase digestion can destroy cell

morphology. The structure of the cell is a function of its protein skeleton, which is highly developed in all cell types, especially in cells that must withstand external "stress" such as squamous cells, fibroblasts, and endothelial cells. When cell morphology is destroyed, it is usually due to protease overdigestion.

Primer-Independent Signal in Cytospin Preparations

It is important to stress that the observations listed above were based on work with paraffin-embedded tissue sections. We have studied nonspecific signal in PBMC cytospin preparations. The rate of primer-independent DNA synthesis

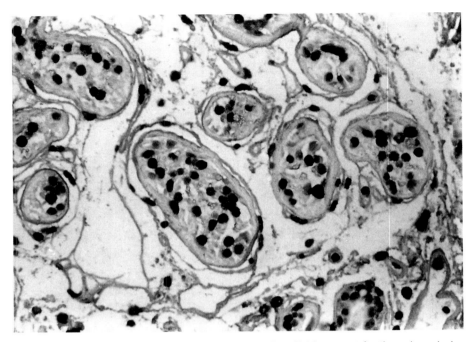

Figure 3-21. *A comparison of* Taq *polymerase and the Stoeffel fragment for the primer-independent signal during* in situ *PCR.* After optimal protease digestion, an intense primer-independent signal is seen if the Stoeffel fragment is used, which is equivalent to that seen with *Taq* polymerase. This suggests that entry of the DNA polymerase is not an important variable at optimal protease digestion times for *in situ* PCR, as the Stoeffel fragment is much smaller in size.

under these conditions (15-hour formalin fixation and 15-minute digestion in 2 mg/ml pepsin) was very low, being much less than 0.1% under optimal protease conditions, as discussed at length in Chapters 5 and 7. What is the basis of this marked disparity? One of the basic differences between the cytospins and paraffin-embedded tissues, as noted above, is that the latter are processed on an automatic machine that sequentially washes the tissue in graded ethanol and xylene and then heats the tissue for 65°C for 4 hours in paraffin wax. The primer-independent signal can be eliminated in tissue sections simply by fixing frozen sections. The signal returned if this fixed, frozen tissue was heated at 65°C for 4 hours. When the cytospin PBMC preparation was heated from 1 to 4 hours at 65°C, the nonspecific detection rate increased to over 90%, although similar results were obtained with shorter heating times and longer protease digestion times. This observation shows

that the primer-independent signal is also related to the protease digestion conditions and fixation time in the cytospin preparations, even with short (several-minute) pretreatments at 65°C (39). It is important that the heating step at 65°C must be with dry heat. The primer-independent signal should be evident after a very short time, even 1 to a few minutes. Similar results may be noted with frozen, fixed tissue (G. J. Nuovo, *unpublished observations,* 1993). Thus, for those doing direct incorporation *in situ* PCR for DNA targets, it is important to be certain that the cells and tissue are *never* exposed to dry heat every for 1 minute. Nonheated tissues and the hot start method *must* be used. I find this easy to do with my aluminum boat method (Chapter 5), as I add all reagents except for the *Taq* polymerase prior to heating of the block. If one is using Perkin-Elmer *in situ* PCR 1000 thermal cycler; one suggestion is to add the reagents minus *Taq* polymerase onto the

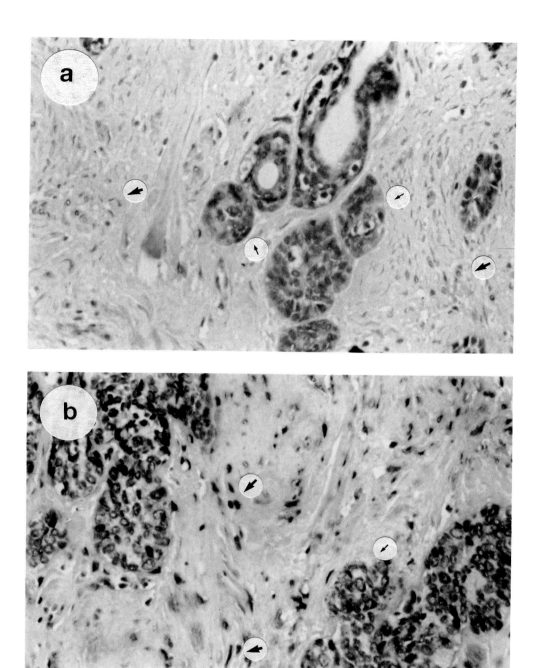

Figure 3-22. *Importance of adequate DNase digestion for the signal evident during RT* in situ *PCR.* The ability to eliminate the nonspecific signal after optimal protease digestion and overnight DNase digestion is critical for RT *in situ* PCR. This elimination permits target-specific cDNA synthesis during RT and specific direct incorporation of the reporter molecule into the PCR-amplified cDNA. **a:** In this example, HPV 18 E7 mRNA was detected by RT *in situ* PCR in the carcinoma cells in this cervical biopsy (*small arrows*). Note how the signal is not evident in the stromal cells (*large arrows*), which would not be expected to be infected by HPV. **b:** Positive control for the tissue in a, in which the carcinoma cells and the stromal cells show the nonspecific signal.

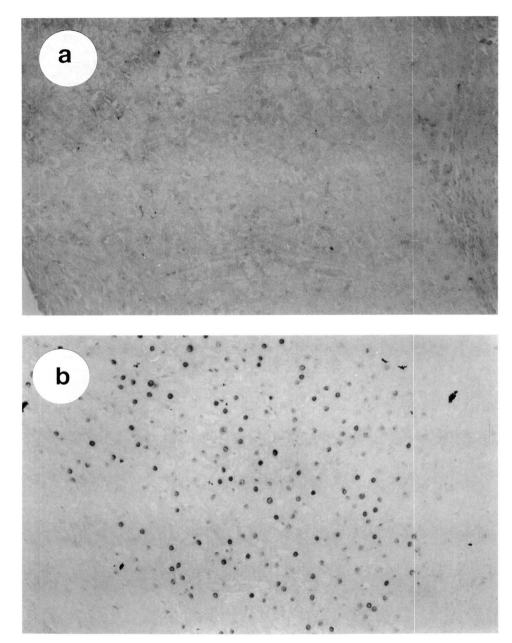

Figure 3-23. *Relationship of the primer-independent signal with DNase digestion to the protease digestion time.* The optimal protease digestion time for this liver biopsy specimen was determined to be 60 minutes. The primer-independent signal was eliminated by overnight DNase digestion after 60 minutes of protease digestion time (**a**). However, if the protease digestion time was decreased to 30 minutes, a strong signal was seen after DNase digestion (**b**), whereas no signal was seen with the serial section that was not digested in DNase (not shown). This enhancement is similar to that described with dideoxy blockage after suboptimal protease digestion time (see Figs. 3-14 and 3-15).

slide before placing it on the heated platen. Chapter 10 describes in detail the Perkin-Elmer *in situ* PCR 1000 thermal cycler.

DNA Repair in Solution Phase PCR

It is clear that, for paraffin-embedded tissues or any cell or tissue exposed to dry heat, primer-independent DNA synthesis is the predominant pathway during *in situ* PCR. We explored the possibility of a primer-independent DNA synthesis pathway during solution phase PCR. In these experiments, total cellular DNA was extracted from both paraffin-embedded and frozen tissues that were fixed for 15 hours in buffered formalin. The DNA extraction process and the electrophoresis protocols are listed in Chapter 2. Solution phase PCR was performed on the extracted DNA with either no primers, target-specific primers, or irrelevant primers, which were chosen such that their target could not be present in the total cellular DNA. The target-specific primers were used to ensure that the DNA was intact. The irrelevant primers were used to study mispriming and primer oligomerization, and the tests with no primers were done to study the primer-independent pathway. The tissue was lymphoid (tonsils and lymph nodes), and the primers were specific for the *bcl-2* gene, which is present as two copies in each cell. Mispriming and primer oligomerization were studied with HPV primers, as this virus does not infect lymphoid cells. These experiments were performed with direct incorporation of ^{32}P-labeled dCTP. After PCR and electrophoretic separation of the DNA synthesized during the reaction, the DNA could be detected by autoradiography after transfer to a filter. The ^{32}P would incorporate into both target-specific PCR product and DNA synthesized secondary to DNA repair, mispriming, or primer oligomerization. The results are provided in Fig. 3-24. Note that no detectable incorporation of the ^{32}P was noted in the DNA extracted from the frozen, fixed tissue if the primers were omitted, although an intense band is noted at the expected size for the target-specific amplification of *bcl-2*. When PCR was done on the DNA extracted from the paraffin-embedded tissues, a diffuse signal was evident when the

primers were omitted but only after prolonged exposure to the radiograph. Clearly, primer-independent DNA repair can occur in solution phase PCR, and, as was noted during *in situ* PCR, it appears to be dependent on heating the tissues during their processing. Interestingly, although a target-specific signal was also seen for the DNA extracted from the paraffin-embedded tissues under hot start conditions, a band at about 50 base pairs, which may represent nonspecific synthesis from mispriming or primer oligomerization, was also evident (Fig. 3-24). That is, the DNA extracted from the frozen, fixed tissue appeared to be less capable of having mispriming and/or primer oligomerization operative during target-specific DNA amplification and, thus, may be more sensitive for low copy targets. Note that primer oligomers were noted despite the use of hot start; this probably reflects the high sensitivity of direct incorporation of a radioactive nucleotide. However, it is evident that mispriming and primer oligomerization *per se* are more intense with solution phase PCR using DNA extracted from paraffin-embedded tissue than frozen, fixed tissue when using equivalent amounts of DNA.

In another experiment to analyze primer-independent DNA synthesis during solution phase PCR, we took highly purified salmon sperm DNA, which is heated to 121°C during processing, as well as nonheated DNA extracted from lymphocytes and exposed it to formalin, ethanol, or acetone with or without bovine serum albumin (BSA). The DNA was then purified, and solution phase PCR was performed without primers and with direct incorporation of ^{32}P-dCTP. As is evident in Fig. 3-25, primer-independent DNA synthesis occurred only if the following conditions were met:

1. Heated DNA
2. Cross-linking fixative (i.e., formalin)
3. Addition of BSA
4. Intact protein–DNA cross-links, as evident by the loss of the signal with protease digestion prior to PCR.

The latter observation likely explains why the primer-independent signal was much weak-

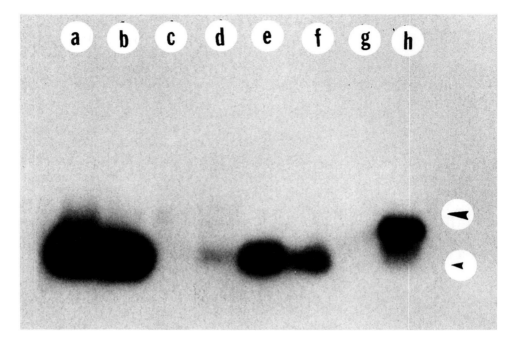

Figure 3-24. *Different DNA synthesis pathways during solution phase PCR.* DNA was extracted from fixed, paraffin-embedded lymphoid tissues (*lanes a–d*) and from tissues that were frozen and then fixed in formalin (*lanes e–h*). Solution phase PCR was done under manual hot start conditions with HPV-specific primers and no DNA (*lanes a* and *e*, primer oligomers); the HPV primers and DNA (*lanes b* and *f*, mispriming and primer oligomers); DNA and no primers (*lanes c* and *g*, DNA repair); or β-globulin-specific primers and DNA (*lanes d* and *h*, target-specific) with incorporation of ^{32}P-dCTP. Each cell would contain two copies of the β-globulin gene, while HPV does not infect lymphoid tissue. Note the intense nonspecific signals in *lanes a, b,* and *e, f*; the greater degree of target-specific amplification in the DNA extracted from the frozen, fixed tissue versus the paraffin-embedded tissue (*lane h* versus *d*); and the lack of detectable primer-independent DNA synthesis (*lanes c* and *g*) after 2 hours of exposure. An equivalent amount of DNA present in *lanes c* and *g* was electrophoresed on a separate gel, transferred to a filter, and then exposed for 2 days. Note that incorporation of the ^{32}P is evident in the DNA extracted from the paraffin-embedded tissue (*inset, lane c*) but not the frozen, fixed tissue (*inset, lane g*). The weakened primer-independent signal likely reflects the protease digestion used in the DNA extraction (compare with Fig. 3-25). The arrowheads mark 300 base pairs (*large arrowheads*) and 50 base pairs (*small arrowheads*) as detected on the ethidium gel; the expected size of PCR-amplified β-globulin DNA is 268 base pairs.

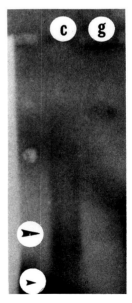

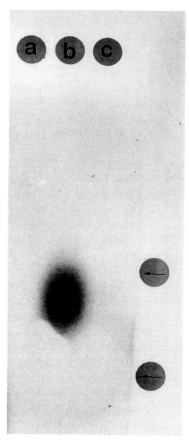

Figure 3-25. *Primer-independent DNA synthesis during solution phase PCR.* DNA was extracted from PBMCs and then fixed for 3 hours in formalin at room temperature (*lane a*), or in formalin and BSA at 68°C (*lane b*), or in formalin at 68°C for 3 hours, precipitated, and then subjected to PCR with direct incorporation using ^{32}P-labeled dCTP without primers (*lane c*). Note that primer-independent DNA synthesis is evident only for DNA that is heated and fixed in formalin in the presence of BSA. The need for intact protein–DNA cross-links is indicated by the loss of this primer-independent signal with protease digestion prior to PCR (data not shown). The *arrows* mark 700 base pairs and 300 base pairs, respectively, as detected on the ethidium gel using a 100 base pair ladder (Research Genetics).

er for the DNA extracted from the paraffin-embedded tonsil tissue (Fig. 3-24), as protease digestion is included in the protocol to extract DNA (as discussed in Chapter 2). These observations lend additional support to the model for DNA repair presented in Fig. 3-5. Specifically, the dry heat induces the gaps in the DNA. The formalin is needed to cross-link the BSA (cellular proteins) with the DNA to prevent separation of the DNA strands during the denaturation step. If too many of these cross-links are lost, the primer-independent signal is lost. This is readily apparent in solution phase PCR (Fig. 3-25) and less apparent with *in situ* PCR, as such protease digestion typically will destroy the tissue morphology. During the annealing step, the *Taq* polymerase fills in the gaps. This model would predict that the primer-independent pathway should be isothermal and not require repeated denaturation and annealing. This is indeed what we have observed (G. J. Nuovo, *unpublished observations,* 1995).

Primer Oligomerization and Mispriming

During In Situ *PCR*

The two nonspecific primer-dependent pathways are depicted in Figs. 3-2 and 3-3. Note that these two pathways—mispriming and primer oligomerization—have one very important feature in common: they each involve the binding of the primer to an area of DNA where there is some, although not complete, homology. Because of this similarity and because they are often operative at the same time during PCR, they are discussed together.

To isolate the relative contributions of primer oligomerization and mispriming to the nonspecific signal found during *in situ* PCR using paraffin-embedded tissue sections, one must be certain that other potential pathways are blocked. As discussed above, two ways to block the primer-independent signal are with overnight DNase digestion or with pretreatment in a solution that contains a dideoxynucleotide. The use of DNase digestion offers an opportunity to study the effect of primer oligomerization because the native DNA should be unavailable for DNA repair or mispriming. However, DNase digestion will clearly not allow for the study of mispriming, as the nontarget DNA would not be available for annealing. To isolate the effect of mispriming, one needs to block with ddTTP under optimal protease conditions or use frozen and then fixed tissues. With the DNA repair mechanism blocked, only the mispriming and primer oligomerization pathways could operate. Then, by comparing the results with those from serial sections treated with DNase (where only primer oligomerization should be operative), the relative contributions of primer oligomerization and mispriming can be determined.

The first set of experiments were done on DNase-treated tissues. To induce primer oligomerization in the amplifying solution and, perhaps, in the cells in the tissue section, the *Taq* polymerase was added prior to increasing the temperature of the block of the thermal cycler. We did not observe any intracellular signal after "cold start" *in situ* PCR and a high stringency wash when irrelevant primers were used on tissues that had been digested in DNase. The irrelevant primers, or those with no possible target match in the tissue tested, were specific for the measles virus nucleocapsid region. There were no histologic changes, such as multinucleated giant cells and cytoplasmic or nuclear inclusions, in the tissue to suggest measles viral infection. These results suggest some hypotheses:

1. Although primer oligomerization can occur in the amplifying solution, the resultant DNA product does not stay inside the cell.
2. Primer oligomerization in the nucleus may occur, but either it does not allow sufficient incorporation of digoxigenin dUTP to be detected or it readily diffuses out of the cell.

To test hypothesis 1, we analyzed the amplifying solution for digoxigenin incorporation. After retrieval of the amplifying solution, it was separated by electrophoresis on an agarose gel. Ethidium staining did demonstrate a smear that was most intense at about 25 to 50 base pairs, suggesting that primer oligomerization did occur in the amplifying solution. The resultant

Southern blot was analyzed for digoxigenin and is shown in Fig. 3-26. Note that strong digoxigenin incorporation is evident in much of the DNA that was synthesized during PCR in the amplifying solution; the DNA smear was very broad, extending from 25 base pairs to over 1,000 base pairs. It is apparent that, although primer oligomerization can occur in the amplifying solution during *in situ* PCR, it apparently does not cause a signal in the nucleus, even though some of the digoxigenin-containing product was less than 50 base pairs in size. It may seem incongruous that these smaller sized sequences do not produce a signal, as one might expect that they should be able to enter the cell. To provide another example of this interesting observation, in another experiment we labeled β-globulin DNA with digoxigenin using solution phase PCR with DNA extracted from human cells as the target. An intense band at the expected size (268 base pairs) was apparent with ethidium staining and detection of the digoxigenin after Southern blot transfer proved that the amplified product incorporated much of the reporter molecule (Fig. 3-26). One microgram of this labeled product was placed in a 10-μl volume over the tissue, overlaid with a coverslip, and then subjected to 20 cycles in the thermocycler. Over 95% of the cells showed no signal, and the remaining cells showed a weak nuclear rimming effect after a high stringency wash (Fig. 3-26). It is apparent that even massive amounts of PCR product in the amplifying solution are easily removed from inside the cell in formalin-fixed tissues if the target is not present in the cells (recall that DNase digestion would destroy the *bcl-2* target).

This inability of large amounts of labeled double-stranded DNA, either from primer oligomerization or when introduced to the amplifying solution, to produce a signal in the cell is not surprising for those investigators who do standard *in situ* hybridization. An in-depth discussion of *in situ* hybridization is provided in Chapter 5. A key point of *in situ* hybridization, which is now discussed, is that large amounts of double-stranded DNA are denatured with the cellular DNA and then conditions are adjusted such that only the target DNA sequences produce a signal. It is important to realize that, in

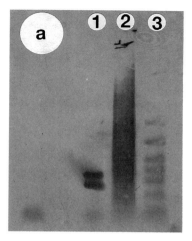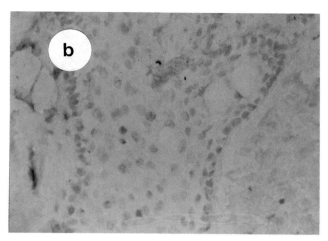

Figure 3-26. *Apparent inability of primer oligomerization to cause a signal during* in situ *PCR. In situ* PCR was performed after optimal protease digestion time and DNase digestion in skin tissue using measles-specific primers. The digestion steps would eliminate DNA repair and mispriming. Thus, any signal should represent primer oligomerization, as this tissue did not contain the measles virus. Under cold start conditions to enhance primer oligomerization, no signal is evident in the tissue section (not shown), although a large amount of DNA synthesis with digoxigenin incorporation was evident in the amplifying solution (**a**, *lane 2*; *lane 1* is the PCR-amplified digoxigenin labeled β-globulin DNA at 268 base pairs; and *lane 3* is a digoxigenin-labeled 100 pase pair ladder with the top band at 800 base pair). In a related experiment (**b**), 1 μg of the digoxigenin labeled amplified cDNA or *bcl-2* DNA was added to the amplifying solution during *in situ* PCR. No detectable labeled product was found in the nuclei after 20 cycles and a post-PCR high-stringency wash. Clearly, *in situ* PCR is similar to standard *in situ* hybridization in that a high-stringency wash will remove labeled DNA that does not have a corresponding high copy target in the cell. This eliminates the need for concern about cross-over contamination during *in situ* PCR.

most conditions, even when the copy number of the target sequence is high, there is a much greater amount of nontarget sequences. Also, the probe DNA would have a propensity to bind or "stick" to other cellular components, primarily proteins that are a major constituent of the cell membrane and cellular cytoskeleton. This would be much more likely for the single-stranded DNA probe than the double-stranded DNA, as the former would be coiled (not linear, such as double-stranded DNA), and thus its bases would be available for hydrophobic interactions and hydrogen bonding with side chains of several of the amino acids that are present in the cellular proteins. There are three important points with regards to the potential causes of background during *in situ* hybridization or PCR *in situ* hybridization:

1. Binding of the single-stranded probe, either to nontarget DNA sequences or to cellular proteins, is similar to mispriming and primer oligomers in the sense that the bonds that keep such complexes together are *much* weaker than those for the probe and target.

2. Double-stranded DNA presents a much larger molecule than single-stranded DNA. A single-stranded 100 base pair DNA molecule is similar to the size of *Taq* polymerase, whereas the double-stranded 100 base pair strand presents a much larger radius, given that it exhibits much more motion than the coiled single-stranded DNA. The point is that single-stranded DNA is certainly freely mobile in the cell after protease digestion; double-stranded DNA's mobility would be more likely to be limited, although even this is probably unlikely under the conditions usually employed during *in situ* hybridization and *in situ* PCR.

3. The wash conditions are critical in determining whether the nonspecifically bound

labeled DNA, be it a probe or from mispriming or primer oligomers, will remain in
the cell or be lost to the overlying solution.

To summarize, during *in situ* hybridization,
large amounts of labeled DNA enter each cell,
but, under the proper conditions, most of it is
washed away and does not create a false signal.
It is important to realize that it is entirely possible to provide conditions that will permit some
of the probe DNA nonspecifically bound to nontarget DNA and cellular proteins to remain attached. This is what creates the *background*. In
the example shown above, persistent binding of
labeled DNA, be it a 100 base pair single-stranded probe, a 200 base pair single-stranded (after
denaturation) amplicon, or a range of labeled
DNA from 50 to several hundred base pairs produced from primer oligomerization to nontarget
DNA sequences in the nucleus or cytoplasmic
proteins, all will produce background.

To understand how to control background, it
is important to realize that the strength of the
molecular attachment of probe and target is invariably much greater than for probe or any other
DNA sequence and nontarget DNA or probe and
cellular proteins. If one chooses conditions that
disrupt these nonspecific attachments, while permitting probe–target hybridization, then background will be greatly reduced. As discussed in
Chapter 2, this is done by adjusting the *stringency* of the postreaction wash such that the Tm
is above that of the nonspecific binding and
below that of the probe–target complex.

Figure 4-19 on page 154 shows an example
using *in situ* hybridization where the posthybridization wash was purposely chosen *below*
the Tm of the nonspecific binding of the probe
to nontarget DNA and cellular proteins. Note
the strong signal located in the cytoplasm and,
importantly, *not* in the nucleus (where the HPV
target would be located). Note that this background is lost if the posthybridization wash is
chosen above the Tm of the nonspecific binding of the probe. However, these stringent conditions do permit target-specific binding of the
probe as demonstrated in Figure 4-19. In an
analogous fashion, the primer oligomerization
that can occur in the amplifying solution during RT *in situ* PCR *can* produce a false-posi-

tive result if it is not removed from its nonspecific binding sites in the cell with a stringent
post-PCR wash (Fig. 3-27). Note that this background signal localizes to the cytoplasm and
not the nucleus, where the signal from DNA
repair, target-specific genomic amplification,
or mispriming would be evident.

The above discussion explains why background may be eradicated by a high stringent
wash secondary to the relatively weak forces
that bind labeled DNA to nontargets. It does
not explain why nontarget double-stranded
DNA also appears to be easily removed from
a cell while the double-stranded probe–target
complex remains inside. Of course, with *in situ*
PCR, large amounts of target-specific amplicons will be generated. As mentioned in Chapter 1, using formalin fixation and optimal protease digestion, there is no apparent migration
of this double-stranded amplicon (or probe–amplicon complex for PCR *in situ* hybridization)
under conditions where large amounts of labeled double-stranded nontarget-specific DNA
do not stay inside the cell. Although any explanation is highly speculative, these observations may relate to the fact that the target is
rigidly fixed in the nuclear matrix or (for RNA)
cytoplasmic cytoskeleton, protein matrix that
"anchors" the amplicon to this specific site,
making it unavailable for diffusion out of the
cell. In effect, this would serve the same function as a solid support with, for example, solid
phase antibody-mediated antigen capture.

To summarize, the synthesis of labeled DNA
in the amplifying solution during *in situ* PCR,
which could occur from primer oligomerization or target-specific amplification, can produce a background signal in cells that do not
contain the target sequence by, most likely,
binding to cellular cytoplasmic proteins. This
background signal can be eliminated by increasing the stringency of the wash (e.g., 62°C
for 15 minutes at 1×SSC).

The absence of any detectable digoxigenin
dUTP incorporated in the cells due to primer
oligomerization under high stringency wash conditions made it easier to study the effect of mispriming. If one assumes that primer oligomerization is not contributing to a cellular signal,
then any staining evident when nonspecific

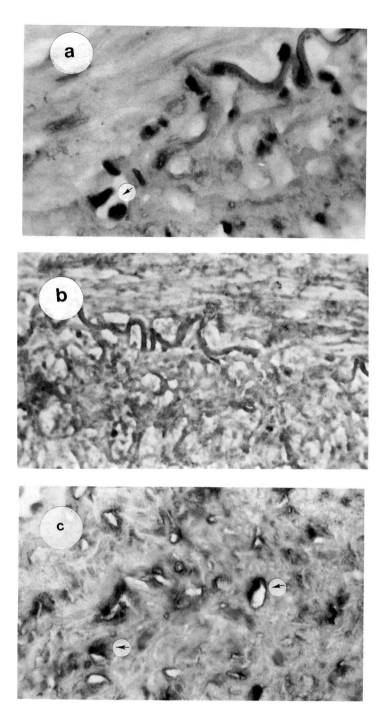

Figure 3-27. *Background is related to post-PCR stringent washes for RT* in situ *PCR.* RT *in situ* PCR was performed on this section of an artery after optimal protease digestion and DNase digestion. **a:** Note the nuclear-based signal (*arrow*) of the positive control (no DNase). **b:** The signal was lost if DNase digestion was done with irrelevant primers and a post-PCR high-stringency wash. **c:** However-er, if this high-stringency wash is omitted, the primer oligomerization that can occur in the amplifying solution can produce nonspecific staining of cell membranes and stromal proteins (*arrows*) that can be confused with a target-specific signal. This problem can be corrected by doing the high-stringency wash, using hot start, or omitting the primers for the negative control; I recommend a high-stringency wash as a basic part of RT *in situ* PCR.

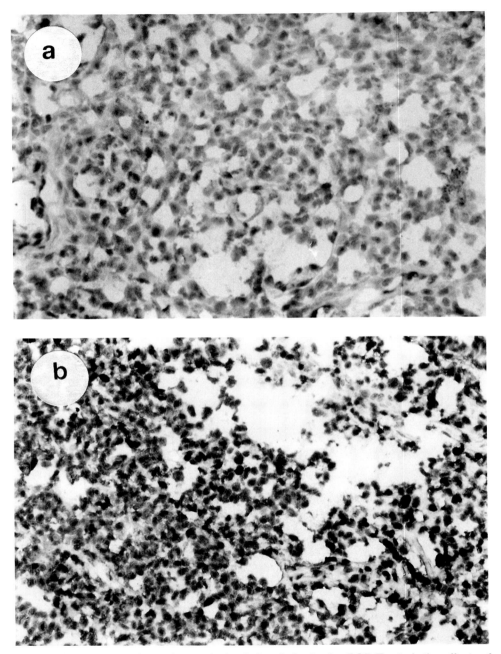

Figure 3-28. *Temperature dependency of mispriming during* in situ *PCR.* To study the effects of mis-priming on the signal during *in situ* PCR, it is essential to block the DNA repair pathway. In this case, this was achieved by using frozen and then fixed tissues that were *not* heated. **a:** No signal is evident in this tonsillar tissue if HPV-specific primers were used with the manual hot start maneuver of *in situ* PCR; the lymphoid tissue of tonsils, which is depicted, would not be expected to be infected by HPV. **b:** Note that a mispriming-derived signal is evident if the *Taq* polymerase is added prior to increasing the reaction temperature.

primers are used after optimal protease digestion and dideoxy blockage (or with frozen, fixed tissue) would presumably reflect mispriming. The results of these experiments are seen in Fig. 3-28. Note that, using frozen, fixed tissue, a signal is evident after *in situ* PCR with irrelevant primers if the *Taq* polymerase is added prior to increasing the temperature of the cycling block (cold start). The signal is nuclear as would be expected given the localization of the nontarget DNA. However, the signal is markedly diminished if the *Taq* polymerase is not added until the temperature of the block reaches 60°C (hot start). This certainly suggests that mispriming is operative during *in situ* PCR of tissue sections if the initial reaction temperature is below the Tm of the mispriming hybridization reaction. The amount of DNA synthesized during *in situ* PCR as determined by digoxigenin incorporation appears to be greater for DNA repair than for mispriming based on the intensity of the relative signals. Nonetheless, one can speculate that the inhibition of mispriming is sufficient to accentuate the relative production of the target-specific product as shown with PCR *in situ* hybridization, which is the next topic of discussion.

Nonspecific DNA Synthesis During PCR In Situ *Hybridization*

Throughout this book the terms PCR *in situ* hybridization and *in situ* PCR are used. The distinction between the two techniques is in their detection processes. In PCR *in situ* hybridization, the PCR product is detected by the use of a labeled probe. Thus, only the target-specific product is detected. In contrast, during *in situ* PCR the product is labeled directly, as it is synthesized within the cell by the use of a reporter molecule in the amplifying solution. Of course, this allows for the detection of both specific and nonspecific DNA. It has been shown that mispriming and a primer-independent pathway, likely DNA repair, can occur during *in situ* PCR. Mispriming can be eliminated by the hot start maneuver, whereas in order to block the DNA repair pathway one must use dideoxy blockage or use tissue that has not been subjected to the prolonged heating that occurs during routine tissue processing. This raises a question about

whether inhibition of mispriming can be beneficial in PCR *in situ* hybridization, where only the target-specific product is detected.

To investigate whether mispriming could reduce the sensitivity of the PCR *in situ* hybridization method, we chose to study SiHa cells. As described above, these cells contain one copy of HPV 16 per cell. PCR was performed with HPV-16-specific primers, which was followed by *in situ* hybridization using a biotin-labeled HPV 16 probe. Using PCR *in situ* hybridization under standard "cold start" conditions, no signal was evident. However, a signal was evident using the single primer pair and PCR *in situ* hybridization if the manual hot start maneuver was employed (see Fig. 5-7). Although it is possible that these data may also reflect enhanced target-specific amplification secondary to inhibition of primer oligomerization in the amplifying solution, this seems less tenable given the apparent absence of this pathway in the cell. Whatever the explanation, it is clear that the hot start maneuver does enhance the sensitivity of PCR *in situ* hybridization. Only with the hot start maneuver is it possible to routinely detect one copy per cell with PCR *in situ* hybridization.

Chemical Hot Start PCR

Although technically not difficult, manual hot start PCR can be somewhat cumbersome, especially if one is analyzing many samples at a given time. Another way to accomplish the same result is by the use of various chemicals (chemical hot start PCR). These methods have fascinating theoretical implications besides obvious practical utility. A simple method involves separating the reaction mixture with the primers from the *Taq* polymerase by use of a wax. The wax would melt at 80°C to allow the *Taq* to mix with the other reagents and then serve as an evaporation barrier during the actual cycling. Such a product is available (AmpliWax, Perkin-Elmer Cetus, Norwalk, CT). A more intriguing technique is to add a reagent to the complete reaction mixture at the onset of PCR, which will inhibit mispriming and primer oligomerization but allow target-specific primer annealing. In nature selective denaturing of DNA at physiological temperature is an obvious requirement for events such as transcription. One such natural method to denature small sequences of a much larger DNA molecule selectively involves relatively small proteins. Two well-characterized single-stranded binding proteins (SSBP) are commercially available and have been used with PCR (34–38). They are gene 32 protein from the bacteriophage T4 and the SSBP from *Escherichia coli*. These proteins have the ability to bind to and selectively cause the separation of a double-stranded DNA molecule. In effect they are lowering the Tm of the specific DNA fragment by interfering with the hydrogen bonding between the base pair matches. It seems plausible that if the proper concentration of SSBP is added to the reaction mixture, the primer–DNA binding that is less homologous (mispriming and primer oligomerization) may be inhibited, but enough target-specific primer binding may still occur owing to its greater number of hydrogen bonds per primer–DNA hybrid. This is illustrated in Fig. 3-29.

We performed experiments with SSBP to determine whether it could enhance the sensitivity of the signal with PCR *in situ* hybridization to one copy per cell. In these experiments all reagents, including the SSBP, primers, and *Taq* polymerase, were added at room temperature. Experiments were done using a wide range of concentrations of the SSBP relative to the primers. The results are listed in Figs. 3-30 and 3-31. Note that the enhanced sensitivity that is the hallmark of hot start PCR was evident without the manual hot start maneuver when an optimal concentration of SSBP was added to the amplifying solution. At a molar equivalent ratio (to total primers) of 1:5, the SSBP may inhibit mispriming without binding so much primer that specific amplification is blocked. The complete blockage of specific amplification at SSBP concentrations near and above the primer concentration is the expected result of primer sequestration. The failure of specific amplification at very low SSBP concentrations should occur if the unwanted side reactions of DNA synthesis overwhelm the specific reaction.

Another system that can block nonspecific DNA synthesis during *in situ* PCR and solution phase PCR is the Uracil-*N*-glycosylase (UNG) technique where dUTP is incorporated into the PCR product. This system is based on the ability of UNG to degrade DNA that is synthesized in the presence of dUTP at temperatures below 55°C. In this manner, UNG can degrade the DNA synthesized at the onset of PCR, which, as described above, may be mostly nonspecific. At temperatures above 55°C, where target-specific amplification would predominate, UNG is not operative. This fascinating system is described in more detail in Chapter 5.

In Cytospin Preparations

The DNA repair primer-independent pathway is not found when routinely processed cytospin cell preparations are used for the *in situ* PCR. As discussed above, cells need to be heated in the absence of an aqueous solution (or in paraffin wax) in order for the primer-independent nonspecific pathway to be evident (Fig. 3-12). Furthermore, as stated above, the primer oligomerization pathway does not produce a detectable signal during *in situ* PCR. It follows that nonspecific DNA synthesis during *in situ* PCR in cytospin preparations can apparently only be generated by mispriming. If this is the case, one would predict that the nonspecific DNA synthesis in cytospin preparations should only be operative under standard or "cold start" *in situ* PCR conditions. This is indeed the case. There are two ways to illustrate this point. First, one can perform *in situ* PCR using cytospin preparations with irrelevant primers. We have done these experiments with a variety of viral-specific primers using cells that did not contain the virus. When *Taq* polymerase was added at room temperature, over 50% of the cells demonstrated a signal. This rate decreased to <0.1% when the hot start modification was used (39).

Another experiment utilized a combination of two different cell types in the cell preparation at, roughly, a 1:1 ratio. The *in situ* PCR was performed with primers that corresponded to a target present in one cell type but ab-

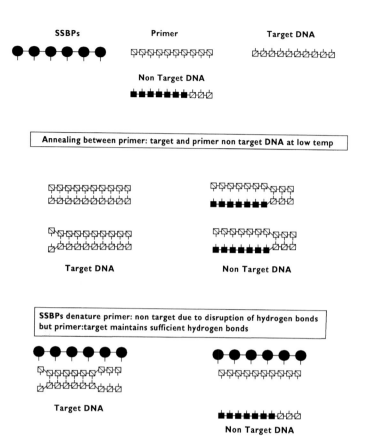

Figure 3-29. *Chemical hot start: proposed mechanism of action of single-stranded binding proteins.* SSBPs may bind to DNA and thus interfere with the hydrogen bond formation between the two hybridized strands. If the hybridized strands have relatively few hydrogen bonds, as would be expected between a primer and nontarget DNA (*right*), this disruption from the action of the SSBPs may be adequate to denature the hybridized DNA. However, disruption of some of the hydrogen bonds of the primer and target may be insufficient to denature these complexes because of the relatively greater number of hydrogen bonds between these completely complementary strands (*left*).

sent in the other cell type. We performed these experiments by mixing SiHa cells and PBMC from an individual with no evidence of HPV infection. HPV-16-specific primers were used, and the *in situ* PCR was performed under standard and hot start conditions. When standard conditions were employed, over 90% of the cells demonstrated a signal. Although the signal could have been either specific or nonspecific in the SiHa cells, it had to be nonspecific in the PBMC. Under hot start conditions, about 50% of the cells had a signal. To determine which

cells were negative, immunohistochemical colabeling with leukocyte common antigen (LCA) was done. The PBMC will label with LCA, but the SiHa cells, which are epithelial, will not. The cells negative by hot start *in situ* PCR with HPV-specific primers did indeed colabel with LCA, demonstrating that only the SiHa cells incorporated the reporter molecule (see Color Plate 2 following p. 242). These observations supported the theory that direct incorporation *in situ* PCR for DNA targets can be performed with unheated cytospin preparations but not

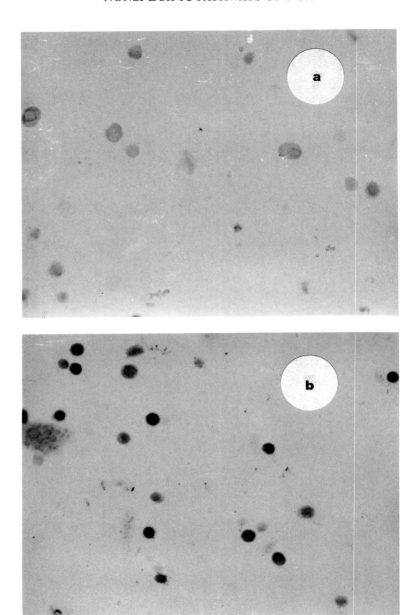

Figure 3-30. *Increased sensitivity of SSBP-mediated PCR* in situ *hybridization*. In the experiments summarized here, all reagents, including the *Taq* DNA polymerase and the SSBP, were added to each sample prior to elevating the temperature of the block of the thermal cycler. **a:** No hybridization signal is evident in SiHa cells, which contain one copy of HPV 16 per cell after PCR *in situ* hybridization analysis with a digoxigenin-labeled HPV 16 probe if no SSBP were added (data not shown) or if the SSBP is added at a molar equivalent ratio to primer of 1:210. A signal is evident with the manual hot start modification (see Fig. 5-7). **b:** A hybridization signal is evident if SSBP is added at a ratio of 1:21 in a parallel experiment done on the same glass slide. This signal presumably is due to the increase in the amount of HPV-16-specific DNA synthesis as a consequence of the inhibition of the unwanted primer-independent pathways by the SSBP.

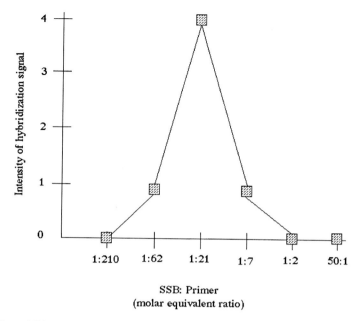

Figure 3-31. *Effect of SSBP concentration on the detection of HPV 16 DNA by PCR* in situ *hybridization without the manual hot start modification.* The presence and intensity of the hybridization signal evident with the addition of SSBP at different molar equivalent ratios to the total primer concentration (2 μM) are depicted. The signal intensity was visually graded from 0 (no signal) to 4 (intense) without knowledge of the SSBP concentration.

with paraffin-embedded tissue sections, in which the DNA repair pathway will produce extensive nonspecific signal.

Nonspecific Primer-Dependent DNA Synthesis During Solution Phase PCR

These data were discussed earlier in this chapter with regard to DNA repair. They are summarized here for completeness. Recall that the mispriming pathway was examined with the HPV-16-specific primers and DNA extracted from the lymphoid tissues, which do not contain HPV, whereas primer oligomerization was studied by omitting the cellular DNA from the reaction. In all experiments, ^{32}P-labeled dCTP was directly incorporated into the PCR product, which was detected by autoradiography after transferring the DNA to a

filter. The following observations were made (Fig. 3-24):

1. Primer oligomerization and mispriming produced signals at about 25 to 50 base pairs.
2. The signals for primer oligomerization and for mispriming were reduced by the hot start maneuver and by the use of fresh, unfixed samples.
3. The signals for primer oligomerization and for mispriming without hot start are intense and can be eliminated by hot start if the target is present. (Fig. 3-24).

It is interesting that, although nonspecific DNA synthesis can be inhibited with the hot start maneuver in solution phase PCR, it can still be detected if the more sensitive ^{32}P detection system is used, but only if the primers do not correspond to a target in the sample (Fig 3-24). Compare this to Fig 3-24 (*lane h*) or Fig.

3-8 where the hot start eliminated mispriming or primer diners when the target was present, presumably target-specific amplification reduces the availability of the primers for mispriming or primer oligomerization.

Target-Specific Amplification

During In Situ *PCR*

A simple way to study specific versus nonspecific amplification during *in situ* PCR is to use target-specific primers and a tissue in which some cells contain the target and others do not. For example, the malignant cells in cervical cancers contain HPV DNA, whereas the stromal cells in the tissue do not. As would be expected, both the cancer cells and the stromal cells demonstrated a signal after RT *in situ* PCR with HPV-18-specific primers in paraffin-embedded cervical tissues if the DNase step is omitted (Fig. 3-23). The signal in the stromal fibroblasts and endothelial cells must represent nonspecific synthesis (i.e., DNA repair), whereas the signal in the cancer cells presumably reflects a combination of DNA repair and target-specific DNA synthesis. The signal localizes to only the malignant epithelial cells if the DNase step is performed and RT *in situ* PCR is done for the HPV transcripts (Fig 3-23).

The relationship between protease digestion and formalin fixation time was discussed at length at the beginning of this chapter. Fortunately, the same relationship holds for target-specific incorporation of the reporter nucleotide and RT *in situ* PCR, as discussed at length in Chapter 7.

To differentiate the DNA target-specific signal (as compared with the cDNA with RT *in situ* PCR) from the primer-independent signal in tissue sections, one must block the DNA repair nonspecific pathway. As detailed above, this can be accomplished in two ways. First, one can pretreat the tissues in a dideoxy-containing solution after optimal protease digestion. Second, one can use frozen tissues that are

fixed in 10% buffered formalin after cryostat sectioning. Both types of experiments were done using cervical cancer and vulvar condyloma tissues. The results were equivalent. Specifically, with the hot start maneuver only target-specific direct incorporation was observed using HPV-specific primers during *in situ* PCR. This was demonstrated, because the signal localized exclusively to the epithelia known (based on the histologic findings) to contain the virus (Fig. 3-32). HPV causes specific cytological changes that are often easy to see on histologic examination of the tissue, making it very well suited for these types of analyses with *in situ* PCR.

Clearly, these observations demonstrate that one can obtain target-specific amplification of DNA in tissue sections. However, it is very important to be aware of the limitations of each technique:

1. The range of proper protease digestion time with dideoxy blockage in paraffin-embedded tissues is narrow; at either end of this range one will obtain a false-positive signal, and thus I do not recommend its use.
2. With the frozen fixed tissue, one must employ the hot start maneuver. The hot start step is *not* needed for RT *in situ* PCR, as the DNase step after optimal protease digestion eliminates all the potential nonspecific pathways.

In Cytospin Preparations

The target-specific amplification of DNA during *in situ* PCR in cytospin cell preparations is discussed above (see section on primer oligomerization and mispriming). A review of the data regarding SiHa cells mixed with the PBMC and then subjected to *in situ* PCR with HPV-16-specific primers will remind us that the hot start maneuver is critical to ensure target-specific incorporation during PCR. At the risk of overemphasizing a key point, this statement is true only if the cytospin preparation has *not* been exposed to dry heat.

During Solution Phase PCR

The final topic is the target-specific pathway during solution phase PCR. Although this has been discussed in various sections of this chapter, it may be useful to review the key points:

1. Assuming the target is present along with nontarget DNA, the detection threshold of PCR for the specific target under standard conditions is about 2,000 to 5,000 copies.

2. However, if the hot start maneuver is used, the detection threshold decreases to 1 to 10 copies.

3. DNA extracted from tissue that has been heated will show a relatively lesser degree of target-specific amplification than DNA extracted from tissue that has not been heated during the paraffin-embedding tissue process (Fig. 3-24). Thus, as is true with Southern blot and dot blot hybridization, PCR is best done using unfixed cells or tissue rather than paraffin-embedded material, assuming one has a choice.

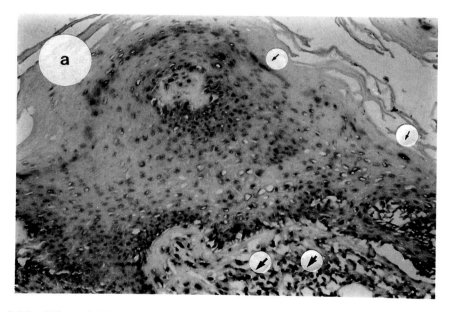

Figure 3-32. *Differential DNA synthesis during* in situ *PCR in tissues pretreated with a dideoxynucleotide in a vulvar wart that contained HPV 6.* **a:** A signal was noted in this paraffin-embedded vulvar wart fixed for 4 hours after 10 minutes of protease digestion. Note that the signal, evident without primers, is present in the epithelium (*small arrows*) and stromal cells (*large arrows*); HPV DNA is not present in stromal cells. **b:** The signal was lost if the tissue was blocked with ddTTP. **c:** After dideoxy blockage, the signal localized to the granular cells during *in situ* PCR if HPV-6-specific primers were used; note the absence of the stromal signal. These latter two features are useful measures of the target-specific localization of the signal.

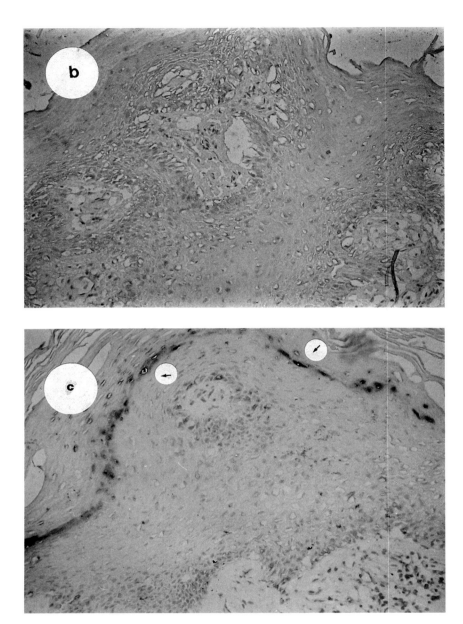

Figure 3-32. *Continued.*

REFERENCES

1. Lawyer FC, Stoffel S, Saiki RK, Myambo KB, Drummond R, Gelfand DH. Isolation, characterization, and expression in *E. coli* of the DNA polymerase gene from the extreme thermophile, *Thermus aquaticus*. *J Biol Chem* 1989;264:6427–6437.
2. Saiki RK, Gelfand DH, Stoffel S, et al. Primer-directed enzymatic amplification of DNA with a thermostable DNA polymerase. *Science* 1988;239:487–491.
3. Innis MA, Gelfand DH, Sninsky JJ, Whote TJ. *PCR protocols. A guide to methods and applications.* San Diego: Academic Press; 1990.
4. Bauer HM, Ting Y, Greer CE, et al. Genital human papillomavirus infection in female university students as determined by a PCR-based method. *JAMA* 1991;265:472–477.
5. Greer CE, Lund JK, Manos MM. PCR amplification from paraffin-embedded tissues: recommendations on fixatives for long-term storage and prospective studies. *Cold Spring Harbor Symp Quant Biol* 1991;1:46–50.
6. Nuovo GJ. HPV DNA in genital tract lesions histologically negative for condylomata: analyses by *in situ*, Southern blot hybridization and the polymerase chain reaction. *Am J Surg Pathol* 1990;14:643–651.
7. Nuovo GJ, Hochman H, Eliezri YD, Comite S, Lastarria D, Silvers D. Human papillomavirus DNA in penile lesions histologically negative for condylomata: analysis by *in situ* hybridization and the polymerase chain reaction. *Am J Surg Pathol* 1990;14:829–836.
8. Brandsma JL, Lewis AJ, Abramson A, Manos MM. Detection and typing of papillomavirus DNA in formaldehyde-fixed paraffin-embedded tissue. *Arch Otolaryngol Head Neck Surg* 1990;116:844–848.
9. Higuchi R, Kwok S. Avoiding false positives with PCR. *Nature* 1989;339:237–238.
10. Lynas C, Cook SD, Laycock KA, Bradfield JWB, Maitland NJ. Detection of latent virus mRNA in tissues using the polymerase chain reaction. *J Pathol* 1989;157:285–289.
11. Mariette X, Gozlan J, Clerc D, Bisson M, Morinet F. Detection of Epstein-Barr virus DNA by *in situ* hybridization and polymerase chain reaction in salivary gland biopsy specimens from patients with Sjogren's syndrome. *Am J Med* 1991;90:286–294.
12. McDonnell JM, Mayr AJ, Martin WJ. DNA of human papillomavirus type 16 in dysplastic and malignant lesions of the conjunctiva and cornea. *N Engl J Med* 1989;320:1442–1446.
13. Riou G, Favre M, Jeannel D, Bourhis J, LeDoussal V, Orth G. Association between poor prognosis in early stage invasive cervical carcinomas and nondetection of HPV DNA. *Lancet* 1990;1171–1174.
14. Shibata D, Fu YS, Gupta JW, Shah KV, Arnheim N, Martin WJ. Detection of human papillomavirus in normal and dysplastic tissue by the polymerase chain reaction. *Lab Invest* 1988;59:555–559.
15. Stetler-Stevenson M, Crush-Stanton S, Cossman J. Involvement of the bcl-2 gene in Hodgkin's disease. *J Natl Cancer Inst* 1990;82:855–858.
16. Syrjanen S, Saastamoinen J, Chang F, Ji H, Syrjanen K. Colposcopy, punch biopsy, *in situ* DNA hybridization, and the polymerase chain reaction in searching for genital human papillomavirus infections in women with normal pap smears. *J Med Virol* 1990;31:259–266.
17. Tidy JA, Parry GCN, Ward P, et al. High rate of human papillomavirus type 16 infection in cytologically normal cervices. *Lancet* 1989;i:434.
18. Young LS, Bevan IS, Johnson MA, et al. The polymerase chain reaction: a new epidemiological tool for investigating cervical human papillomavirus infection. *Br Med J* 1989;298:14–17.
19. Chadwick EG, Yogev R, Kwok S, Sninsky JJ, Kellogg DE, Wolinsky SM. Enzymatic amplification of the human immunodeficiency virus in peripheral blood mononuclear cells from pediatric patients. *J Infect Dis* 1989;160:954–959.
20. Escaich S, Wallon M, Baginski I, et al. Comparison of HIV detection by virus isolation in lymphocyte cultures and molecular amplification of HIV DNA and RNA by PCR in offspring of seropositive mothers. *J AIDS* 1991;4:130–135.
21. Horsburgh CR, Ou C, Jason J, et al. Concordance of polymerase chain reaction with human immunodeficiency virus antibody detection. *J Infect Dis* 1990;162:542–545.
22. Nuovo GJ, MacConnell P, Forde A, Delvenne P. Detection of human papillomavirus DNA in formalin fixed tissues by *in situ* hybridization after amplification by PCR. *Am J Pathol* 1991;139:847–854.
23. Faloona F, Weiss S, Ferre F, Mullis K. Direct detection of HIV sequences in blood: high gain polymerase chain reaction. In: *Proceedings of the sixth international conference on AIDS.* San Francisco: Humana Press; 1988, Abstract 1019.
24. Erlich HA, Gelfand D, Sninsky JJ. Recent advances in the polymerase chain reaction. *Science* 1991;252:1643–1650.
25. Nuovo GJ, Gallery F, MacConnell P, Becker J, Bloch W. An improved technique for the detection of DNA by *in situ* hybridization after PCR-amplification. *Am J Pathol* 1991;139:1239–1244.
26. Frohman MA, Dush M, Martine GR. Rapid production of full length cDNAs from rare transcripts: amplification using a single gene specific oligonucleotide primer. *Proc Natl Acad Sci USA* 1988;85:8998–9002.
27. Newton GG, Graham A, Hepinstall LE. Analysis of any point mutation in DNA: the amplification refractory mutation system (ARMS). *Nucleic Acids Res* 1989;17:2503–2516.
28. Mack D, Sninsky JJ. A sensitive method for the identification of uncharacterized viruses related to known virus groups. Hepadnavirus model systems. *Proc Natl Acad Sci USA* 1988;85:6977–6981.
29. Melchers WJG, Schift R, Stolz E, Lindeman J, Quint WGV. Human papillomavirus detection in urine samples from male patients by the polymerase chain reaction. *J Clin Microbiol* 1989;27:1711–1714.
30. Shibata DK, Arnheim N, Martin WJ. Detection of human papilloma virus in paraffin-embedded tissue using the polymerase chain reaction. *J Exp Med* 1988;167:225–230.
31. Wright PA, Wynford-Thomas D. The polymerase chain reaction: miracle or mirage? *J Pathol* 1990;162:99–117.
32. van den Brule AJC, Meijer CJL, Bakels V, Kenemans P, Walboomers JMM. Rapid detection of human papillomavirus in cervical scrapes by combined general primer-mediated and type-specific polymerase chain reaction. *J Clin Microbiol* 1990;28:2739–2743.
33. Nuovo GJ, Darfler MM, Impraim CC, Bromley SE. Occurrence of multiple types of human papillomavirus in genital tract lesions: analysis by *in situ* hybridization

and the polymerase chain reaction. *Am J Pathol* 1991; 58:518–523.

34. Schwartz G. Single stranded binding proteins and PCR. *Nucleic Acids Res* 1990;18:1079.
35. Panaccio G, Lew G. PCR and lambda phage single-stranded binding proteins. *Nucleic Acids Res* 1991;19:1151.
36. Chase G, Willimas G. Single stranded DNA binding proteins required for DNA replication. *Annu Rev Biochem* 1986;55:103–136.
37. Williams KR, et al. SSBP. Limited proteolysis on the *Escherichia coli* single-stranded DNA binding protein. *J Biol Chem* 1983;258:3346–3355.
38. Wickner SH. DNA replication proteins of *E. coli*. *Annu Rev Biochem* 1978;49:421–428.
39. Chou Q, Russell M, Birch DE, Raymond J, and Bloch W. Prevention of pre-PCR mispriming and primer dinerization improves low copy number amplification. *Nucleic Acids Res* 1992;20:1717–1723.
40. Nuovo MA, Nuovo GJ, MacConnell P, Steiner G. Analysis of Paget's disease of bone for the measles virus using the reverse transcriptase *in situ* polymerase chain reaction technique. *Diagn Mol Pathol* 1993;1:256–265.
41. Nuovo GJ, Lidonocci K, MacConnell P, Lane B. Intracellular localization of PCR-amplified hepatitis C cDNA. *Am J Pathol* 1993;17:683–690.
42. Nuovo GJ, Gallery F, Hom R, MacConnell P, Bloch W. Importance of different variables for optimizing *in situ* detection of PCR-amplified DNA. *PCR Method Appl* 1993;2:305–312.
43. Nuovo GJ, Forde A, MacConnell P, Fahrenwald R. *In situ* detection of PCR-amplified HIV-1 nucleic acids and tumor necrosis factor cDNA in cervical tissues. *Am J Pathol* 1993;143:40–48.
44. Nuovo GJ. *In situ* hybridization protocols. In: Choo KHA, ed. *Methods in molecular biology.* San Diego: Humana Press; 1993;48–105.
45. Nuovo GJ. PCR *in situ* hybridization. *Clini Immunol Newslett* 1992;12:106–112.
46. Nuovo GJ. *In situ* detection of DNA after polymerase chain reaction amplification. In: Celis JE, ed., *Cell biology: a laboratory handbook.* Orlando: Academic Press; 1993:477–487.
47. Nuovo GJ. The clinical utility of detection of human papillomavirus DNA in the lower genital tract. *Infect Medicine* 1995;11:172–183.
48. Nuovo GJ. *In situ* hybridization. In: Damjanov I, Linder J, eds. *Anderson's textbook of pathology.* 10th ed. San Diego: Academic Press; 1995:239–251.
49. MacConnell P, Nuovo GJ. RT *in situ* PCR for the detection of viral RNA and mRNAs. In: Siebert PD, Larrick JW, eds. *Reverse transcriptase PCR.* San Diego: Academic Press; 1994.
50. Nuovo GJ. PCR *in situ* hybridization. In: Wiedbrauk DL, Farkas DH, eds. *Molecular methods for viral detection.* San Diego: Academic Press; 1994:237–259.
51. Simsir S, Nuovo GJ. PCR and RT PCR *in situ* hybridization: applications in viral detection. *Trends Biotechnol.*
52. Nuovo GJ, Gallery F, MacConnell P. Analyisis of nonspecific DNA synthesis during *in situ* PCR. *PCR Method Appl* 1994;4:342–349.

4

In situ Hybridization

As discussed in Chapter 2, *in situ* hybridization is one of the basic molecular hybridization techniques. The key feature distinguishing it from the other methodologies of filter hybridization and PCR is that the sample DNA is detected directly in the intact cell rather than being extracted from the cell before testing. This cell-based detection makes the assay particularly attractive to the pathologist who is used to examining tissues. However, *in situ* hybridization is a relatively insensitive test, and the results are usually negative when the copy number per cell is low (i.e., less than ten per cell), as in point mutations or occult and latent viral infections. In these cases one must use either filter hybridization analysis or PCR to detect the viral genome (Fig. 4-1) (1–6). For example, although 30% to 40% of cervical tissues suspect at colposcopy for human papillomavirus (HPV) infection, though lacking the diagnostic histologic features, will be positive for HPV DNA using Southern blot hybridization; the detection rate for such tissues by *in situ* hybridization is only 2%. The lower detection rate for the *in situ* analysis presumably reflects the low copy numbers of HPV present in these "nondiagnostic" tissues (3,5). A misconception about *in situ* hybridization is that radiolabeled probes (usually ^{35}S or ^{3}H) must be used to maximize its sensitivity. Although this statement may have been true 5 or more years ago, dramatic advances in nonisotopic labeling and, more importantly, detection systems have greatly enhanced the sensitivity of *in situ* hybridization using such common labels as biotin and digoxigenin (7–10). Although reported detection thresholds vary depending on who is making the claim, most would agree that at least ten DNA or RNA copies per cell are needed for

the target to be detectable by standard *in situ* hybridization (6,8,10–12). In the experience of this author and many other investigators, it is not correct to state that *in situ* hybridization can routinely detect one DNA or RNA copy per cell. Fig. 4-2 shows the results of *in situ* hybridization using biotin-labeled probes with three different cervical cancer cell lines that contain 1, 25, and 600 copies of HPV DNA per cell, respectively. The one copy of HPV 16 DNA per SiHa cell was detectable only after PCR *in situ* hybridization.

A general discussion of the protocols and applications of *in situ* hybridization is presented in this chapter. Special emphasis is placed on the use of oligoprobes for *in situ* hybridization. These are small (20 to 40 base pair) probes that can be used for PCR *in situ* hybridization. To generate an oligoprobe, a DNA sequence internal to the sequence of the two primers used for PCR is chosen. This eliminates the possibility that the signal detected after PCR *in situ* hybridization may be derived from the primers themselves (i.e., primer oligomerization). However, their small size does not make them, in general, useful for standard *in situ* hybridization, as they are associated with a narrow window between target-specific signal and background.

THE KEYS TO SUCCESSFUL *IN SITU* HYBRIDIZATION

Slide Preparation

Considering the number of steps required for *in situ* hybridization before one can directly visualize small segments of DNA or RNA deep in the nucleus or cytoplasm of a cell, it is inter-

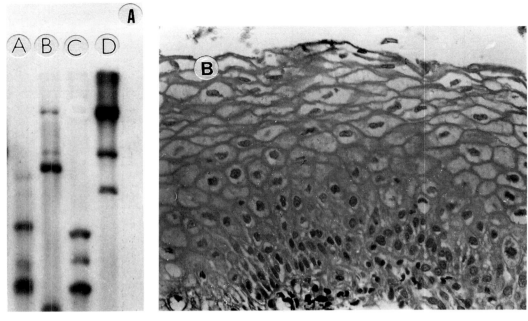

Figure 4-1. *Different detection thresholds of filter hybridization and* in situ *hybridization analyses.* HPV DNA was detected in this cervical biopsy specimen by Southern blot hybridization (**A**, *lane B*). The cervical tissue lacked the histological features of an HPV infection (**B**). As is true for most of the cervical tissues that lack the histological features of a low-grade squamous intraepithelial lesion (SIL), HPV DNA was not detectable by *in situ* hybridization. One explanation for this observation is that the copy number of HPV in the infected cells is below the ten copies per cell threshold of *in situ* hybridization (also see Fig. 2-19).

esting that a major technical advancement had nothing to do with the dynamics of probe entry or hybridization but simply with the preparation of the glass slide. When we started doing *in situ* hybridization about 7 years ago, it was routine to pretreat the slides with poly-L-lysine or a solution of glue (13–16). Although this worked better than no pretreatment where most sections would fall off during the *in situ* procedure, in our experience the sections would, at best, remain on the slide about 75% of the time. Larger sections and *in situ* tests that required high stringency washes, such as RNA *in situ* hybridization, were especially prone to poor tissue adherence. It certainly is a most unpleasant moment to come to the end of a 24-hour *in situ* experiment only to see the tissue "flapping in the breeze" and ultimately be lost. Organosilane, a chemical used in industry to treat glass, solved this problem. A rapid and inexpensive pretreatment of the slides with a solution containing silane improved tissue adherence to over 99%,

even when using the demanding high temperature incubations and washes characteristic of PCR *in situ* hybridization or RNA *in situ* hybridization. The protocol I use for silane coating slides is listed in Protocol 4-1. However, because silane-coated slides can be readily and inexpensively purchased from a variety of vendors and because silane is a toxic chemical that must be used in a fume-flow hood, I recommend that one consider purchasing the slides rather than personally preparing them. I have used silane-coated slides up to 5 years after pretreatment with no apparent loss of tissue adherence.

Protocol 4-1: A Simplified Silanization Protocol to Improve the Adherence of the Tissue to the Glass Slide

Slide cleaning

1. Wash slides in 2N HCl for 5 minutes.
2. Rinse in distilled water for 1 minute.

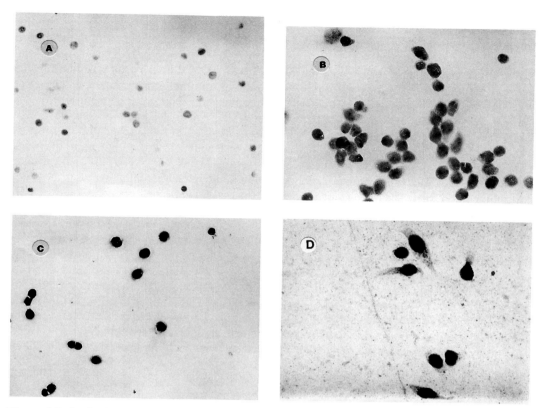

Figure 4-2. In situ *hybridization analysis of HPV DNA in three different cervical carcinoma cell lines and comparison with PCR* in situ *hybridization.* The cervical carcinoma cell lines SiHa (**A**), HeLa (**B**), and Caski (**C**) contain 1, 25, and 600 copies of HPV DNA, respectively. Using standard *in situ* hybridization analysis and biotin-labeled probes, no signal was evident with SiHa cells, a weak signal was noted with HeLa cells, and an intense signal was visible with the Caski cells. Note the intense signal evident in the SiHa cells if PCR *in situ* hybridization is performed, demonstrating a several hundredfold increase in the copy number of HPV 16 after amplification (**D**).

3. Rinse in high-grade acetone for 1 minute and air dry.

Silanization

1. Wash slides in a 2% solution of organosilane in high-grade acetone for 1 minute with gentle agitation.
2. Rinse slides in high-grade acetone for 1 minute and air dry.
3. Store at room temperature in box for ≥5 years.

Fixative

Initially much of *in situ* hybridization was done using unfixed, frozen tissue sections. The use of frozen sections obviated the need for processing paraffin-embedded tissues and, in some instances, protease pretreatments. However, tissue morphology was, at best, only fair when compared with paraffin-embedded sections and was at times barely recognizable. Indeed, some improvement was noticed in the intensity of the *in situ* hybridization signal when frozen tissues were pretreated with protease, but morphological interpretation was next to impossible (10, 17). Furthermore, it is difficult to place multiple frozen tissue sections on one slide. It is highly advantageous to have three to four sections on one silane slide to permit comparative analysis, including the critical positive and negative controls that are necessary to evaluate the results of standard *in situ* hybridization and *in situ* PCR. Clearly it would be preferable to use paraffin-embedded tissues for *in situ* hybridization analyses, as morphology is preserved and one may study archival material. One reason the initial results for *in situ* hybridization studies of paraffin-embedded tissues were so variable and thus somewhat discouraging was that different tissue fixatives were used. Some fixatives are well suited for *in situ* hybridization, and test results are comparable with those obtained with unfixed tissues. Other types of fixatives may destroy the hybridization signal depending on the amount of time the tissue is exposed to the fixative (15,18–22).

Buffered formalin (pH 7.0) is an excellent fixative for *in situ* hybridization. Acceptable fixation times can be several hours to several days to obtain reproducibly strong hybridization signals. Compared with buffered formalin, unbuffered formalin is associated with a reduction of about 50% in the intensity of the hybridization signal (15,20). When fixatives that contain

heavy metals, such as mercury (e.g., Zenker's solution) or picric acid (e.g., Bouin's solution) are used, the effects on the *in situ* hybridization signal are very dependent on the length of time of fixation. A 2-hour fixation in Bouin's solution has minimal effect on the intensity of the hybridization signal. However, intermediate results are seen after 8 hours of fixation, and the *in situ* hybridization signal can be completely eradicated after 15 hours (overnight) of Bouin's fixation (Fig. 4-3) (15,20). This marked reduction in the intensity of the hybridization signal is associated with another interesting effect. The signal is lost at high stringency even when one is certain that the probe and target are completely homologous (15,20). As shown in Fig. 4-4, this loss in the hybridization signal at high stringency when tissues are used that have been fixed in Bouin's solution does not occur if the tissues are fixed in buffered formalin. Recall from previous discussions that a decrease in Tm is expected for an HPV probe–target complex as the degree of homology decreases. It follows

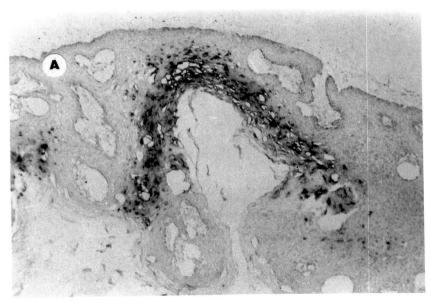

Figure 4-3. *Effect of different times of fixation in Bouin's solution on the intensity of the* in situ *hybridization signal.* A vulvar condyloma that had a high copy number of HPV 6 DNA as determined by Southern blot hybridization analysis was subdivided and fixed in Bouin's solution for 2 hours (**A**), 8 hours (**B**), and 15 hours (**C**). The intensity of the signal with *in situ* hybridization after 2 hours fixation was strong, whereas it was intermediate after 8 hours fixation and markedly decreased after 15 hours fixation.

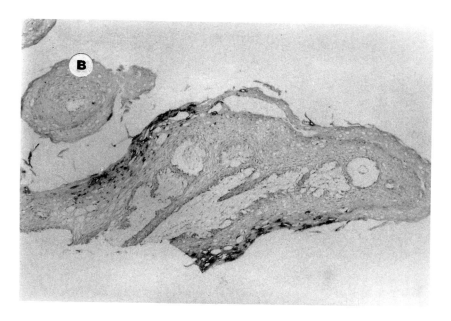

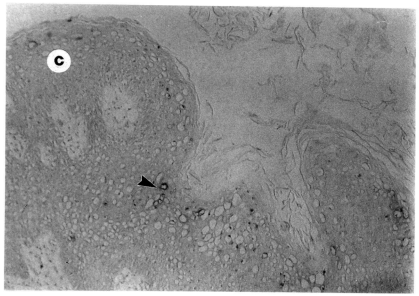

Figure 4-3. *Continued.*

that the heavy metal or picric acid may be causing conformational alterations in the DNA such that complete base pair matching is no longer possible (Fig. 4-5). Figure 4-5 also depicts DNA degradation, another effect of fixation with heavy metals and picric acid not noted after fixation with buffered formalin. However, this effect cannot *per se* explain the decreased hybridization signal, because DNA degradation is evident after 2 hours of fixation in Bouin's solution when the hybridization signal is still unaffected (15,20).

Many people who are attempting to use PCR *in situ* hybridization have asked me if they can

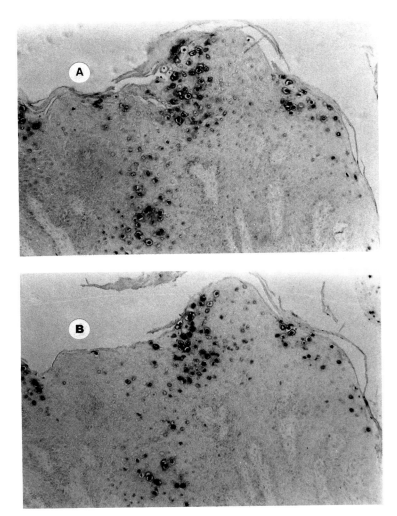

Figure 4-4. *Effect of tissue fixation on the hybridization signal seen at varying stringencies with a homologous probe.* The hybridization signal seen at low stringency (**A**) in a vulvar condyloma fixed overnight in 10% buffered formalin was evident with an HPV 6 biotin probe was not diminished at high stringency (**B**). The hybridization signal was eliminated at high stringency (**C**) if the tissue was fixed overnight in Bouin's solution (compare with Fig. 4-3C, done at low stringency).

use frozen, unfixed tissue. Although such tissues can be used for standard *in situ* hybridization, they are not acceptable for PCR *in situ* hybridization. The reason for this, as is discussed in Chapter 5, is that much of the PCR product migrates out of the cell into the amplifying solution. However, PCR *in situ* hybridization can be successful if one prepares cryostat sections from the frozen tissues on silane slides and then fixes the slide with the tissue in 10% buffered formalin for 4 to 15

hours. In my experience, one also obtains better results with standard *in situ* hybridization, especially with regard to the morphological detail, if frozen tissues are fixed after preparing cryostat sections.

In addition to buffered formalin, there are other types of cross-linking fixatives, such as paraformaldehyde and glutaraldehyde. The mechanism of these fixatives is similar to that of formalin in that it inactivates degradative cellular enzymes by cross-linking these and

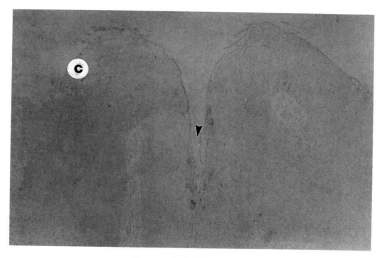

Figure 4-4. *Continued.*

other proteins to themselves and to DNA and RNA. This complexing with RNA may protect the molecule from RNase degradation. This is an important issue in RT *in situ* PCR and standard RNA *in situ* hybridization. In my experience, many investigators are very concerned that RNA is easily degraded in fixed tissue sections. The cross-linking fixatives are superior in protecting the RNA from degradation during tissue processing. However, careful tissue handling is always important. After protease digestion, care should be taken to prevent RNase contamination (e.g., wear gloves at all times), as the protective effect of the protein–RNA complexes has been disrupted. With regard to standard *in situ* hybridization, the protocols listed below are for testing tissues that have been fixed in 10% buffered formalin or some other cross-linking fixative.

Due to recent governmental concern with the potential health hazards of formalin, the use of formalin substitutes for tissue processing has been promoted. I have tested fixatives that are based in alcohol, although proprietary concerns of the companies involved preclude a detailed list of the ingredients. One can obtain good signals with such fixatives (e.g., Histochoice) for *in situ* hybridization. However, the protease digestion step must be reduced

or eliminated to avoid destroying tissue morphology and decreasing or losing the signal. Furthermore, in my experience, these fixatives do not give the robust signals that can be achieved with the use of cross-linking fixatives for *in situ* PCR.

To summarize tissue processing:

1. Fix tissues in 10% buffered formalin for 8 hours to 3 days.
2. Embed the tissue in paraffin.
3. Place three 4-μm sections on a silane-coated glass slide.

Protease Digestion

To allow penetration of the probe into the tissue, the paraffin wax must first be removed. This can be done by placing the slides in xylene for 5 minutes followed by a 5-minute wash in 100% ethanol. The slides can then be air dried and are now ready for the protease digestion solution.

Most fixatives exert primary effects on the cellular proteins either by linking them to other macromolecules such as nucleic acids (buffered formalin) or by denaturation (ethanol) and in this way render inactive native degrading enzymes (15,22–24). However, these effects may hinder access of the probe to the target nucleic acid mol-

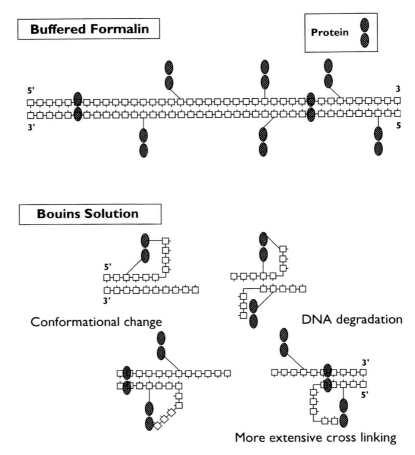

Figure 4-5. *Proposed mechanism of action of different fixatives on DNA.* Formalin-based fixatives such as buffered formalin and Bouin's solution cause complexes between native proteins and nucleic acids. It has been documented that fixatives that contain picric acid such as Bouin's lead to marked degradation of the DNA (15). It is theorized that there is a concomitant conformational change in the DNA in Bouin's fixed tissues that renders its nucleotides less able to hybridize to homologous DNA. This may explain the weakened hybridization signal evident with Bouin's fixed tissues and loss at high stringency with a homologous probe.

ecule. Different methods have been used to facilitate probe entry, including treatment with various chemicals such as HCl, photofluor, and sodium sulfite (12). However, most of the interest has focused on pretreatment with protease.

An arbitrary but useful way to approach the different protease treatments one may use with *in situ* PCR and standard *in situ* hybridization is to separate those that may be activated by low pH, such as pepsin and trypsin, from those that are active at physiological pH, such as proteinase K. Agents like pepsin offer the advantage of rapid and strong inhibition of activity by simple ad-

justment of the pH from 2.0 to 8.5, which is the optimal pH for PCR. This is especially useful in PCR *in situ* hybridization, in which residual protease activity could inactivate the *Taq* polymerase.

Determining the proper concentration of the protease and the optimal digestion time requires some trial and error. Insufficient protease treatment may result in a diminished or completely absent hybridization signal (Fig. 4-6). Too much protease treatment is easily recognized as the tissue morphology will be destroyed (Fig. 4-7). In my experience, pepsin pretreatment (2 mg/ml) for 20 to 30 minutes works well for tissues fixed for 8 hours to several days in that a hybridization signal is obtained and overdigestion of the tissues rarely occurs. Indeed, as discussed in detail in Chapter 6, tissues fixed in 10% buffered formalin for 8 to 72 hours can usually withstand 60 minutes of digestion in pepsin or trypsin (2 mg/ml) with good preservation of morphology. This is one reason I recommend relatively long fixation times. Another reason, much more apparent with RT *in situ* PCR, is that the window of optimal protease digestion for this technique is much larger with tissues fixed for 1 to 3 days than for tissues fixed for 4 to 8 hours.

Given the importance of this issue, a comparative study was done using tissues fixed in buffered formalin for 4 hours, 8 hours, 15

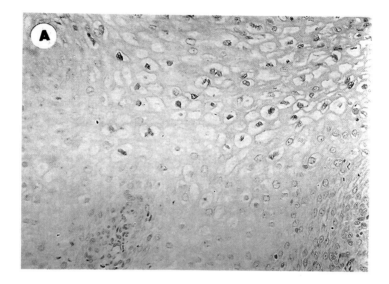

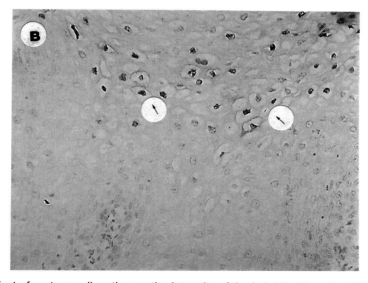

Figure 4-6. *Effect of protease digestion on the intensity of the hybridization signal.* With no protease pretreatment, a weak hybridization signal was evident in this low-grade cervical SIL, which contained HPV 6, using a biotin-labeled probe (**A**). A strong signal was evident in the serial section when the hybridization was preceded by treatment of the tissue in trypsin at 2 mg/ml for 30 minutes (**B**). (See also Figs. 4-8 to 4-11 for additional information on relationship of the hybridization signal with *in situ* hybridization and the protease digestion time.)

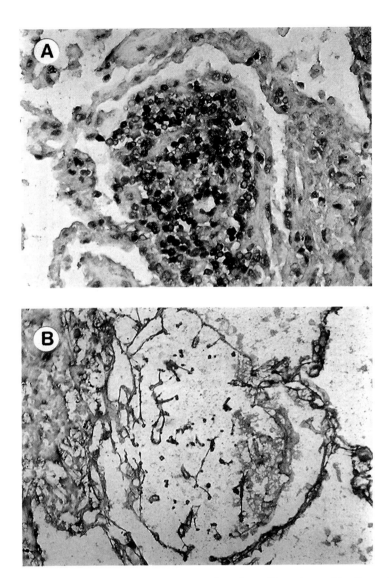

Figure 4-7. *Destruction of tissue morphology by overdigestion with protease.* The tissue is from a biopsy of lung. The tissues in **A** and **B** were fixed in Histochoice, which is an ethanol-based fixative. Note the strong signal with the repetitive *alu* probe with no protease digestion (**A**). If the tissue is digested in pepsin (2 mg/ml for 30 minutes), the signal is lost due to the destruction of the tissue (**B**). Note the loss of tissue morphology. The tissue in **C** was fixed in 10% buffered formalin. No signal was evident without protease digestion (not shown, but see Fig. 4-6). After 30 minutes protease digestion, a strong signal is evident with the *alu* probe (**C**). However, the tissue was overdigested after 90 minutes of protease digestion (not shown). Ethanol-fixed tissues are easily overdigested with protease. Formalin-fixed tissues are more resistant but can also be overdigested, especially if fixed for <4 hours.

hours, 24 hours, 48 hours, and 1 week. These were subjected to standard *in situ* hybridization using a biotin-labeled repetitive *alu* probe. The *alu* sequence is common in human DNA, comprising about 5% of the total cellular DNA in human tissues, and is adequate to produce a strong signal with standard *in situ* hybridization. Optimal protease digestion conditions would be evident as an intense hybridization signal in most cells using the *alu* probe. The

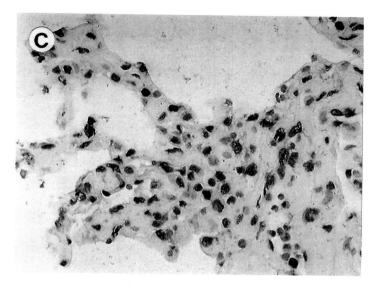

Figure 4-7. *Continued.*

data for these experiments are provided in Table 4-1. Representative photographs are provided in Figs. 4-8 through 4-11. Note the following important points:

1. For tissues fixed in buffered formalin, either no signal or only a weak signal is evident if the protease step is omitted before *in situ* hybridization.
2. The optimal protease digestion time is remarkably constant over a wide range of fixation times using 10% formalin. This is in marked contrast to the comparable results with *in situ* PCR, as discussed at length in Chapters 3 and 7.

3. For most tissues fixed in buffered formalin, 30 minutes of digestion in pepsin will produce an optimal signal with minimal chance of overdigestion as defined by poor morphology. The exception to this statement is tissue fixed for 1 to 4 hours.

Overdigestion in the protease solution will result not only in poor morphology but also a concomitant loss of the hybridization signal. Two common causes of overdigestion of tissues during *in situ* hybridization are (i) short-term (4 hours or less) fixation in 10% buffered formalin or fixation in low percent (2% to 4%) formalin or paraformaldehyde and (ii) diges-

Table 4-1. *The effect of protease digestion time on the signal with standard* in situ *as a function of the time of fixation in 10% buffered formalin*[a]

Fixation time	Protease digestion time (min)				
	0	**5**	**10**	**15**	**30**
4 Hours	1+[b]	1+	3+	3+	Overdigested
6 Hours	1+	1+	2+	3+	—
8 Hours	0	0	1+	3+	3+
16 Hours	0	0	1+	2+	3+
24 Hours	0	0	1+	2+	3+
48 Hours	0	0	1+	2+	3+
1 Week	0	0	0	1+	3+

[a]Pepsin was used at 2 mg/ml at 37°C. The probe was the biotin-labeled repetitive *alu* sequence.
[b]The signal was graded as 0, 1+ (1%–25% of the cells with a weak to moderate signal), 2+ (26%–50% of the cells with a moderate to strong signal), or 3+ (>50% of the cells with a moderate to strong signal).

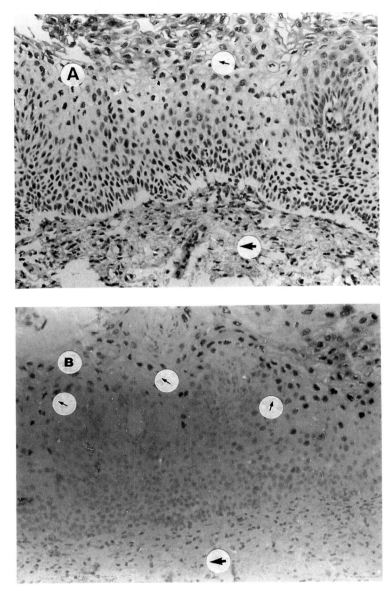

Figure 4-8. *Positive control for* in situ *hybridization.* A cervical biopsy specimen that contained a low-grade SIL positive for HPV 31 was hybridized with a biotin-labeled human DNA probe made from the repetitive *alu* sequence that constitutes about 5% of the DNA in the human genome. **A:** All cells had a detectable hybridization signal using this positive control probe for *in situ* hybridization. Such positive controls help to determine if variables such as protease time, hybridization conditions, and the detection steps are optimized. Note that the hybridization signal is present in both the epithelial cells (*small arrow*) and the stromal cells (*large arrow*). **B:** Compare this distribution with that obtained when the serial section was probed with a biotin-labeled HPV 31 probe. In this case, only the superficial squamous cells that show the crowding, halos, and nuclear atypia of an SIL demonstrate a hybridization signal (*small arrows*); the stromal cells (which HPV does not infect) are negative (*large arrow*).

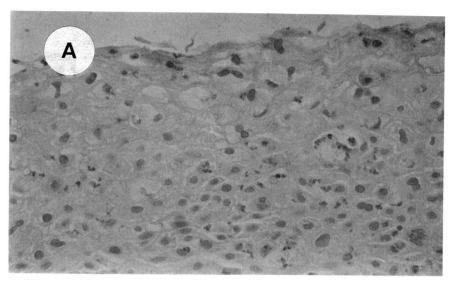

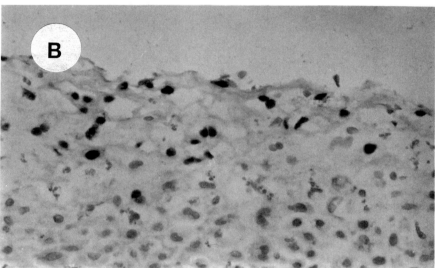

Figure 4-9. *Importance of adequate protease digestion on the hybridization signal with* in situ *hybridization.* This vulvar low-grade SIL was shown to contain HPV 11 DNA by Southern blot hybridization. However, no signal was evident after 12 minutes of protease digestion (pepsin, 2 mg/ml) using a genomic HPV 11 probe and *in situ* hybridization (**A**). However, a strong signal became evident if the protease digestion time was increased to 20 minutes (**B**). For the great majority of tissues fixed in 10% buffered formalin, the optimal protease digestion time using pepsin at 2 mg/ml will be between 20 and 35 minutes.

tion with proteinase K (1 mg/ml). Although proteinase K is an acceptable protease for *in situ* hybridization, overdigestion is more common than with pepsin or trypsin. Overdigestion can occur when proteinase K is used for PCR *in situ* hybridization, and I prefer to use pepsin or trypsin for *in situ* hybridization or RT *in situ*

PCR–PCR *in situ* hybridization. There have been various reports that one protease is superior to others. Indeed, we have noted that digestion in proteinase K sometimes gives a more intense hybridization signal than that with the serial section digested with trypsin (Fig. 4-12). This is not invariable, and I view the various

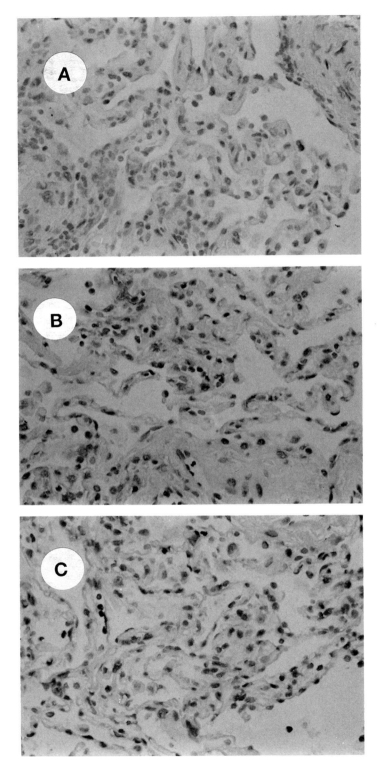

Figure 4-10. *Relationship of the signal with* in situ *hybridization and formalin fixation: short fixation times.* The tissue is a lung biopsy specimen fixed in 10% buffered formalin for 6 hours. Using the repetitive *alu* probe, a weak signal was evident after 10 minutes of protease digestion (**A**). The signal was optimal at 20 minutes of digestion (**B**); a similar signal intensity was evident after 30 minutes of protease digestion (**C**). Protease digestion times of >60 minutes destroyed the tissue morphology (not shown).

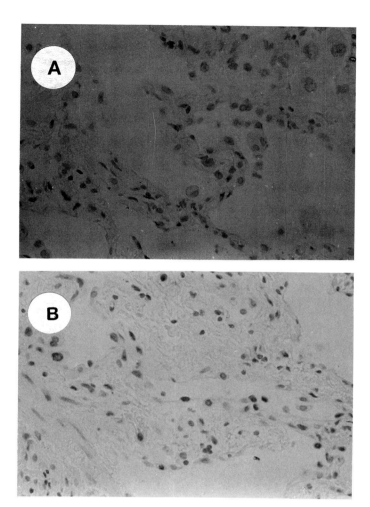

Figure 4-11. *Relationship of the signal with* in situ *hybridization and formalin fixation: long fixation times.* The tissue is a lung biopsy specimen from the same case shown in Fig. 4-10. However, this tissue was fixed in 10% buffered formalin for 15 hours. Using the repetitive *alu* probe, no signal was evident after 10 minutes of protease digestion (**A**). A weak signal became evident at 20 minutes of digestion (**B**). The signal became intense after 30 minutes of digestion (**C**), and the intensity remained strong after 40 minutes (**D**) and 50 to 60 minutes (**E**) of protease digestion. Tissues fixed for at least 15 hours typically are resistant to 1 hour of protease digestion.

protease treatments as equivalent. It is recommended that the investigator choose one of the protease treatments and use it extensively in order to become familiar with its nuances.

The specific type of tissue also can be a factor in protease overdigestion. Some tissues, such as kidney, lymph nodes, and placenta, seem to be more sensitive to protease than others, such as skin, skeletal muscle, and brain tissue.

The final topic in this section is the inactivation of the protease in the digestion solution. This is easily accomplished. One first inactivates the pepsin or trypsin by flooding the slide with a solution of 0.1 M Tris HCl (pH 7.4) and 0.1 M NaCl. If one prefers, the slides can be placed in a 50-ml Copeland jar, which contains this solution. Either method will dilute the pepsin, and any residual pepsin will be inactive at the increased pH. After 1 minute, pour off the Tris solution and flood the slides with 100% ethanol. After 1 minute, place the slides in a rack and dry at 37°C for 5 minutes.

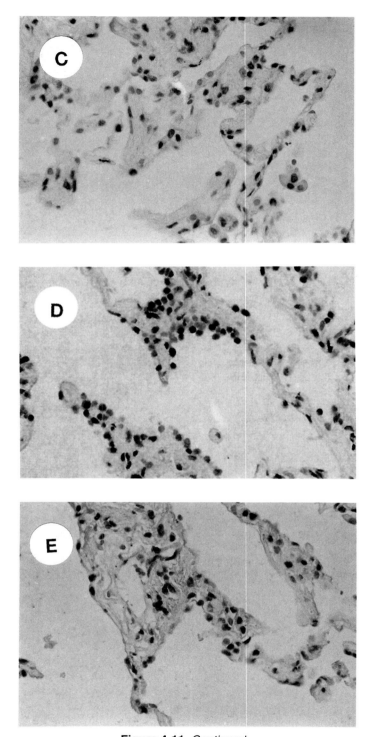

Figure 4-11. *Continued.*

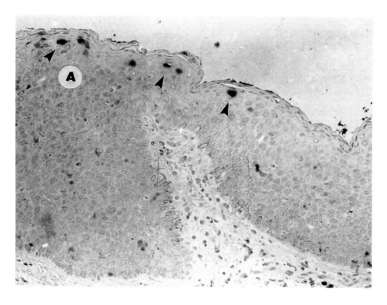

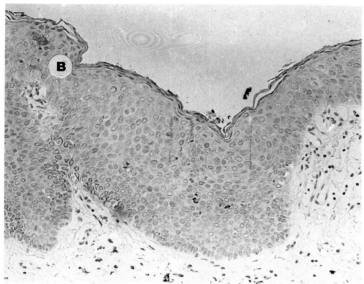

Figure 4-12. *Effects of different protease treatments on the* in situ *hybridization signal after prolonged fixation in 10% buffered formalin.* A stronger hybridization signal is evident in these serial sections of a cervical low-grade SIL when digestion was done with protease K at 1 mg/ml for 15 minutes (**A**, *arrowheads*) than with trypsin at 2 mg/ml for 15 minutes (**B**). The probe is biotin-labeled HPV 51 DNA. Although in this case a stronger signal was evident after proteinase K digestion, the two protease treatments are best viewed as equivalent. An enhanced signal with proteinase K digestion implies tissue that has been fixed for a long time (>1 day). Increasing the digestion time using pepsin or trypsin to 30 minutes should yield an equivalent signal. The signal became strong in this case if the trypsin digestion was increased to 30 minutes (see Fig. 4-9 for an equivalent result).

To summarize protese digestion:

1. Remove paraffin with 5 minutes in xylene, 5 minutes in 100% ETOH, then air dry.
2. Digest in pepsin solution at 37°C for 25 minutes (pepsin solution = 9.5 ml H_2O, 0.5 ml 2 NHCl, and 20 mg pepsin or trypsin); 1-ml aliquots of the pepsin can be stored at −20°C for 1 week and thawed when needed; use immediately after thawing).
3. Wash in 0.1 M Tris HCl and 0.1 M NaCl for 1 min, 100% ETOH, then air dry.
4. For human tissues, test adequacy of protease digestion with a positive control probe (e.g., repetitive *Alu* sequence).

Probe Synthesis

Full-length probes are usually synthesized by either random priming or nick translation. The basics of these two labeling systems are depicted in Figs. 4-13 and 4-14. I have found that each of these systems yields excellent results with full-length probes using DNA templates that range in size from several hundred to over 10,000 base pairs. Many excellent kits are commercially available and can easily be found in the catalogues of the companies specializing in molecular biology reagents (see Appendix). It is important to realize that neither random primers nor nick translation would yield adequately labeled or sized probes if used with oligonucleotides. The shortest DNA sequence that can be labeled with nick translation or random primers, in my experience, is about 100 base pairs. For smaller fragments I recommend that one use

the 3′ tailing kit, as is discussed below.

Two important concepts to discuss with regard to synthesizing probes from large DNA templates are the specific reporter molecule and the size of the resultant probe. The reporter molecule is the labeled nucleotide that one wishes to incorporate into the probe as it is synthesized. Although many different labels have been tested, this section deals with biotin and digoxigenin, two common nonisotopic reporter nucleotides, and the radioisotope-tagged nucleotides ^3H and ^{35}S. Table 4-2 summarizes the advantages and disadvantages of these systems. It is not my purpose to advocate one system over the others. The decision to use a system is dependent on several factors, such as prior experience, preference for color versus grains, and other individual needs and preferences. Indeed, as discussed in Chapter 7, it may be advantageous to use both a nonisotopic label and an isotope in order to label two different RNAs or DNAs in a given cell.

Several good studies have examined the relationship of the size of the probe and the quality of the signal achieved with *in situ* hybridization. These studies have suggested that for tissues fixed in either glutaraldehyde or paraformaldehyde that smaller (about 70 base pairs) probes gave the best results. Although this is valuable information, in my experience the importance of probe size can be minimized by changing the protease digestion time. This relates to the concept of probe entry, as discussed in detail in Chapter 3. Nonetheless, it is recommended that some of the synthesized probe be placed on a

Table 4-2. *Pros and cons of different reporter molecules used for* in situ *hybridization*

Label	Shelf life	Time[a]	Background	Other
Biotin	>5 Years	1 Day	Low-high[b]	Most common of commercial labels
Digoxigenin	>5 Years	1 Day	Low	Not present in tissues
^{35}S	90 Days	3–14 Days	Low to high	Background highly variable
^3H	12 Years	30–60 Days	Very low	Requires expensive emulsion (also ^{35}S)

[a]Time required for completion of *in situ* hybridization testing.
[b]Tissues such as liver and kidney can have high levels of endogenous biotin.

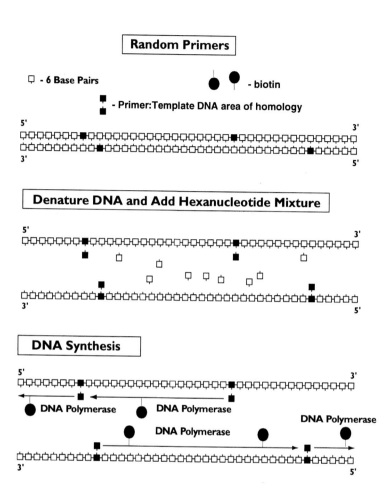

Figure 4-13. *Different labeling strategies for making large (>100 base pair) DNA probes: random primers.* In this technique, the DNA is denatured after which a large number of distinct hexanucleotide primers are added with the dNTPs (one is typically labeled, e.g., with biotin) and DNA polymerase. In a process analogous to the first cycle of PCR, the primers bind to regions of sufficient homology and dictate the synthesis of DNA sequences that will incorporate the labeled nucleotide. Note that many of the hexanucleotides do not find a matching region. The use of a large number of hexanucleotides increases the probability that some will find regions of sufficient homology to initiate DNA synthesis.

Southern blot transfer (see Chapter 2 for relevant protocols). By detecting the reporter molecule, the size of the probe can be determined, and the degree of incorporation can be semiquantitated.

When making probes by random primers or nick translation, I recommend labeling 100 to 500 ng of template DNA. For biotin or digoxigenin labeled probes I recommend the following purification protocol.

Protocol 4-2: Purification of Probes

1. After synthesis, add 2 μl of 0.5 M EDTA to stop reaction.
2. Increase reaction volume to 200 μl.
3. Add 25 μl of 3 M sodium acetate.
4. Add 900 μl of 100% ethanol stored at 20°C.
5. Vortex very well, then store at –70°C for 30 minutes or at –20°C for 2 to 15 hours.

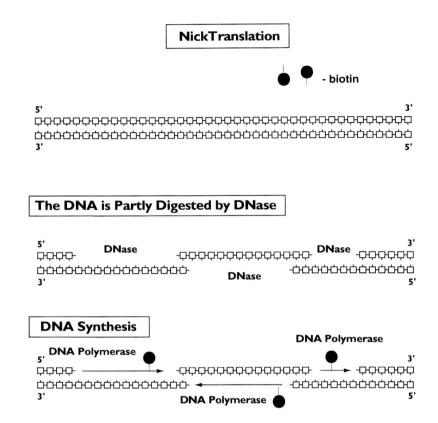

Figure 4-14. *Different labeling strategies for making DNA probes: nick translation.* In this technique, the controlled activity of DNase creates areas where the double-stranded DNA becomes single-stranded. These areas serve as initiation points of DNA synthesis by DNA polymerase in which labeled nucleotides may be incorporated. Note that neither primers nor denaturation is needed for this technique. Furthermore, note the similarity of nick translation with the primer-independent DNA repair mechanism that is postulated to be operative during *in situ* PCR when using paraffin-embedded, formalin-fixed tissue (see Fig. 3-5).

6. Centrifuge at 15,000 rpm for 15 minutes.
7. Decant ethanol, dry, and resuspend pellet in 25 μl using sterile water.
8. Store at 4°C.

To summarize probe synthesis:

1. Label from 100 to 500 ng of template DNA.
2. Purify with ethanol precipitation; then resuspend in 25 μl sterile water.
3. Check size and incorporation with Southern transfer.

Brief mention should be made of the large number of probes that can now be purchased commercially. Probes to most DNA viruses, many RNA viruses, and a very large number of human genes, especially oncogenes, are readily available with a variety of radioactive and nonradioactive labels (see Appendix).

Probe Cocktail and Hybridization

The *in situ* hybridization protocol is summarized in Protocol 4-3:

Protocol 4-3. The Protocol for *in situ* Hybridization

Tissue preparation

1. Place several 4-μm paraffin-embedded sections on a silane-coated glass slide.
2. Wash slides in xylene for 5 minutes.
3. Wash slides in 100% ethanol for 5 minutes.
4. Add 100 μl of protease (pepsin, 2 mg/ml in 0.01N HCl) to tissue section for 30 minutes at room temperature.
5. Inactivate protease by washing in 0.1 M Tris (pH 7.5) and 0.1 M NaCl for 1 minute, wash in 100% ethanol for 1 minute, and air dry.

Probe cocktail (add together the following ingredients)

1. 50 μl deionized formamide
2. 30 μl 25% dextran sulfate
3. 10 μl 20 × SCC
4. 10 μl of the probe (stock solution of 1 to 10 μg/ml)

Note that for oligoprobes decrease formamide to 10 μl and add 40 μl of water.

Denaturing of probe and target DNA

1. Vortex probe cocktail.
2. Add 5 to 10 μl of the probe to a given tissue section.
3. Overlay with plastic coverslip cut slightly larger than tissue section.
4. Place slide on hot plate, 95° to 100°C, for 5 minutes.
5. Remove bubbles over tissue gently with a toothpick.

Hybridization and washing

1. Place slides in humidity chamber at 37°C for 2 hours.
2. Remove coverslips (hold down one end with fingernail and lift off cover slip with toothpick).
3. Wash slides in a solution of 0.2% bovine serum albumin and 0.2 × SSC at 60°C for

10 minutes (reduce temperature to 45°C and increase salt to 1 × SSC for oligoprobe).
4. Wipe off excess wash solution, mark outer part of slide with hydrophobic pen, and place slide in humidity chamber. *Do not let slides dry out.*

Detection

1. For biotin system, add 100 μl streptavidin–alkaline phosphatase conjugate to each tissue section in humidity chamber.
2. Incubate for 20 minutes at 37°C.
3. Wash slides at room temperature for 3 minutes in a solution of 0.1 M Tris HCl (pH 9 to 9.5) and 0.1 M NaCl (detection solution).
4. Place slides in detection reagent solution to which NBT/BCIP has been added (with Digene kit, add 50 μl of each to 20 ml detection solution).
5. Incubate slides for 30 minutes to 1 hour, checking results periodically under microscope.

Counterstain and Coverslip

1. Wash slides for 1 minute in distilled water.
2. Counterstain for 5 minutes in nuclear fast red solution.
3. Wash slides twice, for 1 minute each time, in distilled water.
4. Wash slides for 1 minute in 100% ethanol, and then place in xylene.
5. Cover slip using permount and glass coverslip; view under microscope.

Note that there are few components in the probe cocktail mixture. Several years ago most investigators (including ourselves) included many more reagents. As with so many methodologies, experience has shown which reagents are really needed and which may be excluded.

Briefly, the purpose of the components of the probe cocktail is to denature the target and probe DNA and proceed to hybridization under conditions that permit robust probe–target annealing but do not allow excessive probe–non-target hybridization. The function of the formamide and relatively low salt concentration is to facilitate denaturing of the probe and target DNA at 100°C, which is about 40°C above the Tm of homologous hybridized DNA (see discussion in Chapter 2). During the hybridization step, the relatively high formamide and low salt concentration should disfavor the nonspecific binding of the probe with cellular proteins and nucleic acids while not interfering with probe–target binding, assuming a hybridization temperature of 37°C. Because RNA–RNA hybrids have relatively higher Tms than DNA–DNA hybrids, I increase the hybridization temperature to 50°C when doing RNA–RNA *in situ* hybridization. I also heat the probe and target RNA prior to hybridization at 75°C for 10 minutes to eliminate any secondary structure in the RNA molecules. Dextran sulfate is commonly used to increase the effective concentration of the probe. Bromely et al. (25) have done extensive work correlating the concentration of the probe and the intensity of the hybridization signal under a wide variety of conditions. As noted in Protocol 4-3, the probe concentration is listed as 0.1 to 1 μg/ml. This amount is rarely associated with background problems for the non-isotopic-labeled probes. However, if background is a problem, the concentration of the probe may be decreased tenfold with minimal sacrifice of the hybridization signal (see section on troubleshooting, below) (25). It should be emphasized that the relationship of the concentration of the probe to background is far more critical with the smaller oligoprobes. As discussed below, this is related to the much smaller size (15 to 40 base pair) of the oligoprobes relative to the larger (100 to 250 base pair) probes made from full-length clones of DNA or cDNA.

I strongly suggest placing three tissue sections on each silane-coated glass slide. This arrangement is advantageous, because three separate hybridization reactions can be done on serial tissue sections. Not only is this a more efficient process, it allows one to do comparative analyses on the same area or often the same cells present in a serial section. For example, one can use one section to analyze the tissue for HPV DNA and the other two sections as the positive and negative controls by using the labeled *alu* probe and the plasmid probe, respectively. Another example would be determining the optimal protease digestion by using the *alu* probe and digesting the three tissue samples for various times (Fig. 4-15). To facilitate placing three different probe cocktails on one glass slide, polypropylene coverslips cut to size can be used. I purchase these as autoclavable polypropylene bags from Fisher Scientific. The sheets can be cut into sizes of 3 to 4 cm and autoclaved. A sterile needle can be used to separate the two sides of the plastic bag after autoclaving, and then smaller coverslips, usually from 3 to 8 mm, can be cut for individual sections. For RNA work, use just the inner part of the bag, as this would not have been exposed to handling. An aliquot of only about 5 μl of the probe cocktail is needed for small biopsy specimens of 2 to 5 μm. During the denaturing step, small bubbles may form under the coverslip. To minimize these bubbles, either decrease the size of the coverslip or increase the amount of the probe cocktail. Because these bubbles may cause small areas of false-positive signal (Figs. 4-16), it is recommended that one gently remove them after the denaturing step by pushing them with a toothpick to the edge of the coverslip.

The final issue is the length of the hybridization time. Initially, overnight hybridizations were the rule. However, a shorter time (2 hours) gave similar results and allowed one to complete the entire assay in 1 day. We performed a series of experiments to correlate the strength of the hybridization signal with the time of hybridization from 0 to 120 minutes. These data are presented in Table 4-3.

It is evident that hybridization times of 15–30 minutes are not adequate for *in situ* hybridization, especially for targets of low copy number. This is interesting in light of the discussion in Chapter 3 (Figs. 3-19 and 3-20) about the relationship of the protease digestion time and signal with *in situ* hybridization versus *in situ* PCR. The data just presented add

Table 4-3. *The relationship of the hybridization time to the intensity of the signal with standard* in situ *hybridization*

Hybridization time	Intensity of signal[a]
2 Hr at 37°C	Intense
1 Hr at 37°C	Moderate
30 Min at 37°C	Moderate
30 Min at 67°C	Weak
15 Min at 37°C	Weak

[a]Intensity of signal reflects both the number of positive cells and the intensity of the colorimetric reactions. These results were obtained with a repetitive *alu* probe and an HPV-6-specific probe; the tissue was a vulvar wart that contained HPV 6 at about 100 to 200 copies per infected cell.

additional weight to the argument that reagent diffusion is not the key variable in understanding the relationship between protease digestion and formalin fixation times with *in situ* PCR. The rationale is that 15 minutes is certainly ample time to wash nonspecifically bound probe out of the cell with a high stringency wash. The need for 2 hours of hybridization must reflex some other phenomenon, perhaps the time course of the equilibrium of probe–target annealing.

To summarize the hybridization steps:

1. Add 5 to 10 μl of the probe cocktail (50 μl of formamide + 30 μl 25% dextran sulfate + 10 μl of 20 × SSC + 10 μl of probe [stock solution of 1 to 10 μg per ml]) to each tissue section.
2. Cover with polypropylene coverslip cut to size.
3. Perform two to three reactions per slide.
4. Heat to 95° to 100°C for 5 minutes.
5. Place slides in humidity chamber at 37°C for 2 hours.

Posthybridization Wash

After the hybridization step, one has probe DNA that is hybridized to the target as well as to nontarget molecules such as DNA, RNA, and proteins. First, the coverslip is removed, and then the tissue sections are washed to remove the nonspecific bound probe. To remove the coverslips, one can hold the edge of the coverslip and remove it with a toothpick.

Due to the background problems inherent with ^{35}S-labeled probes and, to a lesser extent, probes labeled with ^{3}H, the posthybridization wash is a key step when radioactive probes are used. Probe that had nonspecifically bound to cellular membranes and nucleic acids could easily produce enough background to render the slide not interpretable after typical exposure times. Obscuring background is much less of a problem when using the most common nonisotopic systems—biotin and digoxigenin. Hence, the washing step with its function of removing the probe that is bound to molecules other than the target is much simplified. The concept is straightforward: Reaction conditions foster disruption of the weaker and fewer hydrogen bonds between the probe and nontarget molecules without sacrificing the target-specific hybridization signal by keeping the Tm below that of the probe–target complex. The conditions of the posthybridization wash are listed in Protocol 4-3, above. Note that low salt and relatively high temperatures are used rather than other agents such as the relatively expensive formamide.

The wash conditions listed in Protocol 4-3 are for the larger probes generated from DNA templates that are >200 base pairs. One important difference between oligoprobes and these full-length probes is that the latter usually produce a more intense hybridization signal due to the greater number of labeled nucleotides that can be incorporated into them

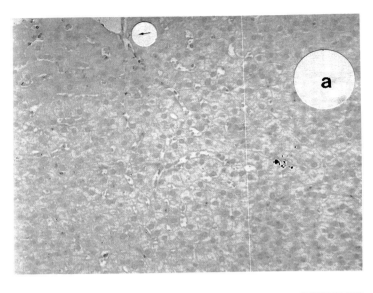

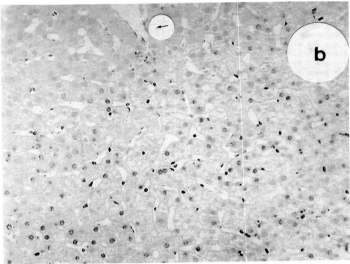

Figure 4-15. *Performing multiple hybridizations on the same glass slide using polypropylene cover-slips.* By using plastic coverslips (Fisher Scientific, autoclavable polypropylene bags) cut to size, one can do multiple separate hybridization reactions by placing many serial sections on the same silane-coated glass slide. This time- and reagent-saving step allows one to demonstrate on one slide what the optimal protease digestion time was for this liver tissue fixed with 10% buffered formalin for >24 hours. Note that no signal was evident with no protease digestion (**a**), a weak signal was evident after 20 minutes of digestion (**b**), and an intense signal was noted after 30 minutes of digestion (**c**). These are serial sections separated by only 4 μm. Thus, one can do comparative analyses on the same cells; the *arrows* mark a blood vessel evident in each section as a "landmark" of the region that is being photographed. These data reinforce the statement that 30 minutes of digestion in pepsin or trypsin (2 mg/ml) is adequate for most tissues. This scheme of doing multiple reactions on a glass slide is also graphically depicted in (**d**).

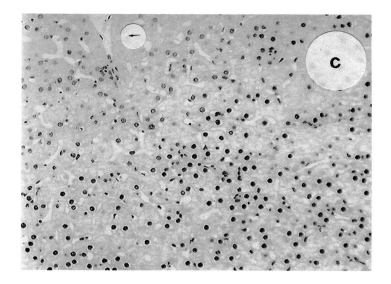

**In situ hybridization - multiple hybridizations on
the same silane coated glass slide**

1. Place several sections on one slide

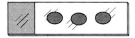

**2. Add probe cocktail, cover with polypropylene
coverslips cut to size**

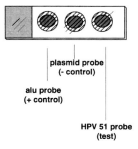

plasmid probe
(- control)

alu probe
(+ control)

HPV 51 probe
(test)

d

Figure 4-15. *Continued.*

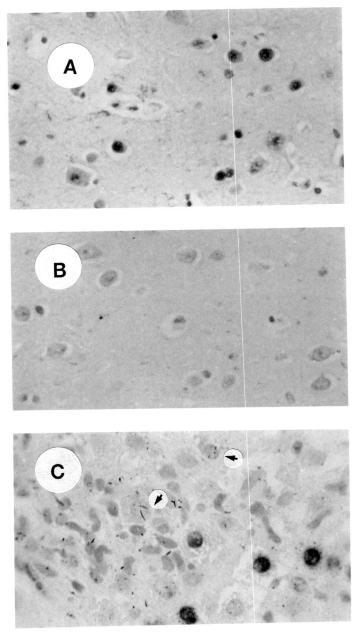

Figure 4-16. In situ *hybridization artifacts.* One artifact that may be evident with *in situ* hybridization is due to bubbles that form over the tissue during the denaturing step. The probe may precipitate over this area and produce a nonspecific signal (**A**). Note that many diverse cells in this brain tissue show a signal with an HIV-1-specific probe; the tissue was from a patient who did not have AIDS. This problem can be eliminated by removing these bubbles after the denaturing step (**B**). Another problem that may be encountered is the precipitation of the crystals of NBT/BCIP. These may be rod shaped or round. When over nuclei, they can be incorrectly interpreted as signal (**C**, *arrows*). This problem can usually be corrected by heating the buffer to which the chromogen is added or decreasing the concentration of the chromogen.

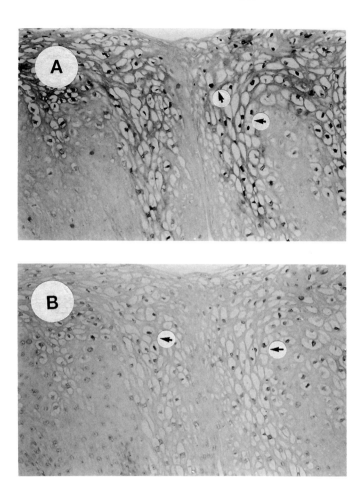

Figure 4-17. *The disparity in the sensitivities and specificities of "full-length" probes versus oligoprobes in standard* in situ *hybridization.* This cervical biopsy specimen contained HPV 6 DNA. Note the intense signal when a series of 150 to 200 base pair HPV 6 probes made from a 600 base pair region by the random primers method is used under low-stringency conditions (**A,** arrows mark area of positive cells). The signal is much weaker if the serial section is analyzed with a series of seven oligoprobes (each 20 base pairs long) specific for an equivalent region of HPV 6 (**B**). The intense signal was maintained if the tissue depicted in A was washed under high-stringency conditions but was lost for the corresponding tissue treated with the oligoprobe (not shown).

relative to an oligoprobe and their greater size, which translates to a greater Tm for the probe–target complex. (Fig. 4-17; see Chapter 5 for additional discussion). Also, at low stringency conditions oligoprobes tend to produce more background than full-length probes (Fig. 4-18). Another difference between the oligoprobe and larger full-length probe relates to the actual conditions of the posthybridization wash. Because the full-length probes are much larger, the difference in the Tms between the probe–target hybridization and the probe–nontarget "stickiness" is *much* greater than the disparity between the signal and background noise for an oligoprobe (see Fig. 5-15). The practical implication is that, when full-length probes are used, it is easy to achieve a temperature for the posthybridiza-

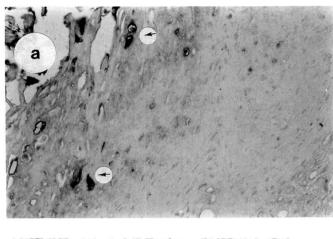

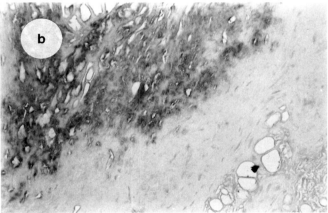

Figure 4-18. *Disparity of signal-to-background ratio between oligoprobes and full-length probes in standard* in situ *hybridization.* The tissue is from a finger cancer that contained HPV 16. At low stringency (42°C, 2 × SSC 10 min), a signal with minimal background is noted with the full-length (nick translation, 8,000 base pair template) probe (**a**, *arrows*). However, high background but minimal signal is evident with the oligoprobe (six 20 base pair probes) tested on a serial section (**b**). At high stringency (68°C, 0.2 × SSC 10 min), the strong signal persisted with the full-length probe (**c**). The background was lost with the oligoprobe at high stringency, but no signal was evident (**d**); the dark material at the surface of the tissue is ink.

tion wash at which the specific signal persists and the background signal is lost. However, these conditions could easily be too stringent for the oligoprobe (Figs. 4-17 and 4-18). One must reduce the stringency until one reaches the narrow window above the Tm of the background hybridization yet below the Tm for the oligoprobe–target annealing. Thus, Protocol 4-3 lists separately the posthybridization wash conditions for oligoprobes. This topic is discussed in much greater detail in Chapter 5, which deals with PCR *in situ* hy-

bridization, for two reasons: (i) oligoprobes are an important part on PCR *in situ* hybridization, and (ii) it is not recommended that one use oligoprobes for standard *in situ* hybridization because they are associated with a smaller signal-to-background ratio than the larger full-length probes. In PCR *in situ* hybridization the amplification step greatly increases the signal-to-background ratio with the oligoprobe.

To summarize the posthybridization wash (for full length-probes):

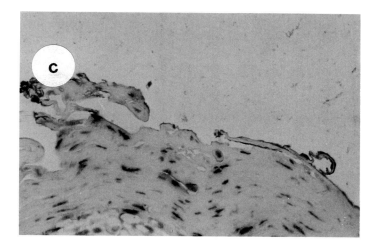

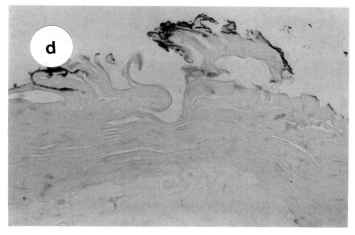

Figure 4-18. *Continued.*

1. Remove the coverslip.
2. Place the slides in 0.2 × SSC with 0.2% bovine serum albumin at 60°C for 10 to 15 minutes.
3. Remove the slides. Avoiding the tissue section, wipe off the excess wash solution from the slide with a Kleenex, and circle the tissue sections with a hydrophobic pen. Do not let the tissue section dry out.
4. Add alkaline phosphatase conjugate.

Detection System

After the posthybridization wash one is left with a complex of target and probe containing labeled nucleotides. Although this section deals only with biotin- and digoxigenin-labeled nucleotides, as noted above, many other labeling systems have been studied. It has been my experience, and apparently the experience of many others, that ^{35}S–, ^3H–, or ^{32}P-labeled probes offer no large advantage over these nonradioactive systems, especially with regard to sensitivity. The reader is referred to the literature for more specific information on radioactive detection systems, nonisotopic systems that are not based on biotin or digoxigenin, and other investigators' protocols for biotin (26–45).

The key component of the biotin and digoxigenin systems is the enzyme alkaline phosphatase, which will be attached to the probe–target complex. For biotin this is readily accomplished with a streptavidin–alkaline phosphatase conjugate. An advantage of this system is that any immunohistochemistry laboratory will have extensive experience with such conjugates and thus be familiar with the nuances of its use. For the digoxigenin system, one employs an antibody against digoxigenin that can be conjugated to the alkaline phosphatase.

Many commercial kits are available for the detection of biotin. Recently, several companies have introduced to the market so called amplified detection systems for biotin. These are based on a molecule that binds to biotin and contains additional biotin sites that can thus increase the numbers of streptavidin and, ultimately, alkaline phosphatase per probe–target complex. The net effect is that each original biotin site on the probe–target complex is replaced by as many as five biotin sites, which, theoretically, increases the number of alkaline phosphatase molecules— whose activity actually produces the signal five-fold. I have tested two such systems that were developed by Enzo and Biogene. In my experience, these are excellent systems that offer a definite although relatively minor increase in sensitivity over other alkaline phosphatase based biotin detection systems. I have noticed an increased background with these "amplified" systems that is easily controlled by reducing the developing time in the chromogen.

When using the digoxigenin system, I recommend that one dilute the antidigoxigenin antibody at 1:150 in the Buffer 1 of the Boehringer Mannheim kit (0.1 M Tris HCl [pH 7.5] and 0.1 M NaCl).

For either the biotin or digoxigenin system, add 50 to 100 μl of the detection reagent to the slide. Incubate at 37°C for 20 to 30 minutes in a humidity chamber. Make certain that the incubator is level so the detection reagent does not gravitate to one side and dry out over some of the tissue section(s).

A wide variety of chromogens are available to localize the probe–target complex. These different chromogens allow one to select a blue, red, or yellow precipitate (other colors are becoming available) that is either water soluble or insoluble. Chromogens that fluoresce due to the activity of alkaline phosphatase are also available, as are ones that yield dark black grains due to gold- or silver-containing complexes. A commonly used chromogen is 5-bromo-4-chloro-3-indolylphosphate in the presence of nitroblue tetrazolium (NBT/BCIP), which yields a blue precipitate.

The choice of counterstain depends largely on the chromogen used. For NBT/BCIP we prefer a pale pink nuclear counterstain called nuclear fast red. For a red precipitate such as new fuschin (DAKOPATTS), a 1% hematoxylin counterstain may be used. A comparison of these two colorimetric schemes is shown in Color Plate 1.

A brief comment is in order concerning another detection system. Horseradish peroxidase systems are often used in immunohistochemistry. In a direct comparative study between a ^{35}S system and two nonradioactive systems (one using alkaline phosphatase and the other horseradish peroxidase), it was shown that the ^{35}S system and alkaline phosphatase systems were equivalent, and both were much superior to horseradish peroxidase (**6**). Whether improvements will be made for systems based on horseradish peroxidase remains to be seen.

To summarize the detection step:

1. Add 50 to 100 μl of the alkaline phosphatase conjugate to the tissue section.
2. Place at 37°C for 20 to 30 minutes in a humidity chamber.
3. Wash slides at 37°C in a solution that contains 0.1 M Tris HCl (pH 9.5) and 0.1 M NaCl for 1 to 3 minutes.
4. Add NBT/BCIP chromogen for 30 to 60 minutes.
5. Check results periodically under a microscope.
6. Counterstain with nuclear fast red for 2 to 5 minutes; wash in water, 100% ethanol, then xylene.
7. Cover slip with permount.

Troubleshooting

The most common problem encountered with the use of nonradioactive detection systems is excessive background. Background may be defined as the presence of a staining reaction with a specific probe in areas of the tissue where the signal should not be present (for example, in normal endocervical cells or in basal cells with a probe for HPV) or, more commonly, in parts of the cell (i.e., cytoplasm) where the target should not be present. A common definition of background would be a staining reaction when the labeled plasmid vector is employed (the plasmid is the vehicle used to clone the probe of interest). In my experience, the most reliable measure of background is to use the probe (not the plasmid control) with a tissue similar to that being studied that does not have the target of interest, as determined by solution phase PCR. Although the plasmid control may provide useful information, especially for probes derived from plasmid-containing clones, probes may differ widely in their propensity for background noise, and the most reliable measure of background is to use the probe itself on a proven nontarget tissue.

Background is the result of nonspecific binding of the probe to nontarget molecules. Two simple and logical ways to deal with background are to decrease the concentration of the probe and/or to increase the stringency of the posthybridization wash. The result of doing the latter is depicted in Fig.4-19. If background is a problem with a full-length probe, try decreasing the probe concentration by tenfold. If the problem persists, increase the temperature of the wash to 65°C and increase the wash time to 20 minutes. Methods for dealing with background when using oligoprobes are presented below. Background may also relate to the purity and concentration of the probe. This is illustrated in Fig. 4-20. Although repurifying the probe can solve this problem, simply diluting it by a factor of 1:10 to 1:50 is often sufficient to remove the background and still retain the target-specific signal.

Background can also relate to the purity of the chromogen. This is particularly important with NBT/BCIP (see Fig. 6-15). Of the various products I have tested, the NBT/BCIP from Digene Diagnostics has been the most problem free with regard to background staining. The chemicals in NBT/BCIP may form small crystal-like precipitates (Fig. 4-16). When these precipitates appear round and are located over a cell, they may mimic a signal. This problem can be avoided by heating the buffer to which the NBT/BCIP is added to 37°C before adding the chromogen. If the problem persists, try decreasing the amount of NBT/BCIP that is added to the substrate buffer.

Another potential problem that may hinder interpretation of test results is poor tissue morphology. For formalin-fixed tissues, loss of morphology is due to overtreatment with the protease solution (Fig. 4-7). Decreasing the time of protease digestion or decreasing the protease concentration tenfold will solve this problem.

Occasionally tissue sections may fall off the slide. If the rate of loss is greater than 5% of the tissue sections, the problem rests with incorrect silanization of the slides. Make sure silane-coated slides were used. If slide preparation appears to be the source of the problem, then carefully repeat the protocol (Protocol 4-1) for silanization. Silane-treated slides are now commercially available (e.g., ONCOR, Gaithersburg, MD). The other reason for tissue sections to fall off is that water was trapped under the paraffin; baking the slides at 60°C for 1 hour should prevent this. Finally, very hard or dry tissue sections embedded in paraffin may come off even with silane-coated slides. A good histotechnologist will quickly recognize this problem and may be able to solve it by re-embedding the tissue.

The most obvious potential problem encountered when using *in situ* hybridization is the absence of a hybridization signal. In this author's experience with testing for the presence of HPV, a common finding when asked to review HPV-negative *in situ* hybridization results that "should be HPV positive" is that the tissue was incorrectly diagnosed as condyloma/squamous intraepithelial lesion and, thus, *should* be HPV negative by *in situ* hybridization (this is discussed in detail in Chapter 8). A flow chart type of protocol for dealing with a negative hybridization signal with a full-length probe is provided in Fig. 4-21. Note that the foundation of this flow chart is

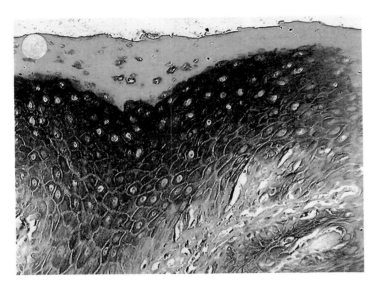

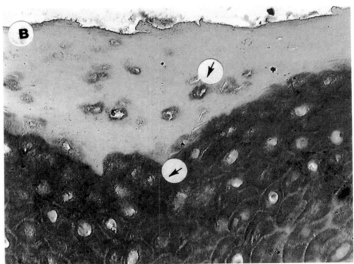

Figure 4-19. *Background versus signal with* in situ *hybridization: the importance of the posthybridization wash and localization.* The tissue is a vulvar lesion negative for HPV. Note the large amount of background evident with the HPV 6/11 probe (**A**) if the posthybridization wash was done for 5 minutes at 20°C in a solution with 1.5M NaCl (very low stringency). Also note that the background localized to the cytoplasm (at higher magnification, **B**), reflecting nonspecific binding of the probe to cellular proteins. However, HPV DNA typically localizes to the nucleus. Furthermore, the cells that appear positive lack the cytological changes of HPV infection. Thus, a knowledge of the expected localization of the signal helps to identify this as background. The background was eradicated if the posthybridization wash was 15 minutes at 60°C in a solution that contained 15 mM NaCl (high stringency, **C**). Note the nuclear signal and lack of cytoplasmic staining in this cervical SIL that contained HPV when analyzed with a biotin-labeled probe of HPV 51 after a high-stringency wash (**D**).

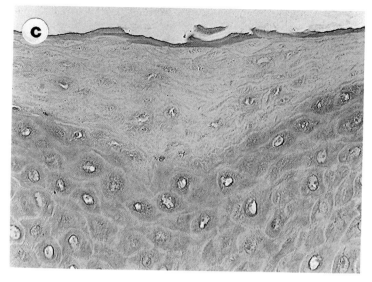

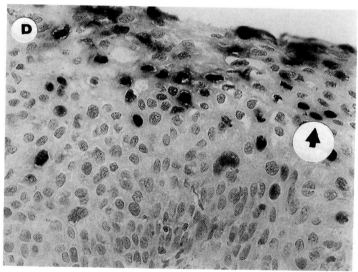

Figure 4-19. *Continued.*

the use of the positive control probe. Again, it is strongly recommended that one employ the positive control probe on each tissue tested by placing multiple sections on a glass slide. Although each factor listed can be responsible for a false-negative result, in my experience the most common causes are *inadequate protease digestion* (including omitting the protease step or using an inactive protease) and an *inactive alkaline phosphatase conjugate.*

OLIGOPROBE: DEFINITION AND PREPARATION

As discussed in Chapter 2, an oligoprobe is a labeled short segment of single-stranded DNA. Its function is to detect the complementary target-specific DNA or RNA. For PCR *in situ* hybridization the probe is designed to detect the amplified product. As is evident from Fig. 5-11, the probe corresponds to a region of

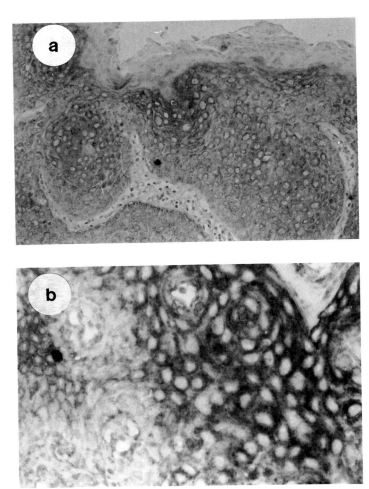

Figure 4-20. *Background versus signal with* in situ *hybridization: the importance of the purity and concentration of the probe.* The lesion is a low-grade cervical SIL that contains HPV 51. Note the high background at very low stringency (300 mM NaCl at 25°C) with the HPV 6/11 probe (**a**). The cytoplasmic localization of the background is evident at higher magnification (**b**). The background is not evident under the same conditions if the HPV 51 probe is used (**c**); note the hybridization signal that is present in some cells (*arrows*). Different probes may vary greatly in the amount of background they can cause, especially under low-stringency conditions. The background with the HPV 6/11 probe was greatly reduced when the concentration of the probe was diluted 1:10. This is evident in another lesion that did contain HPV 6 (**d**); note the target specific signal evident in some nuclei (*arrow*) and that the cytoplasmic background was lost. A logical strategy for high background with full-length probes is to increase the stringency of the posthybridization wash and reduce the concentration of the probe by 1:10 if the probe concentration is >50 ng/ml.

the amplified product internal to the two primers. In this way, the oligoprobe cannot detect primer oligomerization, which is one of the three competing, nonspecific pathways in PCR (see Chapter 3). Also note that, unlike a full-length double-stranded probe, the oligoprobe will detect only one of the two amplified strands.

There are many ways to label an oligoprobe. This discussion will focus on the addition of digoxigenin dUTP to the oligoprobe. The protocols are similar for adding other reporter mol-

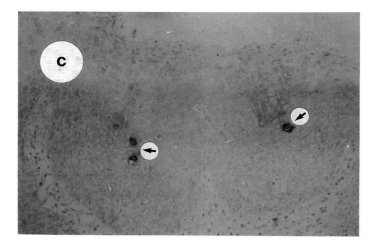

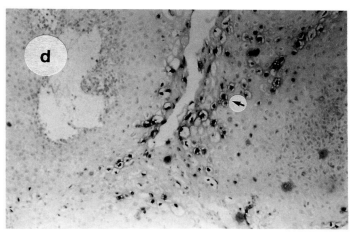

Figure 4-20. *Continued.*

ecules such as ^{3}H, ^{35}S, or biotin, for example. The three common ways to add digoxigenin dUTP to the oligoprobe are (i) random primers; (ii) 3′ end labeling; and (iii) 3′ tailing.

The random primers method is described above (see Fig. 4-13). The key aspect of this method is the use of multiple hexanucleotides. By using many of these hexanucleotide primers, one increases the probability that several will have sufficient homology to the oligoprobe as well as a 3′ match to direct the synthesis of a DNA segment complementary to the probe. As the complementary DNA fragments are being synthesized, about 1 digoxigenin dUTP is added for every 20-nucleotide sequence that is syn-

thesized. There are, however, several drawbacks to the random primer approach. First, the DNA segments made are often much smaller than the oligoprobe that serves as the template for DNA synthesis. As the probe size decreases, the risk of denaturation of the probe–target complex increases. Or, to express it in terms of the Tm, the decrease in probe size is associated with a corresponding decrease in the Tm; a 5 base pair decrease in size decreases the Tm by 8°C for a 20 base pair probe (called 20mer). The second problem relates to the number of digoxigenin dUTP nucleotides that can be added to the probe made from the random primers. If the probe is less than 20 base pairs or the DNA

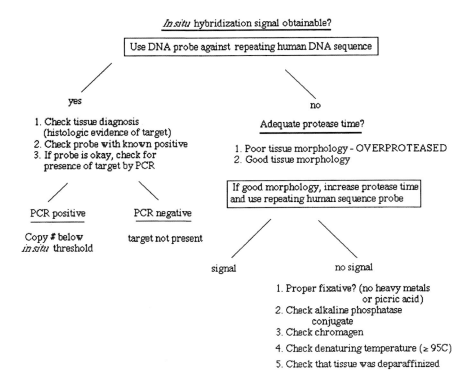

Figure 4-21. *Flow chart for a negative result with* in situ *hybridization.* A step-by-step approach to follow if a hybridization signal is not evident after *in situ* analysis. Note the importance of the positive control (the repetitive *alu* sequence) in this flow-chart analysis. See Figs. 4-10 and 4-11 for examples of the importance of the *alu* probe for troubleshooting a negative *in situ* hybridization result.

template has no or few dTTPS, then it is possible that no digoxigenin will be included. Although this is very unlikely when one uses a full-length probe that is often greater than 1,000 base pairs, it is highly possible when using a 20 to 40 nucleotide oligoprobe as the template for the random primers. Although random primers may allow for the synthesis of an effective probe when using large (>40 base pair) oligoprobes, I do not recommend their use. I have had much better success with oligoprobes labeled at the 3' end.

The 3' end labeling and tailing methods are discussed together. They are both based on the ability of the enzyme terminal transferase to add nucleotides to the 3' end of a DNA sequence. For the end labeling method, typically just one nucleotide that is labeled with the digoxigenin-dUTP is added. This can be done

with the use of a ddUTP-digoxigenin molecule. The dideoxy molecule will prevent the addition of other nucleotides, as there will be no carbon 3 OH group for the triphosphate group of a single nucleotide to complex with via a phosphodiester bond. For the tailing method, one adds a mixture of the unlabeled and dUTP-digoxigenin. Depending on the specific unlabeled nucleotides and the ratio of unlabeled to dUTP-digoxigenin, up to five dUTP-digoxigenin molecules per oligonucleotide can be added.

The advantage of the 3' tailing method is immediately apparent. Probes can be synthesized that have five times the amount of dUTP-digoxigenin as compared with the 3' end labeling method. However, the longer "tail" increases the possibility of nonspecific background relative to the 3' end labeling method. Boehringer Mannheim provides through their

Genius 3′ labeling kit the ability to generate oligoprobes that can be end labeled with ddUTP-digoxigenin or "tailed" with dUTP-digoxigenin. Thanks to the kind generosity of Dr. Brian Holaway at Boerhinger Mannheim, we were able to compare the sensitivities and specificities of the oligoprobes labeled by these two different methods. As these results are critical to successful PCR *in situ* hybridization, our findings are presented in Chapter 5. For the purposes of this discussion, the essential points are

1. One should use less formamide when preparing an oligoprobe cocktail mixture or risk losing the signal.
2. The background signal with oligoprobes is very much dependent on the method of generating the probe, the concentration of the probe, the length of time of hybridization and the conditions of the posthybridization wash. Specifically:
   a. The end labeling system for oligoprobes produces less background but less signal than the end tailing method. I do not recommend the end labeling method for oligoprobes.
   b. The signal and background are much more dependent on probe concentration for oligoprobes than when full-length probes are used.
   c. A hybridization time of 15 hours tends to produce high backgrounds with oligoprobes but not with full-length probes.
   d. The posthybridization wash, which eliminates background but preserves signal, is much different for an oligoprobe than for a full-length probe. Specifically,

Stringency 1	Stringency 2	Stringency 3
2 × SSC	1 × SSC	0.2 × SSC
0.2% BSA	0.2% BSA	0.2% BSA
45°C	54°C	54°C
10 minutes	10 minutes	10 minutes.

As shown in Figs. 5-12 to 5-14 and 5-17, nonspecific staining is evident in the testicular tissue with stringency 1 but not with the conditions listed in stringency 2 or 3. The target-specific signal is evident under the conditions in stringency 2 but is lost with stringency 3. Clearly, stringency 2 allows for the proper balance between the target-specific signal and background. Or, to be more specific, the conditions listed as stringency 2 provide for a temperature that is above the Tm of the nonspecific binding of the probe to cellular elements but below the Tm of the oligoprobe–HIV-1 specific PCR product. However, a signal would still be evident with a full-length probe after a posthybridization wash in stringency 3. To determine if a given probe concentration and stringent wash allows for a robust signal with no background with an oligoprobe, I routinely choose a tissue sample that is known to contain the target and another tissue sample known not to have the target. If a signal is noted in the tissue that does not contain the target, I recommend a decrease in the concentration of the probe by one-half until the background signal is no longer evident. If there is no background signal and the target-specific signal is weak, double the probe concentration and re-do the experiments.

Before we leave this area of the target-specific signal versus the background when using oligoprobes for PCR *in situ* hybridization, there is one more important point to stress. The tissue section that contains cells with a target of interest *will also have cells that do not contain the target that can serve as internal negative controls.* For example, in the testes tissue experiments described above, when the spermatogonia are positive for HIV-1 and the Sertoli cells and Leydig cells are also positive, there is an unacceptable level of background. To make such analyses, the cell type expected to have the target of interest must be known as well as the cell types that will not contain the target. However, one should suspect a background signal when a variety of cell types are positive after PCR *in situ* hybridization.

REAGENTS FOR *IN SITU* HYBRIDIZATION

For those who have worked little with *in situ* hybridization, it may be time consuming to find some of the reagents one must use to do the assay. For convenience, the Appendix lists our sources for the reagents used for the *in situ* hybridization technique. It should be made clear that this listing does not imply that the products are superior to other products on the market, but rather lists products we have used, mostly with good results.

THE APPLICATION OF *IN SITU* HYBRIDIZATION

Now that the methodology of *in situ* hybridization has been discussed in detail, let us turn our attention to examples of the utility of this technique. In addition to providing examples of *in situ* hybridization testing for the surgical pathologist and the researcher, this discussion also serves as a prelude to the comparison of *in situ* hybridization and PCR *in situ* hybridization for HPV DNA presented in Chapter 5. It is also hoped that, using the discussion in Chapter 2 as the foundation, it will provide more information for tissue analysis to assist the nonpathologist.

Detection of HPV DNA by *In Situ* Hybridization

Introductory Statements

The detection of infection by HPV provides a good model for examining the pros and cons of *in situ* hybridization analysis. HPV infection ranges from the occult state, where there are no clinical or pathological signs of infection, to genital warts, which may be more than 5 cm in size, to invasive cancers (11,14,40,46–84). There is extensive information on the correlation of the clinical and pathological features of HPV infection. HPV-induced lesions are an all-too-common disease, and tissue samples are readily available. Furthermore, many cell lines that can be readily obtained from the American Type Culture Collection (ATCC) have integrated copies of HPV DNA that range from 1 copy of HPV 16 (SiHa cells), to 20 to 25 copies of HPV 18 (HeLa cells), to 600 copies of HPV 16 (Caski cells).

Histologic Features of SILs

Cellular events during the early stages of HPV infection are not well understood. Specifically, in the cervix, which is the most common site of infection in the lower genital tract, it is unclear whether the basal cell, the metaplastic cell, or the more mature squamous cell is the portal of entry. Once a lesion forms, however, characteristic histologic changes are usually apparent. Although HPV may induce changes in glandular epithelium, most lesions are due to infection of the squamous cells. Pathologists usually divide the histologic changes seen in HPV-induced genital tract warts into two categories (85–87). First, low-grade squamous intraepithelial lesions (SILs) are characterized by crowding of cells, halos around the nuclei, and variation in nuclear size, shape, and chromaticity (see Figs. 7-5 and 7-6). These changes are most evident toward the middle and superficial layers of the epithelium. The basal epithelium either shows minimal hyperplasia with nuclear atypia or is unremarkable. The second category, the high-grade SILs, may show similar changes in the middle and superficial layers of the epithelium, though such changes are usually less marked. These lesions are distinguished from the low-grade SILs by the changes toward the basal layer, where cell crowding, increased mitotic activity, and nuclear atypia are seen.

Correlation of Viral Results with the Pathological Changes

In situ hybridization analyses of HPV-infected tissues have helped us to understand viral distribution patterns in lower genital tract SILs. A few of the more significant findings are listed below.

1. HPV DNA is more abundant in the cells toward the tissue surface that show perinuclear halos and nuclear atypia.
2. HPV DNA is present in much higher copy

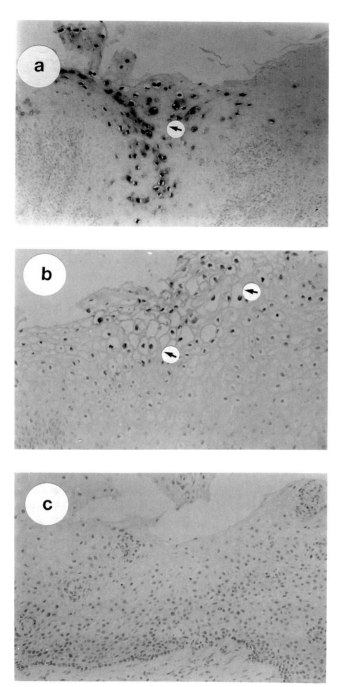

Figure 4-22. *Detection of HPV DNA and proteins in low-grade SILs.* The lesion is a low-grade cervical SIL. Note the many HPV-infected cells toward the surface of the lesion (**a**, *arrow*) (HPV 31 probe).
This is to be expected for a disease that is sexually transmitted. Similarly, the capsid proteins and E4
protein (**b**) were abundant toward the surface (*arrows*), suggestive of the production of intact virions.
Neither E4 nor HPV DNA was detected in the adjacent histologically normal tissue (**c**).

numbers in low-grade SILs than in high-grade SILs and invasive cancers (see Figs. 7-7 and 7-8).

3. The diversity of HPV types is much greater in cervical SILs than in vulvar and penile SILs (3–5,8,9,12,14,17,18,20,22,27,29,35, 36,88–112).

Let us discuss in more detail each of these three observations.

The first two observations are, of course, related because perinuclear halos and nuclear atypia are much more evident in low-grade lesions. When the virus infects a squamous cell one possible consequence is that viral DNA synthesis is "turned on," a process that may be associated with the cytopathic changes listed above. Not only is viral DNA synthesis "turned on," but higher levels of viral RNA and proteins are likewise found in the superficial layers in cells that demonstrate perinuclear halos, nuclear atypia, and cellular crowding (Fig. 4-22). The effect on viral transcription and translation of viral products appears generalized in that the mRNAs corresponding to the different early (E1 to E7) and late (L1 and L2) open reading frames (genes) all appear to be upregulated in these altered cells though to different degrees (11,13,16,35,78,104, 113–117). The observation that the L1 and L2 proteins are present in increased amounts is of interest for two reasons. First, it implies production of intact, and presumably infectious, viral particles. It is obviously favorable for HPV, which is sexually transmitted, to be most abundant and to have complete virions toward the surface of the tissue. Second, immunohistochemical detection of HPV typically uses antibodies against L2, which implies that such assays may not be useful in conditions, such as occult infection or invasive cancers, where late viral gene expression is weak or nonexistent.

A corollary of the increased viral copy number in cells that show perinuclear halos and nuclear atypia is that relatively few viral particles will be present in occult infection where the cell morphology appears normal. It is not surprising, therefore, that HPV DNA is rarely detected by *in situ* hybridization in the setting of occult infection. One needs to use tests such as Southern blot or PCR to detect occult HPV infection (2,72,92,106,118–121).

The third point, the greater diversity of HPV types found in cervical SILs relative to those lesions seen on the vulva and penis, is as fascinating as it is poorly understood. Table 4-4 lists the different HPV types found in low- and high-grade lesions of the vulva/penis and cervix. Note that HPVs 6 and 11 are relatively rare in low-grade cervical SILs, whereas they are detected in 94% of the histologically equivalent lesions of the vulva. Also note that HPV 16, the most common HPV type in genital tract cancers, is, as expected, the most common type in high-grade lesions. HPV 16 is also the most common HPV type in low-grade cervical SILs but is rarely found in low-grade vulvar (and penile) lesions. It can be concluded from the data presented in Table 4-4 that one would need only probes for HPVs 6, 11, and 16 to study vulvar and penile lesions. However, without addition-

Table 4-4. *Distribution (%) of HPV types in cervical and vulvar SILs* [a].

Lesion[b]	HPV 6/11	HPV 16	HPV 18	HPV 31/33/35	HPV others[c]
Cervix					
Low grade	19	32	2	30	17
High grade	0	69	1	25	5
Vulva/penis					
Low grade	94	0	0	4	2
High grade	0	92	0	8	0

Data from Nuovo, ref. 152, and Nuovo (*unpublished observations,* 1992).
[a]Vulvar low-grade SIL is equivalent to condyloma.
[b]Number of lesions studied is 212.
[c]Others are HPVs 42, 43, 44, 45, 51, 52, and 56. These rare types were present in equivalent amounts (each about 2% of the total) in the low-grade cervical SILs.

al probes, one could miss as much as 50% of the HPV types in cervical SILs!

It is not clear why many more HPV types are found in the cervix than are seen in the vulva and penis. Apparently HPVs 6, 11, and 16 have adapted to growth on cutaneous sites more successfully than other types such as HPVs 31, 33, 42, 43, and 51. This adaptation might explain the reason that HPV 16 has been found at other nongenital sites, notably the periungual region of the finger and the conjunctiva (120–125).

Occult Infection by HPV

As mentioned earlier, occult infection is defined as the presence of the virus in the ab-sence of clinical or histologic evidence of the infection. Most studies have focused on the cervix and have demonstrated, with slot blot or Southern blot analysis, that the rate of occult infection is about 10%. When PCR is employed a higher rate of about 30% has, not surprisingly, been found. In our laboratory the rate of occult infection as determined by PCR with consensus primers is about 15% (G.J. Nuovo, *unpublished observations,* 1996). As noted above, studies of occult infection analyzing HPV by *in situ* hybridization have shown that the virus is rarely detected with this technique (1,2,20,70,72,75, 105,116,121,126–132). There are two possible explanations. First, occult infection may escape detection because rare HPV types may be involved that share poor homology with the more common types

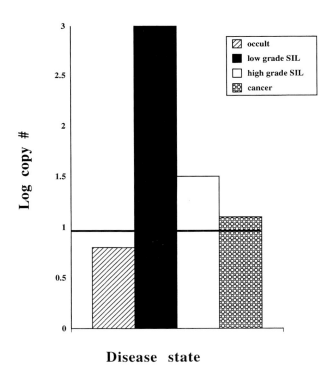

Figure 4-23. *The copy number of HPV relative to disease state.* The number of HPV DNA molecules per cell is strongly related to the disease state. The approximate ranges of viral copy numbers in occult infection, low-grade SIL, high-grade SIL, and invasive cancer are presented using a logarithmic scale. The horizontal line represents the detection threshold of *in situ* hybridization.

included in the probe. However, although rare uncharacterized types have been found, in many instances the more common types such as HPVs 6, 11, and 16 are detected. The second and more tenable explanation is that low numbers of the virus per cell, that is, below the detection threshold of the *in situ* hybridization assay, are characteristic of occult infection. Figure 4-23 illustrates the copy number of HPV as it relates to the "stage" of disease. Note that the number of viral DNA particles per infected cell tends to be less than 20 copies for occult infection and invasive carcinomas (i.e., viral DNA synthesis is not up-regulated). This is an important number because it correlates with the detection threshold of *in situ* hybridization. Figure 4-2 shows that HPV DNA is not detectable in a cervical cancer cell line that contains only 1 copy of the virus per cell, is weakly detectable when 20 copies are present per nucleus, and is intensely positive when 600 copies are present. Thus, if there are 5 copies of HPV DNA per cell in an invasive cancer or in a cell without the morphological features of HPV infection, it will appear negative by the *in situ* assay. It follows that *in situ* hybridization analysis is a poor technique for the study of invasive cancers or occult infection (Tables 4-5 and 4-6), but is as good as Southern blot or PCR for the detection of HPV DNA in low-grade SILs.

The Utility of In Situ *Hybridization* to the Surgical Pathologist for HPV-Related Lesions

Now that some of the basic observations concerning the correlation of HPV DNA detection by *in situ* hybridization and the pathological features of the tissue have been discussed, let us turn our attention to how this information can be used by surgical pathologists in their everyday practice. It is important to consider that many conditions can mimic genital warts clinically and/or histologically. Chronic inflammation, tinea (on cutaneous surfaces), and exaggerated mucosal folds are a few of the conditions that can demonstrate features such as epithelial thickening and nuclear atypia that are also seen in SILs (4,5,67,133,134). Although specific histologic changes associated with HPV-induced SILs have been discussed, it is important to realize that these changes are part of a continuum and that within this spectrum there may be overlap with some non-HPV conditions. It is easy to see the problem this may present to the surgical pathologist. A lesion clinically suspicious of a genital wart may be suggestive but not diagnostic of HPV infection on histologic examination. How does one interpret these equivocal tissues, which, in some studies, comprise up to 40% of genital tract biopsies for suspected genital tract warts (4,5)? Such lesions are sometimes described as borderline or suggestive of SIL. I have had the opportunity to see patients in consult and, although this less-than-certain description may be a reasonable diagnostic approach, it is often very difficult for the patient to deal emotionally with a noncommittal test report for the sexually transmitted genital warts. Furthermore, misdiagnosis of genital tract SILs is a relatively common problem reflecting, in part, the difficulty inherent in interpreting these tissues.

In situ hybridization analysis of equivocal tissue can provide useful information for both

Table 4-5. *Detection rate of HPV DNA by various techniques according to clinical and pathological stages of disease*

	in situ (%)	Southern and slot blot (%)	PCR (%)
Occult (no lesion)	0	10	30
Low-grade SIL	95	95	95
High-grade SIL	70	95	95
Invasive cancers	20	90	90

Data from refs. 61,81,116, and 117 and from Nuovo (*unpublished observations,* 1992).

Table 4-6. *Detection rate of HPV DNA by various techniques in genital tract lesions*

	in situ (%)	Southern and slot blot (%)
Nondiagnostic		
Vulva/penis	10	18
Cervix	1	35
Low grade	95	95
High grade	70	95
Invasive cancers	20	90

Data from refs. 4, 5, 48, 61, 79, and 133 and Nuovo (*unpublished observations,*1992).

the physician and the patient. The typical diagnostic problem for the pathologist is differentiating "nonspecific" changes from low-grade SIL. Recall from Table 4-5 that the detection rate of HPV DNA by *in situ* hybridization in low-grade SILs is 90% to 95% compared with 0% for tissues grossly and microscopically unremarkable. Hence, the test offers high sensitivity and specificity. What is the rate of HPV DNA detection for equivocal tissues taken from patients with clinically visible lesions? This information is provided in Table 4-6. Note that the *in situ* detection rate is much greater for equivocal vulvar and penile tissues than for cervical tissues. What is the reason for this disparity? It likely reflects the observation that cervical low-grade SILs show more conspicuous cytological changes than comparable lesions of the vulva and penis. Whatever the explanation, two diagnostically relevant points may be made from the data presented in Tables 4-4 to 4-6. First, *in situ* hybridization analysis for HPV DNA in equivocal tissues is a reliable way to distinguish mimics from "true" SILs because the detection rate is near 0% for tissues without intraepithelial lesions and over 90% for true SILs. Second, only probes for HPV types 6, 11, and 16 are needed for testing vulvar and penile tissues. However, probes for at least 14 distinct HPV types are needed to test cervical tissue in order to achieve a detection rate for SILs of >90% (Figs. 4-24 and 4-25).

I routinely use *in situ* hybridization analysis for equivocal vulvar and penile tissues because HPV DNA will be detected in about 10% of the cases when the classic histologic changes of a low-grade SIL are not seen (see Fig. 7-15). Because *in situ* hybridization requires at least 20 viral genomes per cell for detection, one may assume that the virus is actively proliferating in the HPV-positive equivocal tissues. This should be contrasted with HPV detection by slot or Southern blot hybridization or PCR. The greater sensitivity of these methods allows viral detection when it may be present in low copy numbers in a quiescent state. In such situations it is unclear if the virus is causing any pathological changes in the tissue. However, if active viral synthesis is occurring, it is feasible that changes such as parakeratosis or papillomatosis noted on pathological examination, even if seemingly nonspecific, may be induced by the specific action of the virus on the tissue.

Histologic Markers of HPV Infection in Equivocal Tissues

About one-fourth of histologically equivocal vulvar and penile biopsy specimens are HPV positive when tested using the highly sensitive PCR technique. Are there definable histologic markers in these equivocal tissues that can distinguish the HPV-positive cases from the HPV-negative ones? This question cannot be answered by conventional PCR or Southern blot hybridization, because the tissue structure is destroyed in preparation for the viral analysis precluding direct correlation of the viral results with the histologic changes (3,4,67,133,134). PCR *in situ* hybridization for intact tissue sam-

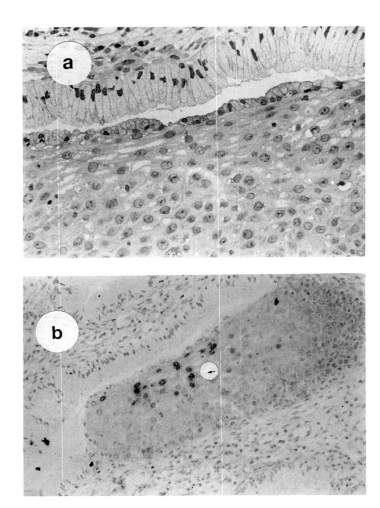

Figure 4-24. *Detection of HPV by* in situ *hybridization in a cervical lesion equivocal for SIL.* This cervical lesion came from a woman with an atypical Pap smear. The histologic features were not diagnostic of an SIL (**a**); note the well-organized appearance and lack of nuclear variability or variably sized and shaped perinuclear halos). HPV was not detected using *in situ* hybridization and probes against HPVs 6, 11, 16, 18, 31, 33, and 35 (not shown). However, a signal was evident if the HPV 56 probe was used (**b**, *arrow*). This illustrates the need for at least 14 distinct HPV probes (see Table 4-3) for the detection of HPV in cervical lesions and the utility of the *in situ* assay in such equivocal cases. It should be stressed that HPV DNA is typically *not* detected by *in situ* hybridization in cervical lesions that lack the histologic features of an SIL (see Fig. 4-25).

ples solves this problem. PCR *in situ* hybridization analyses of equivocal vulvar and penile lesions has shown specific tissue pattern markers of HPV infection such as the epithelial crevice in association with a focally thickened granular layer and focal hyperkeratosis. These findings are of obvious benefit for the pathologist's analysis of such tissues (see Fig. 7-16) and are discussed in detail in Chapter 7.

Detection of Other Viral Nucleic Acids by *In Situ* Hybridization

The *in situ* hybridization methodology is well suited for the study of many viral diseases especially when one considers that probes are readily available for most viruses. Let us now discuss some specific examples with emphasis on the valuable diagnostic information one may

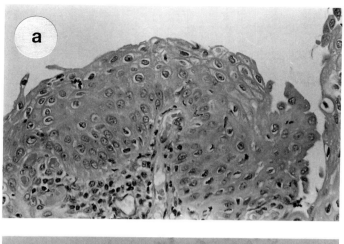

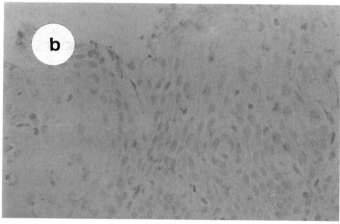

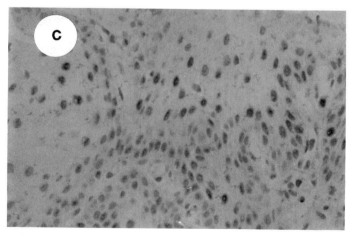

Figure 4-25. *The utility of* in situ *hybridization to the surgical pathologist: HPV.* This cervical lesion was clinically suspicious for a low-grade SIL but lacked the diagnostic histologic features (**a**). Although there is some nuclear variability and atypia, the relative uniformity of the nuclei and presence of nucleoli can be found in a nonspecific reactive condition that can appear on clinical examination to be an SIL. HPV DNA was not detected by *in situ* hybridization using a "consensus" HPV probe (**b**). The negative HPV result in conjunction with the histologic findings suggests that the lesion is not an SIL but rather a mimic. This is very important information for the clinician given the fact that SILs are sexually transmitted and usually ablated. The positive control (*alu* probe) performed on the same glass slide demonstrated a strong signal that shows that the negative HPV result was not due to inadequate hybridization or detection conditions (**c**).

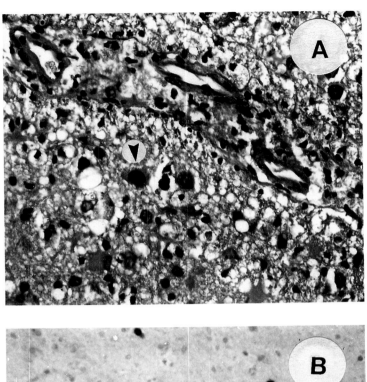

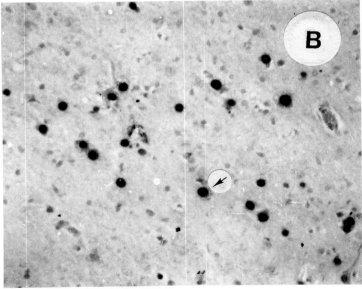

Figure 4-26. *Histologic and molecular analyses of progressive multifocal leukoencephalopathy.* In PML, the nuclei of oligodendroglial cells may be enlarged and have a smudge-like appearance (**A**). These cells contain large numbers of the JC virus (**B**, *arrow*). The virus may also be present in cells that do not show these cytological features and thus can be demonstrated only by *in situ* hybridization. For example, JC viral RNA was detected in some cytologically normal oligodendroglial cells by RT *in situ* PCR (**C**, *arrows*). The signal was not evident if the RT step was omitted (**D**; negative control). The electronmicroscopic appearance of this virus is presented in **E** and **F**.

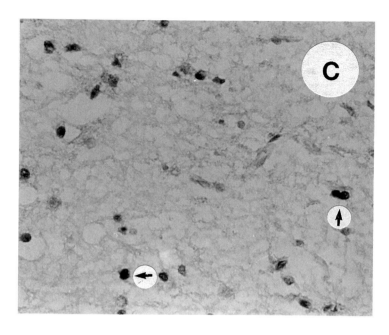

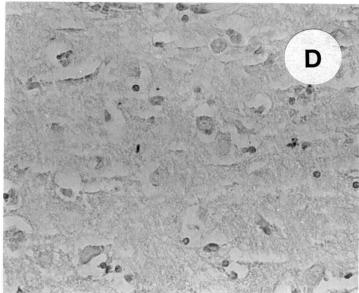

Figure 4-26. *Continued.*

obtain by correlating the histologic changes with the viral test results. One technical point should be clarified before beginning. The only change in the protocol I use for the detection of viral nucleic acids other than HPV is to substi- tute the appropriate probe. There are no further modifications needed. This adaptability great- ly facilitates the use of *in situ* hybridization in the diagnostic pathology laboratory, as the tech- nician need not make any major modification

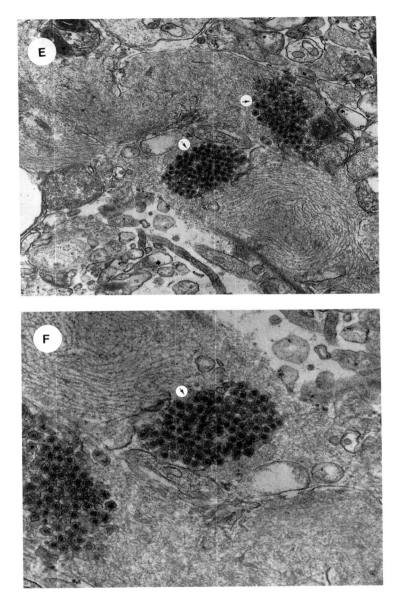

Figure 4-26. *Continued.*

for the detection of different viruses or any specific DNA sequence.

Progressive Multifocal Leukoencephalopathy: the JC Virus

Due to the marked increase in the prevalence of AIDS, the surgical pathologist is now commonly faced with diseases once seen very rarely if at all. Many are infectious diseases, and their histologic characteristics often deviate from those described in the literature for patients who do not have AIDS. A pertinent example for the neuropathologist is progressive multifocal leukoencephalopathy (PML), which is a demyelinating disease seen primarily in the white matter of the brain (38,135–139). The classic histologic change of PML is enlarged oligodendroglial nuclei; inflammation is usually, at most, minimal (Fig. 4-26). PML occurs relatively commonly in AIDS patients, and the disease may have unusual features at both a clinical and pathological level. The disease may be the first sign of immunosuppression in a patient otherwise not known to have AIDS and may present as a focal mass. Neurological complications are very common in AIDS patients and may be due to other diseases such as lymphoma, toxoplasmosis, or other viral infections such as cytomegalovirus (CMV) and herpes simplex virus (HSV). Thus, a focal lesion with recent neurological changes in an AIDS patient may prompt a directed biopsy, and each of these diseases should be included in the differential. On histologic examination, inflammatory cells may be a major component of PML in AIDS patients, and the infiltrate often includes eosinophils (138). This finding is very unusual in PML that is not AIDS related and is responsible for the local mass-like effect. Furthermore, the diagnostic enlarged oligodendroglial nuclei may be difficult to find. The virus that causes PML is a papovavirus related to HPV and is called the *JC virus*. These are the initials of the patient from whom it was initially isolated and should not be confused with the virus/prion that causes Jacob-Creutzfeld disease. The JC virus actively proliferates in PML probably reflecting the immunosuppressed state of the patient and is readily detectable by *in situ* hybridization even when the classical oligodendroglial changes are not evident. Thus, it is possible to make an unequivocal diagnosis of PML even in the setting of an atypical histologic presentation by doing *in situ* hybridization for the JC virus (Fig. 4-26). Because anti-viral therapy is showing some promise for the treatment of PML, a rapid diagnosis has important implications for reducing the morbidity and mortality in AIDS patients with this disease. In this regard, it is of interest that it has been shown that AIDS patients with PML who have lesions with extensive inflammation and rare atypical oligo-

dendroglial cells survive the disease better than those who do not show these histologic features. Given the additional inflammation, some have suggested that other viruses or infectious agents such as CMV, HSV, HIV-1, and toxoplasma may have co-infected tissue with the JC virus. However, *in situ* hybridization analyses for these other organisms was negative (138).

Cytomegalovirus

Cytomegalovirus (CMV) is probably the most common opportunistic viral infection that occurs in patients with AIDS. Several methods are available for the detection of CMV. Viral culture, though sensitive, is time consuming and requires specialized equipment (140). Serological tests also do not give results immediately and are reported to have a relatively low sensitivity, especially in immunocompromised patients (140). Direct and rapid visualization of the virus can be done on cytology specimens and fixed, paraffin-embedded tissue sections using either *in situ* hybridization or immunohistochemistry (31,37,41).

CMV has been detected in a wide variety of organs including the brain, retina, kidney, lung, esophagus, and colon (37,41,32,42,140, 140–144). CMV may induce cytological changes which are unequivocally diagnostic of the infection such as intranuclear eosinophilic inclusions often with clear zones separating them from peripheral chromatin clumping and basophilic cytoplasmic inclusions (Fig. 4-27). When these changes are seen, the virus will always be detectable by *in situ* hybridization or immunohistochemistry; PCR *in situ* hybridization would not be necessary. The hybridization signal is invariably intense, which is indicative of hundreds and probably thousands of viral genomes in the nucleus (Fig. 4-27). However, CMV DNA has been detected in cells which lack these diagnostic features and the hybridization signal in such cells was still often intense. Thus, CMV may actively replicate in cells that lack the characteristic cytological changes of the

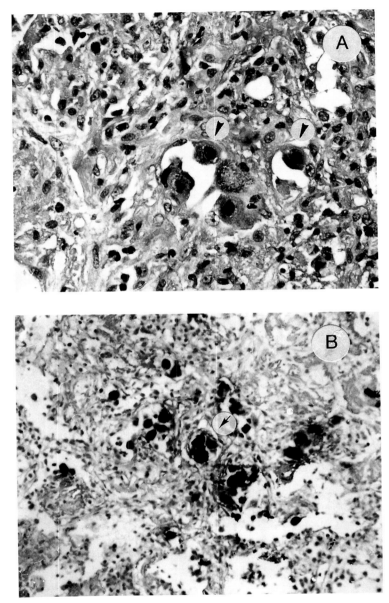

Figure 4-27. *Histologic and molecular analyses of CMV infection.* The diagnostic features of CMV infection are a large nuclear inclusion surrounded by a clear zone and cytoplasmic inclusions (**A**, *arrowheads*). These nuclear inclusions should not be confused with nucleoli, as they are much larger. CMV DNA will be readily apparent in such cells by standard *in situ* hybridization, as they will contain hundreds of viral genomes (**B**, *arrow*).

infection. One study demonstrated that "non-specific" villitis may be due to CMV, because the virus was detected in inflamed villi that did not demonstrate the characteristic cellular inclusions (37).

As mentioned earlier, CMV infection frequently occurs in patients with AIDS. Given that diagnostic cytological changes are not always evident in cells that have relatively large copy numbers of CMV, it is clear that

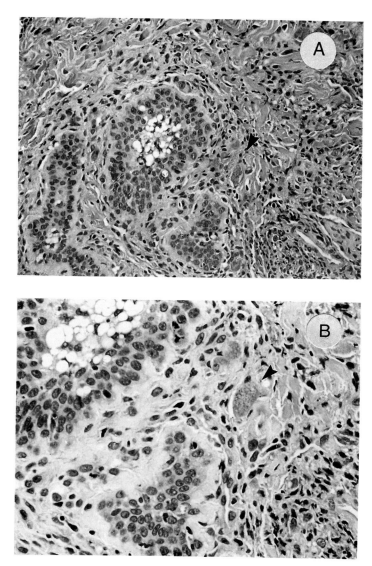

Figure 4-28. *The diagnostic utility of* in situ *hybridization analyses to the surgical pathologist.* This biopsy specimen came from a nonhealing ulcer of the face near the ear (**A**). Note the inflammatory cells, including some with enlarged nuclei (**B**, *arrowhead* corresponds to same area marked with *arrow* in **A**); inclusions were not evident. The clinical impression was herpes simplex infection. However, CMV DNA was detected by *in situ* hybridization (**C**, *arrowhead*).

in situ hybridization may be a significant diagnostic aid (74,144,145). Because specific anti-CMV therapy is now available which may well have serious side effects in patients without CMV infection, it is especially important to make an accurate diagnosis as soon as possible. A brief case report may help illustrate this point: A 40-year-old man at SUNY at Stony Brook, who was HIV-1-positive, presented with a recent history of a draining ulcer on the face. Histological examination revealed intense inflammation

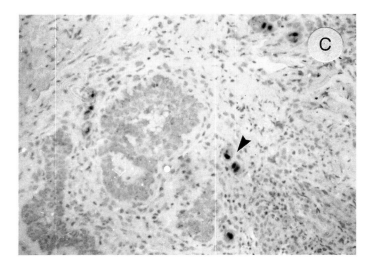

Figure 4-28. *Continued.*

and the presence of viral-like inclusions. The clinical and pathological differential included CMV and HSV, although CMV dermatitis is extremely rare. The antiviral therapy for the two is very different. Gancyclovir is effective against CMV. However, if the patient had HSV gancyclovir, although it may be effective, may cause serious side effects when compared with the less toxic acylovir anti viral therapy used against HSV. In this case *in situ* hybridization demonstrated that CMV, and not HSV, was present and the lesion responded to the anti-CMV medication (Fig. 4-28).

A recent study analyzed lung tissues from AIDS patients with pneumocystis for viruses including HSV, CMV, and adenovirus. It was noted that CMV detection by *in situ* hybridization was common and that these patients had a much greater mortality rate compared with patients with pneumocystis pneumonia who were negative for CMV by *in situ* hybridization or PCR (146). Thus, detection of CMV in a lung biopsy or, perhaps, in a bronchial lavage specimen from a patient with pneumocystis pneumonia may prompt aggressive anti-CMV therapy. This illustrates another clinical utility for the *in situ* assay.

Other Viruses: Epstein-Barr Virus, Herpes Simplex Virus, and Adenovirus

Examples in this next section will demonstrate the widespread applicability of *in situ* hybridization for the detection of various viruses.

Epstein-Barr virus (EBV) is a DNA virus that, like CMV, belongs to the herpes virus family. It has the ability to infect B-lymphocytes and epithelial cells from a variety of sites (30,34,147,148). Infection of B-cells may be manifest as infectious mononucleosis or as a lymphoma. EBV-associated lymphoma is especially common in patients with AIDS and EBV DNA is routinely detected in Burkitt's lymphoma. Although infection of epithelial cells from a variety of sites is being reported, it has been best documented in the epithelium of the nasopharynx where the virus may be isolated in the absence of other disease or in the rare malignant nasopharyngeal carcinoma.

Figure 4-29 demonstrates that EBV DNA is readily detectable in a Burkitt's lymphoma cell line. Figure 4-30 shows the viral distribution of EBV in a "lymphoepithelioma" such as is found in the nasal cavity. Note that the virus localizes only to the epithelial component. We undertook a study to analyze for EBV DNA in a lesion called oral hairy leuko-

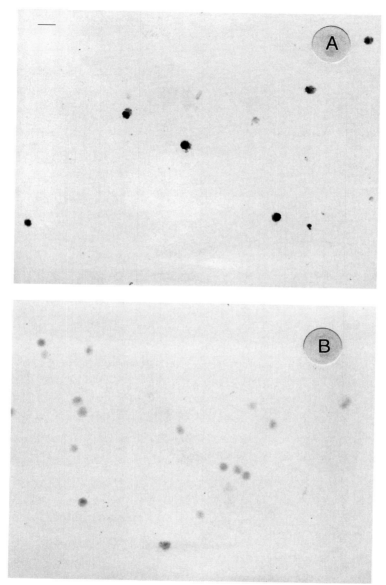

Figure 4-29. *Molecular analysis of two Burkitt's lymphoma cell lines.* EBV DNA was detected in cells from a Burkitt's lymphoma line using a biotin-labeled probe (**A**). The hybridization signal was lost if the EBV DNA was exchanged with biotin-labeled plasmid DNA, which helps demonstrate the specificity of the signal (**B**). However, the region of EBV DNA that is usually the target with *in situ* hybridization, the *Bam*HI internal repeat region 1, is often present in copy numbers of 10 to 20 per cell and may at times be difficult to detect by standard *in situ* hybridization. This was evident (in higher magnification) in the Raji cell line, where only rare cells were EBV-positive with standard *in situ* hybridization (**C**, *arrow*). However, all cells were shown to contain EBV if PCR *in situ* hybridization was performed (**D**). Thus, unlike for productive infection with CMV, for which *in situ* hybridization is adequate, PCR *in situ* hybridization may be needed to determine the exact distribution of EBV in a given tissue section or cellular preparation.

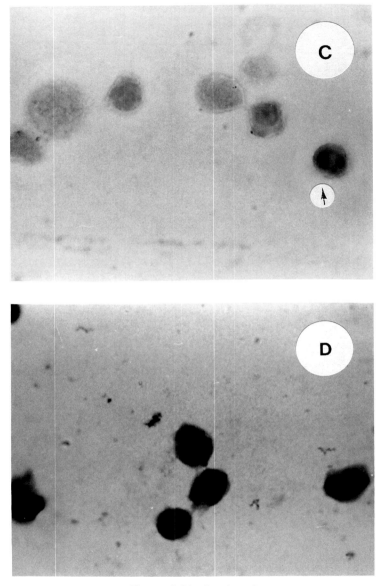

Figure 4-29. *Continued.*

plakia, which is found in people with AIDS. The copy number of the *Bam*HI internal repeat region 1 of the virus is usually present as about 10 copies per cell in latent infection and, thus, may be difficult to detect by standard *in situ* hybridization. Alternatively, larger viral DNA copy numbers are expected with activated infection. Standard *in situ* hybridization can be highly sensitive for EBV if a probe for EBER-1 RNA is employed, given the severalfold amplification of the message that may occur in latent infection. We decided to assay for EBV DNA in this study due to the ubiquitous presence of the DNA in viral infection and the observation that EBER-1 transcripts may be below the detection threshold of stan-

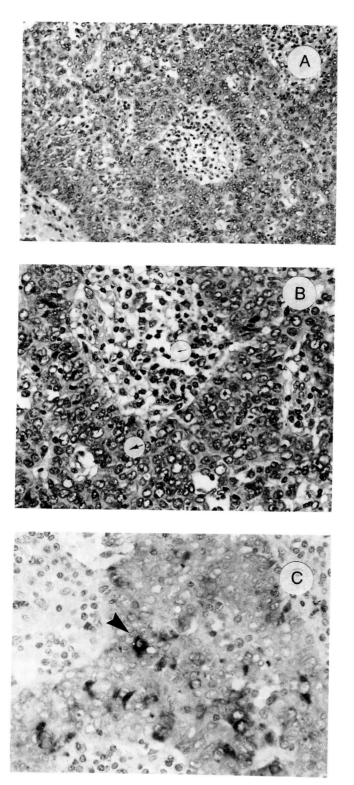

Figure 4-30. *Histologic and molecular analyses of a lymphoepithelioma.* This tumor (**A** and **B**) was detected in the anterior mediastinum and had nests of cells (**B**, *large arrow*) with large, anaplastic nuclei surrounding islands of reactive lymphocytes (**B**, *small arrow*, **A**). EBV DNA was detected in the epithelial areas but not in the lymphoid tissue by *in situ* hybridization (**C**).

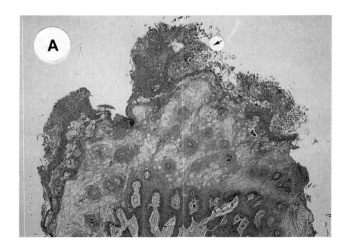

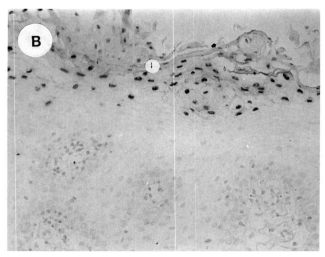

Figure 4-31. *Detection of EBV DNA in oral hairy leukoplakia.* Oral hairy leukoplakia is a lesion on the lateral border of the tongue that occurs in people with AIDS. Note the marked papillomatosis and parakeratosis (*arrow*) evident on histologic examination (**A**). EBV DNA was detected in the superficial cells (*arrow*) of the lesion by standard *in situ* hybridization (**B**). PCR *in situ* hybridization demonstrated that the viral DNA also was present in the basal cells (**C**, *large arrows;* small area indicates superficial cells). Thus, EBV infection in these lesions is equivalent to HPV in cervical SILs, where productive viral infection is evident in the cells toward the surface, whereas the cells toward the basal zone contain quiescent virus detectable by PCR *in situ* hybridization.

dard *in situ* hybridization in certain conditions, such as activated EBV infection. EBV DNA was readily detected in the superficial squamous cells of oral hairy leukoplakia but not in the basal cells as determined by *in situ* hybridization; in this manner, it is analogous to the activated HPV infection typical of low grade SILs (as discussed in Chapter 8). PCR *in situ* hybridization demonstrated that the EBV DNA did extend to the basal epithelial cells (Fig. 4-31).This suggests that infection in the basal cells is latent and is the probable source of the activated viral infection in the superficial squamous cells.

Adenovirus can cause clinically evident disease in the human respiratory tract (146). The

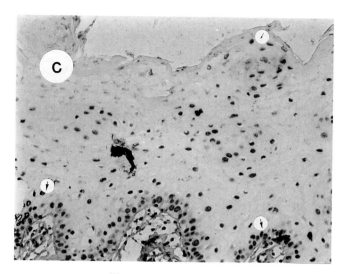

Figure 4-31. *Continued.*

cytological changes associated with adenoviral infection are enlarged nuclei with a smudge-like appearance. As noted above, a recent study analyzed lung tissues from AIDS patients for various viruses. Adenoviral DNA was detected in several lung biopsies from these patients, but only in those who had concurrent pneumocystis pneumonia. An example of the histology of adenoviral pneumonia with the corresponding *in situ* hybridization results is presented in Fig. 4-32.

The herpes simplex virus (HSV) is a very common human pathogen. HSV type 1 is usually found in oral "cold sores," whereas HSV type 2 is associated with genital lesions. In its classical form, the unique cytological changes it may induce are easily identified by the pathologist (32,149–151). These epithelial cell changes include multinucleation, nuclear molding, a homogeneous, glassy nuclear appearance (Fig. 4-33) and, at times, intranuclear inclusions. The virus will always be readily detectable by *in situ* hybridization when these features are evident on microscopic examination. We have seen cases of seemingly "nonspecific" inflammation that were demonstrated to be associated with HSV by *in situ* hybridization analysis (Fig. 4-34). A virus that is related to HSV causes chickenpox—varicella zoster (VZ).

The cytologic changes of VZ are indistinguishable from HSV. A simple way to differentiate these two pathogens is by *in situ* hybridization, because probes can be chosen that do not cross-hybridize with the other virus. Figure 4-35 is an example of a skin lesion that was incorrectly diagnosed as HSV infection due to the multinucleated giant squamous cells; *in situ* hybridization showed an intense signal with a VZ probe and no signal with the HSV probe.

With the AIDS epidemic has come another related virus—human herpes virus type 6. Figure 4-36 shows the nuclear inclusions found in multiple tissues of a child with AIDS who died after an acute illness. *In situ* hybridization demonstrated that the etiologic agent was human herpes virus type 6.

Comparison of *in situ* Hybridization and Immunohistochemistry for the Detection of Infectious Diseases

Brief mention should be made of the comparative capabilities of *in situ* hybridization and immunohistochemistry. Of course, the two techniques differ at a most basic level. *In situ* hybridization seeks to detect a specific DNA or RNA sequence. Immunohistochemistry at-

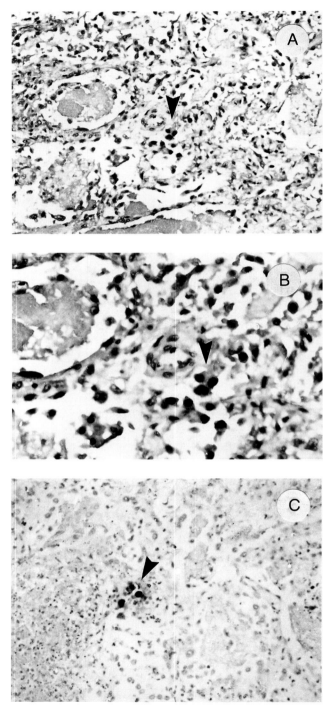

Figure 4-32. *Histologic and molecular analyses of pneumonia in an AIDS patient.* This tissue section was taken from the lung of an AIDS patient whose cause of death included pneumocystis pneumonia. In areas away from the pneumocystis organisms, enlarged nuclei with smudge-type changes were evident (**A, B**). *In situ* hybridization analysis revealed that these cells contained adenovirus (**C**). Infected cells are marked by *arrowheads* in each photo. The large number of such cells and the high copy number of adenovirus suggest that this infection also contributed to the patient's demise.

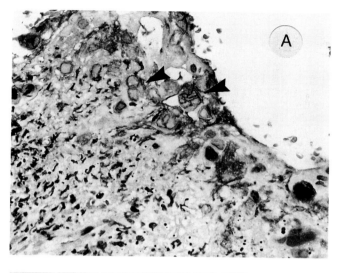

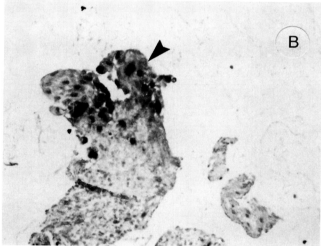

Figure 4-33. *Histologic and molecular analyses of HSV.* This vulvar biopsy specimen was taken from a vesicle that had ulcerated. Note the enlarged epithelial cells with multiple molded nuclei that have a glassy appearance (**A**). *In situ* hybridization analysis revealed that these cells contained HSV (**B**). Viral infected cells are indicated by *arrowheads* in both A and B.

tempts to detect the protein product derived from the DNA–mRNA of interest. Antibody-based technology had a good head start on nucleic acid-based technology, especially for the diagnostic laboratory. This, plus the fact that relatively few diagnostic laboratories use *in situ* hybridization, has perhaps led to a feeling among immunohistochemists that *in situ* hybridization would contribute no more than im-munohistochemistry. One need only look at the literature to notice the conflicting data supporting the superiority of one test or the other for the detection of various viruses (6,28,37, 39,42).

Putting this controversy among investigators aside for a moment, it can be seen that *in situ* hybridization may be the more sensitive technique in situations where relatively little spe-

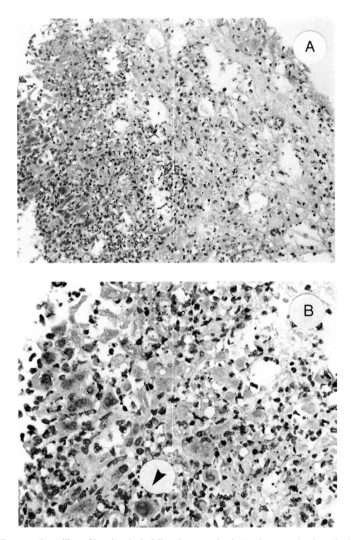

Figure 4-34. *The diagnostic utility of* in situ *hybridization analysis to the surgical pathologist.* This biopsy material came from the duodenum near the ampulla of Vater from a patient who did not have AIDS. The tissue was ulcerated and contained scattered degenerative cells with enlarged nuclei (**A, B**). The marked degeneration hindered interpretation, but in some cells the nuclei appeared glassy (**B**, *arrowhead*). *In situ* hybridization analysis revealed that many of these cells contained HSV (**C**). Isolated HSV in a patient with no evidence of immunosuppression is highly unusual and demonstrates the ability of the *in situ* test to give a rapid, unequivocal diagnosis in a case that presents diagnostic difficulties to the clinician and the pathologist.

cific protein is being produced. One well-characterized example of this is shown in the case of HPV in high-grade SILs. Viral DNA is often present in levels above the detection threshold of about 20 copies per cell, but the virus makes very little capsid protein, which is the antigen that the commercially available antibody is directed against. The end result is a detection rate for high-grade SILs with *in situ* hybridization of about 70% compared with a rate of less than 10% with immunohistochemistry against the capsid (open-reading frame L2) antigen. In

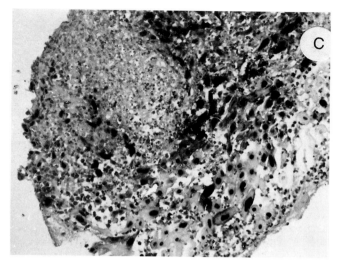

Figure 4-34. *Continued.*

some situations, specific proteins will be abundant and the two tests will yield equivalent results. Two examples would be low-grade vulvar condylomas for HPV and CMV infection where the characteristic inclusions are evident (Fig. 4-37). Another example would be the detection of hepatitis B DNA and core antigen (Fig. 4-38). One more point should be made concerning the relative utility of *in situ* hybridization versus immunohistochemistry: Both assays are based on hydrogen-bond linked complexes (antigen–antibody and DNA–DNA), although other forces such as ionic bonds also play a role. There tends to be greater strength

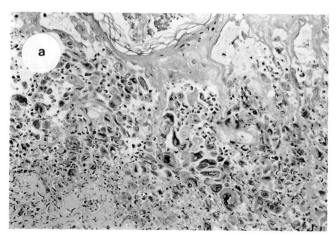

Figure 4-35. *Detection of varicella-zoster by* in situ *hybridization.* This skin biopsy specimen was from a series of grouped vesicles. Note the multinucleated cells with glassy nuclei (**a, b**). The lesion was initially identified as herpes simplex virus infection. However, HSV DNA was not detected by *in situ* hybridization; the *alu* probe gave an intense signal demonstrating that the lesion did not contain HSV (not shown). However, varicella-zoster DNA was detected by *in situ* hybridization (**c**). HSV and varicella-zoster are indistinguishable on histological examination but can be easily distinguished by *in situ* hybridization.

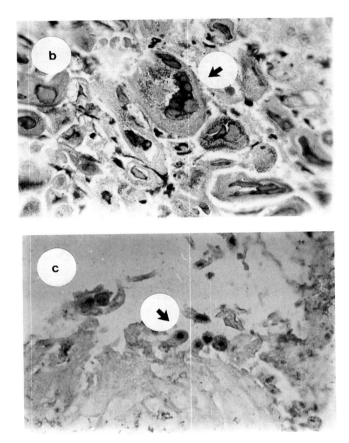

Figure 4-35. *Continued.*

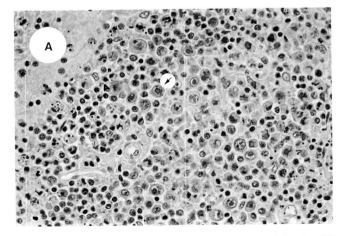

Figure 4-36. *Detection of human herpes virus type 6 by* in situ *hybridization.* The tissue is from the lymph node of a child who died of a systemic illness. Note the cells with the large nuclear inclusions (**A, B,** *arrows*). No HSV, cytomegalovirus, or varicella-zoster viral DNA was detected by *in situ* hybridization (not shown). However, human herpes virus type 6 DNA was detected by *in situ* hybridization (**C,** *arrow*).

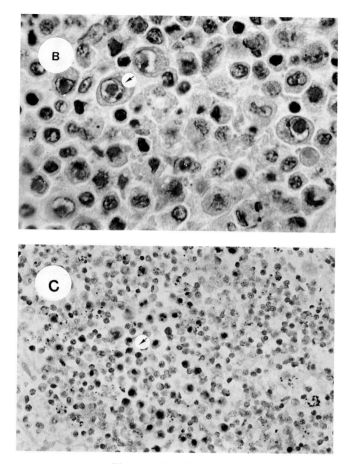

Figure 4-36. *Continued.*

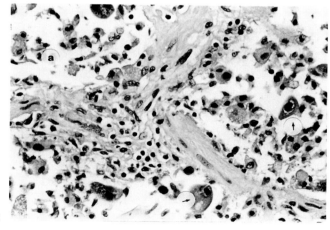

a

Figure 4-37. *Detection of CMV by* in situ *hybridization and immunohistochemistry.* This lung tissue showed the typical CMV inclusions (**a**, *arrows*). The virus was detected in many cells by *in situ* hybridization (**b**, *arrow*) and immunohistochemistry (**c**, *arrows*). The immunohistochemistry assay required proteinase K digestion for an optimal detection. CMV is an example where *in situ* hybridization and immunohistochemistry are equivalent for viral detection. This can be compared with HPV infection, where, for cervical SILs and cancers, *in situ* hybridization is in general a much more sensitive assay.

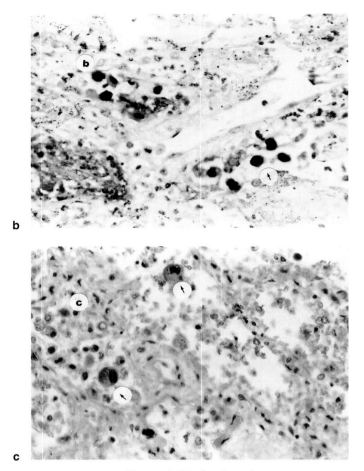

b

c

Figure 4-37. *Continued.*

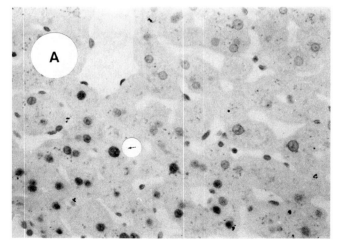

Figure 4-38. *Detection of hepatitis B by* in situ *hybridization and immunohistochemistry.* Hepatitis B DNA was detected in scattered hepatocytes using *in situ* hybridization (**A**, *arrow*). Epitopes against the viral core antigen were detected by immunohistochemistry in a serial section (**B**, *arrow*).

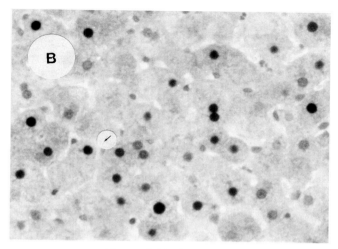

Figure 4-38. *Continued.*

in the nucleic acid complexes because each base pair match will contribute relatively strong hydrogen bonding, whereas less actual complexing occurs per unit volume of molecule with protein–protein bonds. It follows that the difference in developed signal-to-background noise tends to be greater with the *in situ* assay. In my experience, it is easier to reduce background in the *in situ* test while still preserving a strong signal, as compared with immunohistochemical localization.

Let's get back to the controversy over which is better: the immunohistochemical or the *in situ* hybridization technique. My goal is not to resolve this question, but rather to emphasize that the question is very complex and has no simple answer. Clearly, the relative value of one assay over the other will depend in large part on the specifics of the case in question, such as pathology of the lesion, stage of infection, etc. The other point that should be emphasized is the need to be critical when reviewing the literature on this topic. Many different groups have compared the two techniques, with widely varying results. However, in many of these studies, one of the assays was not optimized. For example, studies that claim that immunohistochemical localization of CMV infection is more effective than *in situ* localization of CMV DNA used an AEC-based system for the latter. This system has been shown to be much inferior to the alkaline phosphatase-based systems, at least at the time the studies were done (42). Alternatively, we reported that *in situ* hybridization had a much higher detection rate than immunohistochemistry for CMV in chronic villitis (37). We subsequently learned that our immunohistochemical technique was not optimized. If we used proteinase K digestion instead of trypsin digestion, the two assays became equivalent (152).

In summary, both *in situ* and immunohistochemistry have their place in the diagnostic and research laboratories. Because nonisotopic *insitu* systems are now as sensitive as isotopic-based systems, and because the detection steps are similar for both assays if, for example, one uses biotin probes and biotin-labeled antibodies, the laboratory will find each of these systems to be technically uncomplicated and informative.

REFERENCES

1. deVilliers EM, Schneider A, Miklaw H, et al. Human papillomavirus infections in women with and without abnormal cervical cytology. *Lancet* 1987;i:703–706.
2. Nuovo GJ, Cottral S. Occult infection of the uterine cervix by human papillomavirus in post menopausal women. *Am J Obstet Gynecol* 1989;160:340–344.

3. Nuovo GJ, Darfler MM, Impraim CC, Bromley SE. Occurrence of multiple types of human papillomavirus in genital tract lesions: analysis by *in situ* hybridization and the polymerase chain reaction. *Am J Pathol* 1991; 58:518–523.

4. Nuovo GJ, Hochman H, Eliezri YD, Comite S, Lastarria D, Silvers DN. Detection of human papillomavirus DNA in penile lesions histologically negative for condylomata: analysis by *in situ* hybridization and the polymerase chain reaction. *Am J Surg Pathol* 1990;14: 829–836.

5. Nuovo GJ. Human papillomavirus DNA in genital tract lesions histologically negative for condylomata: analysis by *in situ*, Southern blot hybridization and the polymerase chain reaction. *Am J Surg Pathol* 1990;14:643–651.

6. Nuovo GJ. A comparison of different methodologies (biotin based and ^{35}S based) for the detection of human papillomavirus DNA. *Lab Invest* 1989;61:471–476.

7. Crum CP, Nuovo GJ, Friedman D, Silverstein SJ. A comparison of biotin and isotope labeled ribonucleic acid probes for *in situ* detection of HPV 16 ribonucleic acid in genital pre cancers. *Lab Invest* 1988;58:354–359.

8. Nuovo GJ. A comparison of slot blot, Southern blot and *in situ* hybridization analyses for human papillomavirus DNA in genital tract lesions. *Obstet Gynecol* 1989;74: 673–677.

9. Ostrow RS, Manias DA, Clark BA, Okagaki T, Twiggs LB, Faras AJ. Detection of human papillomavirus DNA in invasive carcinomas of the cervix by *in situ* hybridization. *Can Res* 1987;47:649–653.

10. Walboomers JMM, Melchers WJG, Mullink H et al. Sensitivity of *in situ* detection with biotinylated probes of human papillomavirus type 16 DNA in frozen tissue sections of squamous cell carcinoma of the cervix. *Am J Pathol* 1988;131:587–594.

11. Crum CP, Symbula M, Ward BE. Topography of early HPV 16 transcription in high-grade genital precancers. *Am J Pathol* 1989;134:1183–1188.

12. Nagai N, Nuovo GJ, Friedman D, Crum CP. Detection of papillomavirus nucleic acids in genital precancers with the *in situ* hybridization technique: a review. *Int J Gynecol Pathol* 1987;6:366–379.

13. Crum CP, Nuovo G, Friedman D, Silverstein SJ. Accumulation of RNA homologous to human papillomavirus type 16 open reading frames in genital precancers. *J Virol* 1988;62:84–90.

14. Crum CP, Nagai N, Levine RU, Silverstein SJ. *In situ* hybridization analysis of human papillomavirus 16 DNA sequences in early cervical neoplasia. *Am J Pathol* 1986;123:174–182.

15. Nuovo GJ, Silverstein SJ. Comparison of formalin, buffered formalin, and Bouin's fixation on the detection of human papillomavirus DNA from genital lesions. *Lab Invest* 1988;59:720–724.gamma

16. Nuovo GJ, Friedman D, Silverstein SJ, Crum CP. Transcription of human papillomavirus type 16 in genital precancers. *Cancer Cells* 1987;5:337–343.

17. Lebargy F, Bulle F, Siegrist S, Guellaen G, Bernaudin J. Localization by *in situ* hybridization of γ glutamyl transpeptidase mRNA in the rat kidney using ^{35}S-labeled RNA probes. *Lab Invest* 1990;62:731–735.

18. McAllister HA, Rock DL. Comparative usefulness of tissue fixatives for *in situ* viral nucleic acid hybridization. *J Histochem Cytochem* 1985;33:1026–1032.

19. Moench TR, Gendelman HE, Clements JE, Narayan O, Griffin DE. Efficiency of *in situ* hybridization as a function of probe size and fixation technique. *J Virol Methods* 1985;11:119–130.

20. Nuovo GJ. Buffered formalin is the superior fixative for the detection of human papillomavirus DNA by *in situ* hybridization analysis. *Am J Pathol* 1989;134:837–842.

21. Tournier I, Bernuau D, Poliard A, Schoevaert D, Feldmann G. Detection of albumin mRNAs in rat liver by *in situ* hybridization: usefulness of paraffin embedding and comparison of various fixation procedures. *J Histochem Cytochem* 1987;35:453–459.

22. Nuovo GJ. Comparison of Bouin's solution and buffered formalin fixation on the detection rate by *in situ* hybridization of human papillomavirus DNA in genital tract lesions. *J Histotech* 1991;14:13–18.

23. Dubeau L, Chandler LA, Gralow JR, Nichols PW, Jones PA. Southern blot analysis of DNA extracted from formalin fixed pathology specimens. *Cancer Res* 1986;46:2964–2970.

24. Goelz SE, Hamilton SR, Vogelstein B. Purification of DNA from formaldehyde fixed and paraffin embedded tissue. *Biochem Biophys Res Commun* 1985;130:118–124.

25. Bromley SE, Darfler MM, Hammer ML, Jones-Trower A, Primus MA, Kreider JW. In situ *hybridization to human papillomavirus DNA in fixed tissue samples: comparison of detection methods. Papillomaviruses.* New York: Wiley-Liss; 1990.

26. Cravador A, Herzog A, Houard S, d'Ippolito P, Carroll R, Bollen A. Selective detection of human papilloma virus DNAs by specific synthetic DNA probes. *Mol Cell Probes* 1989;3:143–158.

27. Collins JE, Jenkins D, McCance DJ. Detection of human papillomavirus DNA sequences by *in situ* hybridization in cervical intraepithelial neoplasia and invasive carcinoma: a retrospective study. *J Clin Pathol* 1988;41: 289–295.

28. Alessandri LM, Sterrett GF, Pixley EC, Kulski JK. Comparison of peroxidase–antiperoxidase and avidin–biotin complex methods for the detection of papillomavirus in histologic sections of the cervix uteri. *Pathology* 1986; 18:383–385.

29. Garuti G, Boselli F, Genazzani AR, Silvestri S, Ratti G. Detection and typing of human papillomavirus in histologic specimens by *in situ* hybridization with biotinylated probes. *Am J Clin Pathol* 1989;92:604–612.

30. Mariette X, Gozlan J, Clerc D, Bisson M, Morinet F. Detection of Epstein-Barr virus DNA by *in situ* hybridization and polymerase chain reaction in salivary gland biopsy specimens from patients with Sjogren's syndrome. *Am J Med* 1991;90:286–294.

31. Niedobitek G, Finn T, Herbsy H, Bornhoft G, Gerdes J, Stein H. Detection of viral DNA by *in situ* hybridization using bromodeoxyuridine labeled DNA probes. *Am J Pathol* 1988;131:1–4.

32. Schmidbauer M, Budka H, Ambros P. Herpes simplex virus (HSV) DNA in microglial nodular brainstem encephalitis. *J Neuropathol Exp Neurol* 1989;48:645–652.

33. Ranki M, Leinonen AW, Jalava T et al. Use of Affiprobe HPV test kit for detection of human papillomavirus DNA in genital scrapes. *J Clin Microbiol* 1990;28:2076–2081.

34. Samoszuk M. Rapid detection of Epstein-Barr viral DNA by nonisotopic *in situ* hybridization. *Am J Pathol* 1991;96:448–453.

35. Stoler MH, Broker TR. *In situ* hybridization detection on human papillomavirus DNAs and messenger RNAs in genital condylomata and a cervical carcinoma. *Hum Pathol* 1986;17:250–258.

36. Syrjanen S, Syrjanen K. An improved *in situ* DNA hybridization protocol for detection of human papillomavirus (HPV) DNA sequences in paraffin-embedded biopsies. *J Virol Methods* 1986;14:293–304.

37. Sachdev R, Nuovo GJ, Kaplan C, Greco A. Detection of cytomegalovirus in chronic villitis by *in situ* hybridization. *Pediatr Pathol* 1990;10:909–917.

38. Mori M, Lurata H, Tajima M, Shimada H. JC virus detection by *in situ* hybridization in brain tissue from elderly patients. *Ann Neurol* 1991;29:428–432.

39. Gupka JW, Gupka PK, Rosenshein N, Shah KV. Detection of human papillomavirus in cervical smears. A comparison of *in situ* hybridization, immunocytochemistry and cytopathology. *Acta Cytol* 1987;31:387–395.

40. Eversole LR, Laipis PJ. Oral squamous papillomas: detection of HPV DNA by *in situ* hybridization. *Oral Surg Oral Med Oral Pathol* 1988;65:545–550.

41. Roberts WH, Hammond S, Sneddon JM, Thesing J, Caldwell JH, Clausen KP. *In situ* DNA hybridization for cytomegalovirus in colonic biopsies. *Arch Pathol Lab Med* 1988;112:1106–1109.

42. Robey SS, Gage WR, Kuhajda FP. Comparison of immunoperoxidase and DNA *in situ* hybridization techniques in the diagnosis of cytomegalovirus colitis. *Am J Clin Pathol* 1988;89:666–671.

43. Rotbart HA, Abzug MJ, Levin MJ. Development and application of RNA probes for the study of picornaviruses. *Mol Cell Probes* 1988;2:65–73.

44. Tase T, Okagaki T, Clark BA, Twiggs LB, Ostrow RS, Faras AJ. Human papillomavirus DNA in adenocarcinoma *in situ*, microinvasive adenocarcinoma of the uterine cervix, and coexisting cervical squamous intraepithelial neoplasia. *Int J Gynecol Pathol* 1989;8:8–17.

45. Willett GD, Kurman RJ, Reid R, Greenberg M, Jenson AB, Lorincz AT. Correlation of the histologic appearance of intraepithelial neoplasia of the cervix with human papillomavirus types. *Int J Gynecol Pathol* 1989;8:18–25.

46. Abramson AL, Steinberg BM, Winkler B. Laryngeal papillomatosis: clinical, histopathologic and molecular studies. *Laryngoscope* 1987;97:678–685.

47. Brandsma JL, Lewis AJ, Abramson A, Manos MM. Detection and typing of papillomavirus DNA in formaldehyde-fixed paraffin-embedded tissue. *Arch Otolaryngol Head Neck Surg* 1990;116:844–848.

47a. Burk RD, Kadish AS, Calderin S, Romney SL. Human papillomavirus infection of the cervix detected by cervicovaginal lavage and molecular hybridization: correlation with biopsy results and Papanicolaou smear. *Am J Obstet Gynecol* 1986;154:982–989.

48. Carson LF, Twiggs LB, Okagaki T, Clark BA, Ostrow RS, Faras AJ. Human papillomavirus DNA in adenosquamous carcinoma and squamous cell carcinoma of the vulva. *Obstet Gynecol* 1988;72:63–67.

49. Cullen AP, Reid R, Champion M, Lorincz AT. Analysis of the physical state of different human papillomavirus DNAs in intraepithelial and invasive cervical neoplasia. *J Virol* 1991;65:606–612.

50. Dinh TV, Powell LC, Hannigan EV, Yang HL, Wirt DP, Yandell RB. Simultaneously occurring condylomata acuminata, carcinoma *in situ* and verrucous carcinoma of the vulva and carcinoma *in situ* of the cervix in a young woman. *J Reprod Med* 1988;33:510–513.

51. Ferenczy A, Mitao M, Nagai N, Silverstein SJ, Crum CP. Latent papillomavirus and recurring genital warts. *N Engl J Med* 1985;313:784–788.

52. Firzlaff JM, Kiviat NB, Beckmann AM, Jenison SA, Galloway DA. Detection of human papillomavirus capsid antigens in various squamous epithelial lesions using antibodies directed against the L1 and L2 open reading frames. *Virology* 1988;164:467–477.

53. Gall AA, Saul SH, Stoler MH. *In situ* hybridization analysis of human papillomavirus in anal squamous cell carcinoma. *Mod Pathol* 1989;2:439–443.

54. Griffin NR, Bevan IS, Lewis FA, Young LS. Demonstration of multiple HPV types in normal cervix and in cervical squamous cell carcinoma using the polymerase chain reaction on paraffin wax-embedded material. *J Clin Pathol* 1990;45:52–56.

55. Kashima HK, Kutcher M, Kessis T, Levin LS, DeVilleirs EM, Shah K. Human papillomavirus in squamous cell carcinoma, leukoplakia, lichen planus, and clinically normal epithelium of the oral cavity. *Ann Otol Rhinol Laryngol* 1990;99:55–61.

56. Kadish AS, Burk RD, Kress Y, Calderin S, Romney SL. Human papillomavirus of different types in precancerous lesions of the uterine cervix: histologic, immunocytochemical and ultrastructural studies. *Hum Pathol* 1986;17:384–392.

57. Kawashima M, Favre M, Obalek S, Jablonska S, Orth G. Premalignant lesions and cancers of the skin in the general population: Evaluation of the role of human papillomavirus. *J Invest Dermatol* 1990;95:537–542.

58. Kiyabu MT, Shibata D, Arnheim N, Martin WJ, Fitzgibbons PL. Detection of human papillomavirus in formalin-fixed, invasive squamous carcinomas using the polymerase chain reaction. *Am J Surg Pathol* 1989;13:221–224.

59. Kratochvil FJ, Cioffi GA, Auclair PL, Rathbun WA. Virus-associated dysplasia (bowenoid papulosis?) of the oral cavity. *Oral Surg Oral Med Oral Pathol* 1989;68:312–316.

60. Kreider JW, Howett MK, Leure-Dupree AE, Zaino RJ, Weber JA. Laboratory production in vivo of infectious human papillomavirus type 11. *J Virol* 1987;61:590–593.

61. Lorincz AT, Temple GF, Patterson JA, Bennett AB, Kurman RJ, Lancaster WD. Correlation of cellular atypia and human papillomavirus deoxyribonucleic acid sequences in exfoliated cells of the uterine cervix. *Obstet Gynecol* 1986;68:508–512.

62. MacNab JCM, Walkinshaw SA, Cordiner JW, Clements JB. Human papillomavirus in clinically and histologically normal tissue of patients with genital cancer. *N Engl J Med* 1986;315:1052–1058.

63. McKay M. Subsets of vulvodynia. *J Reprod Med* 1988;33:695–698.

64. Melchers WJG, Schift R, Stolz E, Lindeman J, Quint WGV. Human papillomavirus detection in urine samples from male patients by the polymerase chain reaction. *J Clin Microbiol* 1989;27:1711–1714.

65. Mitao M, Nagai N, Levine RU, Silverstein SJ, Crum CP. Human papillomavirus type 16 infection: a morphological spectrum with evidence for late gene expression. *Int J Gynecol Pathol* 1987;5:287–296.

66. Nuovo GJ, Friedman D. *In situ* hybridization analysis of HPV DNA segregation patterns in lesions of the female genital tract. *Gynecol Oncol* 1990;36:256–262.

67. Obalek S, Jablonska S, Favre L, Orth G. Condylomata acuminata in children: Frequent association with human papillomaviruses responsible for cutaneous warts. *J Am Acad Dermatol* 1990;23:205–213.

68. Ostrow RO, Zachow KR, Niimura M, et al. Detection of papillomavirus DNA in human semen. *Science* 1986;231:731–733.

69. Reid R, Greenberg M, Jenson AB, et al. Sexually transmitted papillomaviral infections I. The anatomic distribution and pathologic grade of neoplastic lesions associated with different viral types. *Am J Obstet Gynecol* 1987;156:212–222.

70. Sato S, Okagaki T, Clark BA, et al. Sensitivity of koilocytosis, immunocytochemistry, and electron microscopy as compared to DNA hybridization in detecting human papillomavirus in cervical and vaginal condyloma and intraepithelial neoplasia. *Int J Gynecol Pathol* 1987;5:297–307.

71. Schneider A, Kraus H, Schuhmann R, Gissmann L. Papillomavirus infection of the lower genital tract: detection of viral DNA in gynecological swabs. *Int J Cancer* 1985;35:443–448.

72. Schneider A, Kirchmayr R, deVilliers EM, Gissmann L. Subclinical human papillomavirus infections in male sexual partners of female carriers. *J Urol* 1988;140:1431–1434.

73. Shah KV, Buscema J. Genital warts, papillomaviruses, and genital malignancies. *Annu Rev Med* 1988;39:371–379.

74. Steinberg BM, Topp WC, Schneider PS, Abramson AL. Laryngeal papillomavirus infection during clinical remission. *N Engl J Med* 1983;308:1261–1264.

75. Sutton GP, Stehman FB, Ehrlich CE, Roman A. Human papillomavirus deoxyribonucleic acid in lesions of the female genital tract: evidence for type 6/11 in squamous carcinoma of the vulva. *Obstet Gynecol* 1987;70:564–568.

76. Syrjanen K, Mantyjarvi R, Vayrynen M, et al. Human papillomavirus (HPV) infections involved in the neoplastic process of the uterine cervix as established by prospective follow-up of 513 women for two years. *Eur J Gynaecol Oncol* 1987;8:5–14.

77. Syrjanen K, Saarikoski S, Vayrnrm M, Syrjanen S, Saastamoinen J, Castren O. Factors associated with the clinical behavior of cervical human papillomavirus infections during a long-term prospective follow-up. The cervix and lower female genital tract. 1989;7:131–143.

78. Taxy JB, Gupta PK, Gupta JW, Shah KV. Anal cancer: microscopic condyloma and tissue demonstration of human papillomavirus capsid antigen and viral DNA. *Arch Pathol Lab Med* 1989;113:1127–1131.

79. Twiggs LB, Okagaki T, Clark B, Fukushima M, Ostrow RS, Faras AJ. A clinical, histopathologic, and molecular biologic investigation of vulvar intraepithelial neoplasia. *Int J Gynecol Pathol* 1988;7:48–55.

80. Waeckerlin RW, Potter NJ, Cheatham GR. Correlation of cytologic, colposcopic, and histologic studies with immunohistochemical studies of human papillomavirus structural antigens in an unselected patient population. *Am J Obstet Gynecol* 1988;158:1394–1402.

81. Walker J, Bloss JD, Liao S, Berman M, Bergen S, Wilczynski SP. Human papillomavirus genotype as a prognostic indicator in carcinoma of the uterine cervix. *Obstet Gynecol* 1989;74:781–785.

82. Wilczynski SP, Bergen S, Walker J, Lia SY, Pearlman LF. Human papillomaviruses and cervical cancer: analysis of histopathologic features associated with different viral types. *Hum Pathol* 1988;19:697–704.

83. Zderic SA, Carpiniello VL, Malloy TR, Rando RF. Urological applications of human papillomavirus typing using deoxyribonucleic acid probes for the diagnosis and treatment of genital condyloma. *J Urol* 1989;141:63–65.

84. Crum CP, Roche JK. Molecular pathology of the lower female genital tract: the papillomavirus model. *Am J Surg Pathol* 1990;14:26–33.

85. Crum CP, Nuovo GJ. The cervix. In: Sternberg SS, Mills JT, eds. *Surgical pathology of the female reproductive system and peritoneum.* New York: Raven Press; 1990.

86. Nuovo GJ, Delvenne P, MacConnell P, Neto C, Chalas E, Mann W. Correlation of histology and detection of human papillomavirus DNA in vulvar cancers. *Gynecol Oncol* 1991;43:275–280.

87. Amortegui AJ, Meyer MP. *In situ* hybridization for the diagnosis and typing of human papillomavirus. *Clin Biochem* 1990;23:301–306.

88. Beckmann AM, Myerson D, Daling JR, Kiviat NB, Fenoglio CM, McDonald JM. Detection and localization of human papillomavirus DNA in human genital condylomas by *in situ* hybridization with biotinylated probes. *J Med Virol* 1983;16:265–273.

89. Burns J, Graham AK, Frank C, Fleming KA, Evans MF, McGee JO. Detection of low copy human papillomavirus DNA and mRNA in routine paraffin sections of the cervix by non-isotopic *in situ* hybridization. *J Clin Pathol* 1987;40:865–869.

90. DelMistro A, Braunstein JD, Halwer M, Koss LG. Identification of human papillomavirus types in male urethral condylomata acuminata by *in situ* hybridization. *Hum Pathol* 1987;18:936–940.

91. Friedrich EG, Wilkinson EJ, Fu YS. Carcinoma *in situ* of the vulva: a continuing challenge. *Am J Obstet Gynecol* 1980;136:830–835.

92. Gal AA, Saul SH, Stoler MH. *In situ* hybridization analysis of human papillomavirus in anal squamous cell carcinoma. *Mod Pathol* 1989;2:439–443.

93. Gupta J, Gendelman HE, Naghashfar Z, et al. Specific identification of human papillomavirus type in cervical smears and paraffin sections by *in situ* hybridization with radioactive probes: a preliminary communication. *Int J Gynecol Pathol* 1985;4:211–218.

94. Gupta J, Pilotti S, Rilke F, Shah K. Association of human papillomavirus type 16 with neoplastic lesions of the vulva and other genital sites by *in situ* hybridization. *Am J Pathol* 1987;127:206–215.

95. Gupta J, Pilotti S, Shah KV, DePalo G, Rilke F. Human papillomavirus-associated early vulvar neoplasia investigated by *in situ* hybridization. *Am J Surg Pathol* 1987;11:430–434.

96. Jacquemier J, Penault F, Durst M, et al. Detection of five different human papillomavirus types in cervical lesions by *in situ* hybridization. *Hum Pathol* 1990;21:911–917.

97. Kettler AH, Rutledge M, Tschen JA, Buffone G. Detection of human papillomavirus in nongenital Bowen's disease by *in situ* hybridization. *Arch Dermatol* 1990;126:777–781.

98. Milde K, Loning T. Detection of papillomavirus DNA in oral papillomas and carcinomas: application of *in situ* hybridization with biotinylated HPV 16 probes. *J Oral Pathol* 1986;15:292–296.

99. Nuovo GJ, MacConnell P, Forde A, Delvenne P. Detection of human papillomavirus DNA in formalin fixed tissues by *in situ* hybridization after amplification by PCR. *Am J Pathol* 1991;139:847–854.

100. Nuovo GJ. Determination of HPV type by *in situ* hybridization analysis: a comparative study with Southern blot hybridization and the polymerase chain reaction. *J Histotech* 1992;15:99–104.

101. Padayachee A, van Wyk CW. Human papillomavirus (HPV) DNA in focal epithelial hyperplasia by *in situ* hybridization. *J Oral Pathol Med* 1991;20:210–214.

102. Pilotti S, Gupta J, Stefanon B, dePalo G, Shah KV, Rilke F. Study of multiple human papillomavirus related lesions of the lower female genital tract by *in situ* hybridization. *Hum Pathol* 1989;20:118–123.

103. Pilotti S, Rilke F, Shah KV. Immunohistochemical and ultrastructural evidence of papilloma virus infection associated with *in situ* and microinvasive squamous cell carcinoma of the vulva. *Am J Surg Pathol* 1984;8:751–756.

104. Pao CC, Lai CH, Wu SY, Young KC, Chang PL, Soong YK. Detection of human papillomaviruses in exfoliated cervicovaginal cells by *in situ* DNA hybridization analysis. *J Clin Microbiol* 1989;27:168–173.

105. Schneider A, Meinhardt G, Kirchmayr R, Schneider V. Prevalence of human papillomavirus genomes in tissues from the lower genital tract as detected by molecular *in situ* hybridization. *Int J Gynecol Pathol* 1991;10:1–14.

106. Syrjanen S, Syrjanen K, Mantyjarvi R, et al. Human papillomavirus (HPV) DNA sequences demonstrated by *in situ* hybridization in serial paraffin embedded cervical biopsies. *Arch Gynecol* 1986;239:39–48.

107. Syrjanen SM, Syryjanen K, Lamberg MA. Detection of human papillomavirus DNA in oral mucosal lesions using *in situ* DNA hybridization applied on paraffin sections. *Oral Surg Oral Med Oral Pathol* 1986;62:660–667.

108. Syrjanen SM, Syrjanen KJ, Lamberg MA. Detection of human papillomavirus DNA in oral mucosal lesions using *in situ* DNA hybridization applied on paraffin sections. *Oral Surg Oral Med Oral Pathol* 1986;62:660–667.

109. Syrjanen S, Saastamoinen J, Chang F, Ji H, Syrjanen K. Colposcopy, punch biopsy, in situ DNA hybridization, and the polymerase chain reaction in searching for genital human papillomavirus infections in women with normal pap smears. J Med Virol 1990;31:259–266.

110. Vallejos H, DelMistro A, Kleinhaus S, Braunstein JD, Halwer M, Koss LG. Characterization of human papilloma virus types in condylomata acuminata in children by in situ hybridization. Lab Invest 1987;56:611–615.

111. Wolber R, Dupuis B, Thiyagartnam P, Owen D. Anal cloacogenic and squamous carcinomas: comparative histologic analysis using in situ hybridization for human papillomavirus DNA. Am J Surg Pathol 1990;14:176–182.

112. Doorbar J, Evans HS, Coneron I, Crawford LV, Gallimore PH. Analysis of HPV-1 E4 gene expression using epitope-defined antibodies. *J Virol* 1988;825–833.

113. Jenison SA, Firzlaff JM, Langenberg A, Galloway DA. Identification of immunoreactive antigens of human

papillomavirus type 6b by using Escherichia coli expressed fusion proteins. *J Virol* 1988;62:2115–2123.

114. Chin MT, Hirochika R, Hirochika H, Broker TR, Chow LT. Regulation of human papillomavirus type 11 enhancer and E6 promoter by activating and repressing proteins from the E2 open reading frame: functional and biochemical studies. *J Virol* 1988;62:2994–3002.

115. Nuovo GJ, Crum CP, Silverstein SJ. Papillomavirus infection of the uterine cervix. *Microbial Pathogenesis* 1987;3:71–78.

116. Bauer HM, Ting Y, Greer CE, et al. Genital human papillomavirus infection in female university students as determined by a PCR-based method. *JAMA* 1991;265:472–477.

117. Nuovo GJ, Nuovo MA, Cottral S, Gordon S, Silverstein SJ, Crum CP. Histological correlates of clinically occult human papillomavirus infection of the uterine cervix. *Am J Surg Pathol* 1988;12:198–204.

118. Shibata D, Fu YS, Gupta JW, Shah KV, Arnheim N, Martin WJ. Detection of human papillomavirus in normal and dysplastic tissue by the polymerase chain reaction. *Lab Invest* 1988;59:555–559.

119. Tidy JA, Vousden KH, Farrell PJ. Relation between infection with a subtype of HPV 16 and cervical neoplasia. *Lancet* 1989;i:1225–1227.

120. Moy RL, Eliezri YD, Nuovo GJ, Zitelli ZA, Bennett RG, Silverstein SJ. Squamous cell carcinoma of the finger is associated with human papillomavirus type 16 DNA. *JAMA* 1989;261:2669–2673.

121. Eliezri YD, Silverstein SJ, Levine RU, Nuovo GJ. Occurrence of human papillomavirus DNA in cutaneous squamous and basal cell neoplasms. *J Am Acad Dermatol* 1990;23:836–842.

122. McDonnell JM, Mayr AJ, Martin WJ. DNA of human papillomavirus type 16 in dysplastic and malignant lesions of the conjunctiva and cornea. *N Engl J Med* 1989;320:1442–1446.

123. Stone MS, Noonan CA, Tschen J, Bruce S. Bowen's disease of the feet. Presence of human papillomavirus 16 DNA in tumor tissue. *Arch Dermatol* 1987;123:1517–1520.

124. Nuovo GJ, Pedemonte BA. Human papillomavirus types and recurrent genital warts. *JAMA* 1990;263:1223–1226.

125. Nuovo GJ, Babury R, Calayag P. Human papillomavirus types and recurrent cervical warts in immunocompromised women. *Mod Pathol* 1991;4:632–636.

126. Byrne MA, Wickenden C, Coleman DV. Prevalence of human papillomavirus types in the cervices of women before and after laser ablation. *Br J Obstet Gynaecol* 1988;95:201–202.

127. Colgan TJ, Percy ME, Suri M, Shier RM, Andrews DF, Lickrish GM. Human papillomavirus infection of morphologically normal cervical epithelium adjacent to squamous dysplasia and invasive carcinoma. *Hum Pathol* 1989;20:316–319.

128. Gallahan D, Muller M, Schneider A, et al. Human papillomavirus type 53. *J Virol* 1989;63:4911–4912.

129. Riva J, Sedlacek T, Cunnane, Mangan C. Extended carbon dioxide laser vaporization in the treatment of subclinical papillomavirus infection of the lower genital tract. *Obstet Gynecol* 1989;73:25–30.

130. Roman A, Fife K. Human papillomavirus DNA associated with foreskins of normal newborns. *J Infect Dis* 1986;153:855–860.

131. Schneider A, Sterzik K, Buck G, deVilliers EM. Colposcopy is superior to cytology for the detection of early genital human papillomavirus infection. *Obstet Gynecol* 1988;71:236–241.

131. Siegmund M, Wayss K, Amtmann E. Activation of latent papillomavirus genomes by chronic mechanical irritation. *J Gen Virol* 1991;72:2787–2789.

132. Tidy JA, Parry GCN, Ward P et al. High rate of human papillomavirus type 16 infection in cytologically normal cervices. *Lancet* 1989;i:434.

133. Nuovo GJ, Becker J, MacConnell P, Margiotta M, Comite S, Hochman H. Histological distribution of PCR-amplified HPV 6 and 11 DNA in penile lesions. *Am J Surg Pathol* 1992;16:269–275.

134. Nuovo GJ, Gallery F, MacConnell P. Histological distribution of PCR amplified HPV 6 and 11 in vulvar lesions. *Mod Pathol* 1992;5:444–448.

135. Nuovo GJ, Blanco JS, Leipzig S, Smith D. Human papillomavirus detection in cervical lesions histologically negative for cervical intraepithelial neoplasia: correlation with Pap smear, colposcopy, and occurrence of cervical intraepithelial neoplasia. *Obstet Gynecol* 1990; 75:1006–1011.

136. Yogo Y, Kitamura T, Sugimoto C, et al. Isolation of a possible archetypal JC virus DNA sequence from non-immunocompromised individuals. *J Virol* 1990;64: 3139–3143.

137. Telenti A, Aksamit AJ, Proper J, Smith TF. Detection of JC virus DNA by polymerase chain reaction in patients with progressive multifocal leukoencephalopathy. *J Infect Dis* 1990;162:858–861.

138. Hair L, Nuovo GJ, Powers J. Atypical progressive leukoencephalopathy in AIDS patients. *Hum Pathol* 1992;23:663–667.

139. Aksamit AJ, Major EO, Ghatak NR, Sidhu GS, Parisi JE, Guccion JG. Diagnosis of progressive multifocal leukoencephalopathy by brain biopsy with biotin labeled DNA:DNA *in situ* hybridization. *J Neuropathol Exp Neurol* 1987;46:556–566.

140. Shulman HM, Hackman RC, Sale GE, Meyers JD. Rapid cytologic diagnosis of cytomegalovirus interstitial pneumonia on touch imprints from open-lung biopsy. *Am J Clin Pathol* 1982;77:90–94.

141. Myerson D, Hackman RC, Nelson JA. Widespread presence of histologically occult cytomegalovirus. *Hum Pathol* 1984;15:430–439.

142. McClintock JT, Thaker SR, Mosher M, et al. Comparison of *in situ* hybridization and monoclonal antibodies for early detection of cytomegalovirus in cell culture. *J Clin Microbiol* 1989;27:1554–1559.

143. Josey YM, Nahmias A, Naib ZM. Viral and virus-like infections of the female genital tract. *Clin Obstet Gynecol* 1969;12:161–168.

144. Garcia AGP, Fonseca EF, Marques RL, Lobato YY. Placental morphology in cytomegalovirus infection. *Placenta* 1989;10:1–18.

145. Alford CA, Stagno S, Pass RF. Natural history of perinatal cytomegalovirus infection. *Excerpta Med* 1980; 77:125–147.

146. Nuovo M, Gallery F, Nuovo GJ. Association of viral coinfection with pneumocystis pneumonia in AIDS patients. *Diagn Mol Pathol* 1993;2:200–209.

147. Telenti A, Marshall WF, Smith TF. Detection of Epstein-Barr virus by polymerase chain reaction. *J Clin Microbiol* 1990;28:2187–2190.

148. Inoue N, Harada S, Miyasaka N, Oya A,Yanagi K. Analysis of antibody titers to Epstein-Barr virus nuclear antigens in sera of patients with Sjogren's syndrome and with rheumatoid arthritis. *J Infect Dis* 1991;164:22–28.

149. Bruner JM. Oligonucleotide probe for herpes virus: use in paraffin sections. *Mod Pathol* 1990;3:635–638.

150. Iwasaka T, Yokoyama M, Hayashi Y, Sugimori H. Combined herpes simplex virus type 2 and human papillomavirus type 16 or 18 deoxyribonucleic acid leads to oncogenic transformation. *Am J Obstet Gynecol* 1988; 159:1251–1255.

151. Kaufman RH, Bornstein J, Adam E, Burek J, Tessin B, Adler-Storthz K. Human papillomavirus and herpes simplex in vulvar squamous cell carcinoma *in situ*. *Am J Obstet Gynecol* 1988;158: 862–871.

151a. Kjaer SK, deVilliers EM, Haugaard BJ, et al. Human papillomavirus, herpes simplex virus and chemical cancer incidence in Greenland and Denmark. A population-based cross-sectional study. *Int J Cancer* 1988;41: 518–524.

152. Nuovo GJ. Human papillomavirus, herpes simplex virus and chemical cancer incidence in Greenland and Denmark. A population-based cross-sectional study. *Int J Cancer* 1988;41:518–524.

153. Prezioso PJ, Cangiarella J, Lee M, et al. Fatal disseminated infection with human herpesvirus-6. *J Pediatr* 1992;120:921–923.

5
PCR *in situ* Hybridization

The previous chapters describe the theory and methodology of PCR and *in situ* hybridization. Despite the widespread use of both PCR and *in situ* hybridization in the last 10 years, it has proved difficult to combine the two. If this combination could be achieved, DNA would be amplified in intact cells and then visualized with *in situ* hybridization. The first person to report a successful PCR *in situ* hybridization technique was Dr. Ashley Haase. This pioneer work, which employed radioactive probes, multiple primer pairs, and a fixed cell suspension, was described in 1990 (1). Although Dr. Haase's work was an important beginning, the need to use cell suspensions limited the utility of this particular methodology. Furthermore, the apparent need for multiple primer pairs limited the applicability of this PCR *in situ* technique. It is difficult and costly to generate multiple sequence-specific primers for highly polymorphic targets. Clearly, a more useful approach would utilize paraffin-embedded tissues and a single primer pair. The ability to perform PCR *in situ* hybridization with paraffin-embedded tissue has been problematic for several reasons. Target DNA must be exposed without destroying tissue morphology. Optimal concentrations of essential reagents, such as primers, magnesium, and the DNA polymerase, must be determined. Furthermore, if the reaction is to be carried out directly on glass slides, loss of tissue adherence and tissue drying would have to be circumvented.

It is amazing to this writer how quickly the field of PCR *in situ* hybridization has advanced since the first edition of this book in 1992. There are several reasons for this rapid advancement. First, many groups have published protocols and data based on PCR *in situ* hybridization (2–26; see Chapter 1 for a more detailed list). The fact that a variety of groups have published such results demonstrates that the technique is becoming more reliable and reproducible. Second, the search to understand the nature of the HIV-1 virus and to create effective treatments for the epidemic of AIDS has prompted investigators to elucidate the mode of transmission of the disease and to develop better ways to monitor its course and its response to antiretroviral therapy. The natural history of the infection in the lymph nodes and peripheral blood mononuclear cells (PBMCs) and the pathogenesis of several manifestations of HIV-1-related disease, such as AIDS dementia and AIDS-related myopathy, could best be addressed by PCR *in situ* hybridization in conjunction with *in situ* PCR; this is discussed in detail in Chapter 9. The final area that needs to be addressed to make *in situ* PCR a commonly used laboratory tool, in this author's opinion, is the manufacturing of "user friendly" *in situ* PCR dedicated machines and associated kits. I believe that with this development the *in situ* PCR procedure will become as straightforward as are Southern blot or *in situ* hybridization with the many commercially available kits now on the market. I have tested most (perhaps all) of the thermal cyclers now being touted as being useful for *in situ* PCR. Although there is no doubt that the system will be improved upon, in my experience the thermal cycler *in situ* PCR 1000 from Perkin-Elmer is the most user friendly of the group. The workshops I have participated in with people with no experience with *in situ* PCR where we did the technique with this apparatus has demonstrated a success rate of over 80% using the start-up protocol presented in Chapter 6.

The discussion of the detection of PCR-amplified DNA is divided into two parts: (i) direct incorporation with a reporter molecule in which the hybridization step is not done (called *in situ* PCR) and (ii) detection of the unlabeled PCR product with a labeled probe using a hybridization step (called PCR *in situ* hybridization). It will become clear that the two methods require different conditions. More importantly, although it is well suited to the analysis of cytospin or tissue culture preparations, there are limits to the use of *in situ* PCR for analysis of DNA in tissue sections. However, these limitations become strengths in RT *in situ* PCR where PCR-amplified RNA (cDNA) can be detected with direct incorporation of the labeled nucleotide in tissue sections. RT *in situ* PCR is discussed in Chapter 7, including a detailed description of nonspecific DNA synthesis invariably present during *in situ* PCR in paraffin-embedded tissue sections.

Before beginning the discussion, a review of the strengths and weaknesses of PCR *in situ* hybridization is in order. PCR *in situ* hybridization has three major strengths. First and foremost, one can combine the extreme sensitivity of PCR with the cell-localizing ability of *in situ* hybridization. *In situ* hybridization is less sensitive than filter hybridization techniques and PCR (27–77). There have been many studies comparing the sensitivities of these three techniques often with regard to the detection of viruses associated with infectious diseases, particularly human papillomavirus (HPV) and human immunodeficiency virus (HIV-1). These studies have strongly suggested that (i) PCR, filter hybridization, and *in situ* hybridization are of equivalent sensitivities for productive viral infections, such as HPV in low-grade squamous intraepithelial lesions (SILs) and (ii) latent infection, as routinely noted in HIV-1 infection, and occult or subclinical infection can be detected by PCR or filter hy-

bridization but *not* by *in situ* hybridization (27–77). This reflects the lower copy number of virus associated with these specific entities. The reported detection thresholds of the three techniques vary considerably due, in part, to methodological variations. For example, the hot start modification for PCR improves the detection threshold from about 1,000–5,000 copies to 1 to 10 copies, assuming 1 μg of background nontarget DNA (3,78). The detection threshold for filter hybridization is generally reported to be about 1 copy per 100 cells (27–77). Most groups report detection thresholds for *in situ* hybridization of about ten copies per cell. Claims that one copy per cell can be detected by *in situ* hybridization have been made. In our experience, such reports are in conflict with the general inability to detect latent HIV-1 infection, which is associated with one to a few integrated copies of DNA by *in situ* hybridization (21,23,79–86). Interest in PCR *in situ* hybridization has grown out of the experience that the relatively high detection threshold of *in situ* hybridization is a major limiting factor for its usefulness.

The second strength of PCR *in situ* hybridization relates to the issue of sample contamination in solution phase PCR. Sample contamination, which can lead to false-positive results in PCR and has limited its usefulness as a diagnostic test, is not encountered in PCR *in situ* hybridization because the positive signal is localized to specific areas within the cell. Furthermore, exogenous labeled DNA from the amplifying solution is easily removed from the cells with a high-stringency wash, as discussed in Chapter 3.

The enormous amount of information provided relative to the histologic distribution of the amplified product after PCR *in situ* hybridization is its third major strength. For example, the demonstration that PCR-amplified HIV-1 DNA is restricted to the endocervical aspect of the transformation zone in the cervix suggests that this area is its portal of entry (discussed in Chapter 9). Similarly, the demonstration that matrix metalloprotease (MMP)-9 and -2 mRNA, but not tissue inhibitor of metalloprotease (TIMP)-1 and -2 RNA, as evident from RT *in situ* PCR, are found in cancer cells that are deeply invasive but that TIMP expression is strong in early invasive cancer suggests that the ratio of MMP to TIMP expression is an important element in cancer cell aggressiveness (discussed in Chapter 8). Of course, this information is not provided by solution phase PCR, as nucleic acid extraction precludes the ability to localize the amplified product directly to a specific cell type.

The weakness of PCR *in situ* hybridization, in my opinion, relates to problems encountered in both PCR and *in situ* hybridization. Competing pathways in the PCR can limit its specificity and sensitivity. Furthermore, background signal from the complexing of the probe and nontarget molecules during *in situ* hybridization can lead to false-positive results, as is discussed and illustrated in detail below. The need for controls for every slide to ensure that conditions are optimized for PCR and that background is not causing problems for interpretation of the hybridization signal will continue to be stressed in this manuscript.

Note that the methodologies described in this chapter can be used for either *in situ* PCR in cytospin preparations or for PCR *in situ* hybridization for paraffin-embedded tissue sections, except where indicated.

BEFORE PCR

Preparation of the Glass Slide

Paraffin-embedded tissue or a cellular suspension should be placed on a slide pretreated with organosilane, which is discussed in Chapter 4. It is essential to place more than one tissue section or cytospin per slide, as this will allow for multiple and comparative analyses, including the essential negative and positive controls. The demanding condition of repeated temperature elevations for denaturing that characterize PCR *in situ* hybridization makes it advisable to use silane-coated slides. A tissue adherence rate of over 98% is achieved with silane-coated slides compared with about 75% for tissues pretreated with poly-L-lysine or for Sobo-treated slides.

Fixation of Cells and Tissue

The rules for *in situ* hybridization and tissue fixation have been well worked out as described in Chapter 4. Neutral buffered formalin is the fixative of choice, and I recommend a fixation time of 15 hours to several days. Recall that tissues fixed in solutions that contain picric acid or heavy metals such as mercury are not optimal for PCR or *in situ* hybridization (40, 47, 87–90). As would be expected, these fixatives will not support PCR *in situ* hybridization.

An essential requirement of the fixative for the success of the *in situ* amplification of DNA or RNA concerns the localization of the PCR product at the site of synthesis. This clearly is of paramount importance for *in situ* PCR, and this issue generated a great deal of controversy early in the evolution of the technique. To address the problem of the relationship of fixative type and the migration of the PCR product, we studied PBMCs that were isolated from a Ficoll gradient (Histopaque 1077, Sigma Diagnostics, St. Louis, MO). About 2,000 cells were placed on silane-coated glass slides and then fixed in acetone, 95% ethanol, and 10% neutral buffered formalin (10% formalin in 0.1 M sodium phosphate buffer, pH 7.0) or Bouin's solution (75 parts saturated picric acid, 25 parts 40% formaldehyde in water, and 5 parts glacial acetic acid; pH 1.6). It is important to place a relatively large number of cells on the slide in a cytospin preparation to prevent the amplifying solution from migrating away from the cells to the edge of the plastic coverslip. By placing two cytospins on a slide, direct comparisons of paired experimental conditions were done. A pepsin solution of 2 mg/ml in 0.01 N HCl at room temperature was used for protease digestion; the digestion time is 12 minutes unless otherwise indicated. The PCR primers were specific for a region of the proto-oncogene *bcl-2*, which should be detectable in all PBMC, and for the nucleocapsid

Table 5-1. *Sequences of the primers used in the study of effects of fixation chemistry and protease digestion in* in situ *PCR with PBMC[a]*

Target	Sequence	Product size (base pairs)

HPV 16
  Primer 1 nt[a] 110
  Primer 2 nt 559
	5'-CAGGACCCACAGGAGCGACC
	5'-TTACAGCTGGGTTTCTCTAC
		449

bcl-2
  Primer 1 nt 2,779
  Primer 2 nt 3,283
	5'-CATTTCCACGTCAACAGAATTG
	5'-AGCACAGGATTGGATATTCCAT
		504[b]

Measles
  Primer 1 nt 115
  Primer 2 nt 549
	5'-GTGTAATAATATCATGGTTA
	5'-CTCTCCAATCTAAATTCACC
		434

[a]nt, Nucleotide position of primer 5' end in the GenBank sequence. The EBV-specific primers used in this study were published by Saito et al. (9).
[b]Kindly supplied by Dr. Ernest Kawasaki.

region of the measles virus, which would not have a target in the PBMC. Also employed was a Burkitt's lymphoma cell line (ATCC VR-603) that contains Epstein-Barr virus (EBV) DNA. These were mixed with oral squamous cells (from an EBV-negative individual) to demonstrate the specificity of the *in situ* PCR signal when using EBV-specific primers. Primer sequences are listed in Table 5-1.

The technique used in these experiments was direct incorporation *in situ* PCR. The actual methodology, including the hardware and the amplifying solution, is discussed in detail below. Under optimal conditions one would anticipate that each of the PBMC would have an intense signal with the *bcl-2* primers, as they all contain the target of interest and should avidly incorporate digoxigenin dUTP during the PCR phase of the procedure. The alkaline phosphatase-based colorimetric detection used chromagen nitro-

blue tetrazolium (NBT), which, in the presence of 5-bromo-4-chloro-3-indolylphosphate (BCIP), yields a dark purple–blue precipitate as the marker of a positive cell. The counterstain, nuclear fast red (ONCOR, Gaithersburg, MD), stains nuclei and cytoplasm a pale pink and in a black and white photograph will be faintly visible.

In situ PCR was performed in our initial experiments on PBMC fixed for 5 minutes, 15 hours, or 39 hours in acetone, 95% ethanol, buffered formalin, or Bouin's solution to determine the importance of fixation chemistry and duration on the *in situ* detection of PCR-amplified DNA. Each experiment was repeated at least once, and the tabulated values are the mean scores; the range of variation between replicate experiments was 0% to 9%, and the highest standard deviation was 9. The results are compiled in Table 5-2. Figure 5-1 shows

Table 5-2. *The effect of fixation chemistry and duration on the detection of amplified* bcl-2 *DNA in PBMC with no protease digestion*

Fixation time	Detection of *bcl-2*–amplified DNA (% positive cells)			
	Formalin	Acetone	95% ETOH	Bouin's
5 Min	5	2	14	0
15 Hr	0	15	31	0
39 Hr	ND[a]	0	9	ND[a]

[a]Not done.

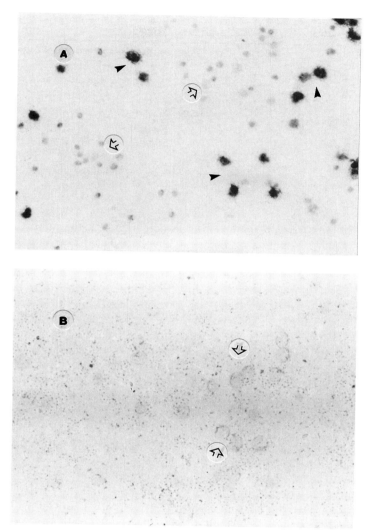

Figure 5-1. *Effect of fixation and protease digestion on detection of amplified* bcl-2 *DNA in PBMC during* in situ *PCR: short fixation time.* These PBMC were fixed for 5 minutes in buffered formalin. A signal was evident in about 25% of the cells after PCR *in situ* with direct incorporation of digoxigenin dUTP (**A;** *arrowheads,* positive cells; *open arrows,* negative cells). No signal was evident if the PBMC were pretreated with trypsin (2 mg/ml) for 15 minutes (**B;** *open arrow,* negative cells). The poor preservation of nuclear detail in B is typical of overdigestion with the protease.

representative photomicrographs. Note that under none of the tested conditions did *all* PBMC have detectable amplified *bcl-2* DNA.

The low and variable detection efficiencies suggested that the fixation conditions may limit cell permeation by a key PCR reagent. To test this hypothesis, the cells were digested with 2 mg/ml of pepsin for 12 minutes prior to *in situ* PCR. The results for *in situ* PCR after protease digestion are listed in Table 5-3. The percentage of positive cells after protease digestion increased to 100% after 15 hours fixation with formalin but decreased to 0% for the acetone- and ethanol-fixed cells as well as for the cells

Table 5-3. *The effect of fixation chemistry and duration on the detection of amplified* bcl-2 *DNA in PBMC with pepsin digestion*

	Detection of bcl-2 amplified DNA (% positive cells)[a]			
Fixation time/pepsin conditions	Formalin	Acetone	95% ETOH	Bouin's
5 Min/2 mg/ml, 12 min	0	0	0	0
5 Min/20 μg/ml, 1 min	1	0	0	—
5 Min/20 μg/ml, 2 min	35	0	0	—
5 Min/20 μg/ml, 5 min	0	0	0	—
15 Hr/2 mg/ml, 12 min	100	0	0	0

[a]Compare these data with those in the first two rows of Table 5-2.

fixed for 5 minutes in buffered formalin (Fig. 5-2). Cells fixed in Bouin's solution did not, as expected, demonstrate a positive signal under any tested reaction conditions.

It was noted that cell morphology was poorly preserved after fixation with acetone, 95% ethanol, or 5 minutes in formalin followed by protease digestion. This suggests that absence of signal may simply reflect loss of the PCR product, as well as many of the other cellular components, out of the nucleus. To address this issue, *in situ* PCR was performed after various fixation times, and the times of protease digestion varied from 1 to 12 minutes with the pepsin concentration decreased to 20 μg/ml and 2 μg/ml. As evident in Table 5-3, no increase in the percentage of positive cells with decreased protease digestion time and concentration was evident for the acetone- or ethanol-fixed cells. However, the positive cells after 5 minutes of fixation in buffered formalin increased from 0% with 12 minutes digestion by 2 mg/ml of pepsin to 35% with a 3-minute digestion by 20 μg/ml pepsin. Note the subsequent decrease to 0% for the formalin-fixed cells if the protease time was increased to 5 minutes, indicating a narrow optimal threshold.

Alternative explanations for the low detection efficiencies in most experiments are that the DNA was amplified and migrated out of the cell or that the fixation conditions blocked *in situ bcl-2* amplification. Obviously, this is a critical distinction. If the first hypothesis is correct one would predict that for the acetone- and ethanol-fixed cells most of the PCR product would migrate to the amplifying solution. If the latter hypothesis is correct, then one would anticipate that the amplifying solution would contain little PCR product after the *in situ* PCR procedure was finished. To test these hypotheses, the amplifying solution was retrieved, its DNA separated on an agarose gel, and the DNA sequences that contained digoxigenin were detected using the antidigoxigenin–alkaline phosphatase conjugate. Furthermore, the DNA was extracted from the fixed cells after *in situ* PCR and run on the gel beside the DNA obtained from the amplifying solution. As is evident in Fig. 5-3, these analyses showed that there was marked *bcl-2*–specific amplification evident in the solution from the cells fixed for either 5 minutes or 15 hours in acetone or ethanol with no protease digestion step, although only rare positive cells were noted with microscopic examination. Interestingly (if not amazingly), no detectable signal was evident in the solution from the cells fixed in buffered formalin for either 5 minutes without digestion (conditions giving 5% positive cells) or, more importantly, 15 hours with protease digestion (conditions giving 100% positive cells). Clearly, these data suggest that *in situ* PCR amplification is occurring in the cells fixed in acetone or ethanol but that most of the product leaves the nucleus and diffuses into the amplifying solution. However, in the cells fixed for 15 hours in buffered formalin and proteased, *all* of the detectable signal localized to the nucleus.

Note that the bands that contained digoxigenin dUTP were evident at 504 base pairs and

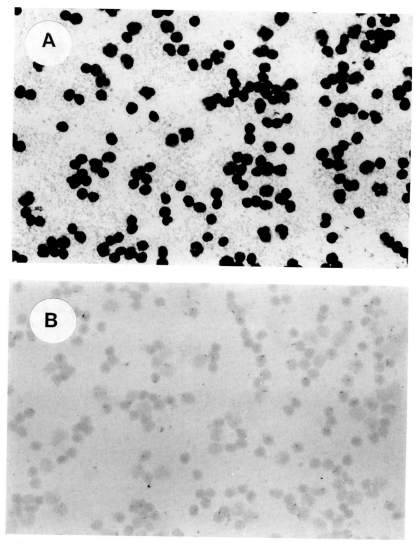

Figure 5-2. *Effect of fixation and protease digestion on detection of amplified* bcl-2 *DNA in PBMC: long fixation time.* The PBMC were fixed for 15 hours in buffered formalin. A weak signal was evident in most cells after PCR *in situ* with direct incorporation of digoxigenin dUTP (not shown). An intense signal was evident in each cell if the PBMC were pretreated with trypsin (2 mg/ml) for 15 minutes (**A**). The signal was eliminated if $MgCl_2$ was omitted from the amplifying solution (**B**); the optimal concentration of $MgCl_2$ in this experiment was 4.5 mM. Note the much better preservation of the cellular detail in B (compare with Fig. 5.1B), indicating that the negative *in situ* PCR result was not due to overdigestion.

hybridized to the probe (Fig. 5-3). This certainly strongly suggests that the bands corresponded to the *bcl-2* target. To demonstrate that the signal seen in cells fixed for 15 hours in buffered formalin and then digested was target specific (as well as the signal seen in the amplifying solution for cells fixed in acetone or ethanol), the digoxigenin-tagged DNA was analyzed for sequences homologous to the internal fragment of the *bcl-2* gene using a ^{32}P-labeled probe and

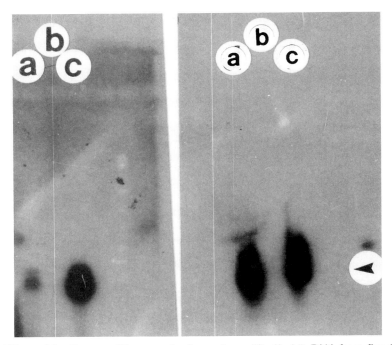

Figure 5-3. *Effect of fixation conditions on the loss of amplified* bcl-2 *DNA from fixed PBMC.* **Left:** Southern blot analysis of the supernatant amplifying solution recovered from selected *in situ* PCR reactions described in Tables 5-2 and 5-3. *Lanes a* report on acetone fixation for 5 minutes (2% positive by *in situ* PCR); *lanes b* on formalin fixation for 5 minutes (5% positive by *in situ* PCR); and *lanes c* on ethanol fixation for 5 minutes without protease treatment (14% positive by *in situ* PCR). The *arrowhead* indicates the position of the 500 base pair band of *Hin*dIII digest of lambda DNA, evident on ethidium staining. Note that a band (in which the digoxigenin has incorporated) of the expected size for the *bcl-2* product is evident in the amplifying solution from the cells fixed in acetone and ethanol but not for the formalin-fixed cells. To demonstrate that the digoxigenin-containing product was indeed the *bcl-2* PCR product, Southern blot hybridization was performed using a ^{32}P-labeled internal oligo-probe. **Right:** Autoradiograph demonstrating that the digoxigenin-labeled PCR product was indeed specific for *bcl-2*. These results suggest that there is migration of the PCR product from the cell to the amplifying solution if one uses denaturing fixatives such as acetone or ethanol. This migration is not evident if the cells are fixed with a cross-linking fixative such as buffered formalin, assuming that the cells have not been overdigested with a protease.

Southern blot hybridization. The digoxigenin-containing bands demonstrated an intense signal with the internal ^{32}P-labeled probe, demonstrating that the DNA did indeed correspond to amplified *bcl-2* gene fragment (9).

Another experiment that demonstrated the difference between ethanol- and formalin-based fixatives with PCR *in situ* hybridization was based on vulvar warts. These lesions contain HPV 6 or HPV 11. We took a vulvar wart that contained HPV 6, divided it into equal parts, and then fixed the tissue for either 6 or 15 hours in 10% buffered formalin or in an ethanol-based

fixative (Histocyte). PCR *in situ* hybridization was then performed using primers specific for HPV 6 and a full-length, biotin-labeled HPV 6 probe. Three observations were evident for the buffered formalin-fixed tissue: (i) the number of positive cells and the intensity of the hybridization signal in the positive cells were much greater after PCR *in situ* hybridization versus *in situ* hybridization; (ii) the signal for both techniques localized, as expected, to the nucleus; and (iii) the optimal protease digestion time for *in situ* hybridization and PCR *in situ* hybridization were each 30 minutes. These were not the observations evident with the tissue fixed in an ethanol-based fixative. Rather, it was observed that (i) the number of positive cells was decreased after PCR *in situ* hybridization versus *in situ* hybridization; (ii) the signal localized to the nucleus after *in situ* hybridization but tended to be cytoplasmic after PCR *in situ* hybridization; and (iii) the optimal protease digestion time for HPV as detected by *in situ* hybridization was 15 to 30 minutes in pepsin; this is in contrast to the results with the *alu* probe, with which optimal results were obtained with no protease digestion (see Chapter 4). The results for the ethanol-fixed tissue are depicted in Fig. 5-4. The cytoplasmic localization of the HPV, a nuclear-based target, and the weakened signal seen after PCR *in situ* hybridization suggests that the cellular integrity is being compromised with the repeated denaturation steps. Presumably, there is concomitant migration of the amplicon in the ethanol-fixed tissue during the PCR step. Alternatively, the results may reflect migration of the amplicon that is not dependent on cellular integrity. It is difficult to understand why two different targets (HPV and the repetitive *alu* sequence) should have such different optimal protease digestion times with ethanol-fixed tissues. It does underscore another advantage of formalin-fixed material: similar optimal protease digestion times for a wide variety of targets, especially if formalin fixation is at least 15 hours.

In summary, these experiments demonstrated that pretreatment with a cross-linking fixative and protease digestion are needed under the conditions defined in this study to detect the target in every cell containing the DNA sequence. The length of fixation treatment is critical. As is discussed in much more detail in the chapter on RT *in situ* PCR, 4 hours of fixation in 10% buffered formalin with protease digestion allows for successful *in situ* PCR. However, longer fixation times allow for a broader window of optimal protease digestion for successful *in situ* PCR. Acetone and ethanol fixatives, which, as Greer et al. (87,88) demonstrated, allow for successful solution phase PCR, led to detection rates of *bcl-2* much below

100% after *in situ* PCR because the PCR product was primarily detectable in the amplifying solution. Thus, neither ethanol nor acetone fixation appears consistently to prevent migration of the amplified product out of the nucleus. In contrast, prolonged formalin fixation creates a "barrier" that greatly inhibits migration of PCR product. Formalin (i.e., formaldehyde) extensively polymerizes proteins and can cross-link nucleic acids (90–103), which probably is the essential step for limiting PCR product diffusion. The extent of migration limitation is striking based on several observations. First, amplified cDNAs corresponding to human and viral mRNAs localize to specific cytoplasmic and nuclear compartments (see Fig. 1-1). Second, amplified HPV 16 DNA is detectable in most paraffin-embedded SiHa cells even after the nucleus is sectioned; presumably some positive cells retain the one copy of HPV 16 after part of their nuclei is removed by the microtome blade. Third, as just described, no amplified product is detectable in the amplifying solution after *in situ* PCR with formalin-fixed, digested cells when all of the cells have intense nuclear staining. Theoretical models to explain the effect of the type of fixative and the migration patterns of the PCR-amplified product are presented in Figs. 5-5 and 5-6.

Formalin cross-linkage apparently can also inhibit entry of at least one key reagent, necessitating a protease digestion step. These effects are evident even after 5 minutes of fixation, as the detection rate under these conditions without proteolysis was about 5% and no product was detectable in the amplifying solution. However, protease digestion did not increase the detection rate to 100% for *in situ* PCR of cells fixed for 5 minutes in formalin. The detection of PCR product in the amplifying solution after longer pepsin digestion for cells fixed for 5 minutes suggested that too few cross-links had been formed to create a robust "migration barrier," although destruction of cell morphology and release of the target into the solution is also likely. It appears that protease digestion may be a necessary step for *in situ* PCR when cross-linking fixatives are used.

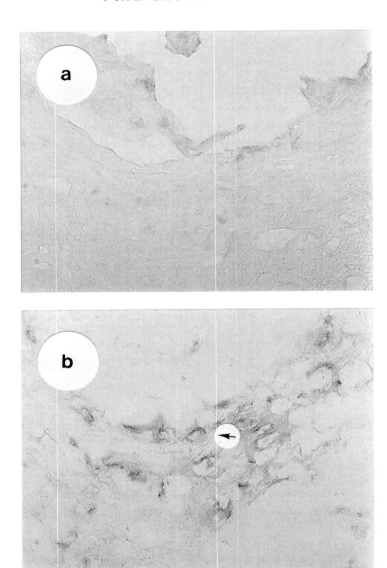

Figure 5-4. *The effect of ethanol fixation on the localization of the signal during PCR* in situ *hybridization and standard* in situ *hybridization.* The tissue is a vulvar wart that contains HPV 6. A weak signal was evident after *in situ* hybridization with no protease digestion (**a**); the signal was stronger after 15 minutes of digestion in pepsin (2 mg/ml), even though tissue morphology was poor (**b**). Note that the signal did not localize well to the nucleus (*arrow*). This is in marked contrast to another target—the repetitive *alu* sequence—where the strongest hybridization signal is seen with no protease digestion and does localize to the nucleus (see Chapter 4). The signal with *in situ* hybridization was stronger if cycling was done without the *Taq* polymerase and localized to the nucleus and cytoplasm (**c**); this suggests a "protease-like" enhancement of the signal with repeated cycling (there was no protease digestion). The signal was not much enhanced after PCR *in situ* hybridization (**d**), again in contrast to formalin-fixed tissue.

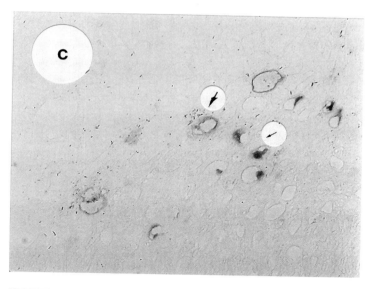

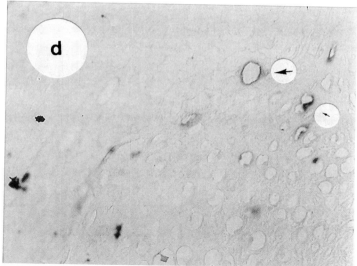

Figure 5-4. *Continued.*

We have compared 5 minute fixation–no protease digestion with 15 hour fixation–15 minute trypsin digestion for the following primers: HPV 16 (in SiHa cells); HPV 18 (in HeLa cells); EBV (in a Burkitt's lymphoma cell line); HPV consensus primers (kindly supplied by Dr. Michele Manos, Cetus Corporation) and Pap smears from women with biopsy-proven cervical SILs; HIV-1 SK38 and SK39 primers (kindly provided by Dr. John Sninsky, Cetus Corporation) and PBMC from patients with AIDS; measles (in measles-infected HeLa cells); and *bcl-2*, as outlined above. In almost all cases results were superior with the longer fixation times and protease step. A notable exception was HIV-1 with which an equivalent colorimetric reaction was evident after 5 minutes of fixation and no protease digestion. The explanation for this difference with HIV-1 detection is not clear, although it is doubtful that it is related to the cell type, as we used lymphocytes in both the EBV and *bcl-2* experiments. It is also doubtful that the explanation involves

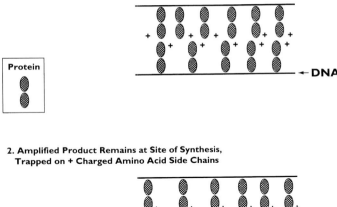

1. Formalin Fixation Creates Protein - DNA Links

Protein

2. Amplified Product Remains at Site of Synthesis, Trapped on + Charged Amino Acid Side Chains

PCR Product

DNA

Figure 5-5. *A proposed model for the apparent lack of migration of the PCR product during* in situ *PCR with formalin-fixed tissues.* The striking localized distribution of the PCR product in RT *in situ* PCR and the apparent inability to detect the product in the amplifying solution after *in situ* PCR in formalin-fixed tissues and cells (see Fig. 5-4) suggests that formalin fixation is inhibiting migration of the PCR product from its site of synthesis. This model proposes that this may reflect a process akin to an ion-exchange type resin where the negatively charged DNA is trapped on the positive charged residues of some of the amino acids.

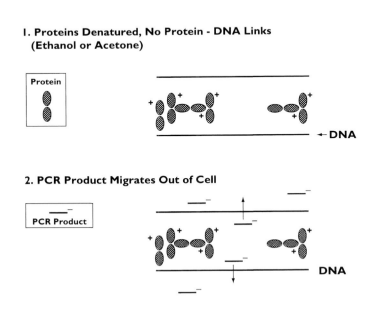

1. Proteins Denatured, No Protein - DNA Links (Ethanol or Acetone)

Protein

DNA

2. PCR Product Migrates Out of Cell

PCR Product

DNA

Figure 5-6. *A proposed model for the migration of the PCR product during* in situ *PCR with ethanol- and acetone-fixed cells and tissues.* Acetone and ethanol fixation support solution phase PCR. However, they do not allow for optimal *in situ* PCR, apparently because some of the product migrates out of the cell. It is speculated that this may reflect the inability of these noncross-linking fixatives to create the migration barrier that is putatively formed after formalin fixation (see Fig. 5-5).

the physical state of the target DNA in the sense that both HIV-1 and HPV 16 in SiHa cells are integrated in the host genome. Other protocols for *in situ* PCR do suggest short fixation times and either no or minimal protease digestion; interestingly, these are usually for the detection of HIV-1 (15,18,19). Although these shorter fixation times will allow for successful *in situ* PCR, I strongly recommend much longer times (8 hours to several days), as they allow for a much broader range of optimal protease digestion time with RT *in situ* PCR and decreases the risk of overprotease digestion. Furthermore, shorter fixation times can give confusing results with the negative controls for RT *in situ* PCR due to varying sensitivities of different cell types to the protease. For example, squamous cells are more resistant to protease than lymphoid cells (Fig. 6-8). With short fixation times and after DNase digestion, the DNA repair-based signal may be lost in the lymphoid cells but still present in the squamous cells. This phenomenon is not evident after prolonged fixation.

To summarize cell and tissue processing:

1. Fix tissues or cells in 10% buffered formalin for 8 hours to several days.
2. Embed the tissue in paraffin or place three cell suspensions on a silane-coated slide. Place at least 1,000 cells per 1-cm area.
3. Place three 4-μm sections on a silane-coated glass slide.
4. Deparaffinize tissue by 5 minute wash in xylene, 5 minute wash in 100% ethanol, and then air dry.

PROTEASE DIGESTION

As is stressed in Chapter 7, which deals with RT *in situ* PCR, the most important variable for successful detection of PCR-amplified cDNA is the protease time. For tissues fixed for 4 to 24 hours in buffered formalin, the optimal protease digestion time for RT *in situ* PCR could vary from 30 to 90 minutes or, rarely, longer. Because different tissues can vary in their optimal protease digestion time even if fixed for the same amount of time, only trial and error

would determine the precise optimal time. This is an important practical consideration, as, for most tissues, one does not know the exact time that the tissue was fixed. This constraint is much less important for PCR *in situ* hybridization. If one would use the same type of tissue for PCR *in situ* hybridization, then 20 to 30 minutes of digestion in the protease (pepsin, 2 mg/ml) would reproducibly give good results even if the fixation time in 10% buffered formalin varies from 8 hours to several days. This is analogous to what was described for standard *in situ* hybridization, as discussed in Chapter 4 (compare the data in Table 4-1 with those in Tables 3-2 and 3-3).

The next issue concerns the type of protease to use. Most of my experience is with pepsin and trypsin because these are the proteases I have used for standard *in situ* hybridization. One reason I prefer pepsin and trypsin is that a simple increase in the pH from 2 to 7 with a DEPC water or Tris solution rinse will greatly diminish the functioning of the protease. Furthermore, in my experience, pepsin or trypsin digestion preserves tissue and cell morphology better than proteinase K, another commonly used protease.

Due to many requests, I have tried digestion with proteinase K for *in situ* PCR and PCR *in situ* hybridization. These tests may provide useful information because the potential depurinating effect of the low pH (2.0) of the pepsin or trypsin digestion could conceivably have contributed to the results noted with the different fixatives and *bcl-2* in the PBMC experiments detailed above. Thus, the experiments with *in situ* PCR and the ethanol and buffered formalin-fixed PBMC were re-done with proteinase K digestion. No differences were observed in the rates of *bcl-2*–positive cells compared with the results of pepsin digestion, including a detection rate of 100% for 15 hour formalin-fixed, proteinase K–digested cells. We have noted similar good results with proteinase K digestion and PCR *in situ* hybridization. My advice is to choose one of these proteases and use it exclusively in order to become familiar with its nuances. Here is an important word of caution to those who use proteinase K.

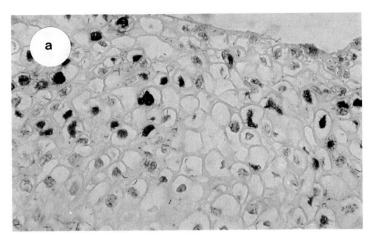

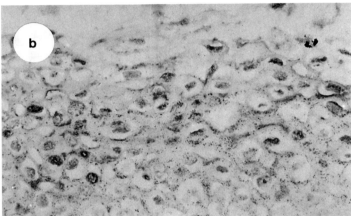

Figure 5-7. *The deleterious effect of "dry heat" on* in situ *hybridization and PCR* in situ *hybridization.* In the first experiment, a cervical SIL that contained HPV 16 was subjected to proteinase K digestion and *in situ* hybridization. A strong signal was evident in many cells (**a**). The signal was markedly reduced if the air-dried slide was subjected to 10 minutes at 94°C after the protease digestion step (**b**). In a similar experiment, SiHa cells were subjected to 15 cycles of PCR; one group of cells was covered by amplifying solution minus the *Taq* polymerase, and the other group was exposed to "dry heat." After the cycling, standard *in situ* hybridization was done using the *alu* probe. A strong signal was evident in the cells that were covered with the amplifying solution (**c**). The signal was lost after repeated exposure to dry heat (**d**). The poor morphological detail evident after dry heat suggests that it has a synergistic effect with protease digestion, enhancing the likelihood of overdigestion. Similar results were noted after PCR *in situ* hybridization. These experiments demonstrate that protease inactivation by dry heat should not be used with either PCR *in situ* hybridization or *in situ* hybridization.

Do not dry heat inactivate the protease after the digestion step. Dry heat will greatly diminish the signal for either PCR *in situ* hybridization or standard *in situ* hybridization (Fig. 5-7). Similarly, for those using the Perkin-Elmer *in situ* PCR thermal cycler 1000, do not leave any of the samples without amplifying solution. This prolonged dry heat will greatly diminish the hybridization signal, even for targets with high copy numbers (Fig. 5-7).

Overdigestion with a protease is easily recognized as loss of cytoplasmic and nuclear detail and occurs with destruction of cellular proteins, which provide most of the skeleton of the

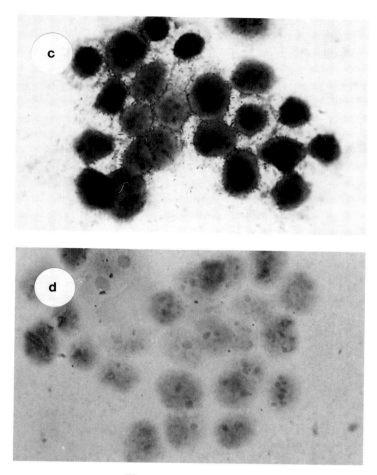

Figure 5-7. *Continued.*

cytoplasm and nucleus in the form of the nuclear matrix. If one uses nuclear fast red as the counterstain, overdigestion by protease can be recognized as the absence of the light pink color in the nucleus and cytoplasm. Instead, one sees the basement membranes forming a prominent labyrinth-type pattern as their glycoproteins are more resistant to the proteases. This problem is more likely to be encountered with tissues that have been fixed for short periods of time (< 4 hours). In such cases, a spectrum of changes will be evident that will correlate with the extent of overdigestion. At the first stages of overdigestion, nuclear-based signals will localize to the cytoplasm (Fig. 5-8). Note that the signal after PCR *in situ* hybridization that corresponds to the HPV 16 DNA in SiHa cells, which is nuclear based, is seen to migrate to the cytoplasm if the protease digestion time is increased from 30 to 60 minutes; note the associated loss of nuclear detail. Clearly, the cytoplasmic membrane is more resistant to protease than the nuclear membrane. After 90 minutes of protease digestion, the signal and cell morphology is completely lost, owing to the loss of the integrity of the cytoplasmic membrane. This simple experiment reminds us that the striking migration of the amplicon with *in situ* PCR evident with cross-linking fixatives is true *only* with optimal protease digestion. Another factor that reflects different stages of over digestion with the protease is evident in biop-

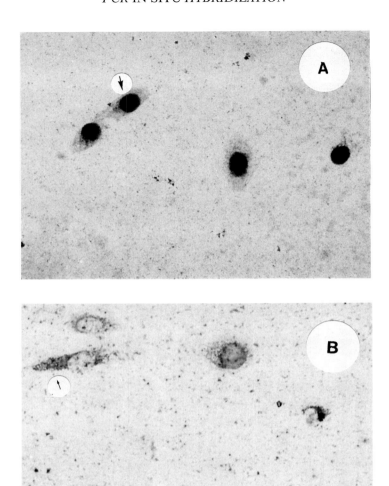

Figure 5-8. *Migration of the amplicon during PCR* in situ *hybridization with formalin-fixed cells and protease overdigestion.* Hot start PCR *in situ* hybridization was done using HPV-16-specific primers in SiHa cells. A strong nuclear-based signal (*arrow*) is seen after 30 minutes of protease digestion (**A**). The signal migrated to the cytoplasm (*small arrows*) if the protease digestion time was increased to 60 minutes (**B**). Note the poor nuclear detail and lack of nuclear signal (*large arrow*) indicative of overdigestion. The signal and cell morphology were both lost after 120 minutes of protease digestion (not shown).

sies fixed for short time periods. At the initial stages of protease overdigestion, the cells toward the center may have no signal and lose their morphology, whereas a signal is evident in the cells at the edge of the tissue (Fig. 5-9). This is seen because the cells toward the edge of the tissue will be more strongly fixed than those in the center with short fixation times, owing to the relatively poor penetrability of formalin. With longer protease digestion times, the signal and the morphologic detail are lost in the cells toward the periphery of the tissue as well (Fig. 5-9). When any evidence of overdigestion is evident, decrease the time of protease digestion by 50% and re-do the experiment.

Insufficient protease treatment is one potential cause of failure to achieve a hybridization signal in PCR *in situ* hybridization. However, in my experience, unless one inadvertently forgets the protease digestion step or uses inactive protease, inadequate protease digestion is an uncommon cause of a lack of a signal with PCR *in situ* hybridization. Alternatively, inadequate protease digestion is the *most* common cause for poor signal with RT *in situ* PCR, as discussed in Chapter 7.

To prepare the protease, it is recommended that one use either pepsin or trypsin at 2 mg/ml (stock solution is 20 mg + 9.5 ml water + 0.5 ml of 2N HCl). After preparing the solution, I freeze 1-ml aliquots and store them at –20°C. The activity of the protease stored at –20°C was studied as a function of time with *in situ* PCR and tissue sections. After 10 days of storage at –20°C, there is measurably decreased activity of the pepsin or trypsin as defined by the amount of protease time required for an optimal signal with nonDNased tissue sections during *in situ* PCR when using paraffin-embedded tissue sections (G. J. Nuovo, *unpublished observations, 1993*). Thus, it is recommended that after one prepares the protease and stores it at –20°C, any remaining protease solution be discarded after 1 week. This restriction does not apply to proteinase K, which maintains its activity for a much longer period of time when stored as a 10× stock solution of 20 mg/ml at either 4°C or –20°C. After thawing the pepsin, use it immediately as its activity decreases when kept at room temperature.

Thus, for PCR *in situ* hybridization, incubate the tissues or cytospins in 2 mg/ml of pepsin or trypsin. Although one can prepare 50 ml of the protease digestion solution, it is more economical to use 300 μl of the solution per slide and place the solution directly on the tissue. The slides may be incubated in a humidity chamber at room temperature. To inactivate the protease, remove the slides from the humidity chamber and hold them vertically to allow the protease solution to run off

the slide. Then flood the slide with 1 ml of a solution of 0.1 M Tris HCl and 0.1 M NaCl (pH 7.5). The slides may then be placed in the humidity chamber and immersed in another 1 ml of the 0.1 M Tris HCl and 0.1 M NaCl (pH 7.5) solution. After 1 minute, flood the slides with 1 ml of 100% ethanol and then air dry.

I am sometimes questioned about residual protease activity after this wash step. This is obviously of potential concern as residual protease activity could destroy the *Taq* polymerase. However, the "solid surface" provided by the glass slide allows one to wash off the protease efficiently and easily. Support of this statement was demonstrated by the ability to amplify a variety of viral target DNAs and RNAs in over 50 consecutive tissues known to contain the target with no evidence of residual protease activity (G. J. Nuovo, *unpublished observations, 1995*).

To summarize protease digestion:

1. Digest in pepsin solution at room temperature for 25 minutes (pepsin solution = 9.5 ml H_2O, 0.5 ml 2 NHCl, and 20 mg pepsin or trypsin; 1-ml aliquots of the pepsin can be stored at –20°C for 1 week and thawed when needed).
2. Wash in 0.1 M Tris HCl and 0.1 M NaCl for 1 minute, 100% ETOH, then air dry.

The Amplifying Solution

During the amplification steps of the PCR *in situ* hybridization technique, one needs to be concerned with the composition of the amplifying solution and with the physical necessities of keeping the solution over the tissue and preventing it from drying out. Concentrations for some of the reagents in the amplifying solution for PCR *in situ* hybridization vary compared with those for standard PCR. The buffer is an exception; one may use the same buffer in PCR *in situ* hybridization as with solution phase PCR. I prefer the buffer included in the GeneAmp kit from Perkin-Elmer. Its composition (of the 10× stock solution) is

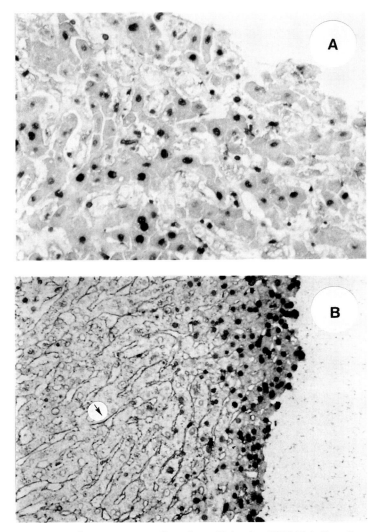

Figure 5-9. *The spectrum of protease overdigestion with* in situ *PCR.* This liver tissue showed an intense nuclear signal with *in situ* PCR after 30 minutes of protease digestion (**A**). After 60 minutes of digestion, the signal was still evident in the cells toward the periphery but lost in the cells toward the center (**B,C**). Note the loss of nuclear detail and prominent basement membranes (**B**, *arrow*) toward the center. This reflects the greater degree of fixation in the cells toward the periphery due to relatively poor diffusion of formalin. No signal is evident after 90 minutes of digestion, and cellular morphology was destroyed (**D**).

100 mM Tris HCl, pH 8.3
500 mM KCl
0.01% gelatin

The most advantageous $MgCl_2$ concentration was determined by subjecting the 15-hour-fixed, pepsin-digested PBMC to *in situ* PCR in 0, 1.5, 4.5, 6.0, and 9.0 mM $MgCl_2$ for seven cycles and 20 cycles each. No signal was evident when the amplifying solution contained no $MgCl_2$ or 9.0 mM $MgCl_2$. A weak signal was evident only after 20 cycles for 1.5 and 6.0

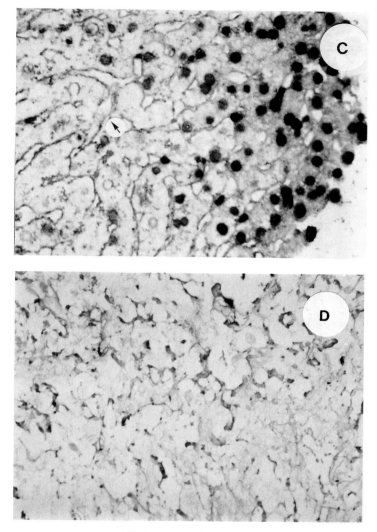

Figure 5-9. *Continued.*

mM $MgCl_2$ compared with the intense signal seen with 4.5 mM $MgCl_2$ (see Fig. 5-2). Thus, for *in situ* PCR with the PBMC and the conditions defined above, 4.5 mM $MgCl_2$ was found to be optimal. We have also found that 4.5 mM $MgCl_2$ gives an intense signal with *in situ* PCR and PCR *in situ* hybridization using a known positive control for the following target-specific primers: HPV 16, HPV 18, HPV consensus primers, HIV-1, HIV-2, measles, EBV, hepatitis C, tumor necrosis factor mRNA, a variety of gelatinase mRNAs, JC virus, and par- vovirus RNA. It appears from these data that 4.5 mM $MgCl_2$ is satisfactory for a wide variety of viral and human RNAs and DNAs when using PCR *in situ* hybridization or RT *in situ* PCR.

A similar optimizing study of *Taq* DNA polymerase concentration showed that a signal was evident with 2.0 U/10 μl of amplifying solution but not with 0.4 or 0.2 U/10 μl. This statement applies to both *in situ* PCR and PCR *in situ* hybridization. Because 2.0 U/10 μl of *Taq* DNA polymerase is about ten times higher than that required for standard PCR, it was reasoned that some of the enzyme might be sequestered on the glass slide. The addition of 1 mg/ml of bovine serum albumin (BSA), which could block enzyme adsorption, resulted in a strong signal even with 0.2 U of *Taq* DNA polymerase/10 μl.

Therefore, the recommended composition of the amplifying solution for PCR *in situ* hybridization is

	Final concentration	Volume (per 50 μl)
Magnesium	4.5 mM	9 μl (25 mM stock)
Buffer (Reaction buffer of the GeneAmp PCR reagent kit, Perkin-Elmer Cetus [PE], Norwalk, CT [PCR buffer II])	10 mM Tris HCl, ph 8.3; 50 mM KCl; 0.001% gelatin	5 μl (PE buffer II)
dNTPs (Prepared by adding 25 μl each of dATP, dCTP, dGTP, and dTTP [each 10 mM stock] and 100 μl water)	200 μM	8 μl (PE dNTP)
Primers	0.5–1.0 μM	3 μl (20 μM stock), (5' and 3' combined)
BSA	0.06%	1.5 μl (2% stock)
Taq polymerase	5 U/50 μl	1 μl
Water		23.5 μl

An important point about the amplifying solution needs to be stressed: Some PCR buffers contain $MgCl_2$. For example, the PCR buffer I from the Perkin-Elmer kit contains 15 mM $MgCl_2$. If this buffer is used, there will be 6 mM $MgCl_2$ in the amplifying solution, which is suboptimal. I have assisted investigators who could not get successful PCR *in situ* hybridization results until it was realized that they were using 6 mM of magnesium in the amplifying solution.

It is at this point that the *in situ* PCR and PCR *in situ* hybridization techniques diverge. Specifically, for *in situ* PCR the labeled reporter molecule is added to the amplifying solution. For PCR *in situ* hybridization this is not done as the label is attached to the probe that is complexed to the amplified PCR product during the hybridization steps of the technique. The optimal concentration of the labeled nucleotide to be used for *in situ* PCR varies markedly with the specific molecule. We have studied optimal conditions for direct incorporation of ^{3}H, ^{32}P, ^{35}S, biotin, and digoxigenin. These data are presented in Chapter 6 and discussed in Chapter 8 because *in situ* PCR is the foundation for the start-up protocol and for the detection of RNAs with the RT *in situ* PCR technique. Suffice it to say at this stage that the optimal concentration of digoxigenin dUTP relative to the concentration of the dTTP is 10 μM/200 μM.

We have adjusted the primer concentration and studied the effects on the signal with PCR *in situ* hybridization. These studies were done with HPV-16-specific primers and low-grade SILs that contain this type of HPV. These studies showed a slight increase in the intensity of the hybridization signal with increasing concentrations from 1 to 10 μM. However, the increase in intensity above 1 μM was minimal, and, given the increased potential for mispriming and primer oligomerization with increasing primer concentration (see Chapter 3), it is recommended to use 1 μM of each of the primers in the amplifying solution.

The Hot Start Maneuver

The final critical point with regard to PCR *in situ* hybridization is that the hot start maneuver *must* be used. The inhibition of mispriming that occurs secondary to withholding an essential ingredient of the PCR reaction until the reaction temperature is above its Tm is required for two important events:

1. Detecting a single-copy target with PCR *in situ* hybridization
2. Using a single primer pair.

Each of these important points is illustrated in Fig. 5-10. The latter point is the next topic of discussion.

Single Versus Multiple Primer Pairs

The topic of diffusion of the amplified product away from its site of origin in the cell has led some investigators to explore the use of multiple primer pairs. Haase et al. (1) described a procedure for PCR amplification that required multiple primer pairs. These primers dictated the synthesis of overlapping fragments that could form a complex of over 1,500 base pairs, which, Haase et al. (1) theorized, would not pass through the nuclear membrane, whereas the individual 450 base pair fragments were membrane permeant. Chiu et al. (22) also described the need for multiple primer pairs in order to obtain a signal with PCR *in situ* hybridization. Our group confirmed these observations using SiHa cells, which contain one copy of HPV 16 DNA, and PCR *in situ* hybridization (Fig. 5-10) (3).

To study the effects of the hot start modification on PCR *in situ* hybridization, formalin-fixed, paraffin-embedded SiHa cells were chosen. This cell line contains one copy of HPV 16 DNA. Five different primer pairs each specific for HPV 16 were used. The sequence of these primers is listed in Table 5-4. Note that each primer pair dictates the synthesis of a fragment of about 500 base pairs. Importantly, each fragment has about a 60 base pair overhang with the adjacent fragment. This will allow for "interamplicon" hybridization. The end result is that each fragment should hybridize to the next and will produce one large fragment whose size will be 1,190 base pairs long.

We compared the results for PCR *in situ* hybridization in the SiHa cells using cold start conditions and primers 1 to 7, hot start conditions and primers 1 and 2, and cold start conditions and primers 1 and 2. As shown in Fig. 5-10, no signal was noted when primers 1 and 2 were used under cold start conditions. A signal was evident when primers 1 to 7 were used under cold start conditions. The strongest signal was obtained if primers 1 and 2 were used under hot start conditions. The question re-

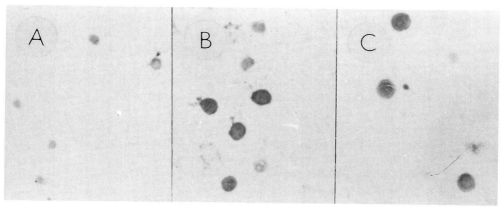

Figure 5-10. *The importance of the hot start maneuver to the sensitivity of PCR* in situ *hybridization.* SiHa cells are derived from a cervical carcinoma, and they contain one copy of HPV 16 DNA per cell. The HPV DNA is not detectable with standard *in situ* hybridization or PCR *in situ* hybridization done under cold start conditions with a single primer pair (**A**). A signal is evident under cold start conditions if multiple primer pairs are used (**C**). However, the signal is stronger if the reaction is done on the same glass slide using a single primer pair and the hot start maneuver to PCR *in situ* hybridization (**B**).

Table 5-4. *Oligoprimers used for amplification of HPV 16 DNA in cells in formalin-fixed tissues*

Primer	Position of first nucleotide	Sequence
PV1 (5')	110	CAGGACCCACAGGAGCGACC
PV2 (3')	559	TTACAGCTGGGTTTCTCTAC
PV3 (5')	501	CCGGTCGATGTATGTCTTGT
PV4 (3')	956	ATCCCCTGTTTTTTTTTCCA
PV5 (5')	898	GGTACGGGATGTAATGGATG
PV6 (3')	1,357	CCACTTCCACCACTATACTG
PV7 (5')	1,300	AGGTAGAAGGGCGCCATGAG

mains: Why is the hybridization signal greater with standard PCR *in situ* hybridization when multiple primer pairs are used? Perhaps decreased permeability of the larger fragment is important, assuming that the degree of fixation of the cells was not adequate to inhibit diffusion of the amplified DNA. Alternatively, and more likely, perhaps increasing the number of primer pairs in standard PCR *in situ* hybridization increases the amount of specific amplification, albeit not as well as a single primer pair with the hot start modification. Whatever the explanation, the observation that PCR *in situ* hybridization signal is greater with a single primer pair and the hot start modification than with multiple primer pairs and standard conditions demonstrates the importance of the hot start modification when analyzing for DNA using PCR *in situ* hybridization. It was emphasized in Chapter 3 that the hot start modification is also essential for detection of DNA targets with *in situ* PCR when using cytospin (nonheated) preparations, again due to inhibition of mispriming. Specific direct incorporation of the reporter nucleotide with hot start *in situ* PCR for DNA targets using tissue sections can also be achieved if one uses frozen, fixed sections that lack the primer-independent DNA repair pathway invariably present in paraffin-embedded sections. It may be useful to restate that the hot start modification is *not* necessary for RT *in situ* PCR. The reason for the latter observation is that DNase digestion, which is the cornerstone of RT *in situ* PCR, eliminates the nonspecific pathways of mispriming as well as DNA repair. Mispriming is apparently the major factor that inhibits target-

specific amplification when the hot start maneuver is not used.

There are a variety of ways to achieve hot start *in situ* PCR. The way I prefer is manual hot start, where all reagents but the *Taq* polymerase are initially placed over the sample. The *Taq* polymerase is added when the aluminum block reaches at least 55°C. Chemical hot start was discussed in Chapter 3 and is summarized later in this chapter.

To summarize the amplifying solution:

1. Use 4.5 mM $MgCl_2$ in the amplifying solution.
2. The recipe for the amplifying solution is

Magnesium	9 μl (25 mM stock)
Buffer (reaction buffer of the GeneAmp PCR reagent kit, Perkin-Elmer Cetus [PE], Norwalk, CT [PCR buffer II])	5 μl (PE buffer II)
dNTPs (prepared by adding 25 μl each of dATP, dCTP, dGTP, and dTTP [each 10 mM stock] and 100 μl water)	8 μl (PE dNTP)
Primers	3 μl (20μM stock) (5' and 3' combined)
BSA	1.5 μl (2% stock)

| *Taq* polymerase | 1 μl |
| Water | 23.5 μl |

3. For PCR *in situ* hybridization and *in situ* PCR for DNA targets (unheated samples), use the hot start maneuver.

THE PCR STEP OF PCR *IN SITU* HYBRIDIZATION AND *IN SITU* PCR

We have discussed the composition of the amplifying solutions that are used for PCR *in situ* hybridization, emphasizing how these solutions differ from those needed for solution phase PCR. In solution phase PCR, one typically adds the sample to the amplifying solution in a 0.5-ml tube and then overlays the solution with mineral oil to prevent evaporation. The thermal conductive properties and close contact between the aluminum heating block and the plastic tube allow for the rapid and effective transfer of heat. For successful PCR *in situ* hybridization, it is necessary to develop an equivalent system for glass slides. In the system that was developed by this author and Ms. Phyllis MacConnell, a plastic coverslip is used to cover the amplifying solution (Figs. 5-11 and 5-12). I use autoclavable polypropylene. The sheets, which are 8.5 by 11 inches, should be cut into smaller sizes of about 4 by 4 inches. Several can be placed inside a plastic box and then autoclaved. The edge can then be cut with scissors and the two sides of the bag gently separated with a sterile needle. The plastic coverslip may be cut to size. For RT *in situ* PCR, place the inner part of each side of the plastic on the sample, as this part would not have RNase from being handled. For most tissue sections, a 1-cm coverslip will suffice. For this sized section, a minimum of 10 μl of amplifying solution should be used. For multiple reactions on a given slide, as is strongly recommended, a hydrophobic pen may be used to separate the different reaction mixtures (Fig. 5-13). This may not be necessary when the sections are placed at least 5 mm apart on the slide. The slide can then be placed inside an aluminum foil "boat," which has two functions.

First, it permits effective and rapid conductivity of heat from the aluminum block of the thermal cycler to the glass slide, although the temperature on the slide 2 will be 2 to 6°C less than on the block (John Atwood, Perkin-Elmer Corp., *personal communication,* 1992). Second, it holds the heated mineral oil over the slide (Figs. 5-11, 5-12). The added oil prevents the amplifying solution from drying out. However, when the coverslip was overlaid with mineral oil the convection currents forming as the oil is heated and then cooled moved the coverslips to and fro. A method was needed to anchor the coverslip onto the slide. Two small drops of nail polish at two ends of the coverslip work well. The nail polish is not affected by the high temperatures and is easily removed after the amplification. It is important *not* to seal the entire perimeter of the coverslip with nail polish or some other adhesive, as the vapor bubbles that form during the denaturing part of the cycle need to escape (Fig. 5-11). This will result in 1- to 5-mm "dead" zones during the PCR step over the tissue that correspond to the bubbles that, of course, lack the amplifying solution. Thus, to summarize, one can do PCR *in situ* hybridization with any standard aluminum block thermal cycler. Materials needed include

1. Several tissue sections on a silane-coated slide
2. An aluminum foil boat (we fashion ours from the large oven liner pans; aluminum wrap tends to leak)
3. Autoclavable polypropylene
4. Nail polish
5. Preheated mineral oil (the oil can be heated in the slots or wells of the thermal cycler).

A commonly asked question concerns the possibility of the amplifying solution diffusing out from under the coverslip. I have studied the mineral oil–amplifying solution interface by adding black dye to the latter. Absolutely no detectable diffusion into the mineral oil was evident throughout the various cycles. Indeed, at times the mineral oil invaginated under the coverslip and "forced" the amplifying solution

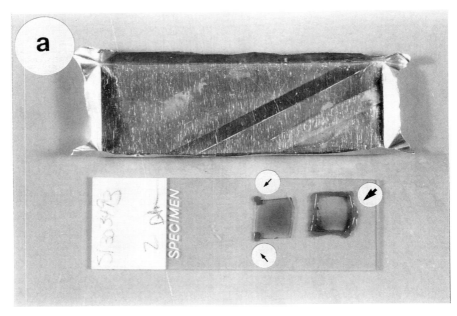

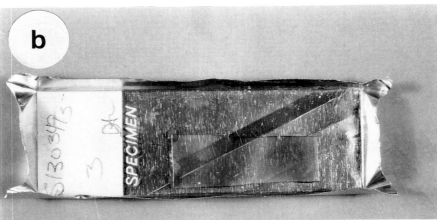

Figure 5-11. *A methodology for doing PCR* in situ *hybridization on the block of a thermocycler: the aluminum boats.* The amplifying solution can be placed over the tissue sections on the silane-coated glass slides. Note how one can perform multiple reactions on the same glass slide by using plastic coverslips cut to size. This allows for the essential positive and negative controls under similar reaction conditions. The coverslip should be anchored with two drops of nail polish (**a**, *small arrows*). Do not encircle the entire coverslip with nail polish, or bubbles will form over the tissue which will prevent amplification in that area; (*large arrow*). By using a larger coverslip, one can do the PCR reaction under one coverslip (**b**). This is especially useful in the start-up protocol and in RT *in situ* PCR. The slides should be placed in an aluminum foil boat (**b**). The boats and slides conduct the heat well, and the boats will retain the mineral oil during the PCR phase of the technique.

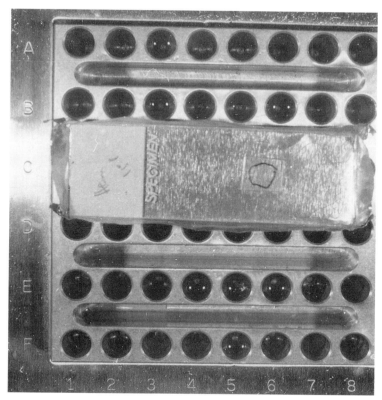

Figure 5-12. *A methodology for doing PCR* in situ *hybridization on the block of a thermocycler: the thermal cycler.* The boat with its slide can be placed directly on the block of the thermal cycler. Drying of the amplifying solution is prevented by adding about 1 ml of heated mineral oil to the boat.

away from an area of the tissue. This was much less likely for large (at least 10-mm) tissue sections or for cytospins that had at least 2,000 cells per 1-cm area. Clearly, the cells in the cytospin or tissue decrease the surface tension of the amplifying solution, which greatly assists in keeping the solution over the specimen. Alternatively, if the cytospin contains too few cells or if the biopsy is too small relative to the size of the coverslip, the amplifying solution may be forced away from the cells toward the edge of the coverslip, and a false-negative result may occur.

As discussed in Chapter 7, DNase digestion, which is the foundation of RT *in situ* PCR, obviates the need for the hot start maneuver. The hot start step is unnecessary because the competing pathway of mispriming that can shift

DNA amplification away from target-specific synthesis is rendered inoperative. Thus, one may add the *Taq* DNA polymerase with the other reagents for RT *in situ* PCR prior to the onset of the PCR step. However, if this procedure is followed for PCR *in situ* hybridization, one will not be able to detect one copy of the target per cell with a single primer pair. Similarly, without the hot start modification for *in situ* PCR with cellular preparations or for frozen, fixed tissues (where the primer-independent pathway is not operative) one will have a high rate of nonspecific incorporation of the reporter molecule. The hot start modification requires withholding the *Taq* DNA polymerase or another key reagent, such as $MgCl_2$, from the amplifying solution at the beginning of PCR. The reagents minus the *Taq* DNA poly-

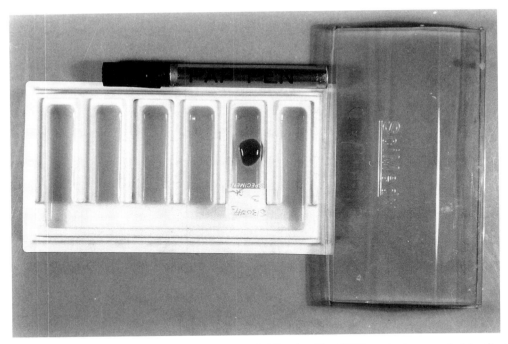

Figure 5-13. *The detection part of PCR* in situ *hybridization.* The PCR product generated *in situ* can be detected after the hybridization step using the digoxigenin-labeled probe by the use of an alkaline-phosphatase-conjugated antibody directed against the digoxigenin. To prevent drying of the antibody solution, which can produce artifactual staining, it is recommended to encircle the tissue using a hydrophobic pen (e.g., "Pap Pen") as well as to use a humidity chamber.

merase are added to the slide, covered with the plastic coverslip, and then anchored with two small drops of nail polish. The slide is then placed in the aluminum boat on the block of the thermocycler. The cycler is programmed to ramp initially to 82°C. When the block reaches 55°C, the edge of the coverslip is gently lifted, the enzyme added in a volume of 1.5 μl per tissue section, the coverslip released, and then the coverslip overlaid with about 1 ml of the preheated mineral oil.

Lifting the coverslip requires some manual dexterity and practice. A common problem initially is that the coverslip curls before the mineral oil overlay can be added. If this occurs, then one is taking too long to add the *Taq* polymerase. This problem can be easily resolved by adding the DNA polymerase when the block reaches 55°C as quickly as possible to each of the sections so that the oil overlay can be added without delay.

There are two alternatives available to those who do not wish to lift the coverslip and add the *Taq* DNA polymerase for the so-called manual hot start maneuver when doing PCR *in situ* hybridization. First, chemical hot start, as described in Chapter 3, can be done using either the *Escherichia coli* single-stranded binding protein (SSBP) or the uracil-*N*-glycosylase system (UNG). The SSBP at optimal concentration inhibits mispriming and primer oligomerization. With the UNG system, the nonspecific pathways are allowed to operate initially, but the resultant DNA that is synthesized is destroyed prior to the initial denaturing step. At temperatures above the Tm of mispriming, UNG does not function, which allows synthesis of the target-specific product.

We examined nonspecific DNA synthesis with the measles primers and PBMC using UNG (kindly provided by Roche Molecular Systems). Because the enzyme can degrade

PCR product containing dUTP, 14 biotin dATP (200 μM) was used in the direct incorporation *in situ* PCR in place of digoxigenin dUTP; the concentration of dUTP was as per the manufacturer's recommendations. As in the experiments with SSBP, all reagents, including the *Taq* DNA polymerase and UNG at various concentrations, were added prior to increasing the temperature of the thermal cycler. The rate of positive cells with the concentration of UNG (1 U) recommended by the manufacturer (Perkin-Elmer Corp.) was greater than 90%, which is equivalent to the nonspecific incorporation rate with *in situ* PCR without the manual hot start maneuver. Similar results were obtained with UNG concentrations from 2 to 5 U per reaction volume. However, the nonspecific detection rate decreased to 50% with 10 U of UNG and to 0% when 20 U of UNG was included in the reaction mixture. This probably relates to adsorption of UNG, as noted with *Taq* polymerase. Recall that the *Taq* adsorption to the glass slide and plastic coverslip can be blocked by BSA, as noted above. The UNG system is technically easier than the manual hot start adaptation to my so-called aluminum boat method. However, it is expensive. Also, if one uses the UNG system for chemical hot start, make certain to remove the solution immediately after the cycling, as the enzyme may degrade the amplicon after the PCR is finished, especially if the slide is brought to room temperature. Another option is to add the *Taq* polymerase to the amplifying solution and preheat this solution to 80°C prior to adding it to the slide. I recommend the latter option to those who are not comfortable lifting the coverslip and adding the *Taq* DNA polymerase. The amplifying solution with the DNA polymerase can be kept in a 0.5-ml GeneAmp tube in a dry bath. The slide is placed in the aluminum boat on the thermal cycler and the temperature of the block set at 60°C. The 10 μl of amplifying solution is then added to each tissue section, the section coverslipped, and the coverslip anchored with two small drops of nail polish. The mineral oil is then added to overlay the surface of the slide. Indeed, this is how the *in situ* PCR thermal cycler 1000 from Perkin-Elmer

achieves hot start, as discussed in Chapter 10. If one is doing direct incorporation of the reporter nucleotide for DNA targets (*in situ* PCR), remember to add the amplifying solution with the *Taq* polymerase immediately *before* placing the slide on the heated assembly tool; even a brief exposure to dry heat can induce the DNA repair pathway, as discussed at length in Chapter 3.

After an initial denaturing step of 94°C for 3 minutes, I recommend 30 to 35 cycles for PCR *in situ* hybridization according to the following protocol: annealing and extension at 55°C for 2 minutes, denaturing at 94°C for 1 minute. The extension stage is omitted because annealing, not primer extension, is the rate-limiting factor in PCR (Dr. Will Bloch, Applied Biosystems, Inc, *personal communication,* 1992). Although the extension step may be useful with very long (>5 kb) targets, in most instances the target is <500 base pairs, and, in my experience, there is no increase in signal by including the 72°C extension step. Indeed, it may be advantageous to omit the extension step as the prolonged times at 72°C may have a deleterious effect on the results for PCR *in situ* hybridization by reducing the concentration of the functional *Taq* DNA polymerase near the end of the 30 to 35 cycles. Although *Taq* polymerase can, of course, withstand high temperatures for extended periods of time, it is very important to realize that it is slowly inactivated at higher temperatures. This problem is accentuated in PCR *in situ* hybridization relative to solution phase PCR, because the much higher surface area to volume ratio of PCR *in situ* hybridization is more likely to heat inactivate with the *Taq* polymerase than with solution phase PCR.

On completion of cycling, the slide is lifted out of the aluminum boat and the coverslip and nail polish removed with a scalpel blade. At this stage, it is best to leave the slide rest vertical for about 1 minute to allow the mineral oil to drain. The remaining oil can be removed by placing the slides in fresh xylene for 5 minutes followed by a 5-minute wash in 100% ethanol. After the slide is air dried, routine *in situ* hybridization may be done (Chapter 4) using the labeled probe.

Protocol 5-1: The Hot Start PCR Step

Note that this protocol assumes one is per-forming PCR *in situ* hybridization on three slides with two reactions per slide:

1. Add the following to a GeneAmp tube
    6.0 μl of the Perkin-Elmer buffer
    11.2 μl of MgCl$_2$ (The GeneAmp buffer, MgCl$_2$ solution [25mM stock stored at 4°C], is from the Perkin-Elmer GeneAmp kit)
    9.2 μl of dNTPs (the dNTPs [prepared by diluting 25 μl of each of the 10 mM stocks of dATP, DCTP, dGTP, and dTTP in 100 μl of sterile water] are from the Perkin-Elmer GeneAmp kit)
    26.6 μl of sterile water
    1.5 μl of 2% bovine serum albumin
    2.0 μl of primer 1 (stock solution 20 μM)
    2.0 μl of primer 2 (stock solution 20 μM)
2. Remove 9.0 μl from the above solution and place in a second GeneAmp tube that is kept on ice.
3. Place 8.0 μl of the amplifying solution over each of the tissue sections (there is enough for 8.2 μl per section, but the 8.0 μl amount is recommended to allow for minor varia-tions in volume).
4. Cover the 8.0 μl with the plastic coverslip; anchor with two small drops of nail polish. Place the slide in the aluminum boat, which is placed on the block of the thermal cycler.
5. Using a soak file of 82°C, start the ther-mal cycler.
6. Add 1.5 μl of the *Taq* DNA polymerase to the 9.0 μl of the solution removed in step 2, mix with the pipette tip, and keep on ice.
7. When the block temperature reaches 55°C, add 1.6 μl of the solution that contains the DNA polymerase to each section by gently lifting the coverslip, then overlay with about 1 ml of the preheated mineral oil stored in the wells or slots of the ther-mal cycler. One should add the *Taq* poly-merase to each of the six sections within 30 seconds in order to prevent curling of the coverslips. Initially, it may be easier to have two people do this manual hot start

maneuver, one to lift the coverslip and the other to add the *Taq*.
8. Abort the soak file, and switch to 94°C for 3 minutes.
9. Cycle at 55°C for 2 minutes and then 94°C for 1 minute for 30 cycles.
10. Remove mineral oil as described above.
11. Perform *in situ* hybridization with the la-beled probe.

THE *IN SITU* HYBRIDIZATION STEP OF PCR *IN SITU* HYBRIDIZATION

General Comments

At this stage, one has a tissue section on a glass slide, and the target DNA of interest has been amplified about 200-fold. The hot start modification greatly inhibited some of the com-peting pathways, especially mispriming, re-ducing the amount of nontarget DNA that was made during the PCR step. In paraffin-embed-ded tissue sections, however, a substantial amount of DNA is made during the PCR step as a consequence of DNA repair. To detect the amplified target-specific DNA and not the DNA made from the nonspecific pathways, a target-specific probe is needed. As discussed at length in Chapter 4, one can use either an oligoprobe or a full-length probe. For standard *in situ* hybridization, the full-length probe is far more advantageous. Its much greater size (100 to 150 base pairs versus 20 to 40 base pairs for an oligoprobe) gives a more intense hybridization signal for two reasons: (i) it con-tains about five times greater label per probe–target complex; and (ii) its longer size greatly increases its Tm, and, thus, the probe–target complex is more stable. Also, the temperature range that separates background from signal is much broader with full-length probes than for oligoprobes. For solution phase PCR, an internal oligoprobe would be used. This is because, as illustrated in Fig. 5-14, the internal oligoprobe would not produce a false-positive signal by detecting DNA synthesized from primer oligomerization.

At this point it may be useful to review the data about primer oligomerization during *in situ* PCR, presented in Chapter 3. It was demonstrated that, with a stringent wash, there was *no* detectable reaction product evident from primer oligomerization in the cell after *in situ* PCR. Thus, it follows that one *can* use a full-length probe, with all its advantages, for detection with PCR *in situ* hybridization. This is a departure from what I recommended in the second edition of this book. My concern then was that most people who do solution phase PCR are not comfortable with the concept that full-length probes are acceptable for detecting the amplicon. Extensive experience has convinced me that primer oligomerization, assuming a high-stringency wash, will not cause a false-positive signal with PCR *in situ* hybridization if a full-length probe is used. The advantages of a full-length probe, as mentioned above, cannot be overstated. Thus, I recommend one of the following strategies:

1. Synthesize a probe of at least 100 base pairs using a second primer pair internal to the primer pair used to generate the amplicon (in effect, a modification of nested PCR, using the internal segment as the probe).
2. Use the full-length probe in all experiments and, in selected runs, the internal oligoprobe to demonstrate the specificity of the former.
3. Use only the full-length probe. As a control, purposely add a large amount of the primer oligomers to the amplifying solution, do PCR, and then do a stringent wash and demonstrate that this is not detected using the full-length probe.

For those who prefer to use the internal oligoprobes, let us discuss some particulars that are important to consider when doing PCR *in situ* hybridization.

Oligoprobe: Definition and Preparation

As indicated in Chapters 2 and 4, an oligoprobe is a labeled short segment of single-stranded DNA. As is evident in Fig. 5-14, the probe is designed such that it corresponds to a region of the amplified product internal to the two primers. Also note that, unlike a full-length double-stranded probe, the oligoprobe will

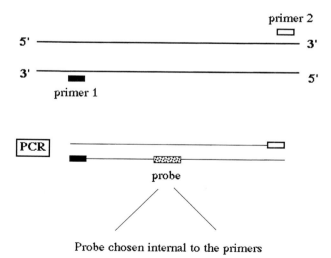

Figure 5-14. *The use of an internal oligoprobe for PCR* in situ *hybridization.* The use an oligoprobe internal to the primers to detect the PCR product eliminates the possibility of detecting product from primer oligomerization. Although this is important in solution phase PCR, it should be appreciated that primer oligomerization apparently does not produce a signal during *in situ* PCR after adequate washing. This allows one to use full-length probes, which have a much greater signal-to-background ratio, with PCR *in situ* hybridization.

detect only one of the two amplified strands.

As discussed in Chapter 4, the most effective way to label an oligoprobe to be used for PCR *in situ* hybridization is by the 3′ tailing method, as per the Genius oligoprobe-labeling kit of Boehringer Mannheim. This is based on the ability of the enzyme terminal transferase to add nucleotides to the 3′ end of a DNA sequence. For the tailing method, one adds a mixture of the unlabeled nucleotides and digoxigenin-labeled dUTP. Depending on the specific unlabeled nucleotides and the ratio of unlabeled to dUTP-labeled digoxigenin, one can add up to 5 dUTP-digoxigenin molecules per oligonucleotide. This gives much greater sensitivity than the 3′ end labeling method, in which only one dideoxy digoxigenin label is added per probe. Let us briefly discuss the rationale behind this statement.

Oligoprobe: Background Versus Signal with the 3′ Labeling Methods

The probe used was the SK19 oligoprobe from Perkin-Elmer that is specific for the *gag* region of HIV-1. The SK19 oligoprobe is 42 nucleotides in size, which makes it large for an oligoprobe. The tissues used were testes and prostate from a man with AIDS. As is discussed in Chapter 9, HIV-1 is routinely detectable in the spermatogonia and their progeny in the testes but is not detectable in the epithelia of the prostate. Thus, any positive signal in the epithelia of the prostate or in cells other than the spermatogonia or their progeny (except for rare macrophages or lymphocytes) must represent nonspecific signal. Two probe cocktails, which are identical except for the way the SK19 oligoprobe was labeled (3′ end labeled or 3′ tailing), were prepared:

Probe cocktail for oligoprobe

1. 10 μl formamide
2. 39 μl sterile water
3. 40 μl 25% dextran sulfate
4. 10 μl 20×SSC
5. 1 μl of the probe

The probe was generated exactly according to the specifications of the Genius labeling kit.

The recipe for the terminal transferase reaction (for oligoprobe tailing) follows:

Synthesis of oligoprobe using 3′ tailing method

1. 4 μl 5× terminal transferase reaction buffer
2. 4 μl CoCl$_2$
3. 1 μl dATP
4. 1 μl digoxigenin dUTP
5. 9 μl SK19 oligoprobe (stock solution contains 100 pmole/100 μl)
6. 1 μl terminal transferase

For 3′ end labeling

1. 4 μl 5× terminal transferase reaction buffer
2. 4 μl CoCl$_2$
3. 1 μl dideoxydigoxigenin dUTP
4. 9 μl SK19 oligoprobe
5. 1 μl terminal transferase
6. 2 μl sterile water

(See Appendix for additional information on the Boehringer Mannheim oligoprobe labeling system.)

Note that for both oligoprobe labeling methods, 9 pmole of the probe is labeled. This is important as the concentration of the oligoprobe may dramatically effect the specificity and sensitivity of the signal, as discussed below. After synthesis, the probe was precipitated using 0.3 M sodium acetate and 2 volumes of 100% ethanol. The pellet was resuspended in 20 μl of sterile water, and 1 μl of this resuspended probe was used per 100 μl of the probe cocktail.

After performing the PCR step using the SK38 and SK39 primers, which correspond to the SK19 oligoprobe, *in situ* hybridization was done on serial sections with the two different probe cocktails. We studied the effects of varying the concentration of the probe, the time of hybridization, and the stringency of the post-hybridization wash on the signal generated with PCR *in situ* hybridization.

Effect of Varying the Concentration of the Probe

The baseline probe concentration of 9 pmole/100 μl is as listed above. We varied the probe concentration from 9 pmole/100 μl to 90 pmole/100 μl. It was noted that the occurrence of nonspecific background signal was strongly related to the probe concentration for the 3' tailed probe in this range. A detectable reaction was evident in the prostatic tissue at the higher concentration of the tailed probe; this must represent the nonspecific background. The background is not evident in the prostatic tissue at the lower probe concentration. The target-specific signal persisted in the spermatogonia with the tailed probe at the lower probe concentration (Fig. 5-15,c). At neither high nor low probe concentration was a signal evident with the end-labeled probe. These data demonstrate that the sensitivity of the tailed probe is greater than the end-labeled probe. However, the specificity of the tailed probe is highly dependent on the probe concentration. *If the concentration of the probe is too high, then a* **high** *rate of false-positive signal will be evident with the tailed probe.* In addition, the false-positive signal with the 3' tailed probe is also highly dependent on the wash conditions, as is now discussed.

Effect of Varying the Stringency of the Posthybridization Wash on the Specificity with the 3' Tailed Probe

As noted above, the nonspecific background is lost, whereas the specific signal is maintained with the tailed oligoprobe if used at a concentration of 9 pmole/100 μl. However, it is important to emphasize that the background with this probe concentration of 9 pmole/100 μl is highly dependent on the stringency of the posthybridization wash. To test this, I varied the stringencies of the posthybridization wash as listed below:

Stringency 1	Stringency 2	Stringency 3
2×SSC	1×SSC	0.2×SSC
0.2% BSA	0.2% BSA	0.2% BSA
45°C	54°C	54°C
10 minutes	10 minutes	10 minutes.

The results of these experiments are given in Fig. 5-15. Note that nonspecific background is evident in the prostate tissue with stringency 1 but not with the conditions listed in stringency 2 or 3. Target-specific signal is evident under the conditions in stringency 2 but is lost with stringency 3. Clearly, stringency 2 allows for the proper balance between the target-specific signal and background. Or, to be more specific, the conditions listed as stringency 2 provide for a temperature that is above the Tm of the nonspecific binding of the probe to cellular elements but below the Tm of the oligo-probe–HIV-1-specific PCR product.

Effect of Varying the Time of Hybridization on the Specificity with the 3' Tailed Probe

After about 2 hours of hybridization, the intensity of the signal reaches maximum and the background is low. With increased times of hybridization, the background signal becomes more evident. After 15 hours of hybridization with an oligoprobe, the background may be so great as to obscure the target-specific hybridization signal. This important point is illustrated in Fig. 5-16.

It is important to stress that the range between background and target-specific signal is much narrower for oligoprobe–target complexes than for the full-length probe–target complexes more typically used with standard *in situ* hybridization, as discussed in detail in Chapter 4. The basis for this statement is illustrated in Fig. 5-17. Note that the ratio of the number of base pairs matches for a full-length probe–target complex versus nonspecific binding of the probe is *much* greater when compared with the equivalent numbers for an oligoprobe. Thus, when one uses a full-length probe, which is usually from 100 to 200 base pairs in size, it is easy to chose a stringency that eliminates the nonspecific signal and maintains the target-specific signal. This is illustrated in Figs. 4-17 and 4-18. Note that an intense signal is evident with the full-length probe using the conditions of stringency 3. The utility of a very stringent wash to eliminate cross-hybridization between related HPV types using full-length probes is seen in Fig. 5-18. The fact that this range is much smaller for oligoprobes means that one must be very careful when choosing the con-

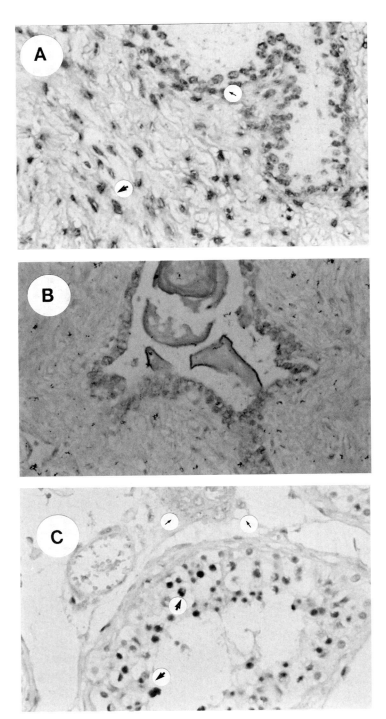

Figure 5-15. *Relationship of background and signal to the stringency of the posthybridization wash using an oligoprobe with PCR* in situ *hybridization.* The tissue is from the prostate of a man who did not have HIV-1 infection. The probe is the tailed digoxigenin labeled SK19 oligomer specific for HIV-1. Under low-stringency conditions (wash no. 1, see text), a signal is evident in most of the cells, including epithelial (**A**, *small arrow*) and stromal cells (**A**, *large arrow*). With increasing stringency of the posthybridization wash, the signal is lost (**B**). However, under these conditions a target-specific signal is evident in the spermatogonia and their progeny (*large arrow*) in the testes of a man who died of AIDS (**C**); note the absence of the signal in the stromal cells (*small arrow*).

ditions that can influence the background signal, such as the oligoprobe concentration and the stringency of the posthybridization wash. I recommend that one use the probe cocktail and stringency protocol (2) listed above. To determine conditions that will produce a robust signal with no background, one should choose a tissue that is known to contain the target and another tissue that does not have the target. If a signal is noted in the tissue that does not contain the target, the concentration of the probe should be decreased by one-half until the background signal is no longer evident. If there is no background signal and the target-specific

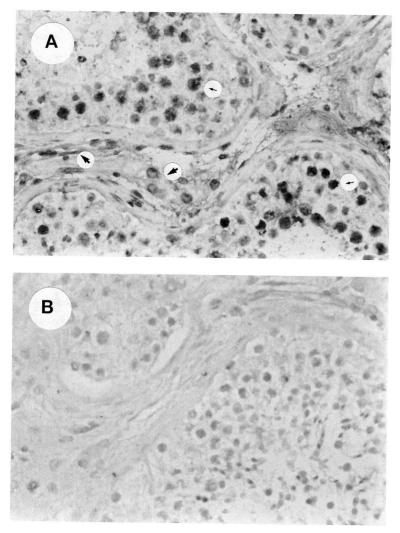

Figure 5-16. *Relationship of background to the time of hybridization using an oligoprobe with PCR in situ hybridization.* The tissue is from the testes of a man who did not have HIV-1 infection. The probe is directed against a region of the EBV genome. If the hybridization time was 15 hours, then strong background was evident in many of the cells (**A**). Again, note that the signal was present in both germ cells (*small arrow*) and stromal cells (*large arrow*). The signal was lost if the hybridization time is decreased to 1.5 hours (**B**). Compare this figure to Fig. 5-15, where the hybridization time was 1.5 hours for each of the tissues.

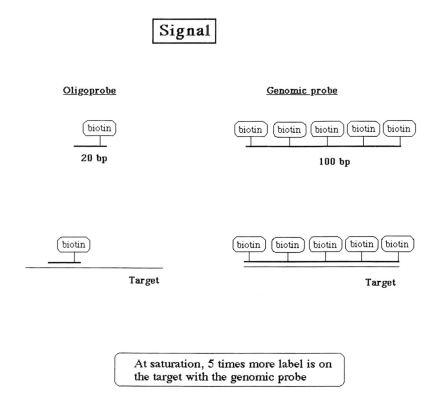

Figure 5-17. *Disparity of results with* in situ *hybridization for oligoprobes versus full-length probes: signal.* A full-length or genomic probe would have more label per probe than an oligoprobe. During hybridization, one typically uses saturating concentrations of the two different types of probe. Furthermore, due to the greater number of hydrogen bonds between the probe and target with full-length probes, these complexes are more likely to remain hybridized at a given stringency compared to the oligoprobe–target complex. Thus, the signal tends to be much stronger for a given target when using a genomic probe rather than an oligoprobe. See Fig. 4-17 for a representation of this phenomenon. This disparity can be overcome by PCR *in situ* hybridization as one amplifies 200-fold the region complementary to the oligoprobe.

signal is weak, double the probe concentration and re-do the experiments.

Before we leave the subject of the target-specific signal versus the background with oligoprobes and PCR *in situ* hybridization, there is one more important point to stress. It is important to remember that any given tissue that contains a target of interest *will have cells that do not contain the target and thus can serve as internal negative controls.* For the testes tissue experiments described above, if the spermatogonia are positive for HIV-1 *and* the Sertoli cells and Leydig cells are also positive, then there is an unacceptable level of background. Of course, one must know which cells have the target of interest and which do not in order to make such analyses. However, one should be aware of the possibility of background signal if a variety of cell types are positive after PCR *in situ* hybridization (Fig. 5-19).

To summarize this section:

1. If using an oligoprobe, use the 3′ tailing method.

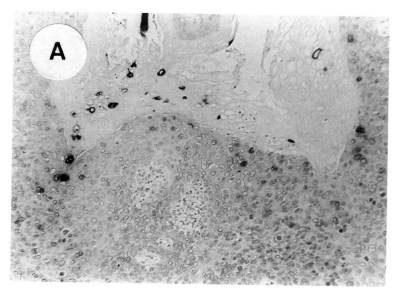

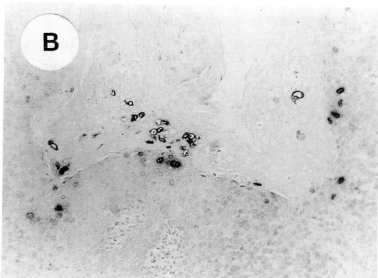

Figure 5-18. *Elimination of cross-hybridization with retention of the signal with a stringent wash using a full-length probe.* The tissue is a vulvar high-grade SIL. A signal is evident at low stringency (42°C, 2×SSC) with an HPV 16 probe (**A**). However, a similar signal is evident using an HPV 31 probe (**B**); the probes are each about 150 base pairs. Note the similar distribution of the signal in these serial sections. This represents cross-hybridization between these two related types and thus precludes the specific determination of the HPV type present in this tissue. At high stringency (68°C, 0.2×SSC) the signal with the HPV 16 probe is still strong (**C**) and the signal with the HPV 31 probe is lost (**D**). This demonstrates that the lesion contains HPV 16. Retention of the signal with the homologous probe is possible under such extreme conditions of stringency with the large probes. This reflects the great disparity between signal and background for full-length probes. However, the signal would be completely lost for the oligoprobe at 68°C and 0.2×SSC. Very high stringency for oligoprobes is about 55°C and 1×SSC.

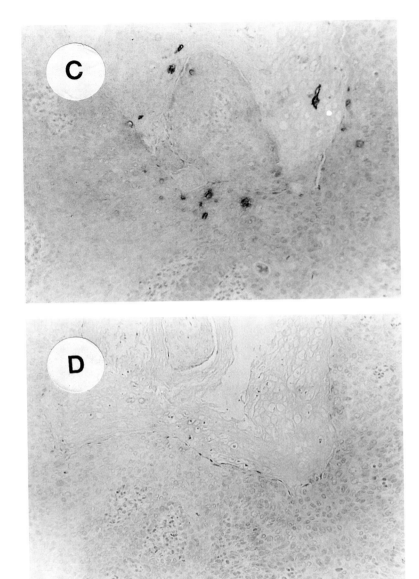

Figure 5-18. *Continued.*

2. The probe cocktail should contain no more than 10% formamide. (The exact composition of the mixture is listed above.)
3. Begin at a probe concentration of 9 nmole.
4. Begin with a 10-minute wash at 50°C using 1×SSC and 0.2% BSA.
5. Preferably, use the full-length probe with PCR *in situ* hybridization. The recipe for the probe

cocktail is listed in Chapter 4. The posthybridization wash should be for 10 minutes at 60°C with 0.2% BSA and 0.2×SSC.

Brief mention will be made of another method to label an oligoprobe, the 3′ amine substitution. This technique allows one to add one reporter molecule to the oligoprobe. If this

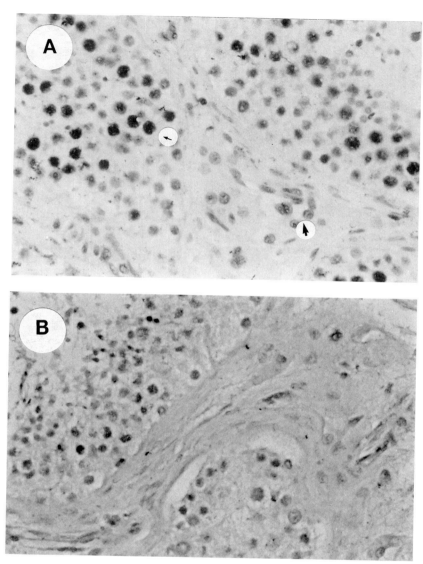

Figure 5-19. *Distribution of the staining for the signal versus background with PCR* in situ *hybridization using an oligoprobe.* The tissue is from the testes of a man who was infected by HIV-1; EBV was not present. **A** shows the signal with an EBV probe after 15 hours of hybridization. Note that background staining is present in a wide variety of cells, including the germ cells (*small arrow*) and stromal cells (*large arrow*). The background was lost if the hybridization time was decreased to 1.5 hours (**B**). Similar results to those in **A** and **B** were obtained if the stringency conditions of the posthybridization wash were 2×SSC/room temperature and 1×SSC/54°C, respectively. **C** shows the signal with the HIV-1 specific SK19 probe after PCR *in situ* hybridization and the corresponding SK38 and SK39 primers after 1.5 hours of hybridization and a posthybridization stringency of 1×SSC/54°C. Note that the germ cells (*large arrow*) were positive, whereas the stromal cells (*small arrow*) were negative. The signal was lost if the stringency conditions were increased to 0.2×SSC/68°C (compare with Fig. 5-16, C and D) or if the *Taq* was eliminated at the lower stringency (**D**).

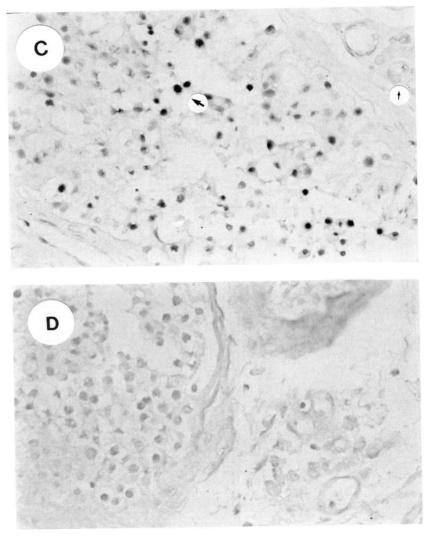

Figure 5-19. *Continued.*

is digoxigenin or a similar substance, then the problems with sensitivity discussed above with the 3′ end labeling also apply. However, one may add a "reporter" enzyme, such as alkaline phosphatase. This obviates the need for the attachment of the enzyme to the probe–target complex in a separate step. However, my preliminary work with this type of probe (attached to SK19 for HIV-1; see Chapter 9) has yielded disappointing results. One concern is that the enzyme may be inactivated in the temperatures required for the hybridization of the probe with the labeled target. It is hoped that additional research in this area will dictate conditions that allow for PCR *in situ* hybridization using such probes.

IN SITU PCR

The remainder of this chapter is devoted to the discussion of direct incorporation of labeled nucleotides that may then be visualized inside the cell, called *in situ* PCR. First the methodology and then the important issue of specific versus nonspecific incorporation of the labeled nucleotide are addressed. As has been stressed throughout this book, this is possible with DNA targets only if the sample has not been heated. Direct incorporation is routine for RT *in situ* PCR methodology, due to the pretreatment of the tissue in DNase, which eliminates the nonspecific native DNA-based signals.

Methodology

The inclusion of a labeled nucleotide in the amplifying solution is the major modification in this technique compared with PCR *in situ* hybridization. Given the technical problems of working with radioactive-labeled nucleotides, especially the time of exposure, background noise, and disposal problems, we have focused on nonisotopic systems. Certainly, it is possible to incorporate radioactive-labeled nucleotides during *in situ* PCR. However, in this section the direct incorporation of digoxigenin dUTP is discussed.

There are only two modifications to the protocol listed above. First, 10 μM digoxigenin dUTP is added to the amplifying mixture. Note that this is at a ratio of 1:20 with regard to the concentration of the dTTP, which competes with the digoxigenin dUTP for incorporation. Second, after the PCR step there is, of course, no need for the *in situ* hybridization step. Rather, the slides are washed at 60°C for 10 minutes with 0.2% BSA and 0.1×SSC. The purpose of this wash is to use the bovine serum albumin to block nonspecific adsorption of the antidigoxigenin–alkaline phosphatase conjugate rather than to remove unwanted probe. Importantly, the wash also removes labelled primer oligomers formed in the amplifying solution that bound to cell components. After this wash, the digoxigenin that has been incorporated into the amplified DNA may be detected according to the following protocol:

Protocol 5-2: Detection of Digoxigenin after *in situ* PCR

Reagent	Conditions	Time (min)
1. Antidigoxigenin antibody–alkaline phosphatase conjugate moiety, (Boehringer	1:150 dilution in Tris (pH 7.5, 0.1 M), 0.1 M NaCl	30

Reagent	Conditions	Time (min)
Mannheim, Indianapolis, IN)	at room temperature	
2. Tris (pH 9.5, 0.1 M), 0.1 M NaCl, and 0.1 M MgCl	Room temperature	2
3. Chromagen	NBT/BCIP at 37°C	5–10

Note the very brief incubation time in the chromagen NBT/BCIP. If no signal is evident after 10 minutes, then it is doubtful that staining will be evident with longer incubation times. In contrast, for PCR *in situ* hybridization, the hybridization signal should *not* be evident in the first 10 minutes. An early signal often means that there will be high background. The signal should be evident in PCR *in situ* hybridization within 15 to 20 minutes and should be maximized by 30 to 60 minutes. The reason is that more label can be incorporated with direct incorporation (where each amplicon has 1 digoxigenin per 20 nucleotides, on average) than with a labeled probe, where the amplicon itself is not labeled. During this time it is important to check the results under the microscope periodically to be certain that the background has not become too great.

Finally, there are other nonisotopic labeled nucleotides that should be suitable for *in situ* PCR. An obvious example is biotin-labeled nucleotides such as biotin-14-dATP and biotin-11-dUTP. Biotin incorporation is commonly used for *in situ* hybridization and immunohistochemistry, and many laboratories have extensive experience with its use. Most of our analyses have employed digoxigenin dUTP. Our preliminary experiments with biotin-14-dATP have shown that a relatively higher concentration to the unlabeled dATP (1:1 ratio) must be used. We have had good results with direct incorporation of tritium, as discussed in more detail in Chapters 7 and 8; ^{32}P and ^{35}S are not to be used for *in situ* PCR, as they are associated with backgrounds that are unacceptably high.

Standard Versus Hot Start Modification

The essential question about *in situ* PCR is: Does the labeled nucleotide incorporate only in target-specific sequences, or does mispriming, DNA repair, or primer oligomerization result in nonspecific incorporation? This issue is addressed at length in Chapter 3.

To summarize the important points concerning *in situ* PCR for DNA:

1. DNA repair is operative in cells and tissue that have been heated to 65°C. This applies to all fixed, paraffin-embedded tissue, as prolonged heating is required for the paraffin embedding. Cytospin preparations are sometimes heated to 65°C when drying. It is essential to know if this has occurred if one is using cytospin material.
2. Primer oligomerization apparently does not produce an intracellular signal during *in situ* PCR.
3. Mispriming invariably occurs during *in situ* PCR but can be blocked with the hot start maneuver.
4. DNA repair is *not* operative in frozen, fixed tissue sections that are not heated and in cytospin preparations that are not heated.

The remainder of this chapter focuses on target- versus nontarget-specific direct incorporation of digoxigenin dUTP during *in situ* PCR. First discussed are cytospin preparations, including experiments in which two different cell populations are mixed and a primer pair is used that is able to amplify a target in only one of the two populations. Second, data obtained when we used "irrelevant primers," primer pairs that could not possibly find specific targets in

the cells being studied, are discussed. The latter is simply accomplished by making primers based on the cDNA of an RNA virus, such as measles, which cannot make its cDNA *in vivo*. Even if the measles virus is present in the cells, unless we do an RT incubation, the cDNA of the virus, which is the target of the primers we would generate, could not be present in the infected cells. The final topic of discussion is *in situ* PCR in tissue sections.

CYTOSPIN PREPARATIONS

Hot Start *in situ* PCR: Two Different Populations

The hot start *in situ* PCR experiments are an outgrowth of those listed in Chapter 4, which involved detection of incorporated digoxigenin dUTP after Southern blot transfer using an HPV-16-specific primer pair and the DNA extracted from SiHa cells. In the current experiments, SiHa cells were mixed with the PBMC of an HPV-negative subject. I used the protocol for hot start (i.e., manual hot start) as outlined above. The term *standard conditions* refers to experiments in which all reagents were added and the sample with reagents covered with a plastic coverslip and then overlaid with mineral oil *before* raising the temperature of the heating block. Whereas SiHa cells might give specific or nonspecific product, amplified DNA from leukocytes must be nonspecific. The digoxigenin would become incorporated into both target-specific and nonspecific amplified DNA.

Color Plate 3 (following p. 242) shows that under hot start conditions with a single HPV 16 primer pair only some of the cells incorporated digoxigenin. The negative cells proved to be the leukocytes, as they reacted with an antibody against leukocyte common antigen in a double-labeling technique (SiHa cells are epithelial cells). Under standard conditions all of the cells, including the leukocytes, incorporated digoxigenin. These results provided reassurance that the hot start modification greatly inhibits the nonspecific DNA synthesis pathways. However, it is important to know if the hot start modification completely eliminated nonspecific uptake. Let us test for this outcome by using the irrelevant primers.

Hot Start *in situ* PCR: Irrelevant Primers

In these experiments, we analyzed PBMC that were part of a study to determine the utility of the *in situ* PCR technique for the rapid detection of HIV-1. The PBMC were fixed and proteased for various times as listed in Table 5-5. HIV-1 DNA was routinely found in CD4-positive PBMC from patients with AIDS. Thus far we have analyzed about 30,000 PBMC from people who are HIV-1 negative by PCR and who lack any of the risk factors for AIDS. Furthermore, we have analyzed about 15,000 PBMC from AIDS patients by *in situ* PCR using primers for measles cDNA. In either instance, any positive cell would presumably represent nonspecific uptake of dUTP. The results of these experiments are listed in Table 5-5. It is important to emphasize that these studies were done under hot start conditions, and the cytospins were air dried and not dried in a heated oven! Note the very low rate of mispriming in general. The rate increased markedly if the hot start modification was not used. Furthermore, the rate increased if the cells were proteased for longer time periods (i.e., overdigested) or if the cells were heated for 4 hours at 65°C. The latter signal was evident even if the primers were omitted (see Figs. 3-10 and 3-12). These data illustrate the importance of the digestion time and slide processing (i.e., heating) for those doing *in situ* PCR with cytospin samples.

The data with the EBV-infected lymphocyte cell line and the squamous cells are reported in Table 5-6. These experiments are similar to those reported above with the cells and the PBMC with an important exception: One can differentiate the two different cell populations on cytologic grounds alone. Note the very low rate of mispriming in the EBV-negative squamous cells but the 100% detection rate with EBV-specific primers in the lymphocytes. These data, as illustrated in Fig. 5-20, demonstrate the utility of mixing experiments using two different cell populations, one that contains the target and one that does not, that can be differentiated on cytologic grounds when doing *in situ* PCR.

Tissue Sections

If one wishes to do *in situ* PCR for DNA in tissue sections, I strongly recommend that they use frozen tissue sectioned on a cryostat and then fixed in formalin. The sections should not be heated under any circumstance. This maneuver eliminates the DNA repair mechanism and allows direct target-specific DNA synthesis if one employs the hot start maneuver.

Table 5-5. *The effect of manual hot start on the* in situ *PCR detection rate using nonsense (measles-specific) primers on PBMCs*

Fixation time/pepsin conditions	Percent positive cells[a]
5 Min/ no protease	0
5 Min/ 20 μg/ml, 2 min[b]	0.02
15 Hr/no protease	0
15 Hr/2 mg/ml, 12 min[b]	0.02[c]
15 Hr/2 mg/ml, 30 min	80

[a] The numbers were based on about 10,000 to 15,000 cells.
[b] The detection rate was 0 if the annealing/extension temperature during cycling was increased from 55°C to 65°C.
[c] The detection rate for 15-hour formalin-fixed cells digested for 12 minutes with pepsin without the manual hot start modification (all reagents added before temperature of block was elevated) was 87%.

Table 5-6. *Effects of different fixatives on the detection of PCR-amplified DNA using EBV-specific primers in a mixture of an EBV-positive cell line (Burkitt's lymphoma) and viral negative squamous cells*

Fixative/time	Detection of amplified DNA (% positive cells)	
	Burkitt's lymphoma	Squamous cells
Acetone/5 min	9	0
Acetone/15 hr	16	0
95% Ethanol/5 min	20	0
95% Ethanol/15 hr	22	0
Formalin/15 hr/protease[a]	100	0

[a]Protease is pepsin at 2 mg/ml for 12 minutes.

To illustrate the utility of this technique, we studied rats that were infected with a DNA virus (adeno-associated virus) that was linked with a gene; this was part of a study of gene therapy. The virus should infect only endothelial cells. Sections of frozen, fixed rat aortas were studied with *in situ* PCR. If hot start *in situ* PCR was done using primers specific for the virus, then a signal was seen in some endothelial cells (Fig. 5-21). As shown in Fig. 5-21, the signal was lost if the primers were omitted or if irrelevant HPV-specific primers were employed. Furthermore, all cell types, including the smooth muscle cells of the media

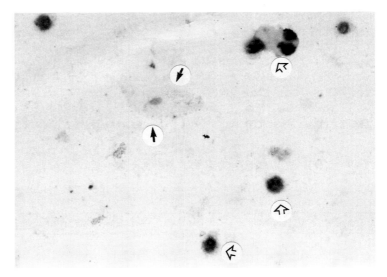

Figure 5-20. *The specificity of* in situ *PCR as demonstrated by cell mixing experiments.* An EBV-positive Burkitt's lymphoma cell line was mixed with viral negative oral squamous cells, fixed for 15 hours in formalin, then digested in pepsin (2 mg/ml) for 12 minutes. With the manual hot start maneuver and EBV-specific primers, all the lymphocytes had a signal with direct incorporation of digoxigenin-labeled nucleotide into the PCR product (*open arrows*). None of the squamous cells, which are easily distinguished cytologically by their ample cytoplasm (*closed arrows*), had nuclei with a detectable signal. Such mixing experiments are a useful control when doing *in situ* PCR or RT *in situ* PCR.

and fibroblasts of the adventia layers, were positive if the hot start maneuver was omitted. Clearly, this is a simpler and more rapid method of detecting this DNA target than using PCR *in situ* hybridization, where an additional hybridization step with the probe would have been needed.

Detection of 3′ Mismatches by *in situ* PCR

Thus far, this book has focused on the importance of homology between the primer and the DNA sequence it anneals to for DNA synthesis in PCR. Hot start PCR took advantage of the relatively poor homology between the

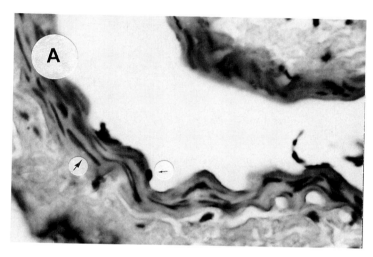

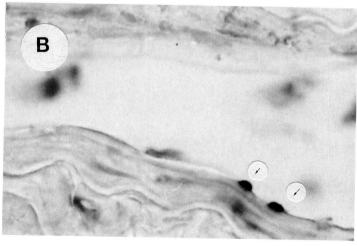

Figure 5-21. *Target-specific direct incorporation hot start* in situ *PCR for a viral DNA target using frozen, fixed tissue.* The tissue is rat aorta. Note the lining endothelial cells (**A**, *small arrow*), smooth muscle media layer (**A**, *large arrow*), and adventia. By using frozen, fixed tissue and the hot start maneuver, one eliminates the DNA repair and mispriming pathways. This allows direct incorporation of the reporter nucleotide during *in situ* PCR. The rat was infected by a DNA virus that infects endothelial cells. The viral DNA was localized by hot start *in situ* PCR to the endothelial cells (**B**); if the hot start maneuver was omitted, all cell types were positive (not shown).

primer and nontarget DNA (mispriming) and primer–primer hybrids (primer oligomerization) for enhancing *Taq*-mediated extension of the primer–target complex. However, homology is not the only factor that is important in determining if there will be *Taq*-polymerase–mediated DNA synthesis. A 3′ match between the primer and target sequence is also an impor-

tant variable for determining whether there will be DNA synthesis during PCR. This can be exploited for the study of point mutations using *in situ* PCR. The rationale is that, even if there is otherwise complete homology between a primer and a DNA sequence, the 3′ mismatch, corresponding to the point mutation, would not allow the normal primer to extend the sequence.

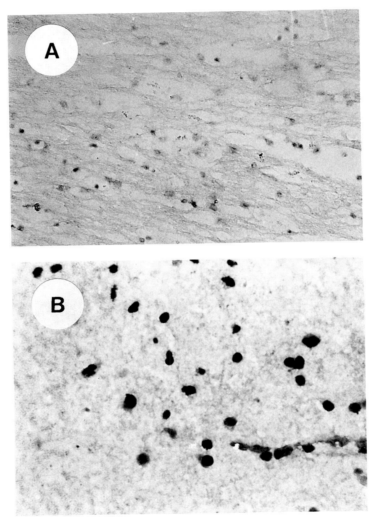

Figure 5-22. *Loss of signal with* in situ *PCR and 3′ primer mismatch.* The tissue was from gerbil brain and was frozen and fixed. Hot start *in situ* PCR was done with a primer pair (for part of the tumor necrosis factor gene) that had one difference: a 3′ substitution of A for T on the sense primer. No signal was evident if the 3′ end had A (**A**), but a strong signal was seen if the 3′ end had T (**B**). This allows one to detect point mutations with *in situ* PCR using hot start and frozen, fixed tissue by choosing primers that have the mutation at their 3′ end.

However, if the primer was modified to include the 3′ mismatch, then the point mutation could be detected.

We undertook a series of experiments to show the utility of hot start *in situ* PCR to detect point mutations. Prerequisite to these studies was the use of frozen, fixed tissues that lacked the primer-independent DNA synthesis pathway. Initially, we chose frozen, fixed sections of gerbil brain and used primers directed against the tumor necrosis factor (TNF) gene. The sequence of gerbil TNF DNA sequence is not known. We chose primers based on a conserved area of the TNF sequence present in the rat and mouse. However, no amplification was evident when we performed solution phase PCR using DNA extracted from the gerbil brain; strong amplification was seen with DNA extracted from mouse tissue. It was reasoned that the problem was not poor homology. To provide evidence to support this hypothesis, we re-did the solution phase PCR at lower annealing temperatures (down to 42°C); no bands were evident on ethidium staining. We then obtained three other primers for each of the two primers where the only difference was the nucleotide at the 3′ end. Thus, we had four different antisense primers and four sense primers that had at their 3′ end either dATP, dCTP, dGTP, or dTTP. Hot start *in situ* PCR was then performed using digoxigenin incorporation and frozen fixed tissue. A signal was evident only with the antisense primer that had C at its 3′ end and the sense primer that had the T at the 3′ end. This explains why the initial primer pair did not work, as the sense primer had an A at the 3′ end (Fig. 5-22).

Following the same rationale, we undertook a study to analyze point mutations in the *ras* gene; these have been associated with a variety of cancers. By doing *in situ* PCR with frozen, fixed tissue and primers that could differentiate between the normal *ras* gene and the mutant gene (with a point mutation), we demonstrated that both cancerous tissue and adjacent, nonmalignant cells contained the *ras* point mutation (G. J. Nuovo, *unpublished observations,* 1993).

Labeled Primers and *in situ* PCR

Direct incorporation of the reporter nucleotide for DNA targets in tissue sections (*in situ* PCR) has required frozen, fixed tissues and the hot start maneuver due to the presence of the DNA repair pathway. It would be highly advantageous if direct incorporation of a labeled *primer* could be performed successfully for DNA targets. This would avoid the hybridization step after PCR and would not suffer from a false-positive signal from DNA repair, as the primer would not participate in the DNA repair pathway. We undertook a series of experiments to address this exciting prospect.

Before describing the data, let us consider some important theoretical aspects that center around the number of reporter nucleotides that one can "bring into" the probe–target or primer–target complex. For standard *in situ* hybridization, assume a probe of 100 base pairs that has one reporter nucleotide per 20 base pairs (thus, five reporter nucleotides per probe–target complex). For *in situ* PCR, assume a 300 base pair amplicon with one reporter nucleotide per 20 base pairs (15 times $2 = 30$ reporter nucleotides per primer-mediated amplicon); we multiply times two, as each strand of the amplicon will be labeled. For primer-mediated *in situ* PCR, assume one reporter nucleotide per primer. Table 5-7 presents the data based on these theoretical considerations. Note the following important points:

1. Several thousand reporter nucleotides must be present in the labeled product in the nucleus for it to be evident as a signal (e.g., HeLa cells with 20 copies per cell and a probe of 8,000 bp would provide 8,000 reporter nucleotides in the nucleus; see Fig. 4-2).
2. The number of reporter nucleotides provided by an oligoprobe may be near the threshold for a signal even after PCR *in situ* hybridization.
3. Direct incorporation of a labeled primer probably would *not* be adequate for a signal to be evident for a 1-copy target; direct incorporation of a reporter nucleotide would yield

Table 5-7. *Relationship between method and amount of labeled nucleotide in nucleus for DNA targets*

	No. of reporter nucleotides per nucleus
Standard *in situ* hybridization	
1 Copy per cell (target 100 base pairs [bp])	5
1 Copy per cell (target 8,000 bp)	400[a]
20 Copies per cell (target 8,000 bp)	8,000[b]
600 Copies per cell (target 8,000 bp)	240,000[b]
PCR *in situ* hybridization (labeled probe)	
Without PCR: 1 copy per cell (target 8,000 bp)	400
With PCR: 1 target to 300 copies (300 bp amplicon in a target of 8,000 bp)	400 + 9,000 = 9,400[c]
With PCR: 1 target to 300 copies (30 bp per probe with 3 labels per probe) (detection of only the amplicon with an oligoprobe)	900
In situ PCR (reporter nucleotide)	
1 to 300 copies (300 bp amplicon)	9,000
100 to 300 copies (300 bp amplicon)	90,000
In situ PCR (labeled primer)	
1 to 300 copies	600
100 to 3,000 copies	6,000

[a]Signal not evident (e.g., SiHa cells and *in situ* hybridization with an HPV 16 probe).
[b]Signal evident (e.g.,HeLa cells and *in situ* hybridization with an HPV 18 probe or Caski cells and HPV 16 probe; see Fig. 4-2).
[c]Assumes a double-stranded probe that covers the entire 300 bp region.

a signal due to presence of nearly 10,000 labels per target-specific sequence.

Given these considerations, it is not surprising that the primer-independent pathway should yield such an intense signal; if one assumes only 10,000 gaps of 300 base pairs in the entire nuclear DNA, then 150,000 reporter nucleotides would be added per nucleus.

We undertook a series of experiments to determine if a signal could be generated using labeled primers. We used HPV 16 primers that had one biotin or digoxigenin per 20mer. The samples were either SiHa cells or paraffin-embedded cervical SILs that contained about 100 copies of HPV 16 per infected superficial cell. No signal was evident with the SiHa cells and direct incorporation of the labeled primer using hot start *in situ* PCR. A weak signal was evident in the cervical SILs that was stronger with the hot start maneuver. We obtained similar results with paraffin-embedded placenta tissues and primers specific for the *bcl-2* gene, present as two copies per cell (Fig. 5-23). The signal

was never as strong as with direct incorporation of the labeled nucleotide, which is consistent with the theoretical data presented in Table 5-7. That is, increasing the copy number from 100 to 3,000 would yield 6,000 reporter nucleotides in the nucleus with a labeled primer versus 90,000 reporter nucleotides with direct incorporation of the labeled nucleotide.

To try to circumvent this problem of sensitivity with labeled primers, we obtained HPV 16 primers that contained *three* biotin moieties per primer; such primers are expensive to obtain and must be over 40 base pairs long. We re-did the experiments with the SiHa cells and the cervical SILs. A signal was seen in only about 10% of the SiHa cells, and the signal with the cervical SILs was still not nearly as strong as with either standard *in situ* hybridization or PCR *in situ* hybridization (Fig. 5-24). Based on the numbers presented in Table 5-7, we theorized that increasing the label per primer threefold and increasing the target number from 100 to 3,000 should yield 18,000 labeled nucleotides per nucleus. Of

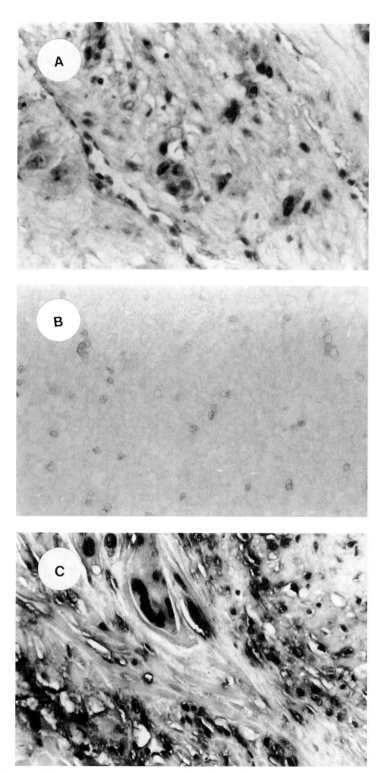

Figure 5-23. In situ *PCR using labeled primers.* The tissue is frozen, fixed human placenta. A signal is evident using digoxigenin-labeled DRB primers and hot start *in situ* PCR (**A**). The specificity of the signal was demonstrated by its absence in nonhuman tissue (**B**, gerbil brain). However, the strength of the signal is weaker than if hot start *in situ* PCR was done using digoxigenin dUTP (**C**).

course, this is much less than the 40,000 labeled nucleotides we would theorize would be present in the nucleus with a 100 copy target and a series of probes that cover the full 8,000 base pair target. Still, a signal is evident with standard *in situ* hybridization and HeLa cells (with about 8,000 labeled nucleotides per nucleus); the signal with the cervical SILs was less than for the HeLa cells. Clearly, we are at a large disadvantage when amplifying rela-

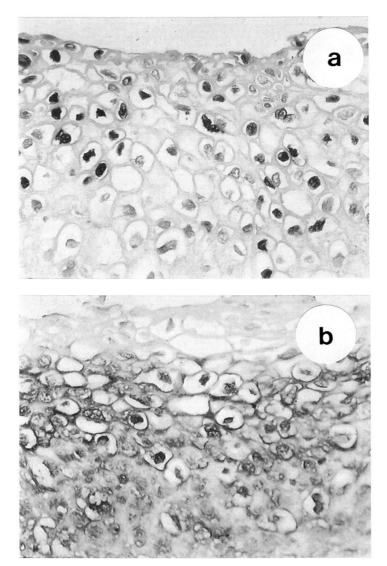

Figure 5-24. *Comparison of intensity of signal with* in situ *hybridization and* in situ *PCR with labeled primers.* **a:** An intense signal is evident with standard *in situ* hybridization in this cervical SIL using an HPV 16 probe (8,000 base pair target = multiple probes of 100 base pairs). **b:** The signal is weaker in the serial section if *in situ* PCR is done using multilabeled primers (three biotin per primer and 450 base pair target), indicating that more label per nucleus can be obtained with the labeled probe.

tively small regions with only a few labels per amplicon as compared with performing hybridizations with labeled probes and targets of several thousand kilobases.

Although it is disappointing that the labeled primers did not yield acceptable results under the conditions just described, it is useful to remember that, by using frozen, fixed tissue and hot start, one *can* achieve intense target-specific incorporation of the reporter nucleotide. Of course, this is of no help with paraffin-embedded tissues in which DNA repair would preclude using reporter nucleotides. We are in the process of attempting to increase the signal with labeled primers using paraffin-embedded tissues by increasing the number of labels per primer and by the use of multiple primer pairs.

REFERENCES

1. Haase AT, Retzel EF, Staskus KA. Amplification and detection of lentiviral DNA inside cells. *Proc Natl Acad Sci USA* 1990;87:4971–4975.
2. Nuovo GJ, MacConnell P, Forde A, Delvenne P. Detection of human papillomavirus DNA in formalin fixed tissues by *in situ* hybridization after amplification by the polymerase chain reaction. *Am J Pathol* 1991;139: 847–854.
3. Nuovo GJ, Gallery F, MacConnell P, Becker J, Bloch W. An improved technique for the detection of DNA by *in situ* hybridization after PCR-amplification. *Am J Pathol* 1991;139:1239–1244.
4. Nuovo GJ, Becker J, MacConnell P, Margiotta M, Comite S, Hochman H. Histological distribution of PCR-amplified HPV 6 and 11 DNA in penile lesions. *Am J Surg Pathol* 1992;16:269–275.
5. Nuovo GJ, Gorgone G, MacConnell P, Goravic P. *In situ* localization of human and viral cDNAs after PCR-amplification. *PCR Method Appl* 1992;2:117–123.
6. Nuovo GJ, Gallery F, MacConnell P. Analysis of the distribution pattern of PCR-amplified HPV 6 DNA in vulvar warts by *in situ* hybridization. *Mod Pathol* 1992;5:444–448.
7. Nuovo MA, Nuovo GJ, MacConnell P, Steiner G. Analysis of Paget's disease of bone for the measles virus using the reverse transcriptase *in situ* polymerase chain reaction technique. *Diagn Mol Pathol* 1993;1:256–265.
8. Nuovo GJ, Lidonocci K, MacConnell P, Lane B. Intracellular localization of PCR-amplified hepatitis C cDNA. *Am J Pathol* 1993;17:683–690.
9. Nuovo GJ, Gallery F, Hom R, MacConnell P, Bloch W. Importance of different variables for optimizing *in situ* detection of PCR-amplified DNA. *PCR Method Appl* 1993;2:305–312.
10. Nuovo GJ. Detection of human papillomavirus RNA in unusual variants of adenocarcinoma of the cervix. *J Histotech* [*in press*].
11. Seidman R, Peress N, Nuovo GJ. *In situ* detection of PCR-amplified HIV-1 nucleic acids in skeletal muscle in patients with myopathy. *Mod Pathol* 1994;7:369–375.
12. Kelleher MB, Duggan TD, Galutira D, Nuovo GJ, Haegert G. Progressive multifocal leukoencephalopathy in a patient with Alzheimer's dementia. *Diagn Mol Pathol* 1994;3:105–113.
13. Nuovo GJ, Becker J, Simsir A, Margiotta M, Shevchuck M. *In situ* localization of PCR-amplified HIV-1 nucleic acids in the male genital tract. *Am J Pathol* 1994;144:1142–1148.
14. Lidonnici K, Lane B, Nuovo GJ. A comparison of serologic analysis and *in situ* localization of PCR-amplified cDNA for the diagnosis of hepatitis C infection. *Diagn Mol Pathol* 1995;4:98–107.
15. Bagasra O, Hauptman SP, Lischer HW, Sachs M, Pomerantz RJ. Detection of human immunodeficiency virus type 1 provirus in mononuclear cells by *in situ* polymerase chain reaction. *N Engl J Med* 1992;326:1385–1391.
16. Nuovo GJ, Margiotta M, MacConnell P, Becker J. Rapid *in situ* detection of PCR-amplified HIV-1 DNA. *Diagn Mol Pathol* 1992;1:98–102.
17. Nuovo GJ, Forde A, MacConnell P, Fahrenwald R. *In situ* detection of PCR-amplified HIV-1 nucleic acids and tumor necrosis factor cDNA in cervical tissues. *Am J Pathol* 1993;143:40–48.
18. Patterson BK, Till M, Otto P, et al. Detection of HIV-1 DNA and messenger RNA in individual cells by PCR-driven *in situ* hybridization and flow cytometry. *Science* 1993;260:976–979.
19. Embretson J, Zupancic M, Ribas JL, Racz P, Tenner-Racz T, Haase AT. Massive covert infection of helper T lymphocytes and macrophages by HIV during the incubation period of AIDS. *Nature* 1993;362:359–362.
20. Embretson J, Zupancic M, Beneke J, Ribas JL, Burke A, Haase AT. Analysis of human immunodeficiency virus infected tissues by amplification and *in situ* hybridization reveals latent and permissive infections at single cell resolution. *Proc Natl Acad Sci USA* 1993;90: 357–361.
21. Nuovo GJ, Gallery F, MacConnell P, Braun A. *In situ* detection of PCR-amplified HIV-1 nucleic acids and tumor necrosis factor RNA in the central nervous system. *Am J Pathol* 1994;144:659–666.
22. Chiu KP, Cohen SH, Morris DW, Jordan GW. Intracellular amplification of proviral DNA in tissue sections using the polymerase chain reaction. *J Histochem Cytochem* 1992;40:333–341.
23. Nuovo GJ, Becker J, Margiotta M, Burke M, Fuhrer J, Steigbigel R. *In situ* detection of PCR-amplified HIV-1 nucleic acids in lymph nodes and peripheral blood in asymptomatic infection and advanced stage AIDS. *J AIDS* 1994;7:916–923.
24. Long AA, Komminoth P, Lee E, Wolfe HJ. Comparison of indirect and direct in-situ polymerase chain reaction in cell preparations and tissue sections. Detection of viral DNA, gene rearrangements and chromosomal translocations. *Histochemistry* 1993;99:151–162.
25. Embelton MJ. RT *in situ* PCR. *Nucleic Acids Res* 1992;20:3831–3834.
26. Nuovo GJ, Gallery F, MacConnell P. Analysis of nonspecific DNA synthesis during solution phase and *in situ* PCR. *PCR Methods Appl* 1994;4:342–349.
27. Nuovo GJ, Cottral S. Occult infection of the uterine cervix by human papillomavirus in postmenopausal

women. *Am J Obstet Gynecol* 1989;160:340–344.

28. Nuovo GJ, Darfler MM, Impraim CC, Bromley SE. Occurrence of multiple types of human papillomavirus in genital tract lesions: analysis by *in situ* hybridization and the polymerase chain reaction. *Am J Pathol* 1991;58:518–523.

29. Nuovo GJ, Hochman H, Eliezri YD, Comite S, Lastarria D, Silvers DN. Detection of human papillomavirus DNA in penile lesions histologically negative for condylomata: analysis by *in situ* hybridization and the polymerase chain reaction. *Am J Surg Pathol* 1990;14:829–836.

30. Nuovo GJ. Human papillomavirus DNA in genital tract lesions histologically negative for condylomata: analysis by *in situ*, Southern blot hybridization and the polymerase chain reaction. *Am J Surg Pathol* 1990;14:643–651.

31. Nuovo GJ. A comparison of different methodologies (biotin based and ^{35}S based) for the detection of human papillomavirus DNA. *Lab Invest* 1989;61:471–476.

32. Crum CP, Nuovo GJ, Friedman D, Silverstein SJ. A comparison of biotin and isotope labeled ribonucleic acid probes for *in situ* detection of HPV 16 ribonucleic acid in genital precancers. *Lab Invest* 1988;58:354–359.

33. Nuovo GJ. A comparison of slot blot, Southern blot and *in situ* hybridization analyses for human papillomavirus DNA in genital tract lesions. *Obstet Gynecol* 1989;74:673–677.

34. Ostrow RS, Manias DA, Clark BA, Okagaki T, Twiggs LB, Faras AJ. Detection of human papillomavirus DNA in invasive carcinomas of the cervix by *in situ* hybridization. *Cancer Res* 1987;47:649–653.

35. Walboomers JMM, Melchers WJG, Mullink H, et al. Sensitivity of *in situ* detection with biotinylated probes of human papillomavirus type 16 DNA in frozen tissue sections of squamous cell carcinoma of the cervix. *Am J Pathol* 1988;131:587–594.

36. Crum CP, Symbula M, Ward BE. Topography of early HPV 16 transcription in high-grade genital precancers. *Am J Pathol* 1989;134:1183–1188.

37. Nagai N, Nuovo GJ, Friedman D, Crum CP. Detection of papillomavirus nucleic acids in genital precancers with the *in situ* hybridization technique: a review. *Int J Gynecol Pathol* 1987;6:366–379.

38. Crum CP, Nuovo G, Friedman D, Silverstein SJ. Accumulation of RNA homologous to human papillomavirus type 16 open reading frames in genital precancers. *J Virol* 1988;62:84–90.

39. Crum CP, Nagai N, Levine RU, Silverstein SJ. *In situ* hybridization analysis of human papillomavirus 16 DNA sequences in early cervical neoplasia. *Am J Pathol* 1986;123:174–182.

40. Nuovo GJ, Silverstein SJ. Comparison of formalin, buffered formalin, and Bouin's fixation on the detection of human papillomavirus DNA from genital lesions. *Lab Invest* 1988;59:720–724.

41. Nuovo GJ, Friedman D, Silverstein SJ, Crum CP. Transcription of human papillomavirus type 16 in genital precancers. *Cancer Cells* 1987;5:337–343.

42. Lebargy F, Bulle F, Siegrist S, Guellaen G, Bernaudin J. Localization by *in situ* hybridization of γ glutamyl transpeptidase mRNA in the rat kidney using ^{35}S-labeled RNA probes. *Lab Invest* 1990;62:731–735.

43. McAllister HA, Rock DL. Comparative usefulness of tissue fixatives for *in situ* viral nucleic acid hybridization. *J Histochem Cytochem* 1985;33:1026–1032.

44. Moench TR, Gendelman HE, Clements JE, Narayan O, Griffin DE. Efficiency of *in situ* hybridization as a function of probe size and fixation technique. *J Virol Methods* 1985;11:119–130.

45. Nuovo GJ. Buffered formalin is the superior fixative for the detection of human papillomavirus DNA by *in situ* hybridization analysis. *Am J Pathol* 1989;134:837–842.

46. Tournier I, Bernuau D, Poliard A, Schoevaert D, Feldmann G. Detection of albumin mRNAs in rat liver by *in situ* hybridization: usefulness of paraffin embedding and comparison of various fixation procedures. *J Histochem Cytochem* 1987;35:453–459.

47. Nuovo GJ. Comparison of Bouin's solution and buffered formalin fixation on the detection rate by *in situ* hybridization of human papillomavirus DNA in genital tract lesions. *J Histotech* 1991;14:13–18.

48. Alessandri LM, Sterrett GF, Pixley EC, Kulski JK. Comparison of peroxidase–antiperoxidase and avidin–biotin complex methods for the detection of papillomavirus in histological sections of the cervix uteri. *Pathology* 1986;18:383–385.

49. Garuti G, Boselli F, Genazzani AR, Silvestri S, Ratti G. Detection and typing of human papillomavirus in histologic specimens by *in situ* hybridization with biotinylated probes. *Am J Clin Pathol* 1989;92:604–612.

50. Mariette X, Gozlan J, Clerc D, Bisson M, Morinet F. Detection of Epstein-Barr virus DNA by *in situ* hybridization and polymerase chain reaction in salivary gland biopsy specimens from patients with Sjogren's syndrome. *Am J Med* 1991;90:286–294.

51. Niedobitek G, Finn T, Herbsy H, Bornhoft G, Gerdes J, Stein H. Detection of viral DNA by *in situ* hybridization using bromodeoxyuridine labeled DNA probes. *Am J Pathol* 1988;131:1–4.

52. Schmidbauer M, Budka H, Ambros P. Herpes simplex virus (HSV) DNA in microglial nodular brainstem encephalitis. *J Neuropathol Exp Neurol* 1989;48:645–652.

53. Ranki M, Leinonen AW, Jalava T, et al. Use of Affiprobe HPV test kit for detection of human papillomavirus DNA in genital scrapes. *J Clin Microbiol* 1990;28:2076–2081.

54. Samoszuk M. Rapid detection of Epstein-Barr viral DNA by nonisotopic *in situ* hybridization. *Am J Pathol* 1991;96:448–453.

55. Stoler MH, Broker TR. *In situ* hybridization detection on human papillomavirus DNAs and messenger RNAs in genital condylomata and a cervical carcinoma. *Hum Pathol* 1986;17:250–258.

56. Syrjanen S, Syrjanen K. An improved *in situ* DNA hybridization protocol for detection of human papillomavirus (HPV) DNA sequences in paraffin-embedded biopsies. *J Virol Methods* 1986;14:293–304.

57. Sachdev R, Nuovo GJ, Kaplan C, Greco A. Detection of Cytomegalovirus in chronic villits by *in situ* hybridization. *Pediatr Pathol* 1990;10:909–917.

58. Mori M, Lurata H, Tajima M, Shimada H. JC virus detection by *in situ* hybridization in brain tissue from elderly patients. *Ann Neurol* 1991;29:428–432.

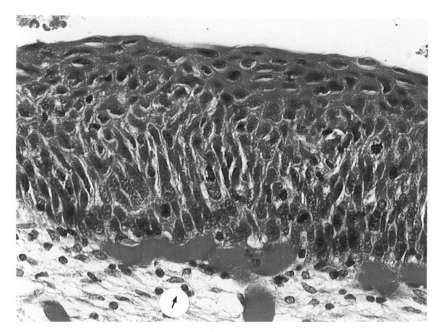

Color Plate 1. *Differential staining of nucleic acids and proteins with the hemoxylin and eosin (H&E) stain.* Nucleic acids yield a dark blue color with the H&E stain and are evident in the nuclei of these squamous cells and the underlying fibroblasts (*arrow*). Any concentrated protein will give a strong pink color with the H&E stain; this is clearly evident in the cytoplasm of the squamous cells, which have ample amounts of the protein keratin.

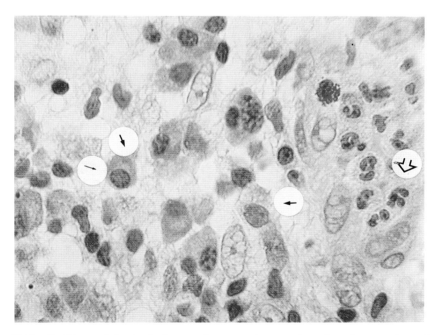

Color Plate 2. *The cytologic features of macrophages, lymphocytes, and neutrophils.* Macrophages have ample cytoplasm that may contain vacuoles, including lysosomes (*small arrow*); their nuclei are either round or have a central groove. Lymphocytes have round, dark nuclei and minimal cytoplasm (*upper left*). Neutrophils have multiple, distinct lobes (*open arrow*). The double *arrows* show the eccentric nucleus and perinuclear clearing of a plasma cell.

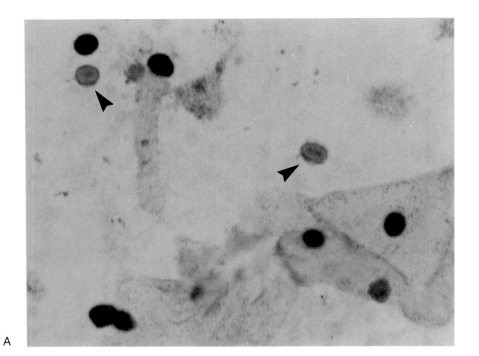

A

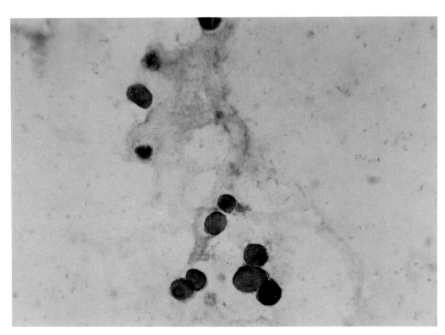

B

Color Plate 3. *Enhanced specificity of direct incorporation of digoxigenin dUTP (dig dUTP) with the hot start modification of* in situ *PCR.* Using a single HPV 16 primer pair with a mixture of SiHa cells and leukocytes, only SiHa cells contained amplified DNA as evidenced by dig dUTP incorporation under hot start conditions; the negative cells were positive for leukocyte common antigen (**A**, *arrows*). Under standard conditions, leukocytes and SiHa cells contained amplified DNA (**B**). Uptake of dig dUTP by the leukocytes must represent DNA synthesis from the unwanted pathways.

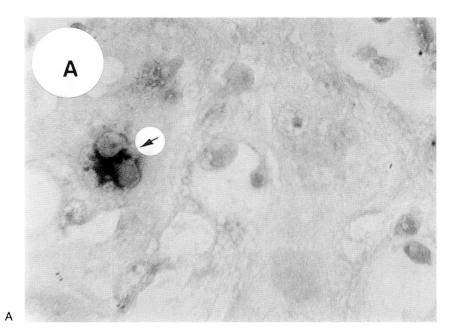

A

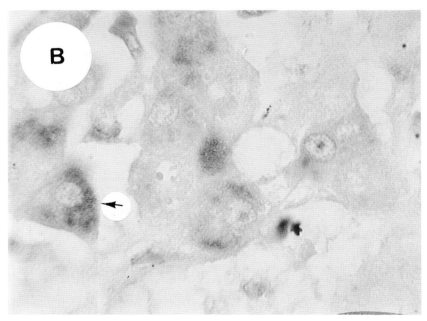

B

Color Plate 4. *Subcellular localization of hepatitis C RNA and proteins.* RT *in situ* PCR for hepatitis C demonstrated that viral RNA was found mostly in hepatocytes, although occasional liver macrophages (Kuppfer cells) and biliary epithelium were infected. The signal for the Kuppfer cells localized to the nucleus and cytoplasm (not shown). The signal in the hepatocytes usually localizes to part of the nuclear membrane (**A**, *arrow*; see also Fig. 1.1). However, at times a cytoplasmic signal that also tends to be centered about part of the nuclear membrane will be evident (**B**, *arrow*). Compare this to the pan-nuclear signal of the positive control (**C**, *arrow*). A hepatitis C protein interestingly was localized by immunohistochemistry to the cytoplasm, directly abutting part of the nuclear membrane (**D**, *arrow;* slide courtesy of Dr. Richard Cartun). This suggests a distinct cellular "roadway" for production of hepatitis C proteins from the RNA. The specific subcellular localization of the signal with RT in situ PCR strongly suggests the specificity of the RNA-based signal.

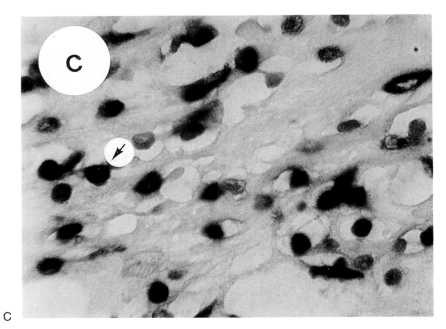

C

D

Color Plate 4. *Continued.*

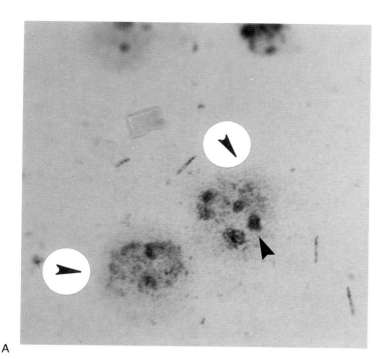

A

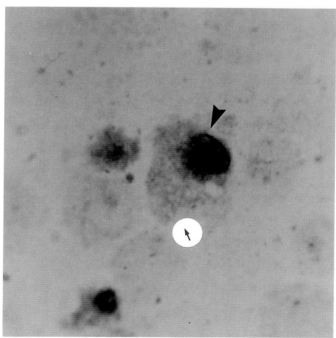

B

Color Plate 5. *Detection of human mRNAs in a megakaryocyte cell line.* The cell line DAMI contains the mRNAs amyloid precursor protein and gelsolin. Analysis of these mRNAs was done after DNase pretreatment by RT *in situ* PCR. Note the different compartmentalizations of the two signals. Amyloid precursor protein PCR-amplified cDNA (**A**) localized to the cytoplasm (*arrowheads* with white background) and to one to three discrete nuclear foci (*arrowhead*) that correspond to the nucleoli; this mRNA was not detected by standard *in situ* hybridization analysis (not shown). Gelsolin PCR-amplified mRNA also localized to the cytoplasm (**B**, *arrow*) and nucleus (*arrowhead*) but appeared to spare the nucleoli. This variable pattern of different mRNAs and, probably, pre-mRNAs likely reflects differing pathways taken by these messages as they are spliced and moved from nucleus to cytoplasm.

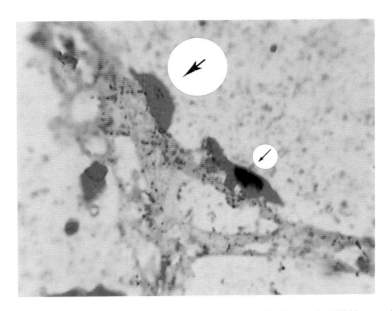

Color Plate 6. *Colocalization of hantaviral RNA and cytokeratin.* Hantaviral RNA was detected by RT *in situ* PCR in many of the cells that were lining the alveoli and that had the cytologic features of pneumocytes. To demonstrate that these cells were alveolar pneumocytes, RT *in situ* PCR for hantaviral RNA was followed by immunohistochemistry for cytokeratin AE 1,3, which would be found only in this cell type. These experiments did show that many of the hantaviral infected cells (blue) colabeled with cytokeratin protein (red) (*small arrow*; note the keratin-positive, hantaviral-negative cell, *large arrow*).

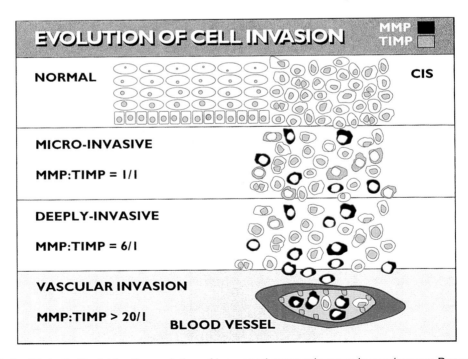

Color Plate 7. *Model for the evolution of increased aggressiveness in carcinomas.* Based on the data derived from cervical cancer tissues and cell lines using RT *in situ* PCR, it is postulated that there is a "natural selection" for cells expressing an MMP and not expressing a TIMP with regard to increased invasiveness and, more importantly, microvascular invasion.

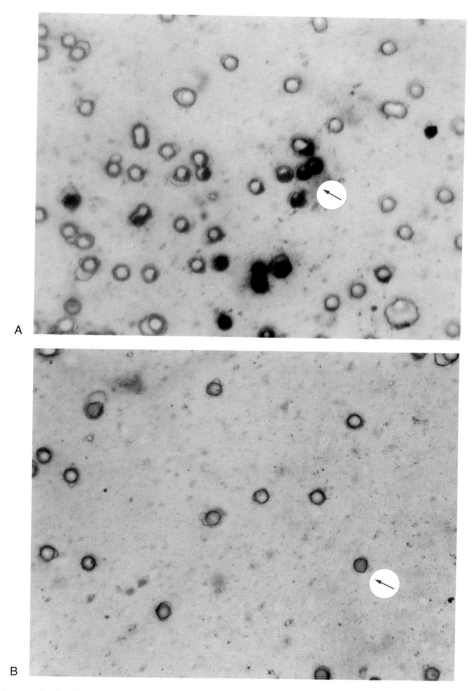

A

B

Color Plate 8. *Analysis of MMP-9 and TIMP-1 PCR-amplified cDNA in the cells that had invaded the matrigel.* MMP-9 mRNA was detected in many of the HeLa cells which had invaded the matrigel (**A**, *arrow*); the signal is blue due to precipitation of NBT/BCIP by alkaline phosphatase immunologically linked to the digoxigenin incorporated into the PCR-amplified cDNA. TIMP-1 mRNA was absent in most of the invasive HeLa cells; the negative pink color is from the counterstain nuclear-fast red (**B**, *arrow*).

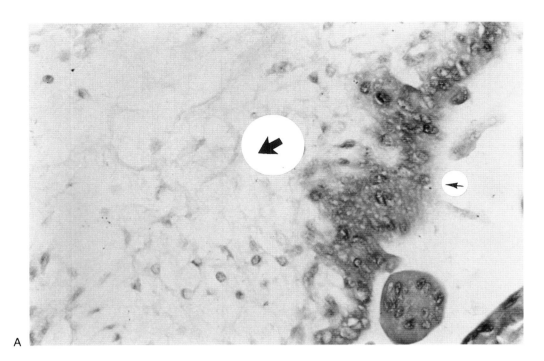

A

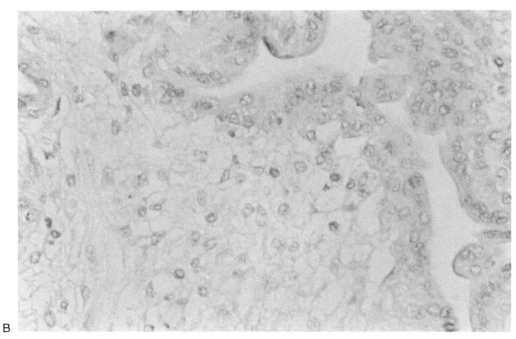

B

Color Plate 9. *Detection of the β–chain of fibrinogen mRNA by RT* in situ *PCR: value of exon-versus intron-specific primers.* The placenta consists of the villi, lined by multinucleated trophoblasts, and the supporting stromal cells. PCR-amplified fibrinogen (β-chain) cDNA was detected in the trophoblasts (**A**, *small arrow*) and not the underlying stromal cells. The signal was lost if the exon-specific primers were substituted with intron-specific primers (**B**).

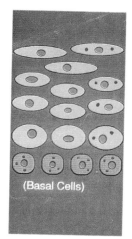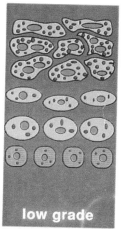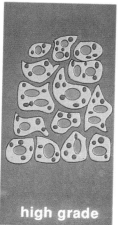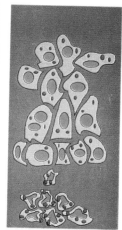

(Basal Cells)

low grade

high grade

HPV INFECTION INTRAEPITHELIAL LESIONS   CANCER

Color Plate 10. *Proposed continuum of HPV infection of the uterine cervix.* This model is based on the results of PCR in situ hybridization of occult HPV infection of the cervix and cervical SILs. In occult infection (*left*), HPV may infect morphologically normal cells that probably are most often undergoing early squamous metaplasia. The virus is represented by the red dots. The virus apparently rarely infects the normal columnar cells. Low-grade SILs are associated with a marked increase in HPV number in the atypical squamous cells, which are located toward the surface. The viral copy number decreases if the lesion progresses to a high-grade SIL or an invasive cancer.

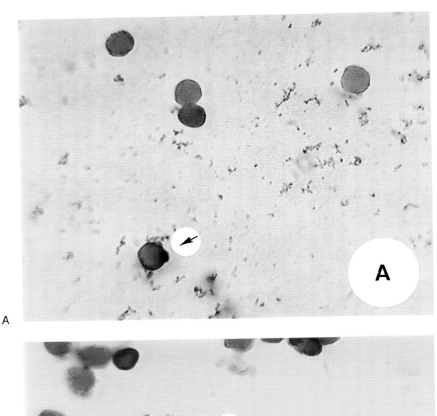

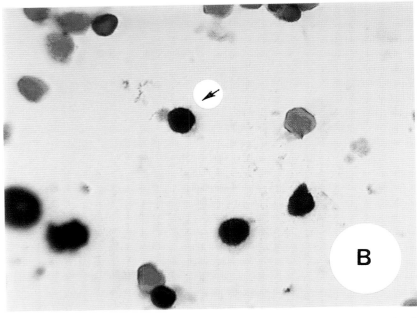

Color Plate 11. *Nuclear versus cytoplasmic localization of HIV-1 DNA as determined by PCR* in situ *hybridization: quiescent versus activated CD4 lymphocytes.* **A:** Quiescent lymphocytes that were infected with HIV-1. A signal was noted in about 10% of these lymphocytes, and it localized to the cell membrane and the thin rim of cytoplasm characteristic of these cells (*arrow*). **B:** In comparison, T-helper cells activated by PHA and then infected with HIV-1 show an over three times percentage of infected cells, and the signal localizes to the nucleus (*arrow*). This observation, readily made with PCR *in situ* hybridization, implies that proviral transport from the surface CD4 receptor to the nucleus is dependent on cellular activation.

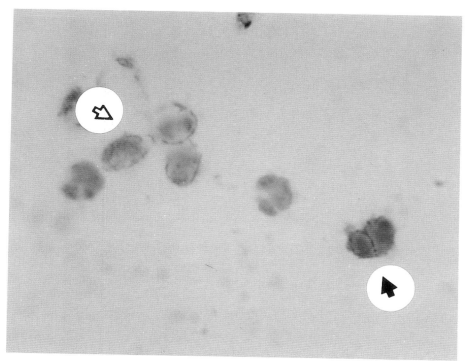

Color Plate 12. *Detection of HIV-1 DNA by* in situ *PCR in PBMC colabeled with CD4 from a patient with AIDS.* Direct incorporation of digoxigenin using a single HIV-1 DNA primer pair is evident as a red color, as the chromogen is new fuchsin (DAKO). The negative cells are light blue due to counterstaining with a 1% hematoxylin solution. After *in situ* PCR, the cells were colabeled for CD4 using immunocytochemistry, which produces a dark rim around CD4-positive cells. Note the several CD4-negative cells, the several HIV-1–negative cells that are CD4 positive (*open arrow*), and the two HIV-1–positive cells that each showed CD4 reactivity (*closed arrow*).

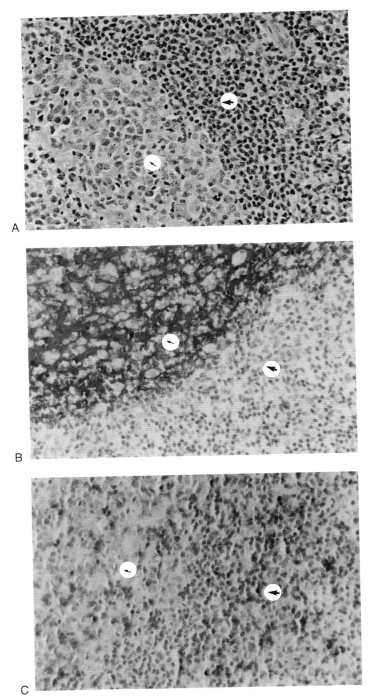

Color Plate 13. *Histologic and immunohistochemical analyses of a lymph node from a patient with asymptomatic HIV-1 infection.* The lymph node from this asymptomatic seropositive individual showed marked follicular hyperplasia and disruption of the mantle zone (**A**, *small arrow,* germinal center; *large arrow,* parafollicular zone). Serial sections show that the CD21+ dendritic cells localized to the germinal center (**B**, red=positive), whereas the CD4+ lymphocytes were commonly seen in the parafollicular zone as well as the germinal center (**C**).

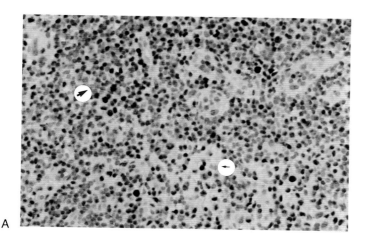

A

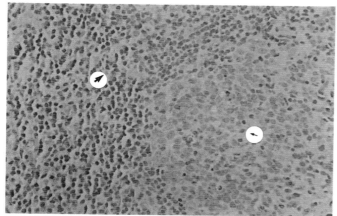

B

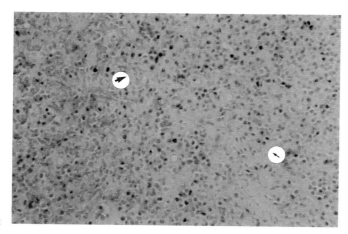

C

Color Plate 14. *Molecular analyses of a lymph node from a patient with asymptomatic HIV-1 infection.* The lymph node depicted in Color Plate 13 was analyzed for viral DNA and RNA. PCR-amplified HIV-1 DNA was detected in many of the cells in the germinal center and parafollicular zones using hot start PCR *in situ* hybridization and the single primer pair SK38 and SK39 or SK145 and SK431 (**A**, blue = positive, pink = negative; the results are for the latter primer pair with the corresponding probe SK102). The signal was lost when PCR *in situ* hybridization was done with irrelevant (HPV-specific) primers, when *Taq* polymerase was omitted, or when the sections were pretreated in DNase. No signal was seen with standard *in situ* hybridization (**B**). HIV-1 RNA was detected by RT *in situ* PCR in a serial section (**C**) but in fewer cells that were positive for HIV-1 DNA. The *small arrows* mark the position of the germinal center. The *large arrows* mark the position of the parafollicular zone.

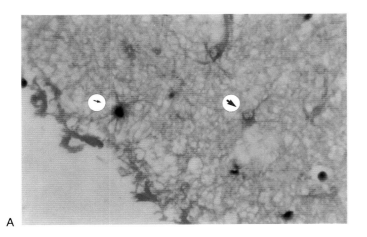

A

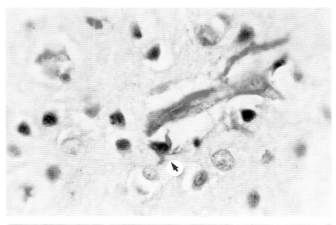

B

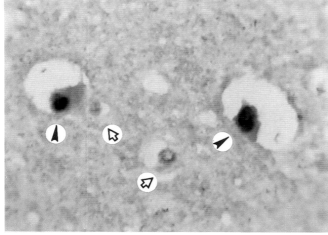

C

Color Plate 15. *Determination of the phenotype of HIV-1–infected cells.* **A:** The phenotype of the cells HIV-1 DNA positive by PCR *in situ* hybridization was determined by immunohistochemical colabeling. HIV-1–positive (dark blue color) astrocytes (GFAP positive, red cytoplasm) were evident throughout the CNS. The *small arrow* marks an HIV-1–positive astrocyte and the *large arrow* a negative astrocyte. **B:** Note the fine branching processes with the GFAP stain, which represents the cytoplasmic processes of the astrocytes. Colabeling with RCA-1 or Mac387 showed that some of the infected cells were microglia/macrophages (*arrow*). **C:** Two HIV-1 DNA-positive cells (*arrowheads*) that show large halos and large nuclei with ample cytoplasm typical of neurons. These cells did colabel with neuron-specific enolase; note the smaller cells that are HIV-1 and neuron specific enolase negative (*open arrows*) have the cytological features (small halos and minimal cytoplasm) of oligodendroglia (no counterstain).

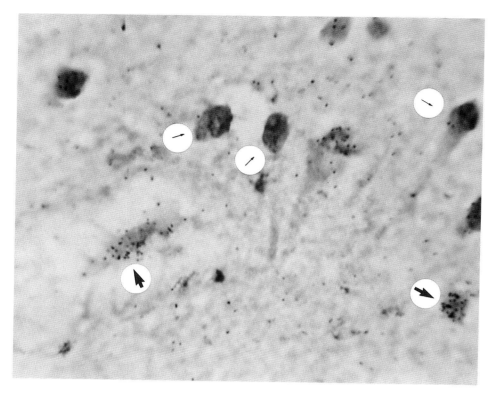

Color Plate 16. *Colocalization of HIV-1 RNA and cytokine mRNA in AIDS dementia.* HIV-1 RNA was detected in many cells in tissues of the cerebrum of a person who died of AIDS dementia (*small arrows,* blue is positive due to NBT/BCIP). The TNF-positive cells were most plentiful in the areas where HIV-1–infected cells were abundant. However, it could not be determined using serial sections if the HIV-1–infected cells were expressing cytokines such as TNF, NOS, MIP-α or MIP-β. Colocalization was done with two separate RT *in situ* PCR reactions to answer this question. TNF mRNA was detected by RT *in situ* PCR using ^{3}H as the reporter system. Note that the TNF-positive cells (large arrows), though in close proximity to the viral infected cells, are HIV-1 negative.

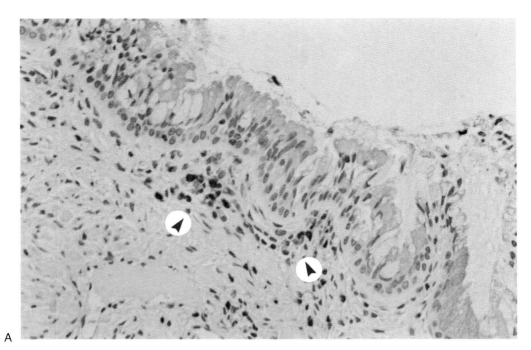

A

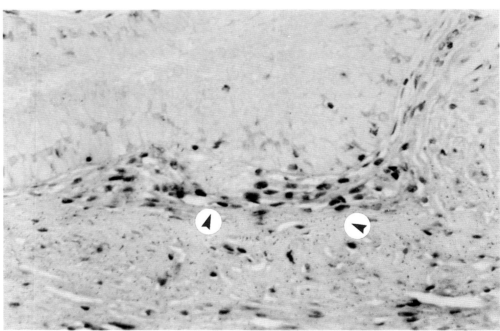

B

Color Plate 17. *Molecular analyses of a cervical tissue from an adult woman with AIDS.* **A:** The endocervical aspect of the transformation zone is evident on immunohistochemical stain for Mac387 (*arrowheads*); note the glandular epithelium and the early squamous metaplasia (*arrows*). These histologic features demonstrate that this is the region of the transformation zone (see more detailed discussion in Chapter 8). **B:** HIV-1 RNA (*arrowheads*) is evident after RT *in situ* PCR in many of the stromal cells at the base of the gland in a distribution similar to the macrophages. Note that the epithelium is negative. Most cells positive for HIV-1 RNA contain PCR-amplified TNF cDNA and PCR-amplified HIV-1 DNA (not shown). The detection of TNF mRNA also suggests that many of the infected cells were macrophages.

59. Gupka JW, Gupka PK, Rosenshein N, Shah KV. Detection of human papillomavirus in cervical smears. A comparison of *in situ* hybridization, immunocytochemistry, and cytopathology. *Acta Cytol* 1987;31:387–395.

60. Eversole LR, Laipis PJ. Oral squamous papillomas: detection of HPV DNA by *in situ* hybridization. *Oral Surg Oral Med Oral Pathol* 1988;65:545–550.

61. Roberts WH, Hammond S, Sneddon JM, Thesing J, Caldwell JH, Clausen KP. *In situ* DNA hybridization for cytomegalovirus in colonic biopsies. *Arch Pathol Lab Med* 1988;112:1106–1109.

62. Robey SS, Gage WR, Kuhajda FP. Comparison of immunoperoxidase and DNA *in situ* hybridization techniques in the diagnosis of cytomegalovirus colitis. *Am J Clin Pathol* 1988;89:666–671.

63. Rotbart HA, Abzug MJ, Levin MJ. Development and application of RNA probes for the study of picornaviruses. *Mol Cell Probes* 1988;2:65–73.

64. Tase T, Okagaki T, Clark BA, Twiggs LB, Ostrow RS, Faras AJ. Human papillomavirus DNA in adenocarcinoma *in situ*, microinvasive adenocarcinoma of the uterine cervix, and coexisting cervical squamous intraepithelial neoplasia. *Int J Gynecol Pathol* 1989;8:8–11.

65. Willett GD, Kurman RJ, Reid R, Greenberg M, Jenson AB, Lorincz AT. Correlation of the histologic appearance of intraepithelial neoplasia of the cervix with human papillomavirus types. *Int J Gynecol Pathol* 1989;8:18–25.

66. Abramson AL, Steinberg BM, Winkler B. Laryngeal papillomatosis: clinical, histopathologic and molecular studies. *Laryngoscope* 1987;97:678–685.

67. Brandsma JL, Lewis AJ, Abramson A, Manos MM. Detection and typing of papillomavirus DNA in formaldehyde-fixed paraffin-embedded tissue. *Arch Otolaryngol Head Neck Surg* 1990;116:844–848.

68. Burk RD, Kadish AS, Calderin S, Romney SL. Human papillomavirus infection of the cervix detected by cervicovaginal lavage and molecular hybridization: correlation with biopsy results and Papanicolaou smear. *Am J Obstet Gynecol* 1986;154:982–989.

69. Carson LF, Twiggs LB, Okagaki T, Clark BA, Ostrow RS, Faras AJ. Human papillomavirus DNA in adenosquamous carcinoma and squamous cell carcinoma of the vulva. *Obstet Gynecol* 1988;72:63–67.

70. Cullen AP, Reid R, Champion M, Lorincz AT. Analysis of the physical state of different human papillomavirus DNAs in intraepithelial and invasive cervical neoplasia. *J Virol* 1991;65:606–612.

71. Dinh TV, Powell LC, Hannigan EV, Yang HL, Wirt DP, Yandell RB. Simultaneously occurring condylomata acuminata, carcinoma *in situ* and verrucous carcinoma of the vulva and carcinoma *in situ* of the cervix in a young woman. *J Reprod Med* 1988;33:510–513.

72. Ferenczy A, Mitao M, Nagai N, Silverstein SJ, Crum CP. Latent papillomavirus and recurring genital warts. *N Engl J Med* 1985;313:784–788.

73. Firzlaff JM, Kiviat NB, Beckmann AM, Jenison SA, Galloway DA. Detection of human papillomavirus capsid antigens in various squamous epithelial lesions using antibodies directed against the L1 and L2 open reading frames. *Virology* 1988;164:467–477.

74. Gall AA, Saul SH, Stoler MH. *In situ* hybridization analysis of human papillomavirus in anal squamous cell carcinoma. *Mod Pathol* 1989;2:439–443.

75. Griffin NR, Bevan IS, Lewis FA, Young LS. Demonstration of multiple HPV types in normal cervix and in cervical squamous cell carcinoma using the polymerase chain reaction on paraffin wax embedded material. *J Clin Pathol* 1990;45:52–56.

76. Kashima HK, Kutcher M, Kessis T, Levin LS, DeVilleirs EM, Shah K. Human papillomavirus in squamous cell carcinoma, leukoplakia, lichen planus, and clinically normal epithelium of the oral cavity. *Ann Otol Rhinol Laryngol* 1990;99:55–61.

77. Kadish AS, Burk RD, Kress Y, Calderin S, Romney SL. Human papillomavirus of different types in precancerous lesions of the uterine cervix: histologic, immunocytochemical and ultrastructural studies. *Hum Pathol* 1986;17:384–392.

78. Chou Q, Russell M, Birch DE, Raymond J, Bloch W. Prevention of pre-PCR mis-priming and primer dimerization improves low-copy-number amplifications. *Nucleic Acids Res* 1992;20:1717–1723.

79. Bagasra O, Hauptman SP, Lischer HW, Sachs M, Pomerantz RJ. Detection of human immunodeficiency virus type 1 provirus in mononuclear cells by *in situ* polymerase chain reaction. *N Engl J Med* 1992;326:1385–1391.

80. Harper ME, Marselle LM, Gallo RC, Wong-Staal F. Detection of lymphocytes expressing human T-lymphotropic virus type III in lymph nodes and peripheral blood from infected individuals by *in situ* hybridization. *Proc Natl Acad Sci USA* 1986;83:772–776.

81. Patterson BK, Till M, Otto P, et al. Detection of HIV-1 DNA and messenger RNA in individual cells by PCR-driven *in situ* hybridization and flow cytometry. *Science* 1993;260:976–979.

82. Pantaleo G, Graziosi C, Demarest JF, et al. HIV infection is active and progressive in lymphoid tissue during the clinically latent stage of the disease. *Nature* 1993;362:355–358.

83. Fox CH, Tenner-Racz K, Racz P, Firpo A, Pizzo PA, Fauci AS. Lymphoid germinal centers are reservoirs of human immunodeficiency virus type 1 RNA. *J Infect Dis* 1991;164:1051–1057.

84. Embretson J, Zupancic M, Ribas JL, Racz P, Tenner-Racz T, Haase AT. Massive covert infection of helper T lymphocytes and macrophages by HIV during the incubation period of AIDS. *Nature* 1993;362:359–362.

85. Hsia K, Spector SA. Human immunodeficiency virus DNA is present in a high percentage of CD4+ lymphocytes of seropositive individuals. *J Infect Dis* 1991;164:470–475.

86. Embretson J, Zupancic M, Beneke J, Ribas JL, Burke A, Haase AT. Analysis of human immunodeficiency virus infected tissues by amplification and *in situ* hybridization revelas latent and permissive infections at single cell resolution. *Proc Natl Acad Sci USA* 1993;90:357–361.

87. Greer CE, Peterson SL, Kiviat NB, Manos MM. PCR amplification from paraffin-embedded tissues: effects of fixative and fixative times. *Am J Clin Pathol* 1991;95:117–124.

88. Greer CE, Lund JK, Manos MM. PCR amplification from paraffin-embedded tissues: recommendations on fixatives for long-term storage and prospective studies. *PCR Methods Appl* 1992;95:117–124.

89. McAllister HA, Rock DL. Comparative usefulness of tissue fixatives for *in situ* viral nucleic acid hybridization. *J Histochem Cytochem* 1985;33:1026–1032.

90. Nuovo GJ. Buffered formalin is the superior fixative for the detection of human papillomavirus DNA by *in situ* hybridization analysis. *Am J Pathol* 1989;134: 837–842.

91. Brutlag D, Schlehuber C, Bonner J. Properties of formaldehyde treated nucleohistones. *Biochemistry* 1977;8:3214–3218.

92. Dubeau L, Chandler LA, Gralow JR, Nichols PW, Jones PA. Southern blot analysis of DNA extracted from formalin-fixed pathology specimens. *Cancer Res* 1986;46:2964–2970.

93. Goelz SE, Hamilton SR, Vogelstein B. Purification of DNA from formaldehyde fixed and paraffin-embedded tissue. *Biochem Biophys Res Commun* 1985;130: 118–124.

94. Tournier I, Bernuau D, Poliard A, Schoevaert D, Feldmann G. Detection of albumin mRNAs in rat liver by *in situ* hybridization: usefulness of paraffin embedding and comparison of various fixation procedures. *J Histochem Cytochem* 1987;35:453–459.

95. Lebargy F, Bulle F, Siegrist S, Guellaen G, Bernaudin J. Localization by *in situ* hybridization of γ-glutamyl transpeptidase mRNA in the rat kidney using ^{35}S-labeled RNA probes. *Lab Invest* 1990;62:731–735.

96. Moench TR, Gendelman HE, Clements JE, Narayan O, Griffin DE. Efficiency of *in situ* hybridization as a function of probe size and fixation technique. *J Virol Methods* 1985;11:119–130.

97. Crum CP, Nuovo GJ. *Human papillomavirus and their relationship to genital tract neoplasms.* New York: Raven Press; 1991.

98. Nuovo GJ, Crum CP. Papillomaviruses and cervical neoplasia. In: Altchek A, Deligdisch L, eds. *Clinical perspectives in obstetrics and gynceology.* New York: Springer-Verlag; 1991:39–54.

99. Nuovo GJ. Human papillomavirus. In: Ehrmann R, ed. *Benign to malignant progression in cervical squamous and glandular epithelium: histology, cytology, and papillomavirus effect.* New York: Igaku-Shoin; 1993:239–263.

100. Nuovo GJ. *Cytopathology of the female genital tract: an integrated approach.* Baltimore: Williams & Wilkins; 1993.

101. Nuovo GJ. *In situ* hybridization protocols. In: Choo K.H.A., *Methods in molecular biology.* San Diego: Humana Press; 1993:98–105.

102. Nuovo GJ. The clinical utility of detection of human papillomavirus DNA in the lower genital tract. *Infect Medicine* 1993;11:172–183.

103. Nuovo GJ. *In situ* hybridization. In: Damjanov I, Linder J, eds. *Anderson's textbook of pathology*, 10th ed. San Diego: Academic Press Inc; 1995:239–251.

6

A Starter's Guide to *in situ* PCR: The Start-Up Protocol

It is assumed that many readers have had minimal or no experience with PCR *in situ* hybridization or RT *in situ* PCR. I have had conversations with a number of scientists either in person or via the telephone who have had many questions about these procedures. As a result of my attempts to answer these questions and through my own experiences, I believe it is important to provide a standard start-up protocol for those wishing to master the technique to detect PCR-amplified DNA and cDNA within intact cells and tissue. I have developed a procedure that, hopefully, will enable the beginner to become proficient with the technique in a relatively short period of time. This so-called start-up protocol is presented with a step-by-step troubleshooting guide. Although some theoretical concepts are presented, the focus is on conducting the tests and on solving problems when things go wrong. The preceding chapters present in-depth discussions of the theory behind the procedures. The sole purpose of the start-up protocol is to learn to amplify and detect DNA in cells. This is a practice exercise rather than an actual detection event, and the PCR-amplified DNA will be *nonspecific* and not dependent on the primer pair. Indeed, much of the amplified product will be primer-independent, reflecting DNA repair. Although this may be disconcerting to some, the process is identical to that used for target-specific amplification. In actuality, the start-up protocol shares many features in common with RT *in situ* PCR. The protocols for target specific-amplification of DNA and RNA are

presented in Chapters 5 and 7, respectively. It is not an overstatement to say that the ability to do this start-up protocol successfully will greatly enhance one's ability to use PCR *in situ* hybridization for the detection of a specific target! Completion of the exercise will demonstrate whether the correct conditions for DNA synthesis have been achieved and will show the results inside intact cells.

I believe the practice exercise can provide even more potential benefit. Specifically, those with little histology experience will gain experience handling tissue sections and/or cellular suspensions on glass slides. Indeed, if the reader has no experience working with tissue samples on glass slides, it would be useful to spend one or two sessions doing standard *in situ* hybridization. If one has access to a pathology laboratory, it would be easy to obtain suitable paraffin-embedded tissue samples. A sample of a vulvar or penile wart would be a good choice because these tissues are invariably intensely positive for human papillomavirus (HPV) DNA. There are several good commercially available kits that contain all the reagents (and positive samples) for HPV detection. I use a kit from Enzo Diagnostics (see Appendix) regularly with good results. Successful detection of HPV or, if preferred, the repetitive *alu* sequence with a biotin- or digoxigenin-labeled probe will, in my experience, be of great assistance to those just beginning with *in situ* PCR.

The preliminary phase of the start-up protocol has two parts:

1. Determining the optimal protease digestion time (the tissue is digested for three different lengths of time, and the time that gives the strongest signal in most of the cells is noted)
2. Using this optimal protease digestion time to demonstrate that the signal is completely eliminated by pretreatment overnight in a solution that contains RNase-free DNase

With these points in mind, let us discuss in a step-by-step manner the start-up protocol for *in situ* PCR.

TISSUE PREPARATION

Methodology

Although *in situ* PCR may be done with cellular preparations or tissue sections, the latter should be used for the start-up protocol. The rationale is that part of the nonspecific signal that is the foundation of the start-up protocol is invariably present in paraffin-embedded, fixed tissues. This component, the DNA repair primer-independent pathway, is usually not present, however, in many cells of a cytospin preparation or cellular suspension unless certain conditions, notably heating after fixing, are used. Place two or, preferably, three tissue sections on the same silane-coated glass slide. Although the type of tissue one uses is not important, tonsillar tissue is a good choice as it is readily available in any surgical pathology laboratory and it contains a diversity of tissue types—epithelial and lymphoid—that can be used to study the pattern of target-specific and nonspecific signal. Of course, if one plans to study a specific type of tissue, such as liver tissue, then that type would be the logical choice for the start-up protocol.

As discussed in Chapter 5, it is essential to use formalin-fixed, paraffin-embedded tissues. If one has access to fresh tissues, it should be fixed from 8 hours to 3 days in 10% buffered formalin prior to embedding in paraffin. The advantage of shorter fixation (≤8 hours) is that short protease digestion times are adequate for an optimal signal (from 3 to 10 minutes of pepsin at 2 mg/ml for tissues fixed for 4 hours). Tissues fixed for 15

hours may require up to 60 minutes of pepsin digestion for an optimal signal with the start-up protocol. The disadvantage of the shorter fixation times is that the window of optimal protease digestion may be very narrow. I have seen instances where tissues fixed for 4 hours will give an optimal signal at 7 minutes of protease digestion and no signal (be overdigested) at 10 minutes using 2 mg/ml of pepsin which, admittedly, is a very high concentration. There is also a higher likelihood with tissues fixed for short time periods that what is determined to be an optimal protease digestion time in one experiment may not be optimal with another run, reflecting the narrow window of optimal digestion and variations in the specific activity of the protease from run to run. For these reasons, I would recommend one use tissues fixed for at least 15 hours. After the tissue sections are placed on the glass slides, they should be baked at 60°C for 15 minutes, although longer baking times (overnight) do not interfere with the *in situ* PCR signal. The baking drives away any water that may be trapped under the paraffin that could cause the tissue to lift off during the procedure, even if one is using silane-coated slides. After the slides are prepared, they may be stored indefinitely at room temperature in a box. I have used tissue sections on slides that were prepared 5 years prior to analysis and obtained successful *in situ* PCR results. Immediately before use, the paraffin is removed by placing the slide in fresh xylene for 5 minutes, followed by 5 minutes in 100% ethanol. The slide is then air dried (Fig. 6-1).

Potential Problems

Incorrect Fixative

It is not an uncommon problem that an investigator fails to use tissue that has been fixed in 10% buffered formalin. A nonpathologist might assume that the tissue has been fixed in formalin when in actuality another fixative was used, and it is difficult to make this distinction after the tissue has been fixed. As discussed in Chapter 4, if the fixative contains picric acid (Bouin's solution) or a heavy metal such as mercury

1. Place 3 Tissue Sections on a Silane Coated Glass Slide

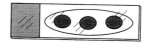

**2. Remove Paraffin with 5 Min. Wash In Xylene,
5 Min. Wash In 100% ETOH, Then Air-Dry**

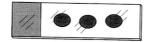

**3. Protease Digest for 30 Min., 60 Min., and 90 Min.
with Pepsin (2 mg/ml)**

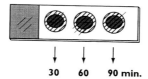

30   60   90 min.

**4. Remove Protease, do in situ PCR for 20 Cycles,
a 3+Signal Denotes Optimal Digestion Time**

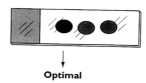

Optimal

Figure 6-1. *Part 1 of the start-up protocol: determining the optimal protease digestion time.* Place three paraffin-embedded tissue sections on one silane-coated slide. The tissue should be fixed in 10% buffered formalin. To determine the optimal protease digestion time, start with 30, 60, and 90 minutes of digestion in pepsin. Then do direct incorporation of the reporter nucleotide (*in situ* PCR). A strong signal in most of the cells, derived from DNA repair, mispriming, and target-specific genomic amplification (by using primers that correspond to a target in the cells), demonstrates the optimal protease digestion time for that tissue. If there is no signal and tissue morphology is poor, re-do the experiments with 5, 10, and 20 minutes of protease digestion; the tissue was likely fixed for <4 hours. If there is no signal and good morphology, try 120 to 150 minutes of protease digestion (though see text for other potential and more likely explanations for this result).

(Zenker's solution), it will *not* allow for successful *in situ* PCR. Picric acid solutions are thought by some to improve nuclear detail and can be recognized by the yellow color of the tissue after fixation. If the tissue has been fixed with a solution that contains picric acid or a heavy metal for at least several hours, the posi-tive control in the start-up protocol will show no signal under any protease condition (see Figs. 4-3 and 4-4 for equivalent result with standard *in situ* hybridization). Types of tissue that are often fixed in either Bouin's solution or B5, both of which contain picric acid, include bone marrow, lymph nodes, and testicular biopsies. Thus, it is better to avoid these tissues for the start-up protocol unless it is certain that they have been fixed solely in 10% buffered formalin.

Poor Tissue Adhesion

Silane-coated slides promote superior tissue adhesion. If the sections fall off more than 5% of the time, the slides may not have been coated with silane or water, and air droplets may have been trapped under the tissue when it was placed on the slide. Although adhesives such as poly-L-lysine or Sobo are adequate for immunohisto-chemistry, it has been found that they do not perform well with PCR *in situ* hybridization. In my experience, loss of tissue from the slide when using these adhesives for PCR *in situ* hybridization can occur more than 50% of the time. Another potential problem with tissue adherence during the start-up protocol is that very hard or poorly fixed sections may fall off even if silane-coated slides are used. The histotechnologist would likely recognize the problem even before the sections are cut; either the tissue needs to be re-embedded, or another tissue must be used in its place.

PROTEASE DIGESTION

Proper protease digestion is *the* most important step for *in situ* PCR in general and for the start-up protocol in particular. Correct protease time is needed for the reagents to have access to the tissue and for the *Taq* polymerase to synthesize DNA robustly within the nucleus. In my experience, insufficient protease time is responsible for *most* of the failures with the start-up protocol in general and within RT *in situ* PCR in particular. Although the data and resultant theories concerning protease digestion and *in situ* PCR are discussed in Chapter 3, it would be useful to summarize some of this information here.

Cross-linking fixatives such as formalin produce their effect, in part, by inactivation of the endogenous catabolic enzymes. This is achieved by formation of covalent bonds between these enzymes and other proteins and with nucleic acids. One can imagine that a resultant complex

three-dimensional labyrinth of proteins and nucleic acids is formed. It was postulated that this labyrinth served as a "solid support ion-exchange type resin" and inhibited migration of the amplified product from the site of origin (see Fig. 5-5). However, it is possible that the protein–nucleic acid links can limit access to the DNA of the different enzymes, such as DNase, *Taq* polymerase, and, when appropriate, reverse transcriptase, that are essential for *in situ* PCR perhaps by preventing access of the target (i.e., DNA gaps, or DNA–RNA target) by the relevant enzyme. This may explain in part the dramatic effect that alteration of the protease time has on both RT *in situ* PCR and the start-up protocol. The key point is that *at certain protease digestion times, one will obtain an optimal signal; at other protease times, the start-up protocol will not be successful!*

A review of the data presented in Tables 5-4 and 5-5 will remind us that *the success of the* in situ *PCR protocol is highly dependent on achieving an optimal balance of times for protease digestion and formalin fixation. One determines the optimal protease digestion time by trial and error.*

With these important points in mind, let us look at how to do the first part of the start-up protocol (Fig. 6-1):

Part 1 of the Start-Up Protocol: Determining the Optimal Protease Digestion Time for *in situ* PCR:

1. Place three tissue sections on one silane slide.
2. Estimate the time of fixation:
   a. If unknown, digest the three individual sections for 30, 60, and 90 minutes with pepsin (2 mg/ml at room temperature).
   b. If known, find the optimal digestion time in Tables 5-4 and 5-5 as a starting point and then add 10 to 20 minutes to this time for the second section and subtract 10 to 20 minutes from the time for the third section.
3. Follow the protocol given below for the *in situ* PCR. Determine which digestion time gives the optimal signal. Write this time

on the blank slides so that it will be used for the second part of the start-up protocol.

If the tissue is too large to place more than one section on a slide, divide the tissue into three parts using a hydrophobic pen and in this manner study the effects of 30, 60, and 90 minutes of protease digestion.

Other Protease Agents

At the behest of many people, I have tried a variety of protease agents, including pepsin, pepsinogen, trypsin, trypsinogen, and proteinase K. Although these are all satisfactory for *in situ* PCR, I prefer pepsin or trypsin for a number of reasons. First, these two are easily inactivated with an increase in pH. Second, as noted above, proteinase K tends to cause overdigestion more commonly than pepsin or trypsin. On the other hand, a stock solution of proteinase K stored at either 4°C or –20°C has a much longer shelf life than pepsin or trypsin which, when frozen at –20°C, begin to lose activity for PCR *in situ* in 1 week (G.J. Nuovo, *unpublished observations, 1993*). I strongly recommend the use of one protease exclusively in order to become familiar with its nuances.

The pepsin solution is prepared by adding 20 mg pepsin + 9.5 ml of water + 0.5 ml of 2N HCl. As noted above, 1-ml aliquots can be frozen and used for up to 1 week. I recommend adding the protease directly to the glass slide and placing the slide in a humidity chamber. For tissue sections of 3 to 15 mm, about 100 μl per tissue section should be used. After digestion, the protease is removed by washing the slide for 1 minute in water, then in 100% ethanol for 1 minute. The slide is then air dried.

Potential Problems

Protease Under- or Overdigestion

This problem has been described above. Because protease digestion is the *key* variable in determining the success of the start-up protocol,

examples of under- and overprotease digestion are given below in the section on interpreting the results.

Residual Protease Activity

Several people have related to me concern about residual protease activity, which, of course, could destroy either the RT or the *Taq* polymerase in the RT *in situ* PCR or PCR *in situ* hybridization techniques, respectively. An advantage of *in situ* PCR relative to solution phase PCR is that the glass slide is a solid support that allows for simple and efficient washes. Thus, even a 1-minute wash in water or a 0.1 M pH 7.5 Tris solution followed by a 1-minute wash in 100% ethanol is enough to remove the protease. Remember, do not dry heat inactivate the protease after the digestion step, as this will have a deleterious effect on the hybridization signal for PCR *in situ* hybridization or standard *in situ* hybridization (see Fig. 5-7).

The optimal protease digestion time is defined as the period that yields an intense signal in at least 50% of the cells. Although we discuss the PCR and detection aspects of the start-up protocol shortly, let us look at some representative data. As shown in Fig. 6-2, the optimal protease digestion time for this liver tissue was 90 minutes. Once you have achieved success with this part of the start-up protocol, congratulations! You have demonstrated that the conditions you are using, including the reagent conditions and detection system, are adequate to synthesize DNA inside the nucleus of a cell.

In the PCR step of the start-up protocol, digoxigenin dUTP will be directly incorporated into the PCR product as it is made in the nucleus. The signal in the nucleus will be mostly nonspecific due to DNA repair and, to a lesser extent, mispriming. I also recommend that one use primers that correspond to a real target in the cells to augment the signal in the non-DNased tissue section. For the purposes of the start-up protocol, suffice it to say that, under optimal conditions, the tissue section should show at least 50% of its cells with an intense nuclear signal; in most cases, over 90% of the cells will have a signal.

THE PCR PART OF THE START-UP
IN SITU PCR PROTOCOL

Methodology

For the PCR part of the start-up protocol, combine the following reagents:

1. 3.0 µl of the GeneAmp buffer (Perkin-Elmer kit)
2. 4.5 µl of 25 mM $MgCl_2$
3. 4.0 µl of the GeneAmp dNTP solution (see the following list)
4. 1.0 µl of primer 1 (20 µM stock solution)
5. 1.0 µl of primer 2 (20 µM stock solution)
6. 0.5 µl of the 1 mM digoxigenin dUTP solution
7. 1.0 µl of a 2% bovine serum albumin solution
8. 14.0 µl of water
9. 1.0 µl of *Taq* polymerase (Perkin-Elmer)

The dNTP solution is made as follows:

1. 25 µl of dATP (10 mM stock solution)
2. 25 µl of dCTP (10 mM stock solution)
3. 25 µl of dGTP (10 mM stock solution)
4. 25 µl of dTTP (10 mM stock solution)
5. 100 µl of sterile water

The 30-µl amplifying solution can then be placed over the tissue sections that are on a glass slide (Fig. 6-3). Although I usually use 20 µl per glass slide, the larger volume may be easier to work with when one is learning the procedure. After placing the solution over each tissue section, cut a plastic coverslip to size and place it over the amplifying solution. To assist the even distribution of the solution over the tissue, gently move the coverslip to and fro with a pair of forceps or a toothpick until the entire tissue section(s) is wet. The heating and cooling that occurs during cycling creates convection currents in the mineral oil that will be used to overlay the coverslip and prevent tissue drying during the PCR. These currents would move the coverslip away from the tissue section. To prevent

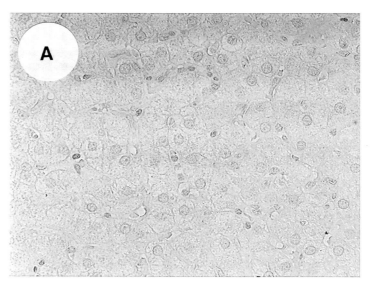

Figure 6-2. *Part 1 of the start-up protocol: optimal protease digestion of 90 minutes.* No signal was evident after 30 minutes protease digestion (**A**). Note the good preservation of tissue morphology, demonstrating that the lack of signal is not due to overdigestion. A signal is evident in rare cells after 60 minutes of protease digestion (**B**). Note that the positive cells are endothelial cells (*small arrow*) and not hepatocytes (*large arrow*); this implies that hepatocytes are more resistant to protease than the endothelium. An intense signal is seen in all cell types after 90 minutes of protease digestion in this serial section tested on the same glass slide (**C**).

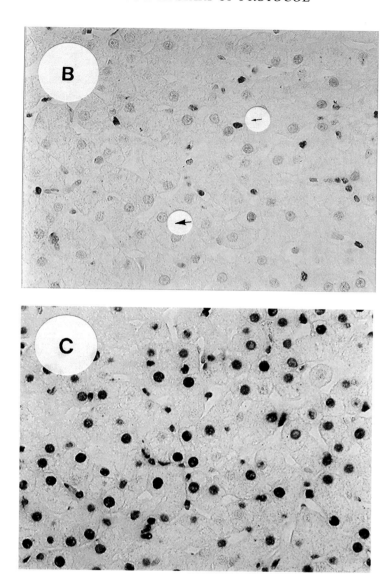

Figure 6-2. *Continued.*

this, anchor two edges of the coverslip to the surface of the glass slide with small drops of nail polish. Do *not* seal the entire perimeter of the coverslip with the nail polish. If the coverslip is completely sealed, the vapor that is released at the denaturing temperature cannot escape, and large bubbles form over the tissue section, preventing amplification in that area (Fig. 5-8). Next, place the slide in an aluminum foil boat made to fit the dimensions of the glass slide with a small margin on all sides. Gently fold the margin edges of the aluminum boat up to prevent the oil from draining off the slide. Place the boat on the block of the thermocycler (Fig. 5-9), which should be programmed as follows:

1. 94°C for 4 minutes (abort, then switch to next cycle)
2. 55°C for 2 minutes, then 94°C for 1 minute

3. 20 Cycles
4. 4°C until one is ready to remove the glass slides from the thermocycler. Note that these thermocycler parameters are for the start-up protocol only.

Mineral oil should be heated in the wells or the slots of the thermocycler or, if one prefers, in tubes in a dry bath kept between 60° and 90°C. When the temperature of the thermocycler reaches 55°C as it ramps to 94°C for the initial denaturing step, add enough mineral oil to fill up the entire aluminum boat. Periodically check the mineral oil during the 20 cycles to make certain that the coverslip is not dry and is still covered with oil. When the cycling is completed, take the slides out of the aluminum foil boats, remove the coverslip, and gently scrape off the nail polish with a scalpel blade. Place the slides standing up on a paper towel for 1 minute to allow the mineral oil to drain. Next, place the slides in xylene for 5 minutes, in 100% ethanol for 5 minutes, and then allow them to air dry.

Potential Problems

The Coverslip Curls

This problem is due to excessive heating of the coverslip. It can be corrected by adding the mineral oil overlay as soon as possible. Specifically, once the temperature of the block reaches 55°C, the coverslip should be covered by the mineral oil.

The Mineral Oil Leaks and the Sections Dry Out

The aluminum boats will occasionally leak. This may be due to flattening of the sides after using the boats several times or to excessive bending of the sides, which may cause small holes. Simply re-adjusting the sides of the boat may stop the leaking; however, sometimes a new boat will have to be made. Leaking boats are rare, and, in our experience, there are no problems with the oil in over 90% of the procedures.

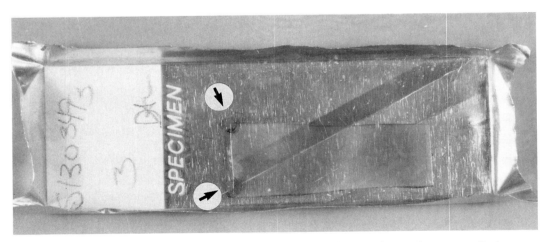

Figure 6-3. *The PCR part of the start-up protocol: using one large polypropylene coverslip.* I recommended placing one coverslip over each of the tissue sections. The coverslip can then be anchored to the glass slide with two drops of nail polish (*arrows*). The use of one large coverslip provides identical reaction conditions for the tissue sections during the PCR step of the start-up protocol. Note that the slide is placed into an aluminum foil boat that is made slightly larger than the size of the silane-coated glass slide. This boat is then placed on the aluminum block of the cycler.

After the Mineral Oil Is Removed the Slide Appears Opaque White Instead of Clear

This appearance is due to contaminated xylene and is easily corrected by changing the xylene and alcohol on a daily basis.

The Thermal Cycler

The PCR part of the start-up protocol illustrates my so-called aluminum boat method and the TC1 from Perkin-Elmer. One can use this aluminum boat method with any aluminum block thermal cycler, including the 480 and 9600 from Perkin-Elmer, or instruments from a variety of other companies, e.g., Coy Laboratories. It is important to stress that the cover of the aluminum block must be closed. Otherwise, the temperature on the glass slide will not reach temperatures adequate for denaturing. If one uses machines with milled down aluminum blocks (where the slide can be placed on directly), I still recommend using the aluminum boat. Otherwise, the slide may reach temperatures that are too high for a prolonged period of time, and the Taq polymerase may become inactive, with a loss of signal. Another alternative is to use the Perkin-Elmer in situ PCR thermal cycler 1000. This is described in detail in Chapter 10. If this machine is used, decrease the initial denaturing time to 3 minutes and subsequent denaturing times to 45 seconds.

THE DETECTION STEP

Methodology

For every 20 nucleotides added by *Taq* polymerase during the amplifying step, approximately 1 digoxigenin dUTP molecule will be present. The detection of digoxigenin-containing products is routine and is based on the protocols listed by Boehringer Mannheim (see Appendix). The following is a modified protocol we have devised to detect digoxigenin-labeled PCR product after *in situ* PCR:

1. Place the slide in a solution of 150 mM NaCl and 0.2% bovine serum albumin (blocking solution) at 50°C.
2. Incubate the slides in this solution for 10 minutes.
3. Remove the slide, wipe away the excess blocking solution, and draw a circle around the tissue section with a hydrophobic pen.
4. Place the slide in a humidity chamber (Fig. 5-10).
5. Before the section dries out, add the antidigoxingen–alkaline phosphatase conjugate. This is made by taking the antidigoxigenin–alkaline phosphatase conjugate available from Boehringer Mannheim and diluting it 1:150 in a solution that contains 0.1 M Tris HCl (pH 7.4) and 0.1 M NaCl. Add 100 μl per slide.
6. Place humidity chamber in an incubator at 37°C for 30 minutes.
7. Place the slide in a solution of 0.1 M Tris HCl (pH 9.5) and 0.1 M NaCl (detection solution) for 1 minute.
8. Place the slide in the detection solution to which NBT/BCIP has been added. If using the NBT/BCIP from Enzo or Digene, add 50 μl of each per 20 ml of detection solution. This solution should be made fresh at the time it is to be used.
9. Stop the reaction after 10 to 15 minutes by placing in water. It is strongly recommended that one view the slide periodically under the microscope during the reaction time. In my experience, a signal is often evident after 5 minutes and becomes maximum by 10 to 15 minutes. Additional time in the solution with the NBT/BCIP will rarely enhance the signal and will usually lead to higher background.

Potential Problems

Drying Out of the Antidigoxigenin–Alkaline Phosphatase Conjugate Solution

The antidigoxigenin–alkaline phosphatase conjugate solution placed on the slide in step 5 of the above protocol may, at times, dry out. This is invariably due to the solution running off the slide into the humidity chamber. This problem can be prevented by using the hydrophobic pen and placing the humidity chamber in a level incubator (Fig. 5-10).

Precipitation of
the NBT/BCIP Solution

When prepared, the NBT/BCIP solution will be light yellow in color. It is to be expected that it will turn a light to medium blue after the slides are added (step 8). However, sometimes the chromagen will precipitate in solution and form large black crystals that appear either tapered or round on the tissue section. This can be prevented by first warming the detection solution to 37°C before adding the chromogen (see Fig. 4-16). Furthermore, we have noted that different sources of NBT/BCIP vary a great deal in their propensity to precipitate. Also, some solutions tend to form dark green precipitates over the tissue sections (Fig. 6-4). Because of these potential problems, I recommend using the NBT/BCIP that is part of the Digene *in situ* kit. This company sells the NBT/BCIP individually.

THE COUNTERSTAIN STEP

The slides should be transferred to the nuclear fast red solution, which can be reused many times. The preference of the investigator will determine the amount of time the slides remain in the counterstain. If one desires to maximize the contrast between the cells with signal and the cells without signal, then a brief time (30 seconds) in the counterstain, which stains nuclei and cytoplasm a pale pink, is indicated. Alternatively, if one wishes to optimize the appearance of the morphology of the tissue, including the negative cells, longer times (3 to 10 minutes) are indicated. I prefer 3 minutes in nuclear fast red. After the counterstain, place the slide in two separate water rinses for 1 minute each. To prepare permanent sections of the tissue, the slides are placed in 100% ethanol for 1 minute and then in xylene. The slide can be mounted using permount mounting medium and a glass coverslip and then be viewed under the microscope. The chromogen and counterstain colors will be retained indefinitely when prepared in this manner.

After determining this optimal protease digestion time, one is ready for the second part of the start-up protocol, which in effect is the prelude to the RT *in situ* PCR technique.

THE DNASE STEP:
THE NEGATIVE CONTROL

Part 2 of the Start-Up Protocol:
Elimination of the Signal with
Overnight DNase Digestion

After determining the protease digestion time that results in the strongest signal in the greatest number of cells after *in situ* PCR, the second and final step of the start-up protocol can be done. The DNase digestion step is an essential part of the start-up protocol as well as being the foundation for the RT *in situ* PCR technique. After the tissue sections have air-dried subsequent to optimal protease digestion, which was determined in part 1 of the start-up protocol, one can apply the DNase solution to one of the two sections (Fig. 6-5). I use the RNase-free DNase from Boehringer Mannheim (see Appendix), although equivalent results have been obtained with the RNase-free DNase solutions from Bethesda Research Laboratories (BRL) and Strategene. Of course, it is important to use an RNase-free DNase when analyzing for RNA.

First, a $10 \times$ buffer is made by adding 70 μl of 3 M sodium acetate, 10 μl of 1 M magnesium sulfate, and 130 μl of DEPC water (Research Genetics, Alabama). This can be stored at -20°C. To prepare the DNase solution, add 1 μl of the $10 \times$ buffer, 1 μl of the DNase solution (10 U per μl), and 8 μl of DEPC water. Place 10 μl of this DNase solution on each tissue section and cover the section with a plastic coverslip. It is important to autoclave the coverslip material prior to use for RNA work. I strongly recommend that the reader use the "double-bag" type of polypropylene plastic so that, after autoclaving, one may cut the plastic to size and then use the inner surface to cover the DNase solution. In this manner, the surface of the plastic that will face the tissue section will not be touched, thus avoiding inadvertent tissue exposure to RNase (the plastic coverslips are discussed in detail in Chapter

5). After adding the DNase solution and covering the tissue sections, the slides should be placed in a humidity chamber and incubated overnight at 37°C.

To inactivate the DNase solution, remove the coverslips, wash for 1 minute in DEPC water, then 1 minute in 100% ethanol, and then allow the slides to air dry. For the start-up protocol one does not have to be concerned about RNase contamination, but for those doing RT *in situ* PCR work, it is important to use sterile toothpicks and gloves when removing the coverslips to minimize the possibility of this potential problem.

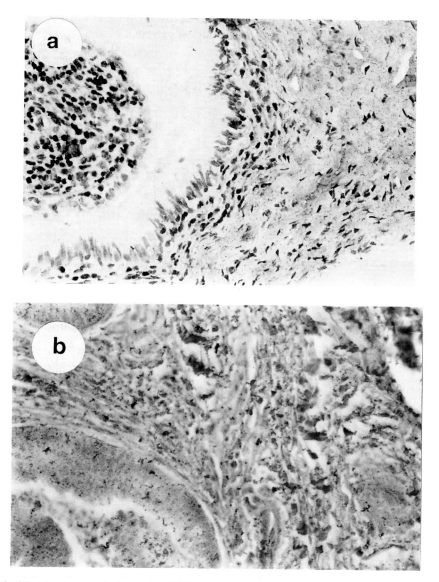

Figure 6-4. *High background with* in situ *PCR due to the chromogen.* The chromogen NBT/BCIP produces an intense and localized dark blue precipitate at the site of *in situ* amplification in the positive control for the start-up protocol (**a**, chromogen from Digene). However, some sources of NBT/BCIP may be associated with a nonspecific and generalized precipitate that masks the signal (**b**) (chromogen from Boehringer Mannheim).

Potential Problems

Inadequate DNase Digestion

The result of inadequate DNase digestion is, of course, the presence of a DNA-based signal after *in situ* PCR. I have had many inquiries from investigators stating that they were experiencing this problem. It is very important to stress that the presence of a DNA-based signal with *in situ* PCR after DNase di-

gestion is *rarely* due to an inadequate DNase concentration or digestion time. Rather, it usually reflects *inadequate protease digestion.* Presumably, there are too many persistent protein–DNA cross-links in the underprotease-digested tissue to allow the DNase adequate access to the entire DNA template. I have done experiments in which a signal was still present after DNase digestion using the 10 U per section described above. Furthermore, the signal persisted even after increasing the con-

1. Place 2 Tissue Sections on a Silane Coated Slide

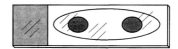

2. Remove Paraffin with 5 Min. Wash in Xylene, 5 Min. Wash in 100% ETOH, Then Air -Dry

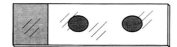

3. Protease Digest Each Tissue for Optimal Time as Determined in Part I

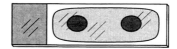

4. Remove Protease with I Minute Wash in 0.1 M Tris HCL (pH 7.5) and 0.1 M NaCl Solution, I Minute in 100% ETOH, Then Air-Dry

Figure 6-5. *Part 2 of the start-up protocol: elimination of the signal by DNase digestion after optimal protease digestion.* In the second part of the start-up protocol, digest two tissues with protease using the optimal digestion time as determined in part 1. Then, incubate one of the two sections overnight with DNase. Remove the DNase, and then do *in situ* PCR. The signal should be strong with the section not treated with DNase and eliminated by the DNase digestion. These represent the essential controls for RT *in situ* PCR.

centration of the DNase to 50 U per section. However, the signal was eliminated with the standard DNase concentration by increasing the time of protease digestion (this is discussed in detail in Chapter 7). This observation again demonstrates that the protease digestion step is the *critical* step for the start-up protocol.

It has been my experience that DNase digestion should be done overnight and that a shorter period of time may be less than adequate. When one considers the large amount of DNA in a nucleus that needs to be digested to eliminate the nonspecific signal, it is not surprising that brief periods of DNase digestion may not completely eliminate the signal. To study this problem, serial tissue sections were digested for the optimal time in protease as defined by an intense signal in over 50% of the cells after *in situ* PCR. The sections on the slide were then digested in the DNase solution for 2, 4, 7, and 15 hours. The

5. Prepare 10 µl of a RNase-Free DNase Solution

6. Place Solution on One Tissue Section, Overlay with Plastic Coverslip

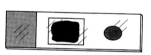

7. Incubate Overnight at 37 C in Humidity Chamber, Remove DNase with 1 Min. Wash in Tris Solution, 1 Min. Wash in 100% ETOH, then Air-Dry

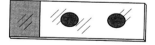

8. Do In Situ PCR for 20 Cycles

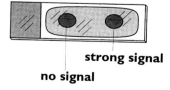

strong signal

no signal

Figure 6-5. *Continued.*

results are shown in Fig. 6-6. Note that the digestions for 2 and 4 hours still produced a signal. However, both 7 and 15 hours of digestion in the RNase-free DNase solution were adequate to render the native DNA non-amplifiable during *in situ* PCR.

Residual DNase Activity

A concern that several people have related to me is that residual DNase activity could destroy either the cDNA made during the RT step or the amplified DNA made by *Taq* polymerase. As stated above, an advantage of *in situ*

PCR over solution phase PCR is that the solid support of the glass slide allows for simple and efficient washes. Thus, even a 1-minute wash in DEPC water followed by a 1-minute wash in ethanol is enough to remove the DNase.

INTERPRETING THE RESULTS

Several scenarios are possible when one views the slide under the microscope.

Desired Result

Part 1: One of the three protease digestion times produces an intense *nuclear-based*

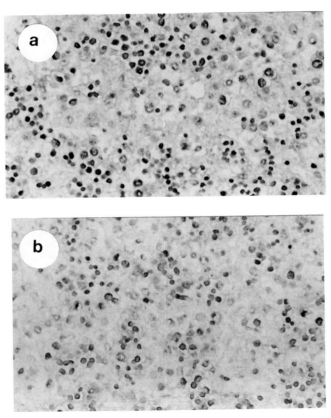

Figure 6-6. *Relationship of the DNase digestion time to the loss of signal in the negative control of the start-up protocol.* This tissue from the spleen was fixed for 15 hours in 10% buffered formalin. After 75 minutes of digestion in pepsin, a strong signal is evident in most of the cells in the positive control (**a**). The signal persisted when the tissue was digested in DNase for 2 hours (**b**) and 4 hours (**c**) but not when the DNase digestion time was 7 hours (**d**).

signal in most of the cells.

Part 2: In *non-DNased tissue*, the protease digestion time determined to be optimal in part 1 again produces an intense nuclear-based signal in most of the cells. In *DNased tissue*, none of the cells show a signal. The negative cells have clearly defined nuclei that stain light pink (Fig. 6-7).

If the above results were obtained, you have demonstrated the ability to amplify and detect PCR product *in situ* and to eliminate it by DNase digestion after adequate protease digestion. Congratulations! You will recall that the signal seen in the non-DNased section is mostly or totally nonspecific, depending on whether the primers used correspond to a specific target present in the tissue. However, the purpose of the start-up protocol is *not* to perform target-specific amplification but to become capable of doing the various steps needed for *Taq* polymerase to function, albeit nonspecifically, within a cell nucleus, to detect this product successfully and to be able to eliminate this signal by DNase digestion. Obviously, once these goals have been achieved, the investigator is ready to move on to the protocols that ensure target-specific amplification.

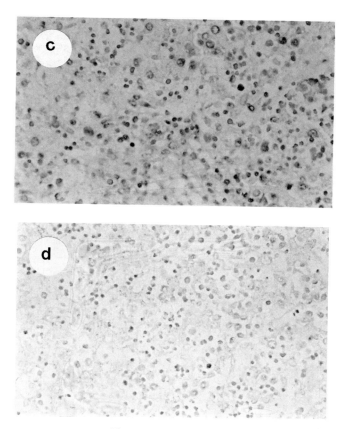

Figure 6-6. *Continued.*

Undesired Result Number 1: Weak to No Signal and Poor Tissue Morphology

This result is caused by overdigestion in the protease solution. A common indicator of poor tissue morphology is that the nuclei do *not* stain well with the nuclear fast red and thus appear ghost-like or are not visible at all. The basement membranes will appear prominent because they are more resistant to protease (Fig. 6-8). This problem is easily corrected. The protease time should be decreased; if the initial times chosen were 30, 60, and 90 minutes, I would recommend re-doing the experiment using 5-, 10-, and 20-minute protease digestion.

Undesired Result Number 2: No Signal; Good Tissue Morphology

This result has many potential causes, the most common of which is underdigestion in the protease solution. Good tissue morphology, defined by the ability of the nucleus and cytoplasm to stain pale pink, demonstrates that the native DNA and RNA are able to bind to the counterstain and, thus, are not overdigested. There are, of course, other possible reasons for a weak signal or no signal in the non-DNased tissue. These include

1. Using tissue not fixed in formalin, especially if fixatives containing picric acid or a heavy metal were used
2. Inadequate silanization of the slide, causing the tissue to fold on itself
3. Incorrect preparation of the amplifying solution, e.g., adding either too little or too much $MgCl_2$
4. Drying of the amplifying solution during the cycling
5. Drying of the antidigoxigenin-alkaline phosphatase conjugate
6. Incorrect pH of the detection solution (i.e., too low)
7. Using either *Taq* polymerase or antidigoxigenin–alkaline phosphatase conjugate that is no longer functional

Before discussing in more detail the most common cause of this problem, let us first discuss the other seven causes listed above.

Tissue Fixative

It may be difficult for the nonpathologist to determine the fixative used for a given tissue. Bouin's solution, which contains picric acid, is occasionally used in some laboratories. This solution will cause the tissue to appear yellow, and, as discussed in Chapters 4 and 5, in such cases the *in situ* PCR will not work under any condition. Unfortunately, tissues that are fixed in heavy metal containing solutions cannot be identified by visual inspection alone. A clue that such a fixative may have been used comes from the tissue type. For example, lymphoid tissue and bone marrow biopsy material may be fixed in solutions that contain either picric acid (though not Bouin's solution, and hence not yellow) or heavy metals, as these allow for better cytological detail and support certain immunohistochemical stains that are useful if lymphoma is in the differential diagnosis. The histology laboratory where the tissues were processed will usually provide information about the fixative used.

There is a simple way to determine if the absence of a signal with the start-up protocol is due to fixation in a solution that contained either picric acid or a heavy metal such as mercury: Consider the two possibilities of a negative result in part 1 of the start-up protocol with regard to the type of fixative used: (i) The tissue was fixed too long in formalin or another type of cross-linking fixative; or (ii) The tissue was fixed in a solution that contained either picric acid or a heavy metal.

Standard *in situ* hybridization can be used to determine which of these two possible explanations is correct. This test will be positive at protease times much *less* than used in *in situ* PCR but will *not* be positive for tissues fixed in either picric acid or certain heavy metals. Thus, one should perform standard *in situ* hybridization with a protease digestion time of 30 minutes. I recommend using the probe specific for the repetitive *alu* sequence, as described in detail in Chapter 4. If a strong signal is present, the tissue was most likely overfixed in formalin or a similar cross-linker and the protease digestion time should be increased (Fig. 6-9). Stated another way, one is very far to the left of the curve de-

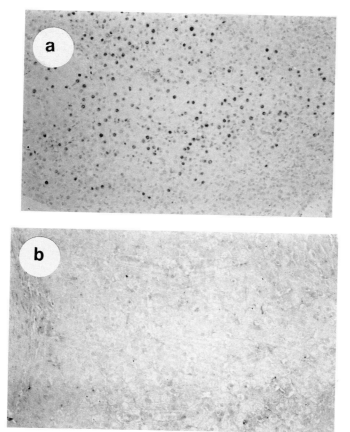

Figure 6-7. *The desired results with the start-up protocol.* This liver tissue was fixed for 15 hours in 10% buffered formalin. Optimal protease time for the start-up protocol was found to be 60 minutes. Note the signal present in most of the cells after 60 minutes of protease digestion (**a**). The signal was eliminated when the tissue was digested overnight in a DNase solution (**b**).

picted in Fig. 6-10. This problem can be rectified by substantially increasing the protease digestion time (see Fig. 3-18). However, if no signal is evident with the *alu* probe, it is likely that the tissue was fixed in either picric acid or a heavy metal and that a signal will not be obtainable with the start-up protocol under any circumstance (see Chapter 4 for a more detailed discussion of the effects of these fixatives on the signal with standard *in situ* hybridization).

It was noted in Chapter 5 that tissue fixed in ethanol- or acetone-based fixatives is not suitable for optimal *in situ* PCR. These fixatives have rarely been used in the preparation of tissue sections in histology laboratories. This, however, may change, as several com-

panies are marketing fixatives based in alcohol as an alternative to formalin, which has come under increased scrutiny due to possible health risks. Various companies have sent to me several alcohol-based and other non-formalin-containing fixatives to be tested for their ability to support *in situ* PCR. This work has demonstrated that these fixatives can be used for tissue successfully tested with *in situ* PCR. There are two notable differences in the process when alternative fixatives are used for the tissue rather than formalin: (i) a signal can be evident without protease digestion and (ii) the signal tends to be weaker and more diffuse than for similar tissues fixed in 10% buffered formalin (Fig. 6-11).

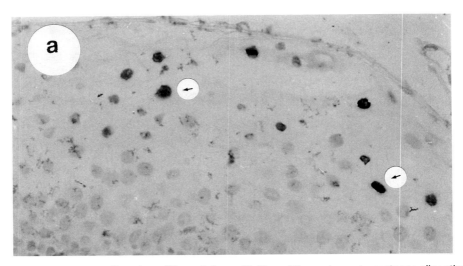

Figure 6-8. *Protease overdigestion: differential sensitivities of tissue types to protease digestion.* Tonsillar tissue consists of a surface layer of squamous epithelium that overlays a large area of lymphoid tissue. This tonsillar tissue was fixed for 4 hours in 10% buffered formalin. A signal was evident in the squamous cells using the start-up protocol after 30 minutes of protease digestion (**a**, *small arrows*). However, note that no signal is evident in the underlying lymphoid tissue (**b**). The poor cellular detail in b shows that the lymphocytes were overdigested in the protease. Lymphoid tissue is among the most sensitive to protease digestion, whereas squamous epithelium is much more resistant, perhaps reflecting the tight junctions that exist between these cells. Liver tissue was fixed for 6 hours in 10% buffered formalin (**c**). No signal was evident when the tissue was digested for 45 minutes in pepsin at 2 mg/ml. Note the poor cytoplasmic and nuclear detail as well as the prominent basement membranes (*arrows*). These features are indicative of protease overdigestion. The basement membranes are much more resistant to protease digestion than cells and thus will remain intact even when the cells are overdigested. Note how a few hepatocytes on the periphery are positive; this is because they are more intensely fixed due to poor diffusion of the formalin.

Inadequate Silanization

Several people have informed me that their tissue sections simply do not stay on the glass slide but rather fold or partly detach. In our experience, the tissue should stay completely intact in over 99% of the cases. Folding or detachment of the tissue is due to poor silanization. It is recommended that one purchase silane-coated slides, which are available from a variety of sources.

Amplifying Solution

Incorrect preparation of the amplifying solution usually indicates one of two specific problems. The first possibility is that too much or too little $MgCl_2$ was added, and the second is that the bovine serum albumin solution was forgotten when relatively small (5 U/50 μl)

amounts of *Taq* polymerase were used. A review of the data and the discussion in Chapter 5 will remind the reader how dependent the signal is on the magnesium concentration. Indeed, omission of the $MgCl_2$ from the amplifying solution is a useful negative control for PCR *in situ* hybridization or *in situ* PCR (Fig. 5-2). The bovine serum albumin is needed, especially when lower amounts of *Taq* polymerase are used, to block the invariable partial adsorption of the enzyme to the plastic coverslip and the glass slide. In the protocol listed above, I recommended using 5 U of *Taq* (1 μl) per 30 μl of total volume. This amount is intended to correct for the addition of too little bovine serum albumin. In actuality, one can use as little as 2.5 U of the enzyme/30 μl but only if the correct amount of bovine serum albumin is added.

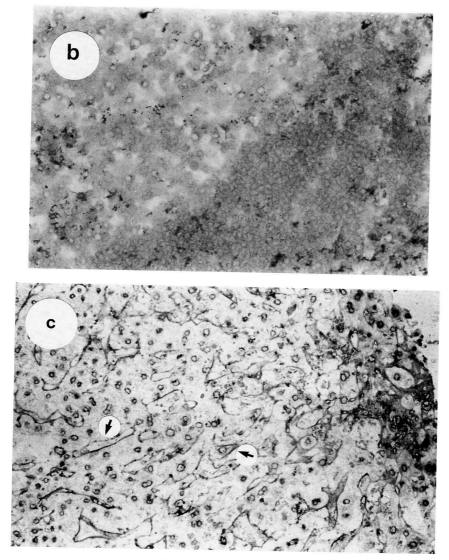

Figure 6-8. *Continued.*

Drying of the Amplifying Solution or the Antidigoxigenin–Alkaline Phosphatase Conjugate Solution

To prevent problems of drying, one should periodically check the slides. Specifically, during the amplifying step of the *in situ* PCR, *gently* touch the plastic coverslip with a toothpick to ascertain if it is still covered with mineral oil. If the oil has drained from the slide, the amplifying solution will dry out within one to two cycles. Similarly, if the antidigoxigenin–alkaline phosphatase conjugate solution used in the detection step runs off the edge of the slide, the tissue section will quickly dry out. Circling the tissue using a hydrophobic pen before adding

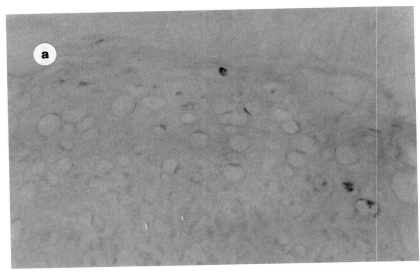

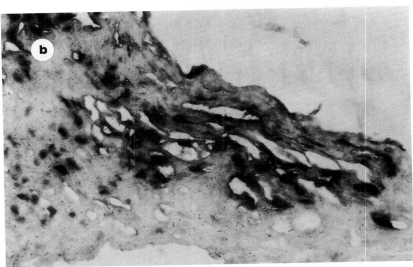

Figure 6-9. *A negative result in both the positive and negative controls for the start-up protocol: determination if the results reflect the tissue fixative or inadequate protease digestion time.* Two skin biopsy specimens each gave a negative result in the positive control for the start-up protocol. Furthermore, the negative control for each was also negative. To determine if this was due to the type of fixative used for the tissue or to an inadequate protease digestion time, standard *in situ* hybridization was done after 30 minutes of protease digestion. No signal was noted for the tissue shown in **a**, whereas a strong signal was noted for the tissue depicted in **b**. Further investigation showed that the tissue in a was fixed in Bouin's solution for at least 15 hours, thus precluding both *in situ* hybridization and *in situ* PCR. The tissue shown in b yielded a signal with the start-up protocol when the digestion time was increased to 2 hours (not shown). One can determine if a negative result with the start-up protocol is due to the type of fixative used or to inadequate digestion time by exploiting the observation that the standard *in situ* signal will be negative with certain fixatives and positive for tissues fixed in formalin at much shorter protease digestion times than needed for *in situ* PCR.

the solution, as well as checking the slides half way through the process, will help to ensure that the solution remains over the tissue.

The Substrate Solution: Incorrect pH of the Chromogen-Containing Solution

Alkaline phosphatase requires a high pH to function optimally. If a negative result is obtained, it is recommended that the pH of this solution be rechecked.

Inactivity of the Taq *Polymerase or the Antidigoxigenin–Alkaline Phosphatase Conjugate*

According to scientists at Perkin-Elmer and Boehringer Mannheim, occasionally an unexpected negative PCR test or digoxigenin detection step is attributed to an inactive reagent. The condition of the *Taq* polymerase, when stored at the correct temperature, is rarely the cause of a negative start-up protocol result. If this is suspected, the status of the *Taq* should be tested with solution phase PCR. Similarly, the antidigoxigenin–alkaline phosphatase conjugate, when stored at the correct temperature, rarely loses its capabilities. However, if the antibody is inadvertently frozen, its activity is markedly diminished. When the amount of solution stored is getting low, I routinely add the remaining solution to a container of fresh solution to help ensure that the antidigoxigenin–alkaline phosphatase conjugate will retain its activity.

Inadequate Protease Digestion

Now that these potential problems have been discussed, let us shift our attention to the most common cause of failure to produce a signal in the non-DNased tissue; inadequate protease digestion.

Recall that the success of *in situ* PCR is highly dependent on the ratio of the times of formalin fixation and protease digestion. Clearly, if the amount of time that a tissue was fixed is known, it is not difficult to ascertain the proper protease digestion time. A problem arises when the fixation time is unknown. Although most archival

specimens from a surgical pathology laboratory are fixed from 4 to 15 hours, there are cases when the fixation time may be extended. For example, tissue that is shipped in the mail prior to processing may be fixed for days. Furthermore, it is not unusual for tissues from autopsies to be fixed for days or even weeks prior to processing. If one does not know the length of fixation time and there is no signal evident with the start-up protocol, I strongly recommend first demonstrating that a strong signal is evident with standard *in situ* hybridization with the positive *alu* probe. Then, re-do part 1 of the start-up protocol using 120, 150, and 180 minutes of pepsin digestion. I also recommend using the DNase digestion as well. If the negative result with part 1 is due to inadequate protease digestion time, *and* the DNase section also gives no signal, then the digestion time must be markedly below the optimal. This statement can be made because a signal will be evident in the DNased section as the protease time approaches the optimal even before a signal is evident with the section not treated with DNase (Fig. 6-10). A negative result at 90 minutes protease digestion in pepsin at 2 mg/ml for *both* the negative and positive controls suggests two possibilities:

1. The pepsin is no longer active.
2. The tissue has been fixed too long for pepsin to work.

Assuming that one has controlled for points 1 through 7 listed above for no signal in part 1, it is most likely that the pepsin is no longer active. This is because it is very difficult to fix a tissue so long as to make even the DNased section negative after 90 minutes of digestion in pepsin. Make certain that the trypsin or pepsin is fresh and that the HCl is added. As described in Chapter 4, the pepsin solution can be stored at −20°C, but it shows a measurable loss of activity after 1 week of storage.

With regard to the second possibility, if the tissue has been fixed for 2 or more days, especially a small or thin biopsy, it may not be possible to obtain a successful result with the non-DNased tissue at any protease time using pepsin or trypsin. When this fixation prob-

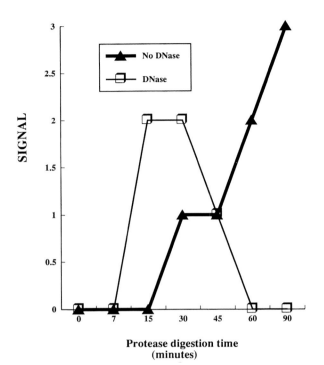

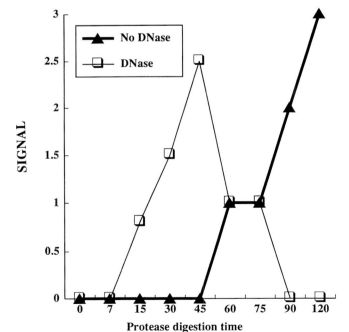

Figure 6-10. *Relationship between the positive (no DNase) and negative (DNase) controls to the protease digestion time with the start-up protocol.* This figure shows how the signal in the negative and positive controls for a skin biopsy fixed for 15 hours (*top*) and 1 week (*bottom*) in 10% buffered formalin varies with the protease digestion time. Note that no signal is evident in either the positive control if the protease digestion time is ≤15 or 30 minutes, respectively. However, with standard *in situ* hybridization a signal will be evident after 30 minutes of protease digestion of tissues fixed for 1 week (see Fig. 6-9). Also note that a signal will be evident with suboptimal protease digestion in the negative control *before* being evident with the positive control. Furthermore, when a signal is evident at suboptimal protease digestion with the positive control, it is usually weaker than for the negative control. It is only at optimal protease digestion that the intense signal with the positive control is seen with no signal for the negative control.

lem appears to be the case, I have learned from experience to try proteinase K digestion. It is important to stress that tissue fixation is generally standardized and that variations from this standard are the exception and are highly unusual. Pepsin or trypsin digestion at 120 minutes will be optimal more than 99% of the time.

Undesired Result Number 3

Part 1: Weak to moderate signal, good tissue morphology

Part 2: In non-DNased tissue, weak to moderate signal, good tissue morphology; in *DNased tissue*, weak to moderate signal typically stronger than the signal evident for the non-DNased tissue, good tissue morphology

These results are caused by underdigestion in the protease solution. The theoretical basis for the stronger signal with the tissue that was digested in DNase is presented in Chapter 3.

For the purposes of this discussion, the key point with regard to this observation is that it demonstrates that the problem *is invariably* inadequate protease digestion and not one of the other seven problems listed above, because none of these would lead to a stronger signal in the DNased tissue with respect to the non-DNased tissue. If this result is obtained it is highly recommended that the protease digestion time be increased by 10 to 20 minute increments until an intense signal is seen with part 1 and the signal is completely eliminated by DNase digestion (Fig. 6-12).

Undesired Result Number 4: Moderate to Strong Cytoplasmic Signal, Weak to Strong Nuclear Signal, Good Tissue Morphology

This cytoplasmic signal is background due to DNA synthesized in the amplifying solution sticking to the cellular proteins. Background signal can be eliminated by increasing the stringency of the wash used after the

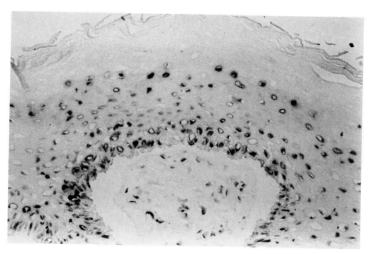

Figure 6-11. *The use of noncross-linking fixatives for* in situ *PCR.* Tissues fixed in 10% buffered formalin are recommended for the start-up protocol. However, due to recent concerns about the long-term health effects of formalin, substitute fixatives are becoming more available on a commercial basis. One such fixative is called Histochoice (Amresco, Inc, Solon, OH). A signal was produced in the positive control for the start-up protocol after 15 hours of fixation in Histochoice. No protease digestion was needed. A smaller percentage of cells showed a signal in the positive control for tissues fixed in Histochoice when compared with the corresponding tissue fixed in 10% buffered formalin. Furthermore, tissues fixed with formalin substitutes were more sensitive to overdigestion with pepsin. See Chapter 5 for a more detailed description of the effect of noncross-linking fixatives on the signal with *in situ* PCR.

in situ PCR, as discussed in detail in Chapter 5. A weak nuclear signal means that the protease digestion time must be increased.

Undesired Result Number 5: Moderate to Strong Cytoplasmic Signal, No Nuclear Signal, Poor Tissue Morphology

This result is due to overdigestion with the protease. As illustrated in Fig. 6-8, protease overdigestion has two stages: loss of a nuclear-based DNA signal to the cytoplasm and then complete loss of signal and cell morphology. Overdigestion can also lead to increased cytoplasmic background. Repeat the experiment after decreasing the protease digestion time by 50%.

A SHORTENED ISOTHERMAL VERSION OF THE START-UP PROTOCOL

The start-up protocol as described above is to prepare the investigator to do RT *in situ* PCR or PCR *in situ* hybridization. One not only determines the optimal protease digestion time for a given tissue and generates the positive and negative controls for RT *in situ* PCR, but one also gets comfortable working with tissue sections on glass slides with the thermal cycler. However, it should be appreciated that there is a much simpler version of the start-up protocol. It may not give one actual experience with the technique used for RT *in situ* PCR, but it does allow one to de-

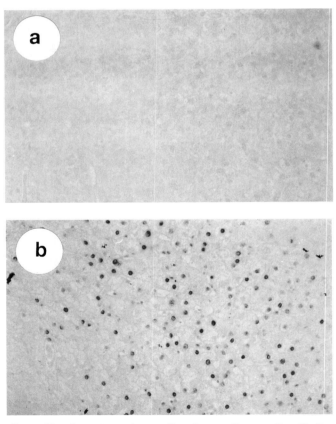

Figure 6-12. *The effect of inadequate protease digestion on the results with the start-up protocol.* If the liver tissue shown in Fig. 6-7 was digested in pepsin for 15 minutes, the signal in the positive control is no longer evident (**a**). Note the presence of a signal in the negative control (**b**). This "paradoxical" enhancement of the negative control (DNase-digested tissue) is typical of tissue that has not been digested for an adequate amount of time in the protease solution.

termine the optimal protease digestion time in *less than 1 hour*. It is based on a simple concept (described in detail in Chapter 3); the signal with the tissue that is not digested in DNase is due mostly to DNA repair. DNA repair is isothermal and provides enormous incorporation of the reporter nucleotide in a matter of minutes. We performed experiments where three tissue sections were digested for different periods of time and then subjected to the amplifying solution plus *Taq* polymerase for 1 to 30 minutes. Amazingly, a strong signal is evident even after 3 minutes of isothermal *Taq*-mediated DNA synthesis but only if the protease digestion time was optimal. This is illustrated in Fig. 6-13. This underscores the large number of gaps that must be induced by heating during paraffin-embedding tissues. I recommend this shortened version of the start-up protocol as an ad-

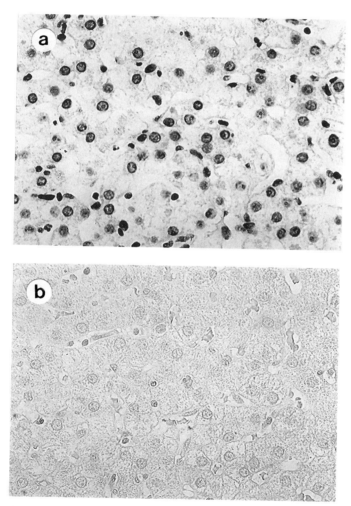

Figure 6-13. *The shortened version of the start-up protocol: rapid isothermal generation of signal from DNA repair.* It was determined using part 1 of the start-up protocol that the optimal protease digestion time for this tissue was 30 minutes. The tissue was digested for 30 minutes. The amplifying solution minus any primer and with *Taq* polymerase was added at 55°C and the reaction allowed to continue for 1 to 30 minutes at this temperature. A strong signal from DNA repair was evident at all time points, even after 3 minutes, although the maximum signal required 7 minutes (**a**). However, no signal was evident if the protease digestion time was suboptimal (15 minutes) after 30 minutes incubation at 55°C (**b**).

junct for the longer version, especially for the investigator who has experience working with tissue section. It certainly is a simple, rapid, and reliable way to determine the optimal protease digestion time for RT *in situ* PCR.

CHOICE OF REPORTER NUCLEOTIDE

Most investigators will prefer to use nonisotopic reporter nucleotides for the start-up protocol. Our experience has shown that digoxigenin dUTP is well suited to the start-up protocol, as the range of digoxigenin dUTP/dTTP that permits successful *in situ* PCR is broad, as evident in Fig. 6-14. I recommend using 10 μM of digoxigenin dUTP to 200 μM of dTTP. Biotin is optimal at a ratio of 1 biotin dATP to 1 dATP; I use 100 μM of each. The optimal ratios of ^{3}H and ^{35}S are presented in Fig. 6-14. However, I do not recommend ^{35}S due to very high background. For those who wish to use ^{3}H, exposure times of 2 to 4 days are adequate. Finally, I have used fluorescene-tagged nucleotides with the start-up protocol. I have not obtained a good signal using darkfield microscopy to detect the fluorescene tag. However, a strong signal was obtained using an antifluorescene–alkaline phosphatase conjugate and the chromogen NBT/BCIP.

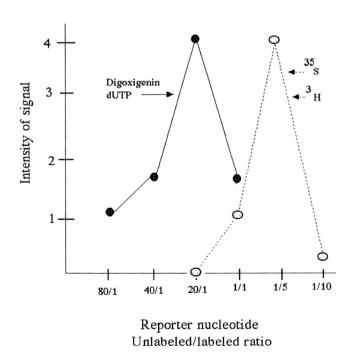

Fig. 6-14. *Optimizing curves for digoxigenin dUTP and several radioactive labeled nucleotides for* in situ *PCR.* The optimizing curves for direct incorporation of digoxigenin, ^{3}H, and ^{35}S during *in situ* PCR. Note that the optimal ratio for digoxigenin is 200 μM dTTP/20 μM digoxigenin dUTP. For ^{3}H, the optimal ratio is 1 μm dCTP and 5 μM ^{3}H dCTP.

7

Reverse Transcriptase *in situ* PCR

In the second edition of this book it was mentioned that perhaps the greatest improvements since the writing of the first edition have been made in the methodology for RT *in situ* PCR. The same could be said about this current edition. The "EZ" RT *in situ* PCR protocol, which uses one enzyme (rTth) and one amplifying solution for both the RT and PCR steps, has greatly simplified the detection of RNA inside intact cells. This, in combination with the better understanding of the mechanisms of the nonspecific signal that may be evident in *in situ* PCR in tissue sections and the ability to eliminate this nonspecific signal reproducibly with overnight DNase digestion, makes it a relatively simple matter to detect *in situ* PCR–amplified RNAs (cDNAs). After one determines the optimal protease digestion time for a given sample, in a matter of a few hours it is possible to detect a given mRNA via the direct incorporation of the labeled nucleotide. I would suggest that RT *in situ* PCR is actually a simpler method both to learn and to perform than standard RNA *in situ* hybridization or PCR *in situ* hybridization, both of which involve hybridization steps.

To appreciate the foundation of RT *in situ* PCR, I believe it is important to review the mechanism of the nonspecific signal in tissue sections before discussing the actual protocols for the *in situ* detection of PCR-amplified cDNA. These protocols are similar to the start-up protocol described in Chapter 5 with the addition, of course, of an RT step. Finally, applications of RT *in situ* PCR are discussed, with emphasis on three RNA viruses—measles, hepatitis C, and hantavirus— and on a variety of human mRNAs, including several of the metalloproteases, gelsolin, amy-

loid precursor protein, and glycoprotein IIB. In Chapters 8 and 9, the detection of human papillomavirus RNAs and HIV-1 RNAs, as well as a variety of cytokine mRNAs by RT *in situ* PCR, are discussed.

THEORY

The theory and practice of PCR *in situ* hybridization is discussed in Chapter 5. It was emphasized that one could *not* do target-specific direct incorporation of the reporter molecule (e.g., digoxigenin dUTP) for DNA targets in paraffin-embedded tissue sections, which is referred to as "*in situ* PCR" in this book. It was discussed that nonspecific DNA synthesis, primarily in the form of DNA repair, invariably would cause a false-positive signal with paraffin-embedded tissue sections. Although DNA repair can be blocked by pretreatment in a solution that contains a dideoxynucleotide, the exacting requirements of correct protease digestion time and the preincubation time with the dideoxynucleotide made this "dideoxy-assisted *in situ* PCR" prone to residual nonspecific false-positive results. This nonspecific signal was reliably and completely eliminated with an overnight digestion in RNase-free DNase if (and only if) the sample was first optimally digested with a protease. Clearly, this would not be of use for the detection of either viral or native DNAs. However, these observations lend themselves very well to the *in situ* detection of RNA viruses or mRNAs using the direct incorporation of the reporter molecule. Specifically, one can first determine which protease

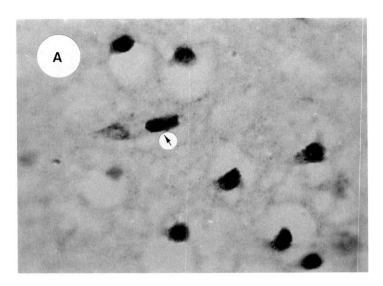

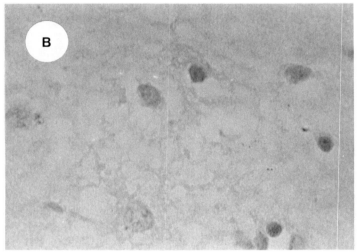

Figure 7-1. *The importance of the negative and positive controls with RT* in situ *PCR.* The tissue is from the CNS of a person who had AIDS dementia. A strong signal was noted in all cell types, including neurons, astrocytes, and oligodendroglial cells with the positive control of RT *in situ* PCR: no DNase digestion (**A**). This demonstrates that the various conditions, including protease digestion time and reagent conditions, were optimal. Note the nuclear localization of the signal (*arrow*; the cytoplasm is not evident), which represents DNA repair and target-specific genomic-based DNA synthesis due to the primers specific for nitric oxide synthetase (NOS). The signal was eliminated by overnight DNase digestion (**B**); this is the negative control. This demonstrates that any signal with the test (after DNase and RT/PCR) will be specific for the cDNA. RT *in situ* PCR was done on the same glass slide as for the mRNA of NOS. A signal was evident in a few cells (**C**). Note the cytoplasmic localization (*arrow*) and the absence of signal in most cell types (as compared with A, the positive control); these are two indicators of target-specific mRNA-based amplification.

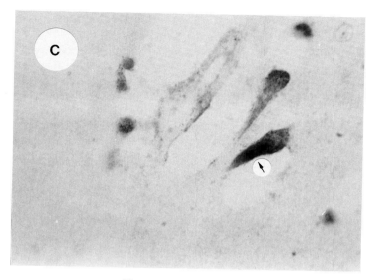

Figure 7-1. *Continued.*

digestion time gives the strongest signal in most cells for the particular tissue or cell sample. The three samples on a single silane-coated glass slide are digested for this optimal time with the protease. Two of the three samples are then incubated overnight in an RNase-free DNase containing solution to eliminate the native nonspecific DNA signal. This is followed by the target-specific synthesis of a cDNA molecule using the enzyme reverse transcriptase (RT) or rTth (Perkin-Elmer). One can then do *in situ* PCR with direct incorporation of the digoxigenin dUTP (or some other reporter nucleotide) using the target-specific primers. To prove that the native DNA-derived signal was eliminated, one uses the tissue sample on the same glass slide that was DNase digested and where the primers were omitted during the RT step; alternatively, irrelevant primers can be employed. Provided that protease conditions were optimal, this section should show no signal and would thus serve as the negative control. Similarly, one could demonstrate that protease digestion for the tissue was optimal and that the PCR and detection steps were working properly with the tissue sample that was not subject to DNase digestion. Under optimal protease conditions, at least 50% of the cells should

demonstrate an intense nuclear signal that thus, would serve as the positive control (Fig 7-1). The relationship between protease digestion, length of fixation time in formalin, and the signal with the positive and negative control are discussed in Chapter 3. The salient points are now reviewed in brief; the reader is referred to Chapter 3 for a more detailed discussion of the important theoretical points.

The Positive Control: Nonspecific DNA Synthesis

The subheading of this section reflects two different perspectives on the results found in the non-DNased tissue section. On the one hand, the ability invariably to see an intense signal in tissue sections with optimal protease digestion pretreatment irrespective of the primers used indicates successful synthesis and detection of DNA within the nucleus—hence, the term *positive control*. The other perspective views the signal derived in this manner correctly as *not* target specific and the possible cause of a false-positive reading when interpreting the RT *in situ* PCR results. Of course, both perspectives are valid.

The Sources of the Signal with the Positive Control

There are four potential DNA synthesis pathways that may be operative inside the cell during *in situ* PCR. These are

1. Target-specific amplification
2. Nontarget primer-dependent amplification (mispriming)
3. Primer oligomerization
4. DNA repair (primer-independent pathway)
(refer to Figs. 3-1 to 3-5 for graphic representation of the four pathways).

Of these, DNA repair is invariably present in paraffin-embedded tissues or any other cell or tissue preparation that has been exposed to dry heat of at least 55°C for ≥1 hour. Indeed, this primer-independent signal may be evident even after several minutes of exposure to such dry heat. DNA repair will usually involve all of the different cell types in a tissue section. In comparison, the target-specific cDNA-based signal for RT *in situ* PCR will rarely involve all cell types unless the target chosen is a "housekeeper" transcript. Thus, the presence of a signal in all cell types after RT *in situ* PCR suggests a nonspecific signal. Alternatively, a signal that is restricted to only one or a few cell types after RT *in situ* PCR suggests a target-specific signal. This simple but important point can be easily demonstrated with viral infections, given the fastidious tropism exhibited by many viruses (see Figs. 7-14 and 7-30, below). This is also evident for human mRNAs. Figure 7-2 shows an example of the latter for matrix metalloprotease (MMP)

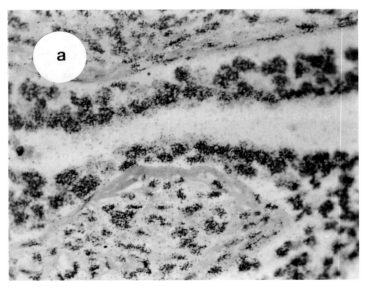

Figure 7-2. *Differential localization of the signal for RT* in situ *PCR versus the positive control.* The signal for the positive control (no DNase) should be evident in all cell types. However, the target-specific cDNA-based signal after DNase digestion and RT *in situ* PCR should be restricted to just those cells that contain the target of interest. This was evident in this section of cervical cancer. Note that the positive control demonstrates a nuclear signal in all cell types, including normal epithelium (**a**). However, RT *in situ* PCR for matrix metalloprotease (MMP-9) mRNA localized to only the invasive cancer cells (*arrow*) and occasional surrounding stromal cells (*open arrow*; note cytoplasmic localization; **b**); the adjacent areas of normal epithelium were negative (**c**,*arrow*). The reporter nucleotide is ^{3}H, hence the black grains. Another example is placenta; the nuclei of all cell types including trophoblasts (*small arrow*) and stromal cells (*large arrow*) were strongly positive in the no-DNase positive control (**d**). After DNase and RT *in situ* PCR for the β-chain of fibrinogen, only scattered trophoblasts were positive (**e**); note the cytoplasmic and perinuclear membrane localization of the signal (*arrows*).

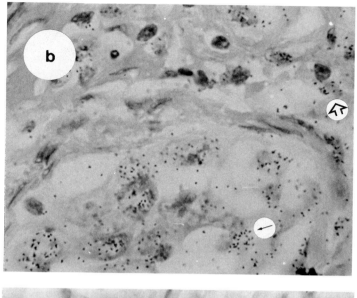

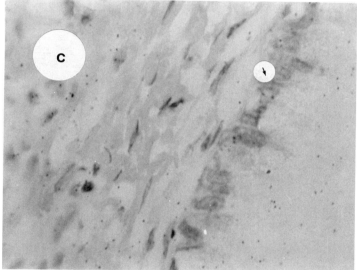

Figure 7-2. *Continued.*

expression in cervical cancer and fibrinogen expression in placenta. Mispriming is another source of DNA synthesis that is operative during *in situ* PCR if the hot start maneuver is not used. In comparison, the hot start method will not inhibit the DNA repair pathway. One can demonstrate the existence of mispriming by using frozen, fixed tissues that lack the primer-independent pathway and primers that do not correspond to any target in the cells in the tissue sample. An example of one such experiment is provided in Fig. 7-3, where no signal is evident with hot start *in situ* PCR using lymphoid tissue and human papillomavirus (HPV)-specific primers (HPV does not infect lymphoid cells). How-

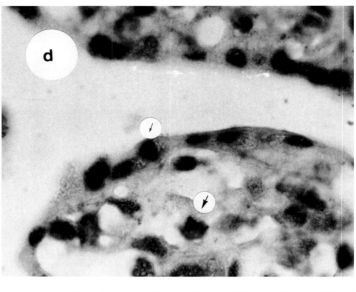

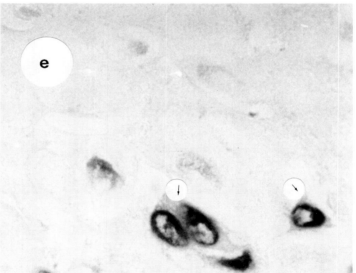

Figure 7-2. *Continued.*

ever, a signal is evident if all reagents including the *Taq* polymerase are added at room temperature. Primer oligomerization does not appear to induce any signal with *in situ* PCR. This can be demonstrated by using paraffin-embedded tissues in which DNA repair and mispriming have been blocked by DNase digestion after optimal protease digestion. If one then does *in situ* PCR using primers that do not correspond to any tar-

get in the cells, no nuclear signal is evident (Fig. 7-4; see also Fig. 3-26). Note how nonspecific *cytoplasmic* staining can be seen if a post-PCR stringent wash is not done (see Fig. 3-27). This, as discussed in detail in Chapter 3, represents nonspecific "stickiness" of the labeled primer oligomers formed in the *amplifying solution* on cytoplasmic proteins and *not* primer oligomerization formed de novo inside the intact cell.

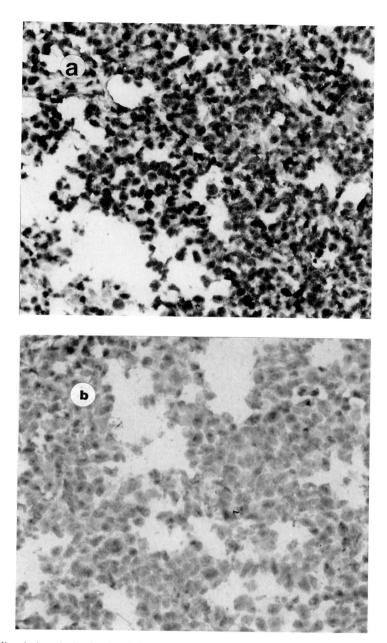

Figure 7-3. *Mispriming during* in situ *PCR.* The tissue is from the tonsil. Frozen and then fixed tissue was used in these experiments. Because the tissue was not heated, the primer-independent signal was not evident. HPV 16-specific primers were used in this study of mispriming, as HPV does not infect lymphoid tissue. Note that a signal is evident after *in situ* PCR if cold start PCR is performed (i.e., all reagents added prior to heating the thermal cycler block)(**a**). However, the signal is eliminated if the hot start maneuver is done (**b**). The hot start maneuver is *not* needed for RT *in situ* PCR, as mispriming and DNA repair are eliminated by DNase digestion after optimal protease treatment. Indeed, cold start contributes to the signal of the positive control via mispriming.

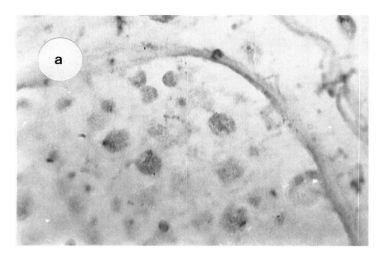

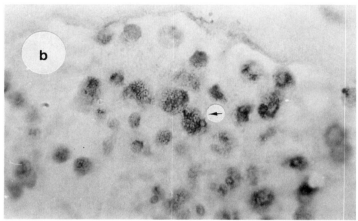

Figure 7-4. *Apparent inability of primer oligomerization to cause a signal during* in situ *PCR.* RT *in situ* PCR was performed after optimal protease digestion time and DNase digestion in this testicular tissue using hantavirus-specific primers. The DNase digestion steps would eliminate DNA repair and mispriming. Thus, any signal should represent primer oligomerization, as this tissue did not contain the hantavirus. Under cold start conditions to enhance primer oligomerization, no signal was evident in the tissue section (**a**), although digoxigenin incorporation secondary to primer oligomerization was evident in the amplifying solution (not shown, though see Fig. 3-26). It is important to stress that this negative result was obtained with a high stringency wash after the PCR step; the lack of the high stringency wash can cause nonspecific attachment of the primer oligomers in the solution to the cellular proteins (see Fig. 3-27). The elimination of these potential causes of background permits a clearly evident target-specific signal for the mRNA of interest, in this case vitronectin mRNA that localized to scattered spermatocytes (**b**, *arrow*); note the reticulated cytoplasmic signal. In comparison, the positive control (no DNase) shows an intense nuclear signal in all cell types (**c**, *arrow*).

This is analogous to one cause of background with standard *in situ* hybridization, as discussed in Chapter 4. Target-specific DNA synthesis is, of course, operative during *in situ* PCR if the primers correspond to a target in the cells in the sample. This can easily be demonstrated using cellular preparations in which two different cell types are mixed, one that contains the target and the other that lacks the target of interest. If hot start (to block mispriming) *in*

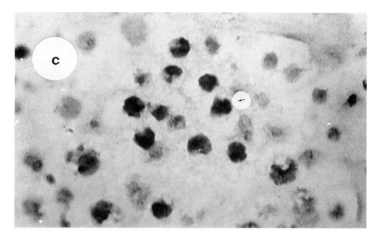

Figure 7-4. *Continued.*

situ PCR is done on the nonheated sample (to avoid DNA repair), then only the cell type that has a target that corresponds to the primers present in the amplifying solution will demonstrate a signal (Fig. 7-5).

It is important to appreciate that the signal in tissue sections undergoing *in situ* PCR due either to DNA repair or to target-specific DNA synthesis is *highly* dependent on the lengths of time of fixation in buffered formalin and of protease digestion. This point is stressed in Chapter 3 and is the focal point of Chapter 6, where the start-up protocol is presented. Figures 7-6 and 7-7 demonstrate this point, which is critical to success with RT *in situ* PCR.

It is not surprising that formalin fixation should be critical to the results of RT *in situ* PCR. The extent of formalin fixation, which cross-links proteins and nucleic acids, has important effects on variables such as probe entry, intensity of the signal, and the requirement for protease digestion in standard *in situ* hybridization (discussed in detail in Chapter 4) (1–16).

The Inhibition of DNA Repair

The primer-independent signal serves a useful function for *in situ* PCR with tissue sections; the signal generated from DNA repair under optimal protease digestion demonstrates successful DNA synthesis inside the nucleus and detection of the resultant labeled product. This observation is the basis of the start-up protocol

presented in Chapter 6. However, because it masks the target-specific signal, clearly one must be able either to eliminate or to block the nonspecific signal to do target-specific *in situ* PCR in tissue sections for either RNA or DNA.

On theoretical grounds, one can envision several ways to prevent or block DNA repair when performing *in situ* PCR. First, DNA could be digested with DNase to the point that it would not support *Taq* polymerase–mediated DNA synthesis. One would predict that prolonged DNase digestion may be needed to render all areas of DNA damage unavailable to synthesis from the activity of *Taq* polymerase. An alternative would be to modify the native DNA such that it could no longer serve as a template for *Taq* polymerase. One such mechanism is the use of dideoxynucleotides, which, when added to the growing DNA chain, block the addition of any more nucleotides (see Fig. 3-15). This technique of preventing the phosphodiester linkage of additional nucleotides to a DNA fragment is commonly used in sequencing DNA. Thus, it would appear feasible that one might be able to block DNA repair during *in situ* PCR by first pretreating the slides in a solution that contains a dideoxynucleotide.

As discussed in Chapter 3, we have been able to prevent DNA repair by both DNase digestion and blockage after the incorporation of a dideoxynucleotide prior to the *in situ* PCR step. However, as is true for the nonspecific DNA repair signal itself, the results

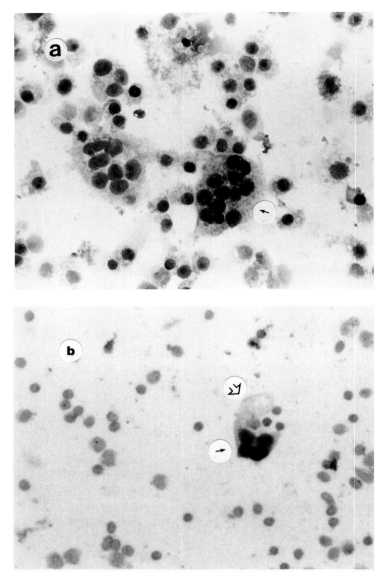

Figure 7-5. *Lack of DNA repair in cytospin preparations.* Measles-infected HeLa cells, which are multinucleated (**a**), were mixed with PBMC, which are uninucleate, from a person with no evidence of measles infection. It is important to stress that the cells were not heated after preparing the cytospin preparation; thus, DNA repair should not be operative. By using the hot start maneuver to block mispriming, a signal is evident after RT *in situ* PCR using measles-specific primers only in the multinucleate cells (**b**, *arrow*). Note the nuclear (*small arrow*) and cytoplasmic (*open arrow*) components of the signal.

one obtains with either DNase digestion or dideoxy blockage are strongly dependent on the length of time the tissue has been fixed in 10% buffered formalin as well as the length of time of protease digestion. Dideoxy blockage, how-ever, is not useful for RT *in situ* PCR. One reason is that the window of optimal protease for blockage of the DNA repair pathway tends to be narrow, making false-positive results from DNA repair likely. More importantly, dideoxy block-

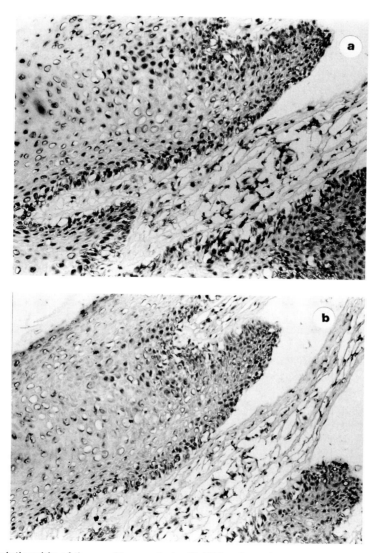

Figure 7-6. *Relationship of the positive control with RT* in situ *PCR to the times of formalin fixation and protease digestion: short fixation time.* The amount of digestion time in pepsin at 2 mg/ml to produce an optimal signal with the positive control increases as a function of the time that the tissue was fixed in 10% buffered formalin. This skin biopsy was fixed for 6 hours. No signal was evident in the positive control if the protease digestion time was 0 to 2 minutes (not shown). The signal became strong after 8 minutes of digestion (**a**) and persisted at 13 minutes of digestion (**b**). However, the tissue morphology was destroyed after 20 minutes of digestion with a concomitant loss of signal (**c**). The high background evident in c is often seen with protease overdigestion, perhaps reflecting the loss of the labeled DNA from the nuclei.

age would not prevent target-specific amplification of the DNA target. This would invariably lead to a false-positive (albeit nuclear) signal for RT *in situ* PCR when one is analyzing for a cellular transcript. However, DNA repair, mispriming, and target-specific DNA synthesis can all be eliminated by DNase digestion *after optimal protease digestion*. Thus, we now focus our attention on DNase digestion for RT *in situ* PCR.

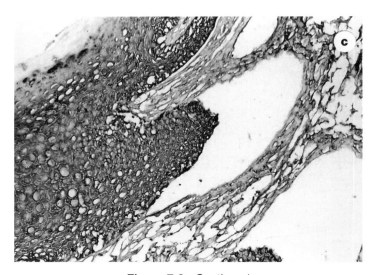

Figure 7-6. *Continued.*

There is one further point to make before reviewing this information, presented at length in Chapter 3. Some investigators have asked me if there might not be an advantage to using frozen, fixed tissues for RT *in situ* PCR. The rationale is that the DNA repair system would not be operative and RNA degradation would be, perhaps, less likely, as one would have strict control over tissue preparation and fixation. I do not recommend the use of frozen, fixed tissues for RT *in situ* PCR. First, DNase digestion will still be needed for cellular genes, for the same reasons as discussed above for dideoxy blockage. Second, it is technically more difficult to place three frozen tissue sections on a glass slide than to place three paraffin-embedded tissue sections. Finally, we have had good success detecting a variety of RNAs that had to be present in tissue using routine surgical biopsies. Such tissues are immediately placed in formalin after the biopsy is performed, and the resultant cross-linking of the RNAs with cellular proteins and nucleic acids likely protects them from RNase digestion until the protease digestion step.

DNase Digestion

Considering the enormous amount of DNA present in the nucleus that could participate in the nonspecific mispriming or DNA repair pathways, one would hypothesize that in order to render the native DNA nonamplifiable, it would have to be exposed for an extended period of time to a high concentration of the DNase. This is schematically depicted in Fig. 7-8. Note in this illustration that a cross-linking fixative such as buffered formalin may protect the DNA from DNase digestion by steric hindrance from the resultant protein–DNA cross-links. This illustration suggests several possibilities about the relationship between the signal after DNase digestion and the length of protease digestion time. Specifically, if the tissue has been fixed for a prolonged time in formalin, extended digestion in protease may be required in order to allow the DNase access to the DNA. Of course, this strong relationship between the times of protease digestion and formalin fixation and elimination of the signal with overnight DNase digestion have been noted. This is discussed in detail in Chapter 3; some of the relevant data are presented again in Table 3-5. Note the following points:

1. When the signal with the non-DNased tissue is optimal (i.e., protease digestion is optimal), no signal is noted after DNase digestion (Fig. 7-1).

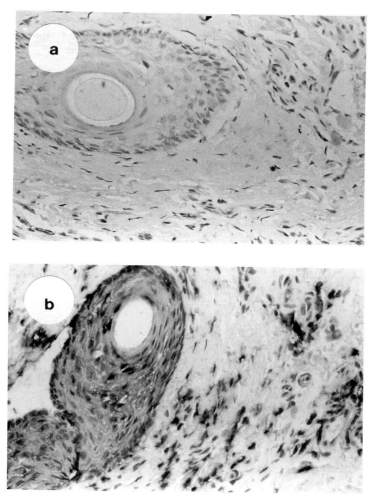

Figure 7-7. *Relationship of the positive control with RT* in situ *PCR to the times of formalin fixation and protease digestion: intermediate fixation time.* This skin biopsy was fixed for 8 hours in 10% buffered formalin. Note that no signal was evident with the positive control if the protease digestion time was 15 minutes (**a**, *arrow*). An optimal signal was evident after 45 minutes of protease digestion (**b**).

2. When the signal with the non-DNased tissue is suboptimal due to inadequate protease digestion, a signal is often present with the overnight DNase digestion and is usually stronger than the signal with the non-DNased tissue (Fig. 7-9).

   The first observation demonstrates that DNase digestion was adequate in rendering the native DNA nonamplifiable. This serves as the basis for the negative control and the test for RT *in situ* PCR. That is, if one is to use direct incorporation of the reporter molecule after the RT step, it is critical to be assured that any resulting signal must be derived from the cDNA because the native DNA has been rendered unavailable for amplification.

   The second observation can be considered a "paradoxical" enhancement of signal with DNase digestion in the setting of inadequate

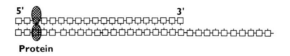

I. Elimination of DNA Repair

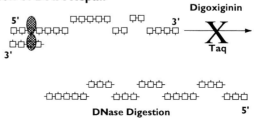

2. Elimination of Mispriming

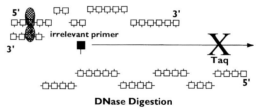

Figure 7-8. *Mechanism of action of DNase digestion.* It is postulated that DNase digestion after optimal protease digestion prevents either repair of single-stranded gaps by *Taq* polymerase during PCR or extension of misprimed oligomers.

protease digestion. The term *enhanced* is used because, as is evident from Table 7-1, when the length of protease time is inadequate, not only is a signal evident in the DNased tissue, but it is often stronger than the signal evident in the serial section on the same glass slide that was not DNased. The fact that a signal is present after DNase digestion with suboptimal protease implies that something is preventing the enzyme from exerting its maxi-

Table 7-1. *Hepatitis C-specific primers and probes used in the study*

	Orientation	Sequence (9)
Primer		
JH51	Antisense	CCCAACACTACTCGGCTA
JH52	Antisense	AGTCTTGCGGCCGCAGCGCCAAATC
JH93	Sense	TCCGCGGCCGCACTCCACCATGAATCACTCCCC
Probe		
Alx89	Sense	CCATAGTGGTCTGCGGAACCGGTGAGTACA
cDNA	—	Nucleotides 8 to 268

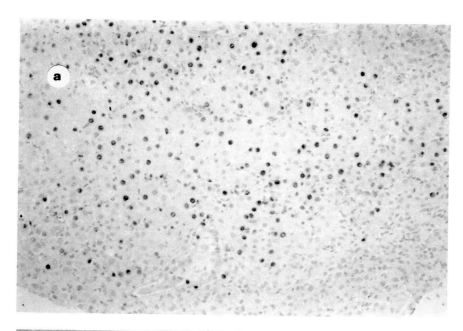

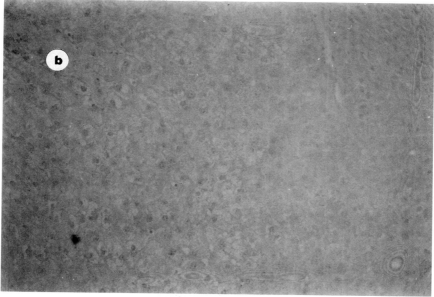

Figure 7-9. *The effect of inadequate protease digestion on the essential controls for RT* in situ *PCR: paradoxical enhancement of the negative control.* This liver tissue was fixed for 15 hours in 10% buffered formalin. Note the nuclear signal present in most cells after 60 minutes of protease digestion (positive control; **a**). The signal was eliminated if the tissue was digested overnight in a DNase solution after the protease pretreatment (negative control; **b**). If the same liver tissue was digested in pepsin for 15 minutes, the signal with the positive control is no longer evident (**c**). However, a nuclear signal is now evident in the negative control (**d**). This "paradoxical" enhancement of the negative control (DNase-digested tissue) is typical of tissue that has not be digested adequately in the protease solution. It is important to be aware of this observation, as it can cause a false-positive result with RT *in situ* PCR. However, the fact that a nuclear-based signal is present with the negative control that is equal to or stronger than the signal with the positive control demonstrates that any signal with the test (DNase and RT) must be nonspecific. This underscores the fact that one *must* have the results with the negative and positive controls to interpret the signal with the test correctly.

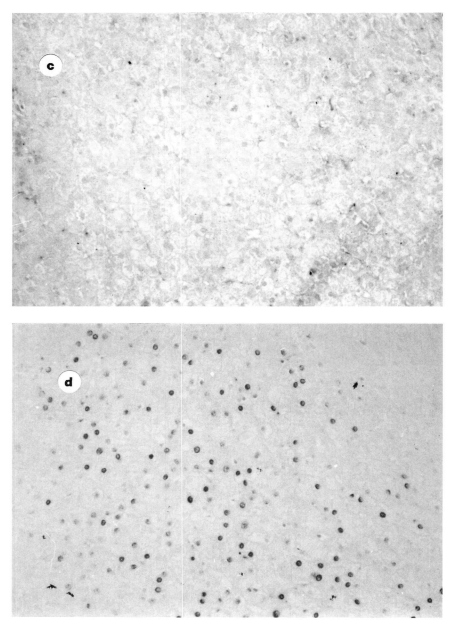

Figure 7-9. *Continued.*

mum activity. How is the DNase able actually to enhance the signal seen with *in situ* PCR under the suboptimal protease digestion? One possible explanation is presented in Fig 7-10. It is speculated that DNase digestion, although blocked from rendering the entire DNA template (with its gaps) incapable of DNA repair due to the steric interference from persistent DNA–protein cross-links, still can either create or extend gaps that can then be filled during the subsequent *in situ* PCR step. Although further testing of this model is

Large number of persistent protein-DNA crosslinks prevent total degradation by DNase

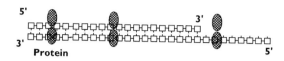

Protein

Enlargement of gap size by DNase digestion and generation of new gaps by DNase digestion

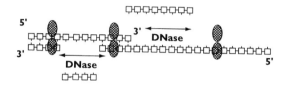

Extension of gaps with incorporation of labeled nucleotide during PCR

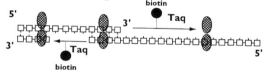

Figure 7-10. *Hypothetical model for the enhancement of the signal in the negative control with inadequate protease digestion.* It is postulated that DNase digestion after suboptimal protease digestion may enhance the signal by creating new gaps and/or increasing the size of the preexisting single-stranded gaps that may be repaired by *Taq* polymerase during PCR.

needed, the important points for RT *in situ* PCR are

1. Under optimal protease conditions, the nonspecific nuclear-based signal should be present in over 50% of the cells in a tissue section.
2. Under the same protease conditions, this signal can be completely eliminated with overnight DNase digestion.
3. These two observations serve as the basis for the negative and positive controls for RT *in situ* PCR. More importantly, because the optimal protease digestion time varies with fixation time and tissue type, one must remember:

It is essential to do the negative and positive control on the same glass slide as the test in RT in situ *PCR.*

Brief mention of two other points should be made. First, we have tried shorter times for DNase digestion. Under optimal protease digestion times, we were unable to eradicate the nonspecific primer-independent signal reliably with *in situ* PCR in tissue sections when the DNase digestion was from 2 to 4 hours. However, the nonspecific signal was eradicated after optimal protease digestion if the DNase digestion time was from 8 to 15 hours (see Fig. 6-6). Second, a common misinterpretation among investigators who have asked me to assist them

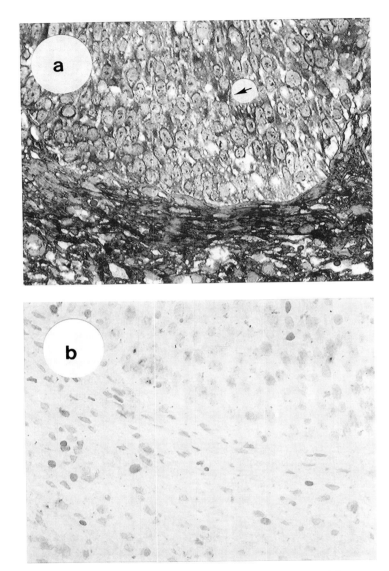

Figure 7-11. *Primer oligomerization in the amplifying solution as a potential cause of background in RT* in situ *PCR: the utility of a high-stringency wash. In situ* PCR was done on this cervical biopsy specimen that did not contain HPV under cold start conditions using HPV-specific primers in order to facilitate the formation of primer oligomers in the amplifying solution. A strong cytoplasmic signal is noted in normal squamous (**a**, *arrow*) and stromal cells (which do not contain HPV; see Figs. 4-6 and 4-9 as examples of the histological distribution of HPV). This background can be eliminated by washing the slide for 15 minutes in 0.2×SSC and 0.2% bovine serum albumin at 60°C (**b**). This background is analogous to that associated with low stringent washes in standard *in situ* hybridization (see Fig. 4-19).

is that the occurrence of a positive signal in the negative control (DNase digested overnight) represents too low a DNase concentration. Assuming one is using 10 U of RNase-free DNase per section, the persistence of a signal in the nega-tive control represents *too short a protease digestion time* rather than an inadequate amount of DNase. Increasing the concentration up to 5× of the DNase will *not* eliminate the nonspecific signal under these conditions. However, increasing the protease digestion time will result in the elimination of the signal (Fig. 7-9).

Summary

For RT *in situ* PCR, I strongly recommend that one use DNase digestion to block the non-specific pathways of mispriming and DNA repair as well as target-specific amplification of the genomic-based sequence. Because each of these pathways is adequately blocked after optimal protease digestion, one can do direct incorporation of the reporter nucleotide after RT *under cold start conditions*. That is, one can add the *Taq* polymerase (or rTth) to the amplifying solution even before increasing the temperature of the thermal cycler. However, recall that under these conditions primer oligomerization can still occur in the amplifying solution. Even though the DNA labeled from primer oligomerization in the amplifying solution does not induce a nuclear signal with RT *in situ* PCR, it can serve as the source of a nonspecific signal by "sticking" to cellular proteins, primarily the cell membrane and basement membrane. This is not surprising to those who do *in situ* hybridization, where one routinely adds large amounts of labeled DNA of from 75 to 150 base pairs and detects signal only in the cells that have the target. It is assumed that the probe enters all cells, but is washed out *after a wash of adequate stringency* in cells lacking the target. When one generates primer oligomers (or DNA synthesized from mispriming) in the amplifying solution, an analogous situation occurs. It follows that a nonspecific signal with RT *in situ* PCR could be generated by avoiding a stringent wash after the PCR step due to the DNA synthesized from primer oligomerization in the overlying solution. This is easily demonstrated, as illustrated in Fig. 7-11. Note how this nonspecific signal localizes to the cytoplasmic membranes. It is due to nonspecific "sticking" of the labeled DNA in the solution and cellular proteins and should not be confused with background signal from DNA repair, which is nuclear based and not affected by any DNA synthesis in the overlying solution. The practical implications for RT *in situ* PCR are clear: *After RT* in situ *PCR, do a stringent wash to eliminate nonspecific binding of labeled DNA in the overlying solution and cellular proteins.*

Other strategies to prevent this source of background are to do hot start and to omit the primers during the RT and PCR step for the negative control. Of these two, I prefer to omit the primers as one of my routine negative controls; this can be used in conjunction with irrelevant primers as another negative control. Also, "cold start" helps accentuate the signal with the positive control and, of course, is technically easier to perform, especially for those using the aluminum boat method.

As a final point, it is unclear why primer oligomerization apparently does not occur in the cell. Whether this relates to sequestration of the primers in the nucleus, ready diffusion of primer oligomers out of the cell with a stringent wash, or other mechanisms requires further study. It is also as interesting as it is enigmatic that primer oligomerization in the amplifying solution did not prevent target-specific PCR in the cell. Primer oligomerization can certainly block PCR in solution phase PCR (L. Haff and J. Atwood, *personal communication,* 1991). It does serve to illustrate that the PCR reaction in the cell is probably shielded from what is occurring in the overlying solution by the natural cellular barriers, primarily the membranes. Thus, the cell and overlying solution should be considered as two separate compartments during *in situ* PCR.

RT *IN SITU* PCR FOR VIRAL TARGETS IN CELLULAR PREPARATIONS

It is important to stress that the above discussions were based on work with tissue sections. If one wishes to use cellular preparations, recall that it is possible to obtain direct incorporation of the reporter molecule with *in situ* PCR for DNA targets under defined conditions, which include the hot start maneuver and defined protease digestion. It follows that one should be able to do target-specific hot start RT *in situ* PCR in cellular preparations (or frozen, fixed tissues) for RNA viruses without the DNase digestion step. To test this hypothesis, we mixed measles-infected HeLa cells and peripheral blood mononuclear cells (PBMCs) from a noninfected individual. The measles-infected cells are easily recognized on microscopic examination due to their large size, intranuclear inclusions, and multinucleation. As is evident from Fig. 7-5, only the measles-infected cells show a signal with RT *in situ* PCR if measles-specific primers are used. It should be stressed that DNase digestion was not done in these experiments. However, I recommend that the reader still perform DNase digestion for RT *in situ* PCR even if cell suspensions or frozen, fixed preparations are being used. In this way, one can do "cold start" PCR and not be concerned about the possibility of DNA repair, which can occur in cytospin preparations if they have been proteased for too long or if they have been inadvertently exposed to dry heat prior to *in situ* PCR. Furthermore, I think it is useful to induce the DNA repair pathway for RT *in situ* PCR, as it serves as a control to demonstrate that the conditions are adequate to support DNA synthesis inside the cell. That is,

1. The signal in the positive control (no DNase using heated samples) demonstrates that one has reached the optimal protease digestion time for that tissue or cellular preparation.
2. The signal in the positive control demonstrates that the user is successfully synthesizing DNA in the nucleus.

Hence, I recommend that those investigators doing RT *in situ* PCR employ paraffin-embedded tissues and DNase digestion. For those using cell suspensions, I recommend heating the slides to 60°C for 15 to 30 minutes after placing them on a silane-coated slide to generate an intense positive control and then using the DNase digestion step to eliminate the possibility of mispriming and DNA repair in the negative control and the test sample.

IMPORTANCE OF THE SPECIFIC LOCALIZATION OF THE SIGNAL WITH RT *IN SITU* PCR

As stressed in this chapter, one cannot interpret RT *in situ* PCR without the negative (DNase, no RT, or RT with irrelevant primers) and posi-

tive (no DNase) controls. No signal with the negative control and an intense *nuclear* signal in the positive control is required before one can confidently analyze the test section. The nuclear localization of the positive control reflects the fact that the DNA repair pathway as well as mispriming and target-specific genomic-based DNA synthesis all occur in the nucleus. Another important principle in the interpretation of RT *in situ* PCR is the specific subcellular localization of the signal. For cellular mRNAs, the signal should localize to the cytoplasm. This can be seen in Fig. 7-12; note the nuclear localization of the signal in the positive control and the cytoplasmic localization of the signal for the test for MMP-9 mRNA in the cancer cells of this cervical squamous cell carcinoma. Also note that the MMP-9 is not evident in the normal cervical epithelium, which is only a few millimeters away from the cancer cells. Figure 7-13 shows another example—in this case for the mRNA that corresponds to map kinase expression in breast cancer. Note that the signal is only evident in the malignant epithelial cells; it is not seen in the surrounding fibroblasts and other stromal cells. These two examples remind us that localization to specific cell types is another hallmark of successful RT *in situ* PCR.

The specific subcellular distribution of RNAs can show much variation, especially for viral RNAs. HIV-1 RNA localizes to the nucleus (described in detail in Chapter 9). Hepatitis C RNA localizes to part of the nuclear membrane (see Figs. 1-1 and 7-14. See also Color Plate 4 following p. 242). Interestingly, an antigen of hepatitis C localizes to the cytoplasm in the area directly adjacent to the nuclear membrane. Measles RNA localizes to the nucleus or cytoplasm, depending if one does the RT step with the sense or antisense strand, as is described later in this chapter. Human mRNAs can also show different patterns. Using the megakaryocyte cell line DAMI and the fibrosarcoma cell line HT1080, we noted either a diffuse cytoplasmic signal (for MMPs and TIMPs in HT1080 cells, see Fig. 1-1) or a reticulated cytoplasmic signal for gelsolin and glycoprotein IIB mRNA (see Color Plate 5 following p. 242 and Fig. 7-15). Interestingly, the PCR-

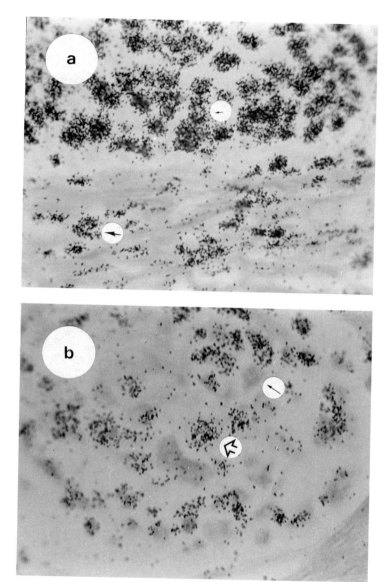

Figure 7-12. *Differential localization of the signal with RT* in situ *PCR: matrix metalloprotease mRNA.* The tissue from a cervical cancer that had invaded a blood vessel. Note the nuclear signal in all cell types (**a**, cancer cells, *small arrow*; stromal cells, *large arrow*) in the positive control (no DNase). A cytoplasmic-based signal (**b**, *open arrow*) is noted after RT *in situ* PCR with MMP-9–specific primers in some of the cancer and stromal cells; note the negative nuclei (b); the adjacent areas of noninvasive carcinoma and normal epithelium including the surrounding fibroblasts, were negative for MMP-9 (see Fig. 7-27). The signals were lost in the negative control (**c**; DNase, RT with irrelevant primers, and high stringent wash). The reporter nucleotide is ³H.

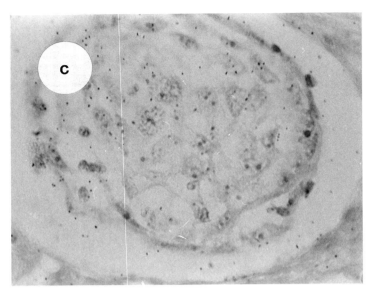

Figure 7-12. *Continued.*

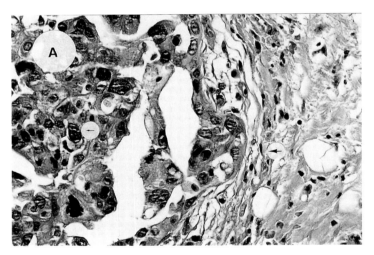

Figure 7-13. *Differential localization of the signal with RT* in situ *PCR: map kinase mRNA.* The tissue from a breast cancer that had metastasized. **A:** Routine H&E stain; the *small arrow* marks the round cancer cells and the *large arrow* the more spindle-shaped stromal cells in A and B. **B:** Note the nuclear signal in all cell types in the positive control (no DNase). **C:** A cytoplasmic-based signal (*open arrow*) is noted after RT *in situ* PCR with map kinase–specific primers in some of the cancer cells; the stromal cells were negative. **D:** The signals were lost in the negative control (DNase, RT with irrelevant primers, and high stringent wash). The reporter nucleotide is digoxigenin.

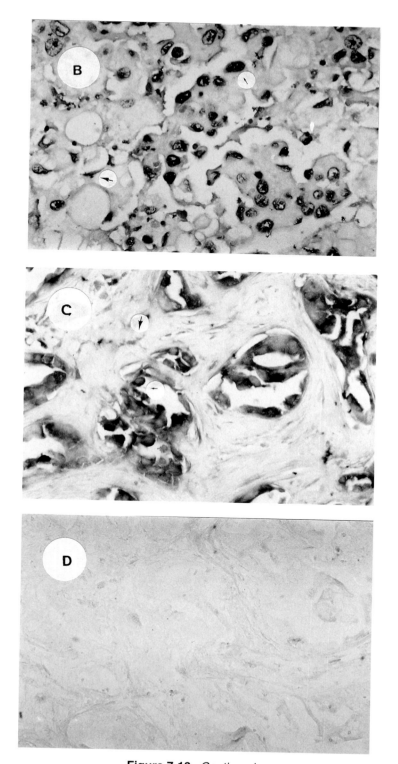

Figure 7-13. *Continued.*

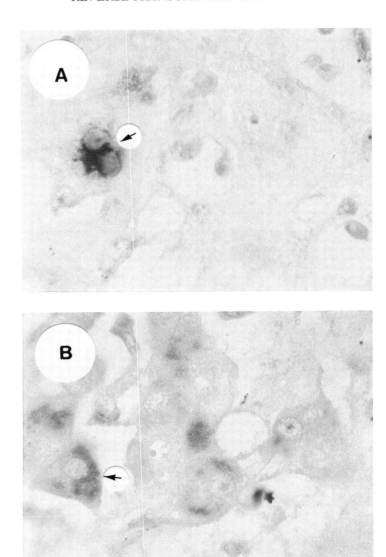

Figure 7-14. *Subcellular localization of hepatitis C RNA and proteins.* RT *in situ* PCR for hepatitis C demonstrated that viral RNA was found in most hepatocytes, although occasional liver macrophages (Kuppfer cells) and biliary epithelium were infected. The signal for the Kuppfer cells localized to the nucleus and cytoplasm (not shown). The signal in the hepatocytes usually localizes to part of the nuclear membrane (**A**, *arrow;* see also Fig. 1-1). However, at times, a cytoplasmic signal that also tends to be centered about part of the nuclear membrane will be evident (**B**, *arrow*). Compare this to the pan-nuclear signal of the positive control (**C**, *arrow*). A hepatitis C protein interestingly was localized by immunohistochemistry to the cytoplasm, directly abutting part of the nuclear membrane (**D**, *arrow;* slide courtesy of Dr. Richard Cartun). This suggests a distinct cellular "roadway" for production of hepatitis C proteins from the RNA. The specific subcellular localization of the signal with RT *in situ* PCR strongly suggests the specificity of the RNA-based signal.

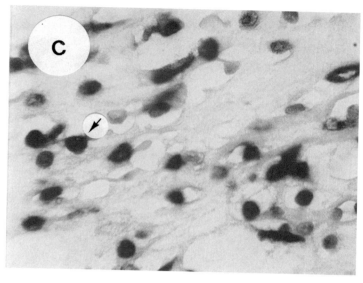

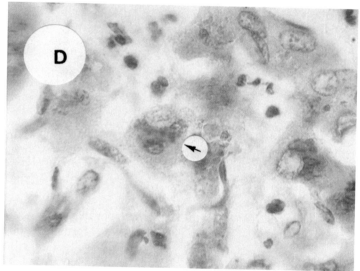

Figure 7-14. *Continued.*

amplified cDNA-based glycoprotein IIB signal also was seen in the nucleus around the nucleoli, whereas another RNA in these same cells, amyloid precursor protein, localized to the nucleoli in these cells. It is presumed that these disparate localization patterns for different RNAs as determined by RT *in situ* PCR in the same cell types reflects the distribution of pre-mRNAs as they are processed from the nucleus to the cytoplasm; this is discussed in more detail below.

In summary, two important variables with regard to the specificity of the signal with RT *in situ* PCR are

1. The signal should localize to the *entire* nucleus with the positive control and, in most cases, show a different pattern, usually cytoplasmic or sometimes part of the nucleus, for the test.
2. A relatively low percentage of the cells in a tissue section should be positive with RT *in*

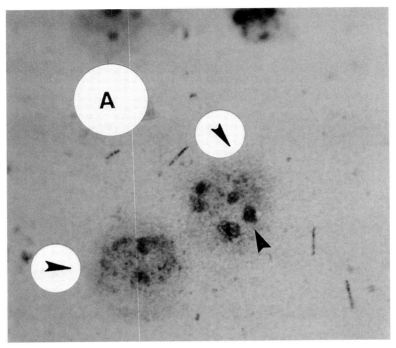

Figure 7-15. *Detection of human mRNAs in a megakaryocyte cell line.* The cell line DAMI contains the mRNAs amyloid precursor protein and gelsolin. Analysis of these mRNAs was done after DNase pretreatment by RT *in situ* PCR. Note the different compartmentalizations of the two signals. Amyloid precursor protein PCR-amplified cDNA (**A**) localized to the cytoplasm (*arrowheads* with white background) and to one and three discrete nuclear foci (*arrowhead*) that correspond to the nucleoli; this mRNA was not detected by standard *in situ* hybridization analysis (not shown). Gelsolin PCR-amplified RNA also localized to the cytoplasm (**B**, *arrow*) and nucleus (*arrowhead*) but appeared to spare the nucleoli. This variable pattern of different mRNAS and, probably, pre-mRNAs likely reflects differing pathways taken by these messages as they are spliced and moved from nucleus to cytoplasm.

situ PCR and the positive cells should be restricted to specific cell types.

In comparison, with the positive control at least 50% of the cells in a tissue sample should be positive, and all different cell types should show staining. An important exception to the latter statement applies to tissue that was fixed for a short period of time; cell types more resistant to protease (e.g., squamous cells and fibroblasts) may show signal with the positive control, whereas other cell types sensitive to protease overdigestion (e.g., lymphocytes) may have no signal.

Figure 7-16 shows a case where the signal with the test was *nonspecific* as evident by a pan nuclear signal for hepatitis C. It is useful to remember that every tissue has its own internal control for interpreting the results with RT *in situ* PCR. It is hoped that the review of the basics of histology in Chapter 2 will assist the nonpathologist in being able to recognize these different cell types.

THE PROTOCOL FOR RT *IN SITU* PCR: THE TWO-STEP PROCEDURE

The most important part of the protocol for RT *in situ* PCR is that *the negative and positive controls should be done on the same glass slide with the actual test.* Alternatively, for large tissue sections for those using the *in situ* PCR thermal cycler 1000 from Perkin-Elmer, the negative and positive controls should be done on

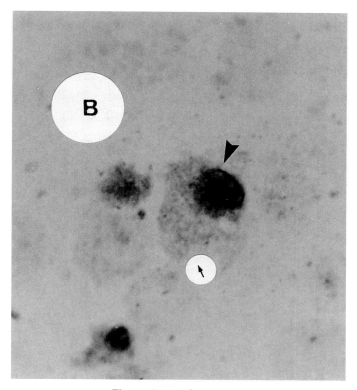

Figure 7-15. *Continued.*

consecutive 4-μm serial sections. This is critical because it provides assurance that the native DNA repair and mispriming pathways have been eliminated (the negative control, DNase, no RT) and that the protease conditions are optimal to amplify DNA inside the cell (the positive control, no DNase). A slide satisfactory for interpretation is defined by the following:

1. No signal is evident in the negative control (DNase, no RT or RT with irrelevant primers).
2. At least 50% of the cells show an intense nuclear signal in the positive control (no DNase).

If these two conditions are not met, then inadequate protease digestion is most likely the problem. The reader is referred to the start-up protocol for a detailed discussion of the interpretation of the different possibilities with the negative and positive controls. Recall that a signal with the negative control means that the experiment should be repeated after increasing the protease digestion time. Alternatively, a weak or no signal with the positive control in conjunction with poor tissue morphology means that the experiment should be repeated after decreasing the protease digestion time. Figure 7-17 depicts the RT *in situ* PCR protocol. Note that after each section is proteased for the amount of time optimal corresponding to the length of fixation in formalin, the top and bottom sections are treated overnight in a solution that contains the DNase. The DNase solution is removed with DEPC-treated water and then 100% ethanol using a sterile technique. Next, one of the two sections digested with DNase is incubated in a solution that contains the RT and the downstream primer. The RT step is followed by direct incorporation *in situ* PCR, preferably with the three tissue sections under the same coverslip to allow the reaction conditions to be

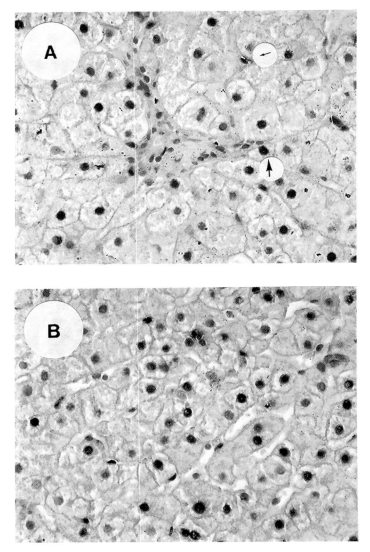

Figure 7-16. *Nonspecific DNA synthesis as a potential cause of a false-positive result with RT* in situ *PCR.* The liver tissue was analyzed for hepatitis C. A strong signal was seen after DNase digestion and RT *in situ* PCR (**A**). However, note that the signal is pan nuclear and involves many different cell types (including endothelial cells, *small arrow*; and hepatocytes, *large arrow*). These two features demonstrate that the signal was nonspecific and due to inadequate protease digestion. Note that the negative control (DNase, no RT) shows a similar result (**B**).

as similar as possible for the negative control, positive control, and the test section. Because digoxigenin dUTP (or some other reporter molecule) is directly incorporated into the PCR product, only 15 to 20 cycles are needed as compared with PCR *in situ* hybridization where 30 cycles are recommended. Indeed, the signal maximizes at about 10 cycles.

At times, it may not be possible to place three tissue sections on the same glass slide because

1. Optimal protease digestion time

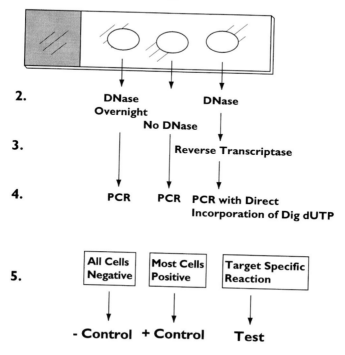

2. DNase Overnight — DNase

No DNase

3. Reverse Transcriptase

4. PCR   PCR   PCR with Direct Incorporation of Dig dUTP

5.

| All Cells Negative | Most Cells Positive | Target Specific Reaction |

- Control   + Control   Test

**6. If the morphology is poor, then less protease
If the - control has + cells, then more protease**

Figure 7-17. *Schematic for RT* in situ *PCR.* A summary of RT *in situ* PCR, which emphasizes the importance of performing the negative and positive controls on the same glass slide as the test run.

the section is too large. For example, brain sections from an autopsy are usually 15 to 20 mm in size, and only one can be placed on a silane slide. In such cases I recommend that the tissue be divided into three parts. One part can be DNased without RT (negative control), the other not DNased (positive control), and the other DNased and treated with RT. If one uses this method it is very useful to have a serial section stained with hematoxylin and eosin (H&E) to determine which part of the slide may be best suited for the DNase and RT step. This is par-

ticularly important when studying cancers, as often one must use large sections with only a relatively small area of cancer.

With these points understood, the following is the recommended protocol for RT *in situ* PCR.

Protocol 7-1

Slide preparation

1. Place three 4-μm sections or three cellular suspensions on a silane-coated glass slide.

2. Deparaffinize tissue section with 5 minutes xylene and 5 minutes 100% ethanol (one does not need to take RNase precautions until after protease digestion); air dry.

3. Digest with trypsin or pepsin (2 mg/ml) at RT for 15 to 90 minutes, depending on the length of time of fixation in formalin.

4. Inactivate pepsin with a 1-minute wash in DEPC water and a 1-minute wash in 100% ethanol; air dry.

   Regarding step 4, I have noted that, if the protease or DNase is removed by washing in water and ethanol in nonsterile Copeland jars, the RNA-based signal may be lost, probably due to RNA degradation. To circumvent this problem, I remove the protease and DNase by simply flooding the slides while horizontal with 1 ml of DEPC water or ethanol that is stored in sterile 50-ml conical tubes; I use sterile 1-ml pipette tips to transfer the DEPC water and ethanol to the slides. These sterile precautions are not needed after the cDNA synthesis step.

Digestion with RNase-free DNase

1. Digest two of the three tissue sections overnight with RNase-free DNase; per each section add
   1 μl of 10× buffer (the buffer is made by adding 35 μl of 3 M sodium acetate, 5 μl 1 M MgSO$_4$, and 60 μl DEPC water).
   1 μl of RNase-free DNase (Boerhinger Mannheim, 10 U/μl)
   8 μl of DEPC water

2. Cover the solution with the inside of the autoclaved polypropylene bag to prevent drying.

3. Place slides in humidity chamber at 37°C overnight.

4. Remove coverslip, wash for 1 minute in DEPC water and 100% ethanol, and air dry.

   The polypropylene bags used in step 2 are best prepared by cutting in 15-cm sheets, placing in plastic container (e.g., empty pipette rack), and then autoclaving. The two layers of the plastic bag may be difficult to separate after autoclaving. They can be separated with a sterile toothpick or needle and then cut to size.

RT step

1. Place on one of the two sections treated with DNase the following solution (these reagents are from the RT PCR kit [Perkin-Elmer]):
   2 μl of MgCl$_2$ (stock 25 mM)
   1 μl of the RT buffer
   1 μl of dATP (stock of each nucleotide at 10 mM)
   1 μl of dCTP
   1 μl of dGTP
   1 μl of dTTP
   1.5 μl of DEPC water
   0.5 μl of 3′ primer (stock solution 20 μM) (one negative control can be obtained by using an irrelevant primer; one example for cellular mRNA would be a primer corresponding to the intron)
   0.5 μl of RNase inhibitor
   0.5 μl RT

2. To prevent drying, coverslip, anchor with 1 small drop of nail polish, place in aluminum boat on block of thermal cycler, and incubate at 42°C for 30 minutes; cover with sterile mineral oil to prevent drying.

3. Remove coverslip, and then remove oil with a 5-minute wash in xylene, followed by a 5-minute wash in 100% ethanol; the sterile technique is no longer necessary.

PCR step

1. For each slide prepare 25 ml solution:
   2.5 μl PCR buffer (the solutions are from the GeneAmp kit [Perkin-Elmer]. The 25-μl volume is adequate for large tissue sections using the aluminum boat method. If the *in situ* PCR thermal cycler 1000 is used, 50 μl should be placed on each of the three sections)
   4.5 μl MgCl$_2$
   4.0 μl dNTP solution (final concentration 200 μM, use GeneAmp kit recipe)
   1.0 μl 2% bovine serum albumin
   0.4 μl digoxigenin dUTP solution (final concentration 10 μM)
   1 μl of primer 1
   1 μl of primer 2 (each stock 20 μM)
   10 μl of water
   0.6 μl of *Taq* polymerase (the *Taq* is added as "cold start"; DNase digestion eliminates

the need for hot start because it eliminates mispriming)

2. Add to slide and cover with one large coverslip; anchor with two small drops of nail polish.
3. Ramp to 80°C, add preheated mineral oil, abort file, and go to 94°C for 3 minutes.
4. Cycle at 55°C for 2 minutes, 94°C for 1 minute, for 15 to 20 cycles.
5. Remove coverslip and polish with scalpel, 5 minutes xylene, 5 minutes ethanol, air dry.
6. Detect digoxigenin using Protocol 6-3.

At the risk of being redundant, permit me to state again the most important point with regard to an inadequate positive and negative control: *The most common cause of a poor or no signal with the positive control and a signal with the negative control during RT* in situ *PCR is inadequate protease digestion.*

THE EZ ONE-STEP RT *IN SITU* PCR PROTOCOL

The protocol listed above demands much actual hands-on time (17). Clearly, it would be highly advantageous if the RT and PCR reactions could be combined under one reaction mixture, with the temperature of the thermal cycler dictating if cDNA synthesis or PCR amplification was occurring. This important advancement was made possible by the rTth enzyme developed by Perkin-Elmer. After an overnight DNase digestion, the one-step RT *in situ* PCR assay, which requires about 4 hours, permits efficient and reproducible detection of RNAs.

Although the enzyme *Taq* polymerase has some RT activity, the level of activity is far below that of conventional RTs, such as that obtained from MMV. Furthermore, the reagent conditions that would support the synthesis of cDNA from RNA by *Taq* polymerase are not conducive to the PCR amplification activity of the enzyme. These problems have been resolved by the modified *Taq* polymerase rTth. Using this enzyme and the reagent conditions described below, one can synthesize cDNA from RNA and then PCR amplify it in one reaction

mixture by varying the time and temperatures of the thermal cycler.

The EZ one-step RT *in situ* PCR protocol is the same as for the two-step procedure through the DNase digestion step. After DNase digestion, perform Protocol 7-2.

Protocol 7-2: The EZ One-Step RT *in situ* PCR Protocol (cDNA Synthesis and PCR Amplification)

1. Prepare the following solution:
   10 μl of the EZ rTth buffer (available in the EZ RT PCR kit [Perkin-Elmer])
   1.6 μl EACH of dATP, dCTP, dGTP, and dTTP, 10 mM stock (available in the EZ RT PCR kit [Perkin-Elmer])
   1.6 μl of 2% (w/v) bovine serum albumin
   1.0 μl of RNasin (available in the EZ RT PCR kit [Perkin-Elmer])
   3.0 μl of primer 1 and primer 2 (20 μM stock of each primer) (omit the primers for the negative control; substitute DEPC water or use irrelevant primers)
   13 μl DEPC water
   12.4 μl of 10 mM MnCl
   0.6 μl of digoxigenin dUTP (1 mM stock)
   2.0 μl of the rTth.
2. cDNA synthesis: 65°C for 30 minutes
3. Denaturation: 94°C for 3 minutes
4. PCR amplification: 20 cycles at 60°C for 1 minute and 94°C for 30 seconds
5. Do stringent wash (0.2×SSC and 0.2% BSA at 60°C for 10 minutes)
6. Detection: incubate with an alkaline phosphatase–antidigoxigenin conjugate (1:150 dilution in 0.1M Tris HCl, pH 7.4, and 0.1 M NaCl) for 30 minutes
7. Chromagen: NBT/BCIP for 10 minutes, counterstain for 3 minutes in nuclear fast red, permount, and coverslip.

In these experiments, the *in situ* PCR 1000 thermal cycler was used (Perkin-Elmer). This employs plastic Amplicovers held over the tissue by a metal Ampliclip placed on the slide by an assembly tool (see Chapter 10).

Figure 7-18 shows some data comparing RNA detection using the one-step RT *in situ* PCR protocol with the two-step procedure.

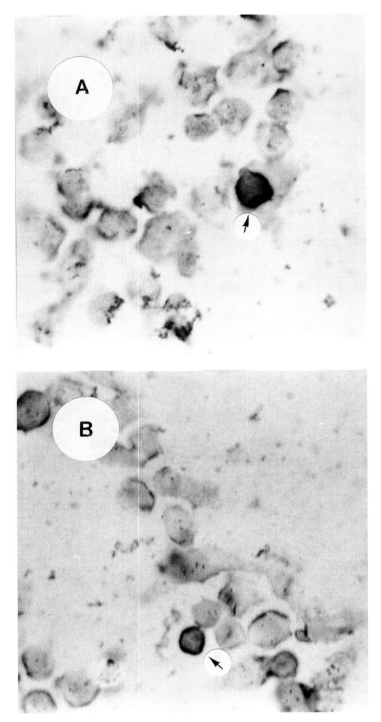

Figure 7-18. *A comparison of the one-step and two-step RT* in situ *PCR techniques.* These HeLa cells were analyzed for TIMP-1 expression. About 10% of cells were shown to express the TIMP-1 mRNA as determined by the two-step (**A**) and one-step (**B**) RT *in situ* PCR protocols; note the cytoplasmic localization of the signal (*arrow*).

APPLICATIONS OF RT *IN SITU* PCR

Some applications of the technique for the detection of RNA viruses and mRNAs are discussed to illustrate important points about performing and interpreting RT *in situ* PCR. Furthermore, these applications show the utility of the methodology, especially in comparison with standard *in situ* hybridization.

Hepatitis C

Hepatitis C is the etiologic agent in most cases of post-transfusion hepatitis (18–45). The identification of viral-specific nucleic acid sequences and antibodies directed against structural and nonstructural epitopes of hepatitis C has greatly facilitated the study of non-A, non-B viral hepatitis. It is now evident that the majority of patients with serological evidence of hepatitis C infection have both clinical and pathological evidence of chronic liver disease. First-generation ELISA tests utilizing C100-3, a nonstructural protein coded by the NS4 region of the viral genome, give relatively high false-positive and false-negative rates; the former is notably evident in cases of autoimmune hepatitis, a group that clinically can be difficult to separate from hepatitis C. Second-generation tests based on recombinant immunoblotting techniques (RIBA®, Chiron Corporation) utilizing additional structural (C22-3 core associated) and nonstructural (C33c, 5-1-1) antigens have improved the sensitivity and specificity of serologic tests compared with the ELISA test. Analysis of cryptogenic chronic hepatitis by RIBA has shown that from 77% to 92% affected are seropositive for hepatitis C compared with <1% in blood donors, suggesting a high exposure rate in the former group (18–45).

Chronic hepatitis secondary to hepatitis C infection may be treated with interferon therapy. Interferon treatment is associated with a wide range of potential untoward effects, and, since it is not effective against other causes of chronic hepatitis, such as autoimmune hepatitis, which may be difficult to differentiate from hepatitis C-related liver disease, it is important to be as accurate as possible in the diagnosis. This need for

accuracy has led to interest in the ability to diagnose the disease on morphologic or molecular grounds and to determine the rate of active liver infection in patients with serologic evidence of exposure to hepatitis C.

Several histological features have been associated with hepatitis C infection of the liver. Common findings include portal lymphoid aggregates, bile duct damage and loss, steatosis, "activated" sinusoidal Kupffer cells and lymphocytes, and hepatocyte necrosis within the limiting plate (chronic active hepatitis). Hepatic fibrosis and regenerating nodules characteristic of cirrhosis have been reported in 44% to 58% of cases. Although in aggregate these histological changes are suggestive of hepatitis C liver disease, they usually do not appear together in a single specimen, and other conditions such as hepatitis B infection and autoimmune liver disease can be associated with the same histological findings. Furthermore, it is unclear which of these changes represents a direct effect of hepatitis C infection and which is a reflection of host response.

Direct localization of hepatitis C RNA in liver by standard cDNA–RNA *in situ* hybridization has suggested that scattered periportal hepatocytes contain the virus but not the inflammatory cells or damaged bile ductal epithelium. One study noted that viral RNA, though detectable *in situ* soon after infection, was not detectable by *in situ* hybridization in the liver of infected chimpanzees 3 weeks after the onset of infection, suggesting that viral copy number decreased as the disease progressed (28). This is not unusual for RNA viruses, as they do not have to synthesize large amounts of RNA to induce disease given the inherent "amplification" function of the viral mRNAs. You may recall from Chapter 4 that, if the viral RNA numbers less than about 10 molecules in a given cell, then it will not be detected by the *in situ* assay. Alternatively, DNA viruses often produce large copy numbers that may be in the thousands in an active infection and thus are easy to detect by standard *in situ* hybridization. It has been suggested that hepatitis C nucleic acids, "inclusions," and antigens are present in both the cytoplasm and nucleus of hepatocytes.

We undertook a study of hepatitis C detection in liver biopsy material using the RT *in situ* PCR technique to determine

1. The detection rates of standard *in situ* hybridization versus RT *in situ* PCR in liver biopsies for hepatitis C
2. The histological distribution of the virus in infected liver tissue
3. The rate of viral infection in the liver in patients with a concurrent positive RIBA test for the virus as well as clinical evidence of chronic hepatitis (43, 45).

Liver biopsy material and concurrent sera analyzed with the RIBA test were available for 42 patients. These cases were obtained from the files of Stony Brook University Hospital. The criteria for selecting patients included a diagnosis of chronic hepatitis during a 1.5-year period in which a second-generation RIBA analysis and a liver biopsy had been performed. Most of the cases were without defined etiologies based on the clinical and pathological findings, although antibodies against hepatitis B core or surface antigens were detected in four cases and a positive antinuclear antibody in three. Biopsies and RIBA tests were prompted by clinical evidence of chronic hepatitis as defined by elevated transaminase levels for longer than 6 months. None of the patients had been treated with interferon prior to biopsy.

Standard *in situ* hybridization was done according to the protocol listed in Chapter 4. In addition to RT *in situ* PCR, RT PCR *in situ* hybridization was also performed on serial sections on the same glass slide used for the standard *in situ* hybridization analysis. As noted in other parts of this book, the distinction between PCR *in situ* hybridization and direct-labeled *in situ* PCR is that the latter technique directly incorporates digoxigenin-labeled nucleotide into the PCR product, whereas with PCR *in situ* hybridization amplified DNA is not directly labeled but is detected with a labeled probe, requiring a separate hybridization step. Thus, in RT PCR *in situ* hybridization the two procedural differences are the omission of digoxigenin dUTP from the amplifying solution and detection of the PCR product using cDNA *in situ* hybridization with the internal 30mer probe (Table 7-1).

The histological features of the 42 tissues varied from minimal portal tract infiltrates to marked portal and lobular inflammation with ductal involvement and fatty changes. Serologic analysis for hepatitis C was positive in 39 of the 42 people who had chronic hepatitis; 2 of 3 who were serologically negative had evidence of hepatitis B infection, whereas there was no defined etiology for the final hepatitis C seronegative person.

An attempt was made to find sequences homologous to the hepatitis C genome using standard *in situ* hybridization. Of the 39 biopsies from patients seropositive for hepatitis C, viral RNA was detected in 9 (23%) using standard RNA–cDNA *in situ* hybridization. The positive cells in these tissues were rare hepatocytes; the signal was most intense at the area of the nuclear membrane (Fig. 7-19). To determine if any additional biopsy specimens contained hepatitis C RNA, serial sections were reanalyzed using RT *in situ* PCR. Hepatitis C RNA was detected in the 9 tissues positive by *in situ* hybridization as well as in an additional 14 cases, for an overall detection rate of 21 of 39 seropositive patients (54%). Each of the three tissues from people seronegative for hepatitis C were negative for the virus with both standard *in situ* hybridization and RT *in situ* PCR. In the nine tissues positive by standard *in situ* hybridization, many more positive cells were detected after PCR amplification (Fig. 7-19). Most of the cells with detectable viral cDNA were hepatocytes. The signal was most intense at the nuclear membrane, and there was occasional cytoplasmic staining. Often, the majority of hepatocytes in a given lobule would be positive, whereas the hepatocytes from an adjacent lobule were negative (Fig. 7-20). Positive Kupffer cells were also readily identified. Rarely, the virus was detected in bile duct epithelium. PCR-amplified viral cDNA was not detected in endothelial cells and only very rarely in lymphocytes, which thus served as internal negative controls (Fig 7-20).

A cell line infected by hepatitis C was also studied (kindly supplied by Dr. Jang Han,

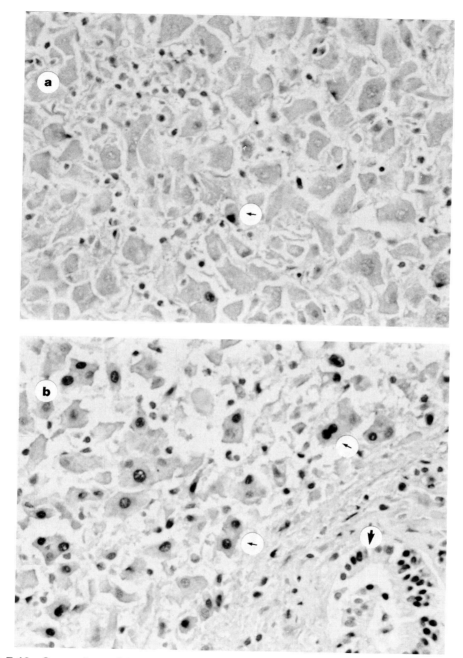

Figure 7-19. *Comparison of detection of hepatitis C by* in situ *hybridization and RT PCR* in situ *hybridization.* Hepatitis C RNA was detected in rare hepatocytes using *in situ* hybridization in this liver biopsy specimen from a patient with chronic hepatitis (**a**). The number of hepatocytes with detectable virus increased markedly when the *in situ* hybridization was preceded by RT and PCR (**b**). Note the presence of the virus in hepatocytes (b, *small arrow*) and bile duct epithelial cells (b, *large arrow*). See Color Plate 5 (following p. 242) and Fig. 1-1 for higher magnification view of localization of hepatitis C RNA.

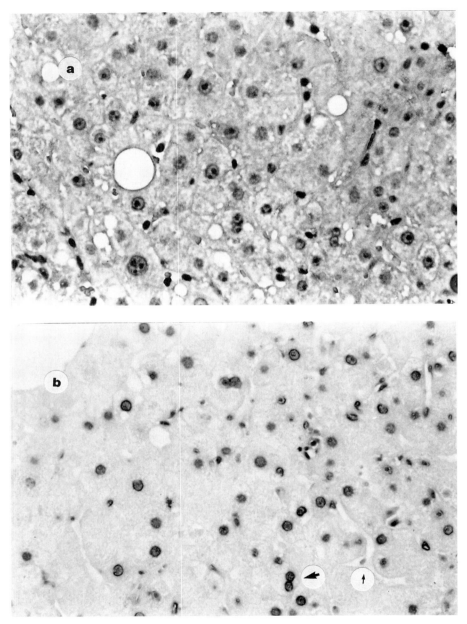

Figure 7-20. *Detection of hepatitis C in a liver biopsy specimen by RT* in situ *PCR.* This liver tissue showed marked portal inflammation and steatosis (**a**). PCR-amplified hepatitis C cDNA was detected in hepatocytes (**b**, *large arrow*, positive hepatocytes; *small arrow*, negative endothelial cells). The signal was lost if the RT step was omitted (**c**); similar negative results were obtained if nonsense (HPV 16-specific) primers were used or if the RT step was preceded by RNase digestion. See Color Plate 5 (following p. 242) and Fig. 1-1 for higher magnification views of localization of hepatitis C RNA.

Figure 7-20. *Continued.*

Chiron Corporation). The infected cell line and a noninfected line were studied without knowledge of which line had been infected by the virus. PCR-amplified hepatitis C cDNA was detected in about 60% of the cells in the infected cell line but in none of the sham-infected cells (46). The signal was present in both the nucleus and the cytoplasm.

Figure 7-20 shows a representative result of the detection of hepatitis C cDNA using the RT *in situ* PCR technique. Included are the essential positive control (omission of DNase step, in which a nonspecific signal reflecting DNA repair and mispriming is evident in the majority of all cell types; see Fig. 7-9) and the negative control (the tissue is digested with DNase, but the RT step is not done or DNase digestion is performed but the RT step is done with nonspecific primers specific for HPV 16 DNA). In Fig. 7-20 the negative control in which no RT step is performed is shown. These controls were performed on the same glass slide with the RT *in situ* PCR test. As another test of the specificity of RT *in situ* PCR, serial sections were examined with RT PCR *in situ* hybridization where the PCR product is not la-

beled *in situ* but rather is detected with an internal digoxigenin labeled probe. With RT PCR *in situ* hybridization the same 21 tissues were positive and the other 18 remained negative. The viral distribution pattern in the positive tissue samples was the same with both RT *in situ* PCR and RT PCR *in situ* hybridization techniques.

The high rate of RIBA positivity seen in this study is not surprising; up to 92% of patients with "idiopathic" chronic hepatitis are RIBA positive, and the antibodies persist in many patients who were initially antibody positive and appear to be unrelated to the course or outcome of disease. Of the patients in this study who were RIBA positive, 46% did not have detectable viral cDNA in their liver biopsies using the RT *in situ* PCR technique. Thus, in the group of patients studied, the RIBA test done in cases of chronic transaminase elevation seemed to produce many false-positive results in relation to the RT *in situ* PCR test. There are several possible explanations for this finding. The most likely is that the viral infection had ended but the antibody response was long lived. Alternatively, the positive RIBA test may have been false positive in the sense that the patient was never infected by the hepatitis C virus. Further prospective studies with serial analyses of liver biopsies and sera for hepatitis C in RIBA-positive patients are needed to address these issues. Another explanation would be that the RIBA-positive patients who did not have the virus detected in their liver biopsies were indeed infected by the virus but, due to the small size of the tissue sample, the RT *in situ* PCR test was negative. However, considering the extreme sensitivity of the RT *in situ* PCR assay and the fact that the positive tissue showed many affected hepatocytes, sampling error seems to be an unlikely cause of a negative RT *in situ* PCR test. Whatever the explanation, it is evident that almost one-half of the patients who are RIBA positive and who have chronic hepatitis do not have evidence of active viral infection in their livers.

Another interesting observation was noted when the detection rate of standard *in situ* hybridization for hepatitis C was compared with the detection rate for RT *in situ* PCR. Although the virus can be detected by standard *in situ* hybridization, it was demonstrated that the detection rate increased markedly after PCR amplification. It follows that in hepatitis C infection of the liver many of the hepatocytes and Kupffer cells contain less than ten viral genomes per cell, as is consistent with the study of Negron et al. (28), which emphasizes the need for the RT *in situ* PCR technique to demonstrate the presence of the virus.

The PCR-amplified viral cDNA in the liver biopsies and the infected cell line was noted in both the nucleus, localizing to the nuclear membrane, and the cytoplasm. Other studies that localized hepatitis C RNA by standard *in situ* hybridization have noted that the virus is usually present in the cytoplasm, although nuclear localization has been described. Although nuclear localization of RNA viruses is not commonly noted, it should be appreciated that the PCR amplification allows the detection of as low as one virus per cell, which may provide a level of detection not possible with other methodologies. The marked distribution of the PCR-amplified viral cDNA at the nuclear membrane suggests a specific geographic relationship of viral transcription with the nuclear matrix, as

has been described for human mRNAs (47–55). Interestingly, the cellular distribution of a hepatitis C-specific epitope as determined by immunohistochemistry was the cytoplasm, abutting the nuclear membrane (Fig. 7-14).

At the time of the writing of this third edition, we have analyzed about 125 additional liver biopsy specimens for hepatitis C, including about 30 from patients who received liver transplants for cirrhosis due to chronic hepatitis C infection. The detection rate of hepatitis C in these additional 125 cases is about 50%. We have not been able to identify any histological criteria that accurately predict which biopsies contain hepatitis C RNA as determined by RT *in situ* PCR. Thus, at this stage, it appears that direct morphologic detection of viral RNA by RT *in situ* PCR is the most reliable method to determine if a case of chronic hepatitis is associated with active hepatitis C proliferation.

We did not define the etiology of the hepatitis in most of the RIBA-positive RT PCR *in situ* negative cases. It is important to note that the initial selection criterion for the patients in the study was an elevated transaminase level, not suspicion of hepatitis C infection. This screening process could have resulted in inclusion of patients with diverse diseases, some of which have histologic overlap with hepatitis C. In most instances, the RIBA test is also used as a screen without history or clinical evidence of hepatitis C, so it is not surprising that patients in the study group might have another basis for chronic inflammation in their liver biopsies.

Interferon therapy is standard therapeutic approach to RIBA-positive patients who have chronic hepatitis assumed on the basis of clinical and pathological findings to be due to hepatitis C. The toxicity that is associated with interferon therapy underscores the need for definitive diagnosis. In this study about one-half of patients with histological evidence of chronic hepatitis and a positive RIBA did not have the hepatitis C genome detectable in the liver. Treatment with interferon may not be appropriate for such patients.

Hepatocellular carcinoma is strongly associated with cirrhosis. Cirrhosis, in turn, is a common occurrence with chronic hepatitis C infection. Because of this, some investigators have suggested that hepatitis C may play a direct etiologic role in cases of hepatocellular carcinoma. Indeed, hepatitis C RNA has been detected by solution phase RT PCR in liver tissues of hepatocellular carcinoma. However, it is not possible to determine if the viral RNA was derived from the cancer cells directly or was a "contaminant" from the bloodstream or surrounding normal hepatocytes.

Dr. G. Lake-Bakkar and I have studied 11 cases of hepatocellular carcinoma for hepatitis C RNA using RT *in situ* PCR. We did not detect viral RNA in the cancer cells. However, we have been able to detect the virus in surrounding nonmalignant hepatocytes, in areas of either chronic hepatitis or cirrhosis. To demonstrate the integrity of RNA in the cancer cells, we detected α-fetoprotein mRNA, which is commonly detected in cases of hepatocellular carcinoma (Fig. 7-21). This suggests that hepatitis C may be a cofactor for hepatocellular carcinoma in the sense that the cellular proliferation that is the hallmark of cirrhosis may predispose the cells to other genetic insults that ultimately lead to the malignant phenotype. However, persistence of the viral genome does not appear to be essential for maintenance of the malignant phenotype. This should be contrasted with HPV, where viral RNA is invariably found in cervical cancer cells (as discussed in Chapter 8).

Measles

Initially, we chose to study HeLa cells infected by the measles virus (kindly supplied by Dr. Eric Spitzer). This choice offered two distinct advantages. First, epithelial cells (including HeLa cells) infected by the measles virus will show characteristic cytological changes easily recognized by light microscopy. Specifically, infected cells become very large and multinucleated and are easily differentiated from other cell types, such as lymphocytes (Fig. 7-22). Second, HeLa cells contain integrated HPV 18 DNA (see Fig. 7-3), which could as-

sist in determining if the initial DNase treatment destroyed the native cellular DNA.

The measles-specific primers were from the nucleocapsid region and were based on the sequence of a clone that was kindly supplied by Dr. William Bellini (56). HeLa cells (ATCC CCL2) were infected with the Edmonston strain of the measles virus (ATCC VR-24) and cultured for 1 to 3 days until the multinucleation characteristic of viral infection became evident. Amplified measles cDNA was detectable in the infected cell line using the RT *in situ* PCR technique. The viral nucleic acid was detectable in each cell that contained the characteristic cytological changes of multinucleation and marked cellular enlargement (Figs. 7-5 and 7-22). Analysis for amplified HPV 18 DNA using type-specific primers was negative, showing that the overnight digestion in DNase did indeed make this, and presumably all, cellular DNA unsuitable for PCR. Note in Fig. 7-22 that the entire nucleus is not positive. Small regions throughout the nucleus and, less conspicuously, in the cytoplasm were negative (this is also evident in Fig. 7-5). This is better appreciated when the cells are viewed with reflective light using confocal microscopy (Fig. 7-22). This is in contrast to the nuclear pattern noted for DNA targets after *in situ* PCR and PCR *in situ* hybridization, which is pan nuclear, i.e., the entire nucleus had detectable signal even when only one integrated copy of DNA was initially present. Interestingly, this nonhomogeneous pattern was also evident using RT PCR *in situ* hybridization for a variety of human mRNAs in the megakaryocyte cell line DAMI, as described previously in this chapter (Fig. 7-15). Although this subcellular localization could represent a diffusion-type artifact, it is conceivable that the pattern represents the specific "tracks" the viral and human mRNAs take in the cell, which, if correct, would suggest that there is minimal diffusion of the PCR product from the site of origin, as supported by the experimental data presented in Chapters 3 and 5. Another observation that supports the contention that there is minimal diffusion of the amplified product is that the specific subnuclear pattern (nucleolar versus perinuclear) is

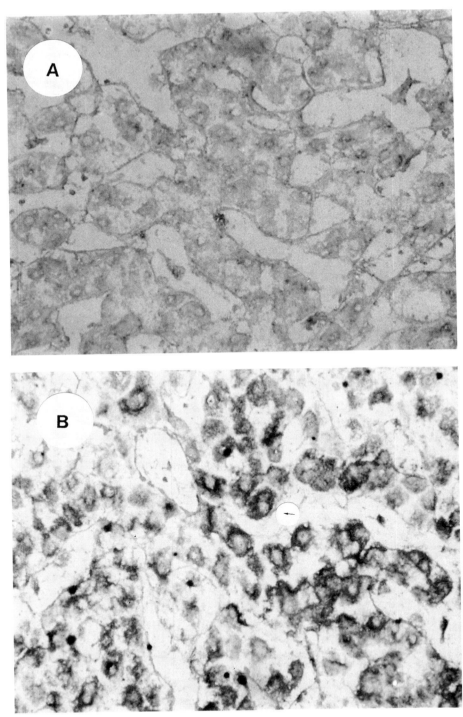

Figure 7-21. *Detection of α-fetoprotein mRNA in hepatocellular carcinoma.* RT *in situ* PCR did not detect hepatitis C RNA in a series of 11 hepatocellular carcinomas (**A**). Although the positive control had an intense signal (not shown), one possible explanation is that the RNA in the tissue had degraded. However, α-fetoprotein mRNA, which is commonly made by hepatocellular carcinoma cells, was readily detected (**B**; note the cytoplasmic localization of the signal).

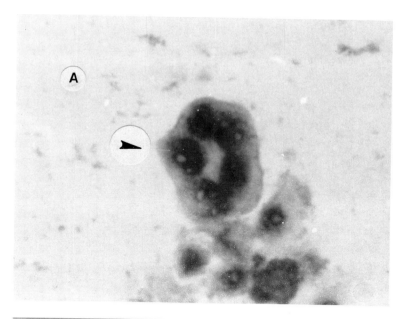

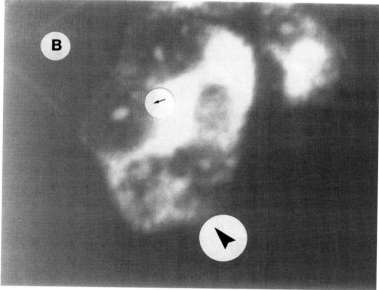

Figure 7-22. *Cytological and molecular analyses of measles-infected HeLa cells.* HeLa cells, which are uninucleate, were infected by the Edmonston strain of the measles virus (ATCC 321). The multi-nucleation characteristic of measles infection is evident in Fig. 7-5. **A:** With RT *in situ* PCR, a signal was evident in the nucleus and cytoplasm of multinucleated cells. Note how the signal is not diffuse but rather appears compartmentalized (*arrowhead*). These cells were next analyzed by confocal microscopy, where the signal appears dark. **B:** The photograph (at ×3,000) highlights the cytoplasmic (diffuse, *arrowhead*) and nuclear localization (distinct, *small arrow*) of the signal obtained with the measles primers and RT *in situ* PCR; the negative area in the nucleus corresponds to the nucleoli (see Fig. 7-23).

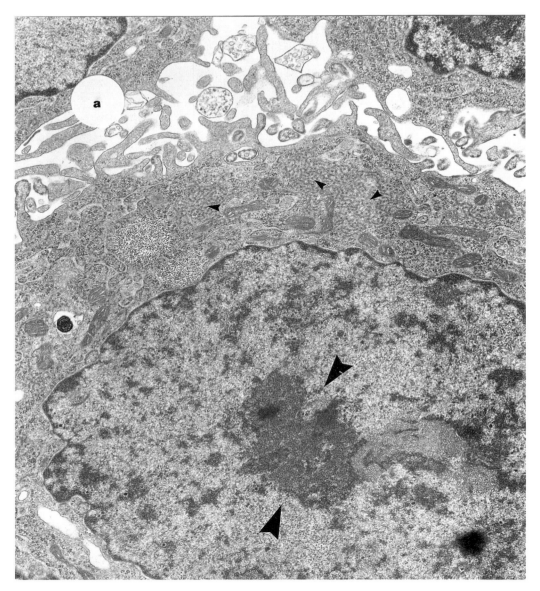

Figure 7-23. *Electron microscopy localization of the measles virus in measles-infected HeLa cells.* The measles virus is easily recognizable in electron microscopy by its tubular appearance. The viral nucleocapsid was present in the nucleus and cytoplasm of the infected cells. This is evident as the criss-crossing tubuloreticular bodies (**a**, *small arrows*, and at higher magnification in **b**). The regions where the virus was not present after RT *in situ* PCR correspond to the nucleoli and intranuclear inclusions (**a**, *large arrows*).

not the same but may vary for a given mRNA when compared with another studied in the same cell line.

    The measles-infected HeLa cells were next studied by electron microscopy. The measles virus is easily identified by electron microscopy due to the characteristic criss-crossing tubuloreticular appearance of its naked nucleocapsid (Fig. 7-23). The viral nucleocapsid localized to the nucleus and the cytoplasm. The virus

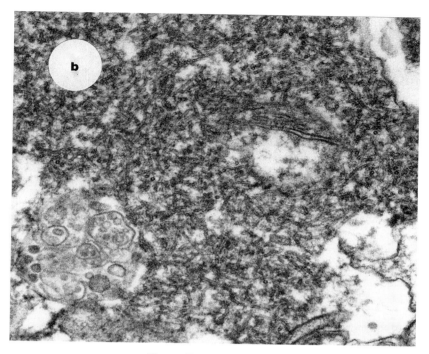

Figure 7-23. *Continued.*

at times was evident in much of the nucleus except in the nucleoli, where the capsid structures were absent (Fig. 7-23). The virus was dispersed throughout the cytoplasm around the cellular organelles. It is evident that this pattern corresponds to that seen with light microscopy after RT PCR *in situ* (Fig. 7-22).

Based on this information gained from the detection of the measles virus in infected HeLa cells, we undertook a study of Paget's disease of bone (56–78). The etiology of Paget's disease of bone is unknown. Epidemiological studies have suggested an infectious etiology. Ultrastructural examination of tissues from Paget's disease of bone and another bony lesion, giant cell tumor of bone, has occasionally revealed virus-like particles, so-called tubuloreticular bodies. Howatson et al. (64) reported that these inclusions were similar to those in cells infected by several viruses including the measles virus and the respiratory syncytial virus (RSV). Such observations have led some investigators to analyze these tissues for a variety of viruses. Mills et al. (66–68) reported that antibodies directed against epitopes of the measles virus and RSV are reactive against tissues from Paget's disease of bone. The presence of measles RNA in most of the osteoclasts, lymphocytes, osteocytes, and fibroblasts of tissues from each of five Paget's disease of bone cases as detected by *in situ* hybridization were subsequently reported (58, 71). However, Ralston et al. (73) were not able to detect the measles virus in 11 cases of Paget's disease of bone using PCR.

We obtained 11 samples of Paget's disease of bone and 2 of giant cell tumor of bone, including one in which the tubuloreticular bodies were evident on ultrastructural examination. All tissues were fixed in 10% buffered formalin after decalcification for 1 to 4 days in a 10% solution of formic acid.

We performed both standard *in situ* hybridization and RT *in situ* PCR and RT PCR *in situ* hybridization for measles cDNA. Furthermore, given the reports of measles-related antigens in Paget's disease of bone, we employed a monoclonal primary antibody against the nucleocapsid region of the Edmonston strain of the measles virus (DAKO-LCA, DAKO-PATTS) and performed immunocytochemistry on the tissue sections and the cell line.

Figure 7-5 depicts a low-power view of the cytological features of measles-infected HeLa cells. Note that approximately 10% of the cells showed the multinucleation characteristic of infection by the measles virus; HeLa cells do not typically demonstrate multinucleation. The nuclei in the multinucleated cells showed prominent basophilic inclusions. Of the uninucleate cells, 56% had similar intranuclear inclusions. Cytoplasmic inclusions were not evident. The measles-infected HeLa cells were analyzed for the nucleocapsid antigen using immunohistochemistry. Detectable antigen was noted in 3% of the cells. Standard *in situ* hybridization was performed with a digoxigenin cDNA probe that corresponded to the nucleocapsid region. A hybridization signal was evident in some of the nuclei in the multinucleated cells. The intensity of the hybridization signal tended to be weak to moderate. None of the uninucleate cells had a detectable hybridization signal using standard *in situ* hybridization. These results were compared with those obtained with RT *in situ* PCR. After RT *in situ* PCR for measles cDNA using primers from the nucleocapsid region, all cells with multiple nuclei had a signal that was more intense than with standard *in situ* hybridization. The PCR-derived signal typically spared one focus per nucleus that corresponded to the inclusion. Of the uninucleate cells, 65% had detectable signal (56, 79). To demonstrate the specificity of direct incorporation, measles-infected HeLa cells were admixed with peripheral leukocytes from an individual with no evidence of measles infection. Only the measles-infected HeLa cells had a detectable signal (Fig. 7-5). This is an important negative control to use when studying cell lines. Furthermore, RT PCR *in situ* hybridization was performed in which only unlabeled nucleotide is incorporated by RT PCR followed by standard *in situ* hybridization using an internal digoxigenin-labeled probe. A hybridization signal is evident under these conditions.

None of the tissues from the cases of Paget's disease of bone or giant cell tumor of bone

demonstrated any antigens that cross-reacted with the monoclonal measles antibody. Similarly, no hybridization signal was evident after standard *in situ* hybridization for the measles virus or after RT *in situ* PCR.

To investigate if the negative results could reflect degradation of nucleic acids after decalcification, standard DNA *in situ* hybridization was done with a biotin-labeled probe for a repetitive human DNA sequence (ONCOR, Gaithersburg, MD). A hybridization signal was evident. To demonstrate that measles cDNA could be made and amplified after decalcification, purified cDNA corresponding to the nucleocapsid region of the measles virus (kindly supplied by Dr. William Bellini) was analyzed by PCR after RT overnight treatment in decalcification solution. Amplified cDNA was evident as detected by Southern blot hybridization. Furthermore, the measles cDNA in the infected HeLa cells was still detectable using the RT *in situ* PCR technique after overnight treatment of the cells in the decalcifying solution.

In summary, the results of this study do not support the hypothesis that Paget's disease of bone is associated with infection by the measles virus. The extreme sensitivity of the RT *in situ* PCR lends support to this argument. These negative results are consistent with a recent report in which measles virus was not detected in eleven cases of Paget's disease of bone using RT PCR.

One line of evidence used to support the hypothesis that measles infection is associated with Paget's disease of bone is the presence of viral-like inclusions. In this study, the inclusions found in measles-infected cells, though tubular, were not straight, but rather criss-crossed extensively compared with the more linear inclusions seen in Paget's disease of bone or giant cell tumor of bone (56).

There are other possible explanations for the negative results noted in this study. The measles virus may have been present but the nucleic acid sequence corresponding to the nucleocapsid region altered or absent. This explanation seems unlikely, as this region is characteristically present in chronic diseases associated with the virus.

"Giant Cell Pneumonitis": Case Reports

This author was sent material from two cases in which the patient died after a fulminant course of pneumonia of unknown etiology. Each demonstrated many multinucleated alveolar lining cells (Fig. 7-24). These cases are now discussed to illustrate the utility of RT *in situ* PCR. In this regard, it should be stressed that, because the patients had died, no sera were available for viral titer studies, nor was fresh, frozen tissue available for virological analyses.

Case 1

A 38-year-old woman came to autopsy at SUNY Stony Brook. She was status postrenal transplant 8 years previously. One month prior to her death, she developed a "flu-like illness." Her condition deteriorated and was marked by a progressively worsening pneumonia unresponsive to antibiotic therapy. The clinical impression was cytomegalovirus pneumonia.

At autopsy, there was marked and extensive pneumonia. A representative section is shown in Fig. 7-24. Note that several of the alveolar lining cells are multinucleated. Although this can occur in a variety of viral infections, such as cytomegalovirus, RSV infection, and herpes infection, it raised the possibility of measles pneumonitis. By using the RT *in situ* PCR technique, we were able to demonstrate that the cause of death was measles pneumonitis (Fig. 7-24).

Case 2

A 3-year-old girl, previously healthy, developed a flu-like illness. Her course was marked by a rapidly progressive pneumonia unresponsive to antibiotic therapy. At autopsy, the histological appearance was similar to that of Case 1. Measles cDNA was not detected by RT *in situ* PCR. However, RSV cDNA was detected and localized primarily to the multinucleated cells (Fig. 7-24).

Pneumonitis of Unknown Etiology in Previously Healthy People

In 1993, Dr. Marvin Kuschner of the Department of Pathology, SUNY, noted at autopsy that several previously healthy people had died from a rapidly progressive pneumonia. Three of these people died in May 1993 at the same time that the outbreak of hantaviral infection was described in the Four Corners region of the United States. Again, no sera or fresh tissue were available from these autopsy cases; hantaviral infection at that stage was best diagnosed by detecting viral-associated antibodies in the sera or detecting viral RNA in fresh tissue using RT PCR. The latter procedure, although sensitive, requires a specialized facility due to the danger of infection by the still viable virus. We had formalin-fixed tissues from these three people and tissues from one other person who died of unexplained pneumonia in October 1993, although he was immunocompromised from chronic steroid use for rheumatoid arthritis. We used tissues from six other people, three who had died of pneumonia of known etiology and three who had no evidence of pneumonia, as controls. These tissues were analyzed for hantaviral RNA by RT *in situ* PCR. Two different primer pairs were used: a "consensus" sequence that can detect any of the five serotypes of hantavirus and a pair specific for the hantavirus that was associated with the hantavirus pulmonary syndrome that caused the epidemic in the Four Corners region in May 1993 (80–90).

PCR-amplified hantaviral cDNA was detected in the lung tissue of the three cases and in none of the six controls using the RT *in situ* PCR technique. In the positive cases, viral RNA was detected in about 20% of pneumocytes and alveolar endothelial cells as determined with the "consensus" and "Four Corners specific" primer pair. The use of different primer pairs is another important check on the specificity of RT *in situ* PCR; demonstration that the same cells are positive in serial sections is strongly suggestive of target-specific cDNA amplification. Infected endothelial cells were identified in a wide variety of other sites, but at rates

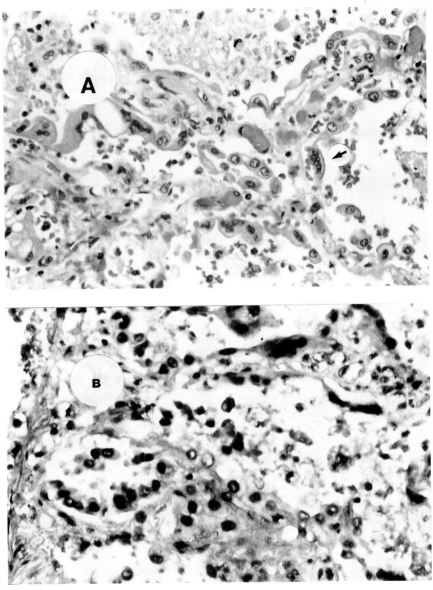

Figure 7-24. *Utility of RT* in situ *PCR in the analysis of giant cell pneumonitis.* The tissue in **A** was from the lung of a woman who was on immunosuppresive drugs to prevent rejection of a renal transplant who died of pneumonia. Note the mutlinucleated cells (*arrow*). These can be found in a variety of viral diseases. Measles infection is documented in **B** by RT *in situ* PCR on the tissue section with primers that correspond to the nucleocapsid region. Another case of giant cell pneumonitis is presented in **C** at much higher magnification; this was from a previously healthy 3-year-old who died of an acute illness. Measles RNA was not detected by RT *in situ* PCR (not shown). However, respiratory syncytial viral RNA was detected in the multinucleated giant cells by RT *in situ* PCR (**D**).

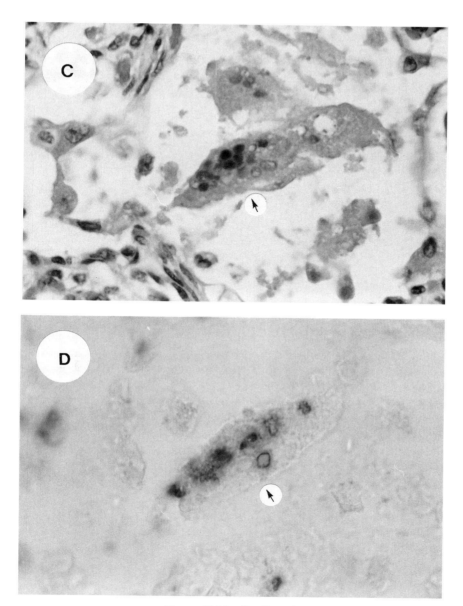

Figure 7-24. *Continued.*

much lower than in the lungs (Fig. 7-25). The selective localization of the viral RNA in many pneumocytes and pulmonary endothelial cells using a highly sensitive PCR-based test demonstrates a correlation between direct viral infection in the lung and the disease process.

Color Plate 6 following p. 242 shows colabeling of hantaviral RNA with keratin; the latter was detected by immunohistochemistry. Colocalization of keratin shows that the infected cell must be an alveolar lining cell, as the other cell types of the alveoli do not make keratin. It has been my experience that such colabeling experiments are best done by performing the *in situ* PCR first, and then the immunohistochemistry. Note that the signal for the latter is red, which is

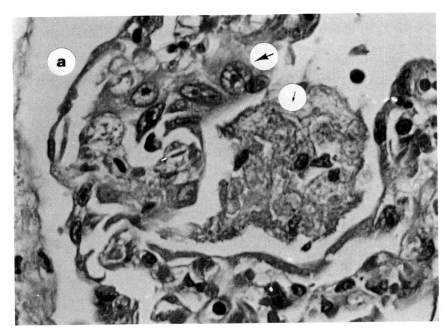

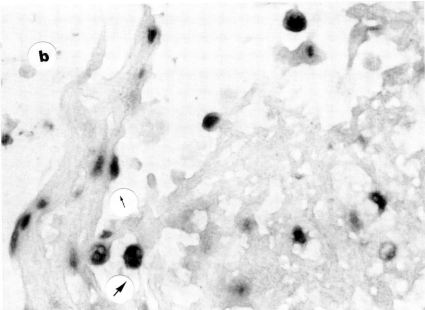

Figure 7-25. *Detection of hantaviral RNA by RT* in situ *PCR.* The tissue in **a** is from the lung of a previously healthy person who died of an acute respiratory disease. Note the alveolar exudate (*small arrow*) and large, atypical alveolar pneumocytes (*large arrow*). In **b**, hantaviral RNA was detected by RT *in situ* PCR in 20% of these cells (*large arrow*) and in a similar percentage of the alveolar endothelial cells (*small arrow*). Infected endothelial cells were found in most organs, but in only about 1% of such cells (not shown). **c** shows the kidney, where atypical renal tubular cells are evident (*arrow*). PCR amplified hantaviral cDNA was detected in some of these cells, shown in **d**.

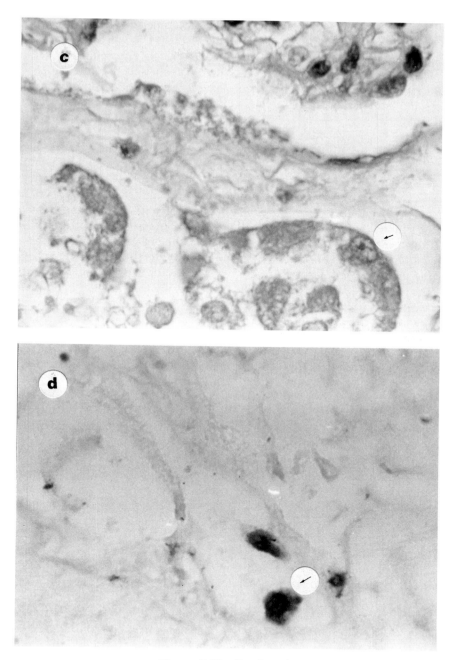

Figure 7-25. *Continued.*

easily differentiated from the blue NBT/BCIP signal of the PCR-amplified hantaviral cDNA. Many antigens are still easily detected after *in situ* PCR; this topic is discussed in more detail in Chapter 9 under the topic of AIDS dementia.

As another control, we attempted to obtain tissues from the Four Corners region. Dr. N. Knolte was kind enough to send us three such samples. We studied them with RT *in situ* PCR without knowing the viral status of the patients.

The RT *in situ* PCR technique correctly identified two cases as hantavirus positive and the other as negative. It is hoped that RT *in situ* PCR will allow for the rapid detection of hantavirus in biopsy and autopsy materials when sera analysis and fresh tissue analysis are usually not possible.

Human mRNAs

Megakaryocytes are cells found in bone marrow and are involved in the syntheses of platelets. We studied the megakaryocyte cell line DAMI for a variety of mRNAs. The experimental protocol was as outlined for the measles virus. Primers specific for three different mRNAs were employed, including amyloid precursor protein (APP), gelsolin (GEL), and glycoprotein IIB (GIIB) (79, 91–100). The inability to amplify native DNA after overnight DNase treatment was documented by primers specific for the human gene *bcl-2*. In each case a signal corresponding to mRNA was noted. Interestingly, the pattern was different for each of the three different mRNAs. As evident in Color Plate 5 (following p. 242), discrete nuclear foci were seen with APP, whereas a "reverse-image pattern" was seen with GEL and GIIB. GEL and GIIB showed an intense and lace-like cytoplasmic signal; no cytoplasmic signal was seen with APP. Electron microscopic evaluation demonstrated that the discrete foci evident with APP were nucleoli. We infer that APP mRNA (presumably at the pre-mRNA stage) localizes to nucleoli, whereas GEL mRNA localizes to the cytoplasm and nucleus but only in non-nucleolar regions.

The signal generated with the human RNAs was most likely derived from transcripts after extensive splicing because the cells were pretreated with RNase-free DNase and, due to the large size of the transcripts, prior to intron splicing (up to 20 kb). One interpretation of the data described above is that the subnuclear localization reflects different geographic "routes" taken by these RNAs as they proceed from pre-mRNA to active message. Discrete localization has been demonstrated by others

for several pre-mRNAs. In this regard it is of interest that U3, one of the snRNAs essential in the splicing apparatus, localizes to the nucleolus, whereas the other snRNAs studied have a perinucleolar distribution. Whether our results indicate differential localization of the RNAs along the nuclear matrix will require further study.

No hybridization signal was evident with standard RNA–cDNA *in situ* hybridization for GEL or APP (79). This suggests that the copy number of these messages per cell is less than 20. A signal was evident for each of these mRNAs after PCR amplification of the corresponding cDNA. A cytoplasmic signal was evident with GEL and GIIB but not with APP. One possible explanation is that the cytoplasmic mRNA for the latter is normally rapidly turned over and degraded. This seems unlikely given the presence of the nucleolar signal and the cytoplasmic signals for the other two RNAs. It is feasible that amplified cDNAs may be more difficult to detect in the cytoplasm relative to the nucleus given the larger volume of the former. Another explanation to consider is that the APP pre-mRNA may have been synthesized and processed in the cell but that under the conditions of this study the end step of transport to the cytoplasm of translationally active message had not occurred. Xing and Lawrence (49) noted a nuclear but no cytoplasmic signal for some pre-mRNAs and speculated that the nuclear matrix may play a role in the release of the active message into the cytoplasm. We are in the process of analyzing this issue using conditions known to induce the synthesis of active message in various cell lines. Preliminary data with proteins inducible with phorbol myristate acetate have shown that a cytoplasmic signal is evident in few cells before stimulation of mRNA synthesis, but, after stimulation, a cytoplasmic signal is evident in most cells using the RT *in situ* PCR methodology (D. French and G.J. Nuovo, *unpublished observations,* 1992). We have also been able to demonstrate that increased invasiveness of Caski cells in the matrigel assay is associated with upregulation of MMP-9 and MMP-2 expression (101).

Gelatinase

An important process in both normal tissue and malignant tumors is the remodeling and infiltration, respectively, of the connective tissue in the stroma (102–105). This function is performed by a variety of enzymes that are typically released in an inactive form and require some event after release, such as proteolytic cleavage, to become active. Because members of the family contain a zinc moiety they are sometimes referred to as *metalloproteases*. We have studied two members of this family—the 72- and 92-kD gelatinases (MMP-2 and MMP-9, respectively)—for their expression in tissues that contain invasive tumors.

The 92-kD gelatinase was examined first in a sarcoma cell line known to produce the corresponding mRNA. The cell line is called HT1080 and was kindly provided by Dr. Deborah French. RT *in situ* PCR was performed using primers specific for the 92-kD gelatinase. If DNase was not performed (the positive control), then an intense signal was evident in the nucleus but not the cytoplasm (see Fig. 1-1). If DNase was done but the RT step omitted, then no signal was seen. When DNase was followed by RT *in situ* PCR after optimal protease digestion time, a cytoplasmic signal was noted (Fig. 1-1). Also note how the nuclear signal is lost. This reminds us that the "internal cellular compartmentalization control" provides an important measure to the specificity of the RT *in situ* PCR technique: the nuclear-based signal for the positive control localizes to the entire nucleus, whereas the RNA-based signal is seen in the cytoplasm, as discussed in detail above. Also note the sharp demarcation between the cytoplasmic (RNA) and nuclear (DNA) signals, suggesting minimal diffusion of the amplicon from its site of synthesis under conditions of optimal protease digestion in these formalin-fixed cells.

PCR-amplified cDNAs that corresponded to the 72- and 92-kD gelatinases were detected in each of 19 invasive tumors that have thus far been studied. The mRNAs localized to the tumor cells and the stromal cells directly around the invasive nests. Interestingly, the stromal cells were negative for the mRNAs in areas away from the invasive tumor. These findings are consistent with those of other investigators who used standard *in situ* hybridization, although we noted that there was often a tenfold or higher increase in the number of positive cells when comparing standard *in situ* hybridization with RT PCR *in situ* hybridization for the 72-kD gelatinase. Perhaps the most intriguing finding in the study was evident in cervical and breast carcinomas. In both cases, areas of *in situ* (noninvasive) cancer are often in the same field with invasive nests of tumor cells. Thus, one can study the differential expression in the invasive versus noninvasive areas of these mRNAs in the same reaction with RT *in situ* PCR. It was apparent from these studies that the noninvasive dysplastic cells usually did not express either mRNA (Fig. 7-26). One can argue that this is strong evidence that the invasive phenotype is associated with the production of these gelatinases, as the highly sensitive RT *in situ* PCR technique may be able to detect even one transcript. Thus, a negative result strongly suggests that specific mRNA is not present. A negative result with standard *in situ* hybridization, with a higher detection threshold of about ten copies per cell, raises the question that a negative result may be due to low production of a given RNA or, for viral infections, DNA molecule.

To address the question of whether MMP or its natural inhibitor (TIMP-1 or -2) expression was associated with clinical prognosis, we compared the RT *in situ* PCR results for cervical cancers with good prognosis (primarily microinvasive cancers with a 5-year survival rate of near 100%) with cervical cancers with poor prognosis (deeply invasive, with a high rate of microvascular invasion) (106). A summary of these data is provided in Table 7-2. Note the following points:

1. MMP is expressed by cancer cells and the surrounding stromal cells of good and poor prognosis.
2. The MMP:TIMP ratio (the percentage of cancer or stromal cells expressing MMP-9 and -2 compared with the percentage of cells expressing TIMP-1 and -2) is about 1 in cervical cancers with good prognosis.

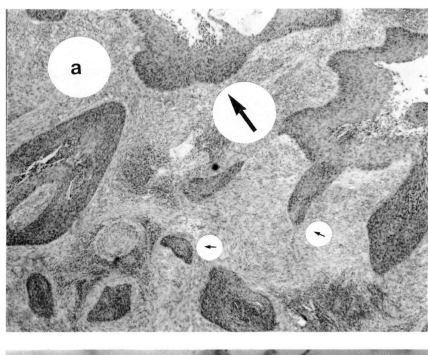

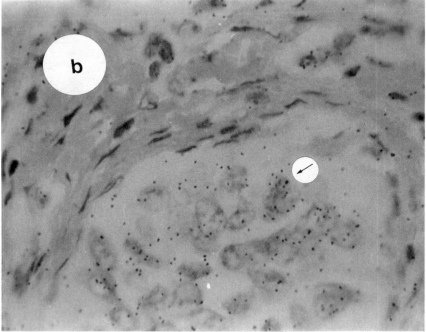

Figure 7-26. *Correlation of MMP-9 expression and the histological features in cervical cancer.* **a** shows a cervical cancer where the noninvasive carcinoma *in situ* component (*large arrow;* also called high-grade SIL) and invasive component (*small arrow*) are evident. PCR-amplified MMP-9 cDNA was detected in the invasive cells (**b**) but not in the carcinoma *in situ* component (**c**).

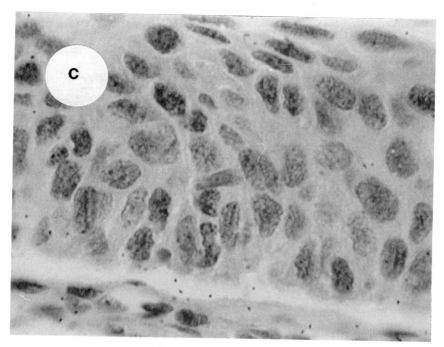

Figure 7-26. *Continued.*

Table 7-2. *A comparison of the pooled MMP to TIMP rations from the cervical cancers with good versus poor prognoses*

	MMP-9 and MMP-2 positive[a]	TIMP-1 and TIMP-2 positive	MMP/TIMP ratio
All cases			
Good prognoses			
Cancer cells	9.7	12.2	0.8
Stromal cells	7.2	7.3	1.0
Poor prognoses			
Cancer cells	11.8	2.2	5.4
Stromal cells	10.0	2.9	3.4
Cases 9, 12, 16			
Areas of low-grade, minimally invasive cancer			
Cancer cells	9.0	12.0	0.7
Stromal cells	6.2	5.4	1.1
Areas of high-grade, deeply invasive cancer			
Cancer cells	11.7	3.0	3.9
Stromal cells	8.8	3.5	2.5
Metastases from cases 10 and 19			
Cancer cells	32.0	1.7	18.8
Tumor in vascular spaces from cases 10 and 19			
Cancer cells	30.1	1.3	23.1
Cell line data			
HeLa	12.0	10.0	1.2
SiHa	6.0	7.0	0.9

[a]The MMP and TIMP data were compiled by adding the percent of cells positive for either MMP or TIMP.(From Nuovo et al., ref. 106, with permission.)

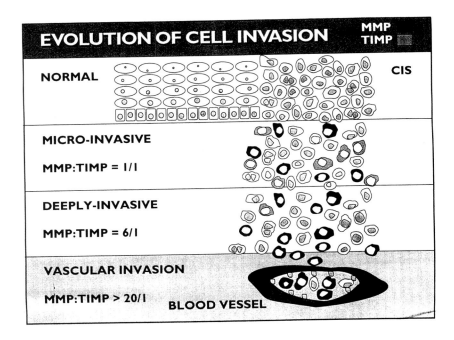

Figure 7-27. *Model for the evolution of increased aggressiveness in carcinomas.* Based on the data derived from cervical cancer tissues and cell lines using RT *in situ* PCR, it is postulated that there is a "natural selection" for cells expressing an MMP and not expressing a TIMP with regard to increased invasiveness and, more importantly, microvascular invasion.

3. The MMP:TIMP ratio is greater than 5:1 in cervical cancers of poor prognosis.
4. The MMP:TIMP ratio is greater than 20:1 in cervical cancer cells that have invaded blood vessels or metastasized to lymph nodes.

This suggests that the evolution of aggressive cancer involves the "natural selection" of cancer cells that can express MMP and not TIMP; a model based on this hypothesis is provided in Fig. 7-27 and Color Plate 7 following p. 242.

One can study the invasive properties *in vitro* by the use of the matrigel system (Collaborative Biosystems, Cambridge, MA). In this assay, a complex matrix of proteins that includes collagen IV (the primary collagen of basement membranes and stroma) are coated on a filter. Cells are grown on top of this filter. If they invade through the matrix, they will anchor to pores present in the filter. This allows for the ready separation of cells that are invasive from those in the same tissue culture specimen that lack this ability. We were able to perform RT *in situ* PCR using HeLa cells (these are invasive but not metastatic in the nude mouse model) and the matrigel assay. This involves fixing the matrigel filter in formalin and then anchoring it to the glass slide. Using RT *in situ* PCR, it was demonstrated that the percentage of HeLa cells that were invasive in the matrigel that expressed MMP-9 and -2 was significantly higher than for their noninvasive counterparts (Figs. 7-28 and 7-29; see also Color Plate 8 following p. 242); however, TIMP expression rates were equivalent. This suggests that matrigel invasion, similar to early *in vivo* invasion, selects for MMP expression, whereas metastatic potential, as noted in Table 7-2, requires both MMP expression and the loss of TIMP transcription.

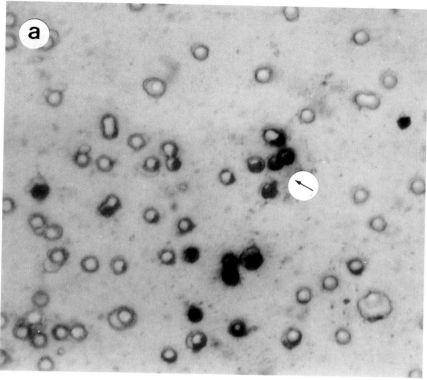

Figure 7-28. *Analysis of MMP-9 and TIMP-1 PCR-amplified cDNA in the cells which had invaded the matrigel.* MMP-9 mRNA was detected in many of the HeLa cells that had invaded the matrigel (**a**, *arrow*); the signal is dark due to precipitation of NBT/BCIP by alkaline phosphatase immunologically linked to the digoxigenin incorporated into the PCR-amplified cDNA. TIMP-1 mRNA was absent in most of the invasive HeLa cells (**b**, *arrow* marks negative cell).

Parvovirus

Parvovirus is a DNA virus that usually infects children or immunocompromised patients (107–115). Its target cell is the nucleated red blood cell. Thus, the clinical syndrome associated with parvoviral infection includes anemia and, in children, erythroblastosis with edema. The infected red cell precursors often show a large, glassy nuclear inclusion that helps to identify the disease process.

Figure 7-30 shows a section from the liver of a child who died of parvoviral infection. Note the groupings of the red cell precursors at low magnification and the nuclear inclusions at higher magnification. An attempt was made to detect parvoviral-specific mRNA using RT *in situ* PCR. As is evident from Fig. 7-30, a signal occurred after RT *in situ* PCR. It showed the same distribution as the red cell precursors. The other cells in the tissue, including hepatocytes and white blood cell precursors, were negative. This finding again highlights two key features of RT *in situ* PCR: (i) the ability to correlate the molecular and histological findings and (ii) the internal negative controls that are built into every tissue section.

Fibrinogen

Fibrinogen production is essential for successful gestation. Although it has been assumed that placental fibrinogen is derived from maternal sources, some clinical data have suggested

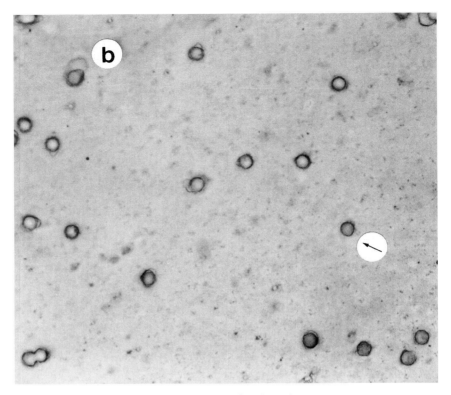

Figure 7-28. *Continued.*

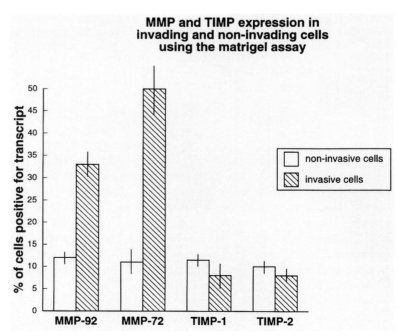

Figure 7-29. *A comparison of the expressions of MMP-92, MMP-72, TIMP-1, and TIMP-2 mRNA as determined by RT in situ PCR in the cells that had invaded the matrigel versus those that were non-invasive.* The matrigel assay allows for a separation of the HeLa cells that invaded into it (about 2%) versus those from the same culture plate that were noninvasive. The results are those of triplicate experiments, with the vertical line representing the SEM.

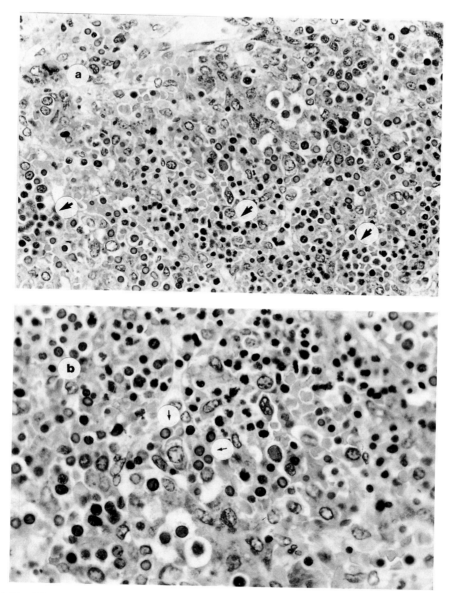

Figure 7-30. *Histological and molecular analysis of parvoviral infection.* The distribution of the red blood cell precursors in the liver with extensive extramedullary hematopoiesis is evident at low magnification (**a**, *arrows*). Note the intranuclear inclusions in the red cell precursors evident at higher magnification (**b**, arrows). Parvoviral mRNA was detected by RT *in situ* PCR in a similar distribution (**c**, *arrows*; and, at higher magnification, **d**).

that cells from the placenta may be able to synthesize fibrinogen directly. To address this question, we used RT *in situ* PCR for each of the three mRNA chains of fibrinogen α, β, and γ. A representative slide is shown in Fig. 7-2.

Fibrinogen mRNA, β-chain, was detected in this placenta from an 18-week gestation in a voluntary termination of pregnancy (116). This and other data derived from this study suggest that the placenta may play a critical role in fibrino-

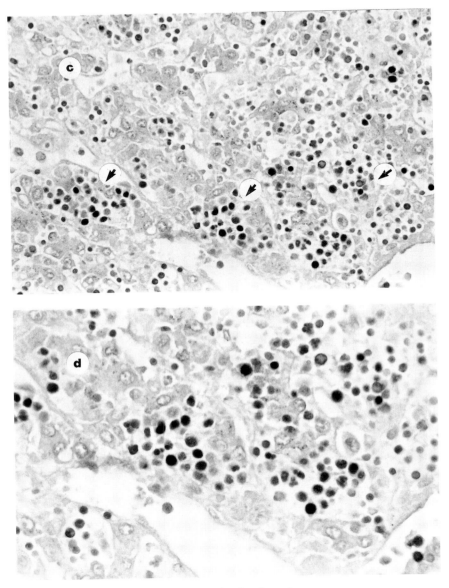

Figure 7-30. *Continued.*

gen dynamics during gestation by direct synthesis of the molecule. Note how the signal localizes to the cytoplasm. The sequence of the β-chain is known. Thus, we were able to do RT *in situ* PCR with a primer sequence specific for the intron; under these conditions, no signal was evident with RT *in situ* PCR (see Color Plate 9 following p. 242). The use of primer pairs that span exons and introns is another very useful control when doing RT *in situ* PCR.

Expression of Other mRNAs

A variety of techniques, including RT PCR and Western blotting, have demonstrated that vitronectin can be detected in spermatids. Pre-

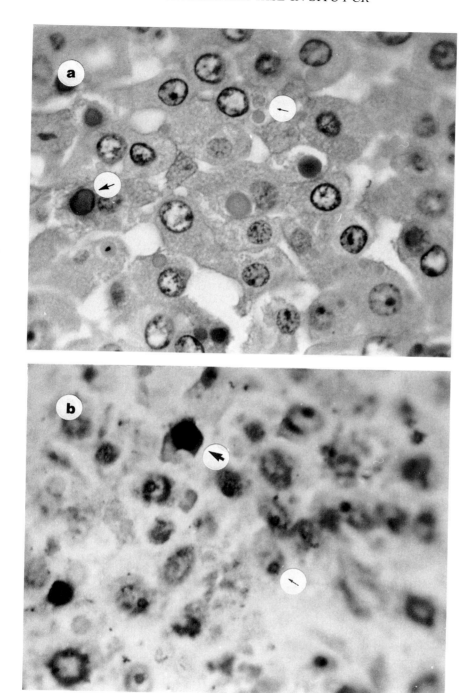

Figure 7-31. *Detection of bacterial RNA by RT* in situ *PCR.* *a:* Lung tissue in which there is a large infiltrate of macrophages. Note the variably sized cytoplasmic inclusions, the Michealis-Guttman bodies,which in this case represent a marker of the etiological bacterial agent *Rotococcus* sp; the smaller ones have a characteristic laminated appearance (*small arrow, large arrow,* larger, more developed Michealis-Guttman body). **b:** PCR amplified rotococcal cDNA was detected in these Michealis-Guttman bodies using RT *in situ* PCR; note the concentric pattern of the signal in the smaller bodies.

cise cellular localization, however, has been difficult. RT *in situ* PCR has shown that expression of vitronectin occurs exclusively in the primary and secondary spermatocytes, suggesting a strict regulation of expression with cell maturation (117) (Fig. 7-4). Similarly, endothelial receptor expression has been detected in the kidney by RT PCR and Northern blot analysis. RT *in situ* PCR demonstrated differential expression of the various endothelial receptor mRNAs in renal tubular cells and stromal cells (118).

Detection of Bacterial RNA by RT *in situ* PCR

We undertook several studies to detect bacterial nucleic acids using *in situ* PCR. It would be highly advantageous to use model systems where there would be an obvious cellular marker for the bacterial RNA or DNA. We chose two such models. The first model was malakoplakia and the second infection by mycobacterial sp.

Malakoplakia is a disease associated with a variety of bacteria. It usually involves the bladder, although any tissue can be involved. The classic histological marker of malakoplakia is the Michealis-Guttman body. This is a cytoplasmic inclusion (Fig. 7-31). The case we studied was a case of malakoplakia in the lung of a man who had AIDS; bacterial culture demonstrated that the etiologic agent was *Rotococcus* sp. We performed RT *in situ* PCR using broad-spectrum bacterial primers kindly supplied by Dr. Charles Steinmann; these primers can detect transcripts from over 95% of bacterial species thus far studied. A signal was evident that localized to the Michealis-Guttman bodies (Fig. 7-31). The one-step EZ RT *in situ* PCR protocol was used; no modifications were needed for detection of the bacterial RNA.

Mycobacteria localize to macrophages; they are usually found in areas where the macrophages and lymphocytes form aggregates, called *granuloma*. The macrophages are often multi-nucleated. Mycobacterial RNA was detected in their target cell, the macrophage, in the typical poorly formed granuloma in the lymph nodes of AIDS patients who had known *Mycobacterium avium-intracellulare* disease. In this study, we

analyzed for the presence of these so-called atypical mycobacteria in cervical lymph nodes of children without AIDS. We were able to demonstrate that about one-half of these cases were associated with mycobacterial RNA; the viral nucleic acid localized to the macrophages (119). Again, the EZ RT *in situ* PCR protocol was used without any modification. It appears that detection of bacterial RNAs can be done following the same principles and protocols as outlined for the detection of human and viral RNAs.

REFERENCES

1. Ansari B, Coates PJ, Greenstein BD, Hall PA. *In situ* end-labeling detects DNA strand breaks in apoptosis and other physiologic and pathologic states. *J Pathol* 1993;170:1.
2. Beckmann AM, Myerson D, Daling JR, Kiviat NB, Fenoglio CM, McDonald JM. Detection and localization of human papillomavirus DNA in human genital condylomas by *in situ* hybridization with biotinylated probes. *J Med Virol* 1983;16:265.
3. Dubeau L, Chandler LA, Gralow JR, Nichols PW, Jones PA. Southern blot analysis of DNA extracted from formalin fixed pathology specimens. *Cancer Res* 1986;46:2964.
4. Fleming KA, Evans M, Morey AL. Optimization of non-isotopic *in situ* hybridization on formalin fixed paraffin-embedded material using digoxigenin labeled probes and transgenic material. *J Pathol* 1992;167:9.
5. Kiyabu MT, Shibata D, Arnheim N, Martin WJ, Fitzgibbons PL. Detection of human papillomavirus in formalin-fixed, invasive squamous carcinomas using the polymerase chain reaction. *Am J Surg Pathol* 1989;13:221.
6. Mark A, Trowell H, Dyall-Smith ML, Dyall-Smith DJ. Extraction of DNA from formalin-fixed paraffin-embedded pathology specimens and its use in hybridization (histo-blot) assays. Application to the detection of human papillomavirus DNA. *Nucleic Acids Res* 1987;17:17–20.
7. McAllister HA, Rock DL. Comparative usefulness of tissue fixatives for *in situ* viral nucleic acid hybridization. *J Histochem Cytochem* 1985;33:1026.
8. Moench TR, Gendelman HE, Clements JE, Narayan O, Griffin DE. Efficiency of *in situ* hybridization as a function of probe size and fixation technique. *J Virol Methods* 1985;11:119.
9. Nuovo GJ, Silverstein SJ. Comparison of formalin, buffered formalin, and Bouin's fixation on the detection of human papillomavirus DNA from genital lesions. *Lab Invest* 1988;59:720.
10. Nuovo GJ. Buffered formalin is the superior fixative for the detection of human papillomavirus DNA by *in situ* hybridization analysis. *Am J Pathol* 1989;134:837.
11. Nuovo GJ. Comparison of Bouin's solution and buffered formalin fixation on the detection rate by *in situ* hybridization of human papillomavirus DNA in genital tract lesions. *J Histotech* 1991;14:13.
12. Nuovo GJ, MacConnell P, Forde A, Delvenne P. Detection of human papillomavirus DNA in formalin fixed tissues by *in situ* hybridization after amplification by PCR. *Am J Pathol* 1991;139:847–854.

13. Stoler MH, Broker TR. *In situ* hybridization detection on human papillomavirus DNAs and messenger RNAs in genital condylomata and a cervical carcinoma. *Hum Pathol* 1986;17:250.

14. Samoszuk M. Rapid detection of Epstein-Barr viral DNA by nonisotopic *in situ* hybridization. *Am J Pathol* 1991;96:448.

15. Gelb AB, LeBrun DP, Warnke RA. Estimation of tumor growth fractions in archival formalin fixed paraffin-embedded tissues using two anit-PCNA/cyclin monoclonal antibodies. *Am J Pathol* 1992;141:1453.

16. Greer CE, Peterson SL, Kiviat NB, Manos MM. PCR amplification from paraffin-embedded tissues: effects of fixative and fixative times. *Am J Clin Pathol* 1991; 95:117.

17. Nuovo GJ, Forde A. An improved system for reverse transcriptase *in situ* PCR. *J Histotech* [*in press*].

18. Nuovo GJ, Gallery F, Hom R, MacConnell P, Bloch W. Importance of different variables for optimizing *in situ* detection of PCR-amplified DNA. *PCR Method Appl* 1993;2:305–312.

19. Bach N, Thung SN, Schaffner F. The histological features of chronic hepatitis C and autoimmune chronic hepatitis: a comparative analysis. *Hepatology* 1992;15: 572–577.

20. Brinton MA. Non-A, Non-B hepatitis. In: Schlesinger S, Schlesinger MJ, eds. *The togaviridae and flaviviridae.* New York: Plenum Press; 1986:327–374.

21. Choo QL, Kuo G, Weiner AJ, Overby LR, Bradley DW, Houghton M. Isolation of a cDNA clone derived from a blood borne nonA, nonB viral hepatitis genome. *Science* 1989;244:359–362.

22. Chou Q, Russell M, Birch DE, Raymond J, Bloch W. Prevention of pre-PCR mis-priming and primer dimerization improves low copy number amplifications. *Nucleic Acids Res* 1992;20:1717–1723.

23. Fagan EA, Ellis DS, Tovy GM, Portmann B, Williams R, Zuckerman AJ. Virus like particles localized in liver in sporadic nonA, nonB fulminant hepatitis. *J Med Virol* 1989;27:76–80.

24. Haase AT, Retzel EF, Staskus KA. Amplification and detection of lentiviral DNA inside cells. *Proc Natl Acad Sci USA* 1990;87:4971–4975.

25. Han JH, Shyamala V, Richman KH, et al. Characterization of the terminal regions of hepatitis C viral RNA: identification of conserved sequences in the 5′ untranslated region and poly(A) tails at the 3′ end. *Proc Natl Acad Sci USA* 1991;88:1711–1715.

26. Kuo G, Choo QL, Alter HJ, et al. An assay for circulating antibodies to a major etiologic virus of human nonA, nonB hepatitis. *Science* 1991;244:362–364.

27. Alter HJ, Purcell RH, Holland PV, Feinstone SM, Morrow SG, Moritsugu Y. Clinical and serological analysis of transfusion associated hepatitis. *Lancet* 1975;ii: 838–841.

28. Negron F, Pacchioni D, Shimizu Y, et al. Detection of intrahepatic replication of hepatitis C virus RNA by *in situ* hybridization and comparison histopathology. *Proc Natl Acad Sci USA* 1992;89:2247–2251.

29. Nuovo GJ, Margiotta M, MacConnell P, Becker J. Rapid *in situ* detection of PCR-amplified HIV-1 DNA. *Diagn Mol Pathol* 1992;1:98–102.

30. Nuovo GJ, Gallery F, MacConnell P, Becker J, Bloch W. An improved technique for the *in situ* detection of DNA after polymerase chain reaction amplification. *Am J Pathol* 1991;139:1239–1244.

31. Scheuer PJ, Ashrafzadeh P, Sherlock S, Brown D, Dusheiko GM. The pathology of hepatitis C. *Hepatology* 1992;15:567–571.

32. Trepo C, Vitvitski L, Hanz O, et al. Identification and detection of long incubation nonA, nonB hepatitis virus and associated antigens or antibodies. *J Virol Methods* 1980;2:127–139.

33. Weiner AJ, Kuo G, Bradley DW, et al. Detection of hepatitis C viral sequences in nonA, nonB hepatitis. *Lancet* 1990;335:1–3.

34. Yamada S, Koji T, Nozawa M, Kiyosawa K, Nakane PK. Detection of hepatitis C virus (HCV) RNA in paraffin-embedded tissue sections of human liver of non-A, non-B hepatitis patients by *in situ* hybridization. *J Clin Lab Anal* 1992;6:40–46.

35. Mitchell LS, Jeffers LJ, Reddy KR. Detection of hepatitis C virus antibody by first and second generation assays and polymerase chain reaction in patients with autoimmune chronic hepatitis types I, II, and III. *Am J Gastroenterol* 1993;88:1027–1034.

36. Cassani F, Muratori L, Manotti P. Serum autoantibodies and the diagnosis of type-1 autoimmune hepatitis in Italy: a reappraisal in the light of hepatitis C virus infection. *Gut* 1992;33:1260–1263.

37. Magrin S, Craxi A, Fabiano C. Hepatitis C virus replication in autoimmune chronic hepatitis. *J Hepatol* 1991;13:364–367.

38. Nishiguchi S, Kuroki T, Ueda T. Detection of hepatitis C virus antibody in the absence of viral RNA in patients with autoimmune hepatitis. *Ann Intern Med* 1992;116: 21–25.

39. Yuki N, Hayashi N, Hagiwara H, Kamada T. Serodiagnosis of chronic hepatitis C in Japan by second-generation recombinant immunoblot assay. *J Hepatol* 1993; 17:170–174.

40. Brown D, Powell L, Morris A, Dusheiko GM. Improved diagnosis of chronic hepatitis C virus infection by detection of antibody to multiple epitope. *J Med Virol* 1992;38:167–171.

41. Hoofnagle JH, DiBisceglie AM, Schindo M. Antiviral therapy of hepatitis C: present and future. *J Hepatol* 1993;17:130–136.

42. Yamamoto H, Hayashi E, Nakamura H, Ito H, Kambe H. Interferon therapy for nonA, nonB hepatitis: a pilot study and review of the literature. *Hepatogastroenterology* 1992;39:377–380.

43. Nuovo GJ, Lidonnici K, MacConnell P, Lane B. Intracellular localization of polymerase chain reaction (PCR)-amplified hepatitis C cDNA. *Am J Surg Pathol* 1993; 17:683–690.

44. Nouri Aria KT, Sallie R, Sangar D, Alexander GJM, Williams R. Detection of genomic and intermediate replicative strands of hepatitis C virus in liver tissue by *in situ* hybridization. *J Clin Invest* 1993;91:2226–2234.

45. Lidonnici K, Lane B, Nuovo GJ. A comparison of serologic analysis and *in situ* localization of PCR-amplified cDNA for the diagnosis of hepatitis C infection. *Diagn Mol Pathol* 1995;4:98–107.

46. Yoo BJ, Selby MJ, Choe J, et al. Transfection of a differentiated human hepatoma cell line (Huh7) with in vitro transcribed hepatitis C Virus (HCV) RNA and establishment of a long term culture persistently infected with HCV. *J Virol* 1995;69:32–38.

47. Fey EG, Krochmalnic G, Penman S. The nonchromatin substructures of the nucleus: the ribonucleoprotein (RNP)-containing and RNP-depleted matrices analyzed by sequential fractionation and resinless section electronmicroscopy. *J Cell Biol* 1986;102:1654–1665.

48. Lawrence JB, Singer RH, Marselle LM. Highly localized tracks of specific transcripts within interphase nuclei visualized by *in situ* hybridization. *Cell* 1989;57: 493–502.

49. Xing Y, Lawrence JB. Preservation of specific RNA distribution within the chromatin-depleted nuclear substructure demonstrated by *in situ* hybridization coupled with biochemical fractionation. *J Cell Biol* 1991;112: 1055–1063.

50. Verheijen R, Van Verrooji W, Ramaekers F. The nuclear matrix: structure and composition. *J Cell Sci* 1989;90: 11–36.

51. Mirkovitch J, Mirault ME, Laemmli UK. Organization of the higher-order chromatic loop: specific DNA attachment sites on nuclear scaffold. *Cell* 1984;39: 223–232.

52. Carmo-Fonesca M, Tollervey D, Pepperkok R, et al. Mammalian nuclei contain foci which are highly enriched in components of the pre-mRNA splicing machinery. *EMBO J* 1991;10:195–206.

53. Zamore PD, Green MR. Biochemical characterization of U2 snRNP auxiliary factor: an essential pre-mRNA splicing factor with a novel intranuclear distribution. *EMBO J* 1991;10:207–214.

54. Wang J, Cao LG, Wang YL, Pederson T. Localization of premessenger RNA at discrete nuclear sites. *Proc Natl Acad Sci USA* 1991;88:7391–7395.

55. Lawrence JB, Marselle LM, Byron KS, Johnson CV, Sullivan JL, Singer RH. Subcellular localization of low-abundance human immunodeficiency virus nucleic acid sequences visualized by fluorescence *in situ* hybridization. *Proc Natl Acad Sci USA* 1990;87:5420–5424.

56. Nuovo MA, Nuovo GJ, MacConnell P, Steiner G. Analysis of Paget's disease of bone for the measles virus using the reverse transcriptase *in situ* polymerase chain reaction technique. *Diagn Mol Pathol* 1993;1:256–265.

57. Heimann A, Scanlon R, Gentile J, MacConnell P, Nuovo GJ. Measles cervicitis: a cytological and molecular biological analysis. *Acta Cytol* 1992;36:727–730.

58. Abelanet R, Daudet-Monsac M, Laoussadi S, Forest M, Vacher-Lavenu M-C. Frequency and diagnostic value of the virus-like filamentous intranuclear inclusions in giant cell tumor of bone, not associated with Paget's disease. *Virchows Arch [A]* 1986;410:65–68.

59. Baslé MF, Fournier JG, Rozenblatt S, Rebel A, Bouteille M. Measles virus RNA detected in Paget's disease bone tissue by *in situ* hybridization. *J Gen Virol* 1986;67: 907–913.

60. Baslé MF, Rebel A, Fournier JG, Russell WC, Malkani K. On the trail of the paramyxoviruses in Paget's disease of bone. *Clin Orthop* 1987;217:9–15.

61. Fornasier VL, Flores L, Hastings D, Sharp T. Virus-like filamentous intranuclear inclusions in a giant-cell tumor, not associated with Paget's disease of bone. *J Bone Joint Surg [A]* 1985;67:333–336.

62. Fournier JG, Rozenblatt S, Bouteille M. Localization of measles virus nucleic acid sequences in infected cells by *in situ* hybridization. *Biol Cell* 1983;49:287–290.

63. Harvey L, Gray T, Beneton MNC, Douglas DL, Kanis JA, Russell RGG. Ultrastructural features of the osteoclasts from Paget's disease of bone in relation to a viral aetiology. *J Clin Pathol* 1982;35:771–779.

64. Howatson AF, Fornasier VL. Microfilaments associated with Paget's disease of bone: comparison with nucleo-capsids of measles virus and respiratory syncytial virus. *Intervirology* 1982;18:150–159.

65. Jacobs TP, Michelsen J, Polay JS, D'Adamo AC, Canfield RE. Giant cell tumor in Paget's disease of bone. Familial and geographic clustering. *Clin Orthoped* 1986;202: 203–208.

66. Mills BG, Holst PA, Stabile EK, et al. A viral antigen-bearing cell line derived from culture of Paget's bone cells. *Bone* 1985;6:257–268.

67. Mills BG, Singer FR. Nuclear inclusions in Paget's disease of bone. *Science* 1976;194:201–202.

68. Mills BG, Singer FR, Weiner LP, Suffin SC, Stabile EK, Holst PA. Evidence for both respiratory syncytial virus and measles virus antigens in the osteoclasts of patients with Paget's disease of bone. *Clin Orthop* 1984;183: 303–311.

69. Mirra JM. Pathogenesis of Paget's disease based on viral etiology. *Clin Orthop* 1987;217:162–170.

70. Mirra JM, Bauer FC, Grant TT. Giant cell tumor with viral-like intranuclear inclusions associated with Paget's disease. *Clin Orthop* 1981;158:243–251.

71. Negoescu A, Mandache E. The ultrastructure of nuclear inclusions in the giant-cell tumor of bone. *Pathol Res Pract* 1989;184:410–417.

72. O'Driscoll JB, Buckler HM, Jeacock J, Anderson DC. Dogs, distemper and osteitis deformans: a further epidemiological study. *Bone Miner* 1990;11:209–216.

73. Ralston SH, Digiovine FS, Gallacher SJ, Boyle IT, Duff GW. Failure to detect paramyxovirus sequences in Paget's disease of bone using the polymerase chain reaction. *J Bone Miner Res* 1991;6:1243–1248.

74. Rebel A, Baslé M, Pouplard A, Malkani K, Filmon R, Lepatezour A. Bone tissue in Paget's disease of bone. Ultrastructure and immunocytology. *Arthritis Rheum* 1980;23:1104–1114.

75. Schajowicz F, Ubios AM, Araujo ES, Cabrini RL. Virus-like intranuclear inclusions in giant cell tumor of bone. *Clin Orthop* 1985;201:247–250.

76. Singer FR. Paget's disease of bone: a slow virus infection? *Clin Orthop* 1980;159:293–296.

77. Singer FR, Mills BG. Evidence for a viral etiology of Paget's disease of bone. *Clin Orthop* 1983;178: 245–251.

78. Welsh RA, Meyer AT. Nuclear fragmentations and associated fibrils in giant cell tumor of bone. *Lab Invest* 1970;22:63–72.

79. Nuovo GJ, Gorgone G, MacConnell P, Goravic P. *In situ* localization of human and viral cDNAs after PCR-amplification. *PCR Methods Appl* 1992;2:117–123.

80. Nichol ST, Spiropoulou CF, Morzunov S, et al. Genetic identification of a hantavirus associated with an outbreak of acute respiratory illness. *Science* 1993;262: 914–917.

81. Hantavirus pulmonary syndrome—United States, 1993. *MMWR* 1994;43:45–48.

82. Duchin JS, Koster FT, Peters CJ, Simpson GL, Tempest B, Zaki S. Hantavirus pulmonary syndrome: a clinical description of 17 patients with a newly recognized disease. *N Engl J Med* 1994;330:949–955.

83. Zaki SR, Greer PW, Coffield LM, et al. Hantavirus pulmonary syndrome: pathogenesis of an emerging infectious disease. *Am J Pathol* 1995;146:552–579.

84. Hjelle B, Jenison S, Torrez-Martinez N, et al. A novel hantavirus associated with an outbreak of fatal respira-

tory disease in the Southwestern United States: evolutionary relationships to known hantaviruses. *J Virol* 1994;68:592–596.

85. Spiropoulo CF, Morzunov S, Feldmann H, Sanchez A, Peters CJ, Nichol ST. Genome structure and variability of a virus causing hantavirus pulmonary syndrome. *Virology* 1994;200:715–724.

86. Puthavathana P, Lee HW, Kang CY. Typing of hantaviruses from five continents by polymerase chain reaction. *Virus Res* 1992;26:1–14.

87. Xiao SY, Chu YK, Knauert FK, Lofts R, Dalrymple JM, LeDuc JW. Comparison of hantavirus isolates using a genus-reactive primer pair polymerase chain reaction. *J Gen Virol* 1992;73:567–573.

88. Song JW, Baek LJ, Gajdusek DC, et al. Isolation of pathogenic hantavirus from white-footed mouse (*Peromyscus leucopus*). *Lancet* 1994;344:1637.

89. Huggins J, Hsiang C, Cosgriff T. Prospective, double blind, concurrent, placebo controlled clinical trial of intravenous ribavirin therapy of hemorrhagic fever with renal syndrome. *J Infect Dis* 1991;164:1119–1127.

90. Nuovo GJ, Simsir A, Steigbigel R, Kuschner M. Analysis of fatal pulmonary hantaviral infection in New York by reverse transcriptase *in situ* PCR. *Am J Pathol* [*in press*].

91. Greenberg JM, Rosenthal DJ, Greeley TA, Tantravah R, Hardin RJ. Characterization of a new megakaryocyte cell line: the Dami cell. *Blood* 1988;72:1968–1974.

92. Rozenblatt S, Eizenberg O, Ben-Levy R, Lavie V, Bellini WJ. Sequence homology within the morbilliviruses. *J Virol* 1985;53:684–690.

93. Yei C, Kristan-Hewlett I, Baker CC, Howley PM. Presence and expression of human papillomavirus references in human cervical carcinoma cell lines. *Am J Pathol* 1985;119:361–367.

94. Hartwig K, Chambers KA, Stossel TP. Localization of gelsolin with actin filaments in cell membranes of macrophages and platelets. *J Cell Biol* 1989;108:467–479.

95. Gardella JE, Gorgone GA, Newman PJ, Frangione B, Gorevic PD. Characterization of Alzheimer amyloid precursor protein transcripts in platelets and megakaryocytes. *Neurosci Lett* 1992;17:100–103.

96. Norrby E, Oxman MV. Measles. In Fields BN, Knipe DM, eds. *Fields virology.* Vol. 1. New York: Raven Press; 1990:1013–1036.

97. Ponte P, Gonzalez-Dewhitt P, Schilling J, et al. A new A4 amyloid mRNA contains a domain homologous to serine proteinase inhibitors. *Nature* 1988;331:525–527.

98. Pontz M, Eisman R, Heidenreich R, et al. Structure of the platelet membrane glycoprotein IIB. *J Biol Chem* 1987;262:8476–8482.

99. Lyman S, Aster RH, Visentin GP, Newman PJ. Polymorphism of human platelet membrane glycoprotein IIB associated with the Baka/Bakb alloantigen system. *Blood* 1990:75:2343–2348.

100. Kwiatkowski DJ, Stossel TP, Orkin SH, Mole JE, Colten HR, Yin HL. Plasma and cytoplasmic gelsolins are encoded by a single gene and contain a duplicated actin-binding domain. *Nature* 1986;323:455–458.

101. Nuovo GJ. The relationship between metelloprotease, their inhibitors, and viral transcripts in the invasive behaviour of cervical cancer cell liner. *J Histochem Cytochem* (submitted).

102. Liotta LA, Steeg PS, Stetler-Stevenson WG. Cancer metastasis and angiogenesis: an imbalance of positive and negative regulation. *Cell* 1991;64:327–336.

103. Monteagudo C, Merino MJ, San-Juan J, Liotta LA, Stetler-Stevenson WG. Immunohistochemical distribution of type IV collagenase in normal, benign, and malignant breast tissue. *Am J Pathol* 1990;136:585–592.

104. Pyke C, Ralfkiaer E, Huhtala P, Hurskainen T, Dano K, Tryggvason K. Localization of messanger RNA for Mr 72,000 and 92,000 type IV collagenases in human skin cancers by *in situ* hybridization. *Cancer Res* 1992; 52:1336–1341.

105. Sato H, Kida Y, Mai M, et al. Expression of genes encoding type IV collagen-degrading metalloproteinases and tissue inhibitors of metalloproteinases in various human tumor cells. *J Cell Biol* 1992;78:342–349.

106. Nuovo GJ, MacConnell P, Valea F, French DL. Correlation of the *in situ* detection of PCR-amplified metalloprotease cDNAs and their inhibitors with prognosis in cervical carcinoma. *Cancer Res* 1995;55:267–275.

107. Mochizuki SM, San Gabriel MC, Nakatani H, Yoshida M, Harasawa R. Comparison of polymerase chain reaction with virus isolation and haemagglutination assays for the detection of canine parvoviruses in faecal specimens. *Res Vet Sci* 1993;55:60–63.

108. Telerman A, Tuynder M, Dupressoir T, et al. A model for tumor suppression using H-1 parvovirus. *Proc Natl Acad Sci USA* 1993;90:8702–8706.

109. Wu H, Rossmann MG. The canine parvovirus empty capsid structure. *J Mol Biol* 1993;233:231–244.

110. Sol N, Morinet F, Alizon M, Hazan U. Trans-activation of the long terminal repeat of human immunodeficiency virus type 1 by the parvovirus B19 NS1 gene product. *J Gen Virol* 1993;74:2011–2014.

111. Cortes E, San Martin C, Langeveld J, et al. Topographical analysis of canine parvovirus virions and recombinant VP2 capsids. *J Gen Virol* 1993;74:2005–2010.

112. Asano Y, Yoshikawa T. Human herpesvirus-6 and parvovirus B19 infections in children. *Curr Opin Pediatr* 1993;5:14–20.

113. Nuesch JP, Tattersall P. Nuclear targeting of the parvoviral replicator molecule NS1: evidence for self-association prior to nuclear transport. *Virology* 1993;196: 637–651.

114. Saller DN Jr, Rogers BB, Canick JA. Maternal serum biochemical markers in pregnancies with fetal parvovirus B19 infection. *Prenatal Diagn* 1993;13:467–471.

115. Bloom ME, Berry BD, Wei W, Perryman S, Wolfinbarger JB. Characterization of chimeric full-length molecular clones of Aleutian mink disease parvovirus (ADV): identification of a determinant governing replication of ADV in cell culture. *J Virol* 1993;67:5976–5988.

116. Galanakis D, Nuovo GJ, Spitzer S, Kaplan C. Demonstration of fibrinogen mRNA in human trophoblasts by reverse transcriptase PCR *in situ*. *Thrombosis Res* 1996;81:263–269.

117. Nuovo GJ, Preissner M, Bronson R. Vitronectin expression in the male genital tract. *Mol Hum Reprod* 1995; 10:2187–2191.

118. Chow LH, Bubramanian S, Nuovo GJ, Miller F, Nord EP. Endothelial receptor expression in the renal medulla identified by *in situ* RT PCR. *Am J Physiol* 1995;269:449–457.

119. April M, Garlich J, Nuovo GJ. Detection of atypical mycobacterial RNA by in situ PCR in cervical odentis. *Otolaryngol* (in press).

8

Applications of PCR *in situ* Hybridization: Human Papillomavirus

Human papillomavirus (HPV) causes warts both on the genital tract and at nongenital sites. Behavioral patterns clearly are an important risk factor for the spread of genital tract warts, given their strong association with the patient's sexual history. The immunological status of the person also plays a role in HPV-related disease, although this is not as well understood. Nongenital warts are often easy to diagnose on clinical examination due to their papillary, firm, and "warty-like" appearance. The diagnosis of genital tract warts, especially on the cervix, may be more difficult, given the problems inherent in colposcopy and the Papanicolaou smear. This difficulty has led to the development and use of more sophisticated molecular techniques for the diagnosis of HPV infection of the genital tract. Management of HPV infection includes a variety of modalities including excision, ablation, and, to a lessor extent, immunotherapy. Therapy for genital tract warts is clearly important because of their documented relationship with cervical cancer. Given that cervical warts are easily removed, cervical cancer may be the best example of a cancer that can be nearly eradicated by simple preventative methods.

HPV is ideally suited for analysis by PCR *in situ* hybridization for several reasons. There is a wealth of information concerning the correlation of histology and HPV DNA detection (1–36). HPV-associated lesions have copy numbers of the virus ranging from one to thousands per cell. There are many carcinoma cell lines that have well-characterized copy numbers of HPV DNA. In addition, there are several intriguing questions about HPV-associated lesions that are perfectly suited for investigation by PCR *in situ* hybridization. For example, do all the cells in an HPV-related lesion actually contain HPV DNA, and is the virus found in the directly adjacent, normal epithelium?

The current understanding of the epidemiology and pathogenesis of HPV is summarized in this chapter, and the utility of *in situ* hybridization and *in situ* PCR for the diagnosis and management of infection by the virus is discussed.

EPIDEMIOLOGY

Genital tract warts are among the most common of the sexually transmitted diseases. The Centers for Disease Control and Prevention estimates that over 1.5 million people in the United States acquired genital tract warts in 1994. This number is, at best, an estimate, as HPV infection is not a reportable disease. It is estimated that over 30 million people are infected with HPV in the United States (37,38).

Many epidemiological studies have compared the importance of different risk factors for cervical HPV/warts and cervical cancer. Although the conclusions vary somewhat from one study to the next, most studies have demonstrated the following:

1. The number of sexual partners rather than the age at first intercourse, parity, or method

of birth control is a pre-eminent factor for the risk of cervical warts and cancer.

2. The number of sexual partners of the male (the so-called high-risk male) is a risk factor for cervical warts and cancer.
3. Cigarette smoking is an important factor for the risk of cervical squamous intraepithelial lesion (SIL) and cancer and appears to have a synergistic effect with the number of sexual partners.
4. The use of condoms may be associated with a decreased risk of acquiring cervical warts (37–45).

The importance of the number of sexual partners as a risk factor is clearly consistent with the notion that HPV is a known sexually transmitted agent. Cigarette smoking may increase the likelihood that dysplastic cells infected by HPV will develop other genetic insults and ultimately progress to either a high grade SIL or cancer.

Additional epidemiological studies have suggested that HIV-1 may increase the likelihood of cervical SIL and cancer. However, since HIV-1 infection is now predominately spread by venereal contact, it is difficult to know if this is a simple coincident association or an actual cause–effect observation. Another point that these studies have highlighted is perhaps the most frustrating. The risk of cervical cancer is correlated with conditions of poverty and no prior Papanicolaou smear or, less likely, an atypical Papanicolaou smear that was not followed up (38). These data highlight the importance of offering yearly Papanicolaou smear screening to poor women who otherwise would not have this test done. However, it can be difficult to reach and treat populations with inadequate access to health care.

Immunological factors play a role in HPV disease. Increased incidence of HPV infection has been associated with immunosuppression due to allografts, AIDS, and, to a lesser extent, pregnancy. It has been suggested that cigarette smoking can contribute to an immunological risk factor for HPV infection by adversely affecting the cervical lymphocytes and Langerhans cells. Of course, cigarette smoke also contains mutagens, which have been found to be concentrated in the cervical mucus.

A final point about the epidemiology of HPV infection concerns HPV types in genital warts in children. HPV 2 is the most common type in nongenital warts in children and adults; this type is not detected in genital warts in adults (46,47). HPVs 6 and 11 are the most common types in cutaneous genital warts and are not found in nongenital cutaneous warts. Finding genital tract warts in children raises the serious question of sexual abuse. Several studies have shown that genital tract warts in children contain either HPVs 6/11 (about 70%) or HPV 2 (30%) (46,47). It is presumed that the HPV 2 positive warts were not acquired from the genital tract of an adult. The source of the virus for lesions which contain HPVs 6 or 11 is from the genital tract, either due to abuse or from the mother during birth. Laryngeal papillomas, which usually contain HPV 11, have been shown to result from HPV infection as the child passed through the birth canal (37,48).

VIROLOGY

General Statements

HPV is, like most pathogens that are sexually transmitted, extremely fastidious in its growth requirements. For the most part, HPV is restricted to squamous epithelium. During their evolution, the over 70 types of HPV thus far identified became well adapted to different specific sites. For example, HPV 2 is the most common type in nongenital warts, but, in adults, it is rarely if ever isolated from genital tract lesions, as noted above. Conversely, HPVs 6 and 11, which are the most common types in vulvar, penile, and perianal warts, are rarely, if ever, encountered at nongenital cutaneous sites. HPV 16 appears to be the most "flexible" HPV type, having been isolated from SILs and cancers of the cervix, penis, vulva, periungual region, and conjunctiva (38,49,50).

Because of the extremely fastidious nature of HPV it is not readily grown in tissue or cell culture. HPV cannot easily be introduced into laboratory animals, despite the fact that papillomaviruses as a family involve most other mammals. This inability to grow HPV readily makes it difficult to identify the virus and its associated effects. It would take tests developed in the field of molecular biology, which can easily identify any specific DNA or RNA sequence, to provide the rapid detection of HPV and enable the investigator to correlate this information with various pathological, clinical, and basic molecular events.

Basic Structure

HPV is a DNA virus with a simple protein coat. It belongs to the papovavirus family, which includes mouse polyoma virus and a group of viruses that can cause CNS disease, including SV40, the BK virus, and the JC virus, which causes progressive multifocal leukoencephalopathy (discussed in Chapter 5). The amount of the covalently closed circular double-stranded DNA present is small, even for a virus, and consists of about 8,000 base pairs. The protein or capsid coat does not have an envelope and is icosahedral and comprised of 72 units or capsomeres measuring 55 μm in diameter.

The small size of about 8,000 base pairs translates into relatively few viral-specific functions. Each function involves a defined part of the total genomic sequence and is responsible for the production of a specific protein. These functional units are referred to as open reading frames (ORFs), because they are "read" as a specific unit by the RNA polymerase. These ORFs are dictated from only one of the two DNA strands (the upper or sense strand) and use 69% of this DNA sequence. Part of the "unread" portion is the upstream regulatory region that is used by the virus to modulate its activity. Two ORFs have been associated with production of the viral protein coat and are referred to as the L1 and L2. The letter L stands for *late*, referring to the observation that the coat or capsid proteins are produced late in the infectious cycle of the virus. Seven other ORFs have been identified and are referred to as the *early* ORFs, E1 through E7. E6 and E7 appear to play essential roles in the evolution of an infected cell into an immortalized cell (one capable of sus-

tained growth in cell culture) and a malignant, invasive cell, as is discussed in more detail below.

The distinct types of HPV are genotypes identified by their nucleic acid sequences, not serotypes, where the basis is the antibody response against one of their proteins. For a particular HPV to be designated as a new type, at least 50% of its genome must be different from all the other types that have thus far been characterized. It is important to realize that this new type will most likely share certain parts of its genome with other of the HPV types, i.e., there will be regions of strong homology. This is particularly true for certain regions of the virus, for example, ORFs L1 and E2, which are well conserved among the different members of the group. The implication of this statement is that a probe for a given HPV type may detect other HPV types. However, whereas the homology between the probe and the target type is complete, or 100%, the homology will be less for a related type. For example, HPVs 31 and 16 share over 70% homology over parts of their respective genomes corresponding to the E6 and E7 ORFs. Therefore, whereas an HPV 16 probe that includes this area will detect HPV 31 at low stringency, it will probably not detect it at high stringency, where near 100% homology is needed for a probe and target to remain hybridized. The clinical implications are twofold: (i) A given probe may detect more than one specific HPV type, especially at low stringency, and (ii) the specific type of HPV in a tissue or cell sample often cannot be determined at low stringency due to the cross-reactivity of two or more types.

With this brief review of some of the basic molecular and clinical aspects of HPV, let us look at the utility of *in situ* PCR in understanding HPV-related pathogenesis.

SiHa CELLS

SiHa cells provide a useful reference for PCR *in situ* hybridization. This is a human cell line that contains one copy of HPV DNA, type 16 (51). Claims that the one copy of HPV DNA can be detected by standard *in situ* hybridization are contrary to most investigators' experiences. Although I have noted a signal with standard *in situ* hybridization and SiHa cells, at most only a few percent of the cells show a signal using large (100 to 200 base pair) probes over the entire 8,000 bp viral sequence. This signal may represent, in part, DNA–RNA hybrids, as certain transcripts, such as the ORF E6, are relatively abundant in this cell line.

Our initial experiments with PCR *in situ* hybridization (52,53) supported the idea, developed by Haase et al. (52) that multiple primer pairs were necessary for successful PCR *in situ* hybridization. These primers dictated the synthesis of overlapping fragments that could form a complex of over 1,500 base pairs, which, they theorized, would not pass through the nuclear membrane, whereas the individual 450 base pair fragments were membrane permeable. The apparent need for multiple primer pairs has limited the applicability of the PCR *in situ* technique because of the high cost and, more importantly, the difficulty of generating multiple sequence-specific primers for highly polymorphic targets. Nonetheless, using standard PCR *in situ* hybridization (i.e., without the hot start modification) and a biotin-labeled genomic probe, we could not detect the one copy of HPV 16 DNA when a single HPV 16-specific primer pair was used (53). However, a hybridization signal was evident after amplification when multiple primer pairs were used (Fig. 8-1).

The importance of the hot start modification had to be understood for success to come with a single primer pair. Recall that multiple reactions may be done on the same glass slide. In this way we were able to ascertain that a hybridization signal could be detected after PCR with a single primer pair using the hot start modification and that the intensity of the signal was greater than that obtained with multiple primer pairs under standard or "cold start" conditions (Fig. 8-2).

An estimate of the degree of target-specific amplification was another useful measure provided by the experiments with SiHa cells. As mentioned previously, there are multiple cervical carcinoma cell lines that have well-defined copy numbers of HPV DNA. Two such lines are HeLa cells, with about 25 copies of HPV 18, and Caski cells, with about 600 copies of HPV 16. Figure 8-3 compares the hybridization signals obtained after PCR with SiHa cells with the nonamplified signal seen with HeLa and Caski cells. Based on these observations, one can estimate that there is about a 200-fold increase in the copy number of native DNA in the cell as a consequence of PCR. Although 200 copies are easily detectable with *in situ* hybridization (4,54,55), this increase appears to be much below what may be obtained with solution phase PCR and has led to the misconception that *in situ* PCR is much less robust than solution phase PCR. However, it is important to realize that the much smaller reaction volume in the nucleus compared with a 0.5-ml tube will greatly impact the amount of DNA that can be synthesized during *in situ* PCR. In solution phase PCR, target amplification usually ends at 10^7 copies due to limiting concentrations of key reagents and the decreased likelihood of primer–target annealing due to the enormous excess of target DNA. This so-called saturating concentration of amplified target (copy number/volume) is, of course, dependent on the volume of the amplification solution. Recall from Chapter 2 that the standard diameter of a cell nucleus is 5 μm, which is several orders of magnitude below that of the 50-μl GeneAmp tube. Thus, the amount or copy number of the amplified target that equals the saturating concentration with *in situ* PCR will be several orders of magnitude below solution phase PCR. It can be calculated that the number of copies that can be made in the nucleus during *in situ* PCR before a saturating concentration of the product is reached is about 1,000 (Dr. Lawrence Haff, Perkin-Elmer, *personal communication,* 1992).

LOWER GENITAL TRACT LESIONS

The Cervix

Before we discuss the histological distribution of HPV DNA in cervical lesions as determined by PCR *in situ* hybridization, it would seem useful to provide a brief discussion of cervical histology for those who are not pathologists. The more general concepts of the differ-

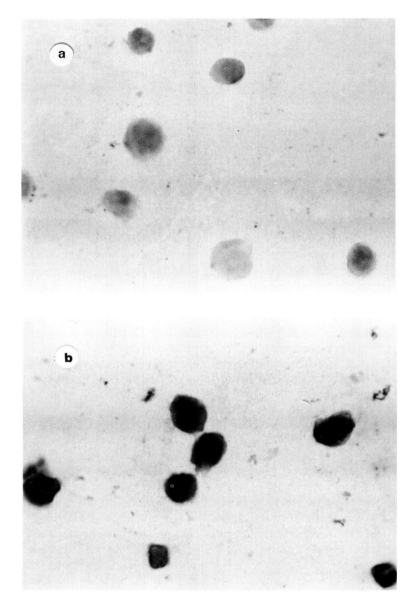

Figure 8-1. *The apparent need for multiple primers for the detection of one HPV DNA copy with standard PCR* in situ *hybridization.* The one copy of HPV DNA type 16 present in SiHa cells was poorly detected if *in situ* hybridization with a biotin-labeled probe was done after amplification with the primer pair PV1 and PV2 (see Table 8-1) (**a**). A hybridization was evident, however, if the *in situ* hybridization was preceded by amplification using the multiple primer pairs PV1 through PV7 (**b**).

ent types of epithelia and stromal cells is provided in Chapter 2.

Two different types of epithelium, columnar and squamous, are found in the cervix (37,56). They coexist at a region called the *trans-* *formation zone,* where the columnar mucous-producing cells are eventually replaced by the squamous cells through a process called *squamous metaplasia.* As the squamous cells mature, they flatten, and their nuclei become smaller. The cells are well organized and evenly spaced from one another (Fig. 8-4).

In the event that HPV infects the cervix and produces a lesion, a set of morphological changes occur that, in their classic form, are easily recognized by the pathologist. The virus short circuits the normal orderly maturation process of cells. As a result, the cells become crowded. Often some nuclei overlap (this does not occur in normal epithelium), and other cells are more widely spaced. The variable cell density is the classic histological change induced by HPV infection. Furthermore, the nuclei no longer become smaller as the cells move toward the surface. Instead, there is marked variation in nuclear size, shape, and color. Multinucleated cells, especially binucleated forms, are often seen, as well as perinuclear halos that also vary in size and shape (Fig. 8-5). When these histological changes that are induced by HPV are noted, the lesion is referred to as a *squamous intraepithelial lesion* (SIL).

Many pathologists divide SILs into two groups. First, there are the low-grade SILs. The histological features toward the middle and surface of the epithelium are as described above. The basal epithelium is minimally altered, either appearing normal or showing mild crowding and nuclear enlargement (Fig. 8-5). Substantial cellular crowding and nuclear atypia in the basal zone in conjunction with increased mitotic activity and atypical mitotic forms characterizes the second group, the high-grade SILs (Fig. 8-6). The abnormal cells characteristic of SILs are usually initially detected on screening the Papanicolaou smear sample of cervical cells (37,56).

Given that the basal changes are an important distinguishing feature of low- versus high-grade SILs, a salient question is, what is the basis of this difference? To understand this important point, it is useful to look at the observations made from experiments in which normal cervical or penile epithelium is transfected by HPV in the laboratory setting. Two changes are evident when normal squamous epithelium is transfected by HPV:

1. An increased rate of growth of the cells, i.e., hyperplasia, with cytologic changes

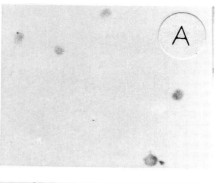

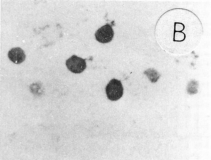

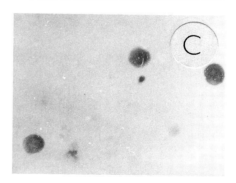

Figure 8-2. *Detection of one HPV DNA copy with a single primer pair and the hot start modification of PCR in situ hybridization. As described in Fig. 8-1, the one copy of HPV16 DNA was poorly detected using PCR in situ hybridization if a single primer pair was used (**A**). However, if the hot start modification of PCR was used where the Taq polymerase was not added until the reaction temperature reached 55°C, then the one copy was detected with PCR in situ hybridization and the single primer pair PV1 and PV2 (**B**). Note that the intensity of the hybridization signal is greater than with multiple primer pairs and standard PCR in situ hybridization (**C**) when the two reactions are done on the same glass slide.*

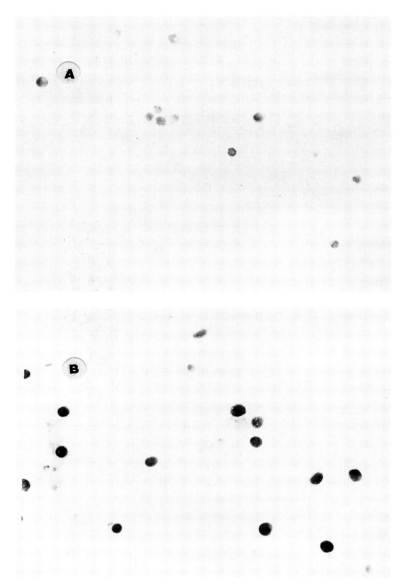

Figure 8-3. *Semiquantitation of the degree of amplification in PCR* in situ *hybridization.* HPV DNA was not detected in SiHa cells if standard *in situ* hybridization was done (**A**). A signal was evident using PCR *in situ* hybridization (**B**). The degree of amplification is about 200-fold based on the non-amplified signal evident with HeLa cells (about 25 copies of HPV 18 per cell; **C**) and Caski cells (about 600 copies of HPV 16 per cell; **D**).

that include perinuclear halos and nuclear atypia.

2. A transformation of the morphology of the cells seen as marked cellular crowding, an increase in the nuclear to cytoplasmic ratio, and more intense hyperchromaticity (57–60).

Over 20 distinct HPV types have been detected in genital tract lesions. Certain types, notably HPVs 6, 11, 42, 43, and 44, are found in low-grade SILs and very rarely in high-grade SILs or invasive cancers. The other types, notably HPVs 16, 18, 31, 33, 35, and 51, are

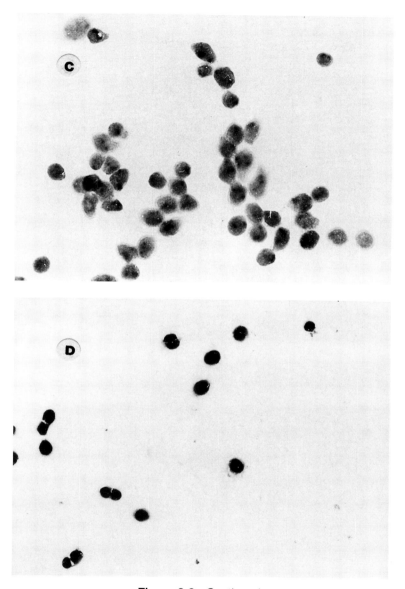

Figure 8-3. *Continued.*

found in low-grade and high-grade SILs as well as invasive cancers. All HPV types are capable of causing the first alteration. As the squamous cells proliferate they will attempt to mature. This is evident on cytologic analysis by an increased amount of cytoplasm and a flattening out of the cell and biochemically by a shift of its metabolism to keratin formation. When these changes occur, it triggers the virus to produce large amounts of its DNA, RNA, and protein. The DNA synthesis of the cell is also increased, which makes the nucleus enlarge, become hyperchromatic and irregular in shape, and, at times, to become binucleate (Fig. 8-7). Although this does not kill the cell, it causes the cytoplasm to swell and the organelles to be

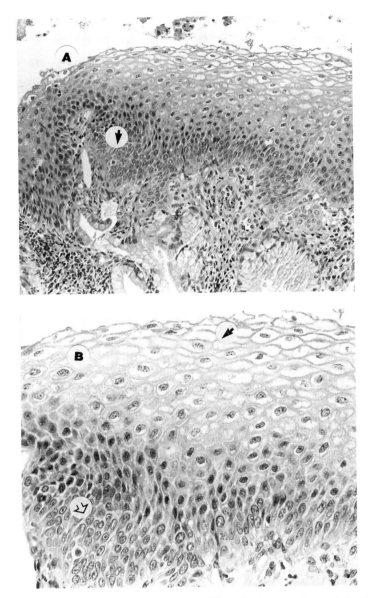

Figure 8-4. *Normal histology of the uterine cervix.* The uterine cervix contains two types of epithelium—simple columnar glandular and stratified squamous. The area where the two come together is called the *transformation zone* (**A**). In this area, through the process of squamous metaplasia, the glandular epithelium is eventually replaced by the squamous epithelium. The transformation zone is the site where most HPV-related lesions of the cervix occur. The area marked by the *arrow* is shown at higher magnification in **B**. Note the well-ordered appearance of the normal mature squamous epithelium and how the cells become more widely separated as they move toward the surface (*arrow*). The *open arrow* depicts the less mature metaplastic cells, which are more densely packed but still well ordered. This is probably the region where HPV initially infects the cervical epithelium in most instances.

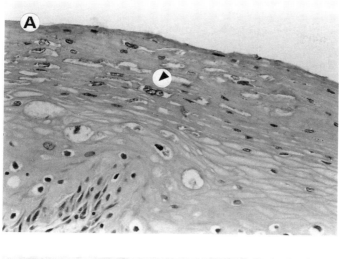

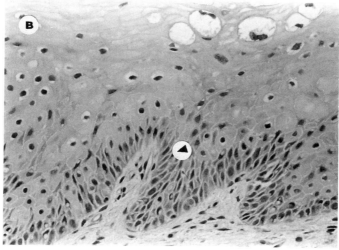

Figure 8-5. *The histology of a cervical low-grade SIL.* One possible outcome of HPV infection of the cervix is a low-grade SIL. Histologically, these lesions are characterized by a disordered arrangement of cells in the middle and superficial zones of the epithelium (compare with Fig. 8-4B). In addition to the variable cell density in the zone, the nuclei show substantial variability in their size, shape, and chromaticity. Binucleate forms are common, as are variably sized and shaped halos around the atypical nuclei (**A**, *arrowhead*). The basal part of the epithelium (**B**, *arrowhead*) is unremarkable except for some mild reactive-type changes.

pushed to the cell perimeter. This is recognized cytologically as a distinct perinuclear halo. Cells that demonstrate perinuclear halos and the nuclear changes just described will usually be strongly positive for viral nucleic acids or proteins when analyzed by *in situ* hybridization or immunohistochemistry, respectively (see Figs. 8-12 and 8-14, below).

Not all HPV types are capable of causing cellular transformation. Unlike the "early" hyperplastic response with halos and nuclear atypia, transformation is not associated with maturation of the squamous cells. As would be expected from the preceding discussion, it is not associated with large amounts of HPV DNA, RNA, or proteins. However, the cyto-

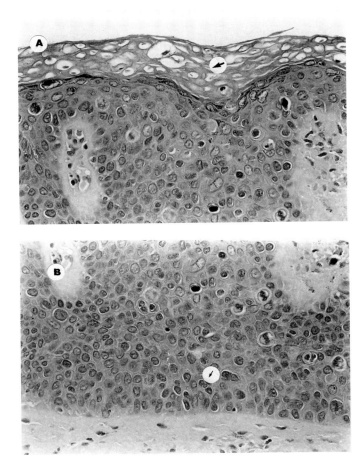

Figure 8-6. *The histology of a cervical high-grade SIL.* Another possible outcome of HPV infection of the cervix is a high-grade SIL. Histologically, these lesions may demonstrate the disordered arrangement of cells and nuclear atypia in the middle and superficial zones of the epithelium that are also seen in the low-grade lesions (**A**); the *arrow* depicts para- and hyperkeratosis, which can also be seen in such lesions although it not a diagnostic feature. However, unlike the low-grade lesions, there is substantial cellular disorganization, nuclear atypia, and mitotic activity in the basal and parabasal layers (**B**, *arrow*).

logic changes are marked and include more overt disorganized growth pattern and intense nuclear hyperchromaticity; perinuclear halos are not evident. It is clear that this transforming effect is, from the viruses' standpoint, a more subtle change in which small amounts of distinct viral proteins, probably from E6 and E7 expression, are interacting with cellular elements to effect the appearance and, more importantly, behavior of the cell. The change in behavior is that the cells may become able to

proliferate indefinitely, a process called *immortalization*. In a sense, the virus can use this pathway to ensure "lifetime" association with the cell that it has infected; indeed, the viral DNA is often integrated into the host DNA (Figs. 8-8 to 8-10).

To summarize, HPV can cause two distinct cytologic changes that most likely occur through two distinct pathways. All types can induce the cells to proliferate and mature, manifested by the halos, nuclear atypia, and crowd-

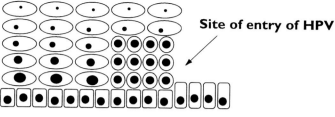

Site of entry of HPV

Mid and Upper Zones
Hyperplasia, Cell Crowding, Halos

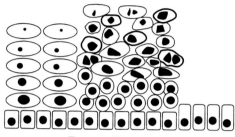

Basal Zone
Minimal Hyperplasia, Crowding

Figure 8-7. *Graphic representation of the effects of HPV on cervical epithelium: early effects.* The initial effects of HPV infection that may be due to any HPV type include hyperplasia, cellular crowding, and marked production of viral proteins and nucleic acids in the more mature squamous cell, which is related to the perinuclear degeneration (halo) (see Fig. 8-11).

Mid and Upper Zones
Hyperplasia, Cell Crowding, More Nuclear Atypia
Less Conspicuous Halos

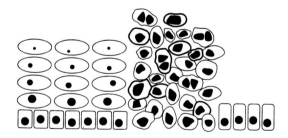

Basal Zone
Basal Hyperplasia, Atypia, Mitotic Figures

Figure 8-8. *Graphic representation of the effects of HPV on cervical epithelium: late effects.* In some HPV infections the less differentiated reserve/metaplastic cell becomes transformed as evidenced by crowding, nuclear atypia, mitotic activity, and atypical mitotic forms. Much less virus is found in such cells in which the viral DNA may integrate into the host genome. This transforming effect, which is an obligatory preinvasive step, can be induced by many (e.g., HPVs 16, 18, 51) but not all HPV types; HPVs 6, 11, and 42 do not appear capable of causing these changes.

Normal Squamous Cells Grown in Laboratory

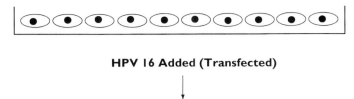

HPV 16 Added (Transfected)

Transformation

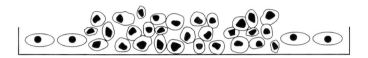

NOTE
1. **Transformation Rate by HPV 16 is About 60%**
2. **Transformation Rate is Higher for HPV 18**
3. **HPVs 6 or 11 Do Not Transform**
4. **Transformed Cells May Stop Proliferating**

Figure 8-9. *HPV infection of the cervix: transformation.* A common event after infection by one of the oncogenic HPV types such as HPV 16 is *transformation.* This is characterized both in the laboratory and *in vivo* by an abnormal crowded growth pattern and cytologically by an increased nuclear to cytoplasmic ratio and hyperchromaticity.

Normal Squamous Cells

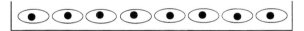

Cells Stop Proliferating by About 10th Growth Cycle

HPV 16 Added (Transfected)
Cells Continued to Proliferate Indefinitely

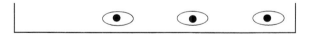

NOTE

1. **HPVs 6 and 11 Can Not Immortalize**
2. **HPV 18 More Efficient in Immortalizing than HPV 16**
3. **Immortalized Cells Can Not Invade**

Figure 8-10. *HPV infection of the cervix: immortalization.* Infection by one of the oncogenic HPV types such as HPV 16 may also induce *immortalization.* This is characterized by the persistent growth of the infected cells. Instead of the cells halting cell division after a certain number of growth cycles, they continue to proliferate. Despite their highly dysplastic appearance, these immortalized cells usually do *not* have the ability to invade local tissues or metastasize.

ing recognized as a low-grade SIL. This may be viewed as the early infectious form the virus uses to spread from one person to another. One reason this is evident in most surgical biopsy specimens is that SILs are most commonly detected in women being screened for disease and thus are being detected early in their evolution. Other types, notably HPVs 16 and 18, can subsequently induce the less-differentiated basal cells to proliferate in a disorganized fashion, show nuclear atypia, and be able, at times, to continue to grow indefinitely. We recognize this as high-grade SIL and the latter change as neoplasia. Although the virus does not need the later pathway to aid in its spread from one person to another, it may be viewed as a way to ensure that the virus will persist in a given person long after the initial infection occurs. The observation that HPVs 6 and 11 cannot cause the second change in cell culture explains why these types are rarely associated with biopsies that show high-grade SIL or cancer.

It is well documented that hyperplasia, transformation, and immortalization can be induced by a wide variety of agents, called *co-carcinogens*. In the cervix, HPV is the primary cocarcinogen in the sense that cervical cancer very rarely forms in the absence of HPV. This is analogous to other sites where one cocarcinogen may predominate. For example, laryngeal cancer rarely occurs in the absence of a history of cigarette smoking. An important "behavioral" change accompanies immortalization. After around 10 to 20 growth cycles normal, hyperplastic, or even transformed cells often stop to proliferate. Because they continue to proliferate, immortalized cells will be susceptible to other co-carcinogens that can further change their morphology and behavior (Figs. 8-10 and 8-11) (2,3,9,16,17,20,23,24,37,54–56,60–85). In the test tube there is no reliable cytologic marker to indicate which transformed cells are immortalized; however, it is clear that when cells are infected with HPV 18 they are more likely to become immortalized than when infected with HPV 16 or most of the other oncogenic HPV types.

Squamous cells immortalized by HPV in the test tube usually do not invade when transplanted into laboratory animals, often immunocompromised (nude) mice. However, the immortalized cells can be induced to have a greater rate of invasive potential if cotransfected with DNA sequences called *oncogenes*. Oncogenes are native DNA sequences that play critical roles in normal growth and development. However, their expression in immortalized cells often leads to the next level in the continuum of abnormal behavior—the ability to invade and metastasize (3,5,7,8,14,23,86–90). An analogous situation likely occurs *in vivo*. HPV infection is the necessary initial event in the evolution of cervical cancer, which, when associated with transformation and immortalization, makes the cells susceptible to oncogene activation that may, in turn, be induced by other carcinogenic events such as cigarette smoke or x-irradiation (91,92).

To summarize, initial HPV infection, when associated with a SIL, is initially characterized by a marked increase in viral DNA, RNA, and protein levels and is manifested cytologically as perinuclear halos, cellular crowding toward the surface, and nuclear variability. We recognize these cytologic changes as a low-grade SIL. The next stage is transformation/immortalization, which affects the more basal cells. These cells show a more drastic degree of a disorganized growth pattern, a greater degree of nuclear variability, and hyperchromaticity that extend to the more superficial aspects. We recognize these changes in a high-grade SIL. The relatively high rate of progression of low- to high-grade SILs, based on prospective studies, is predicted from the laboratory studies cited above. High-grade SILs contain much less virus but, in simplistic terms, the virus is having a much greater effect on the cellular metabolic machinery. Key events in the evolution to a high-grade SIL and cancer include viral integration, which is associated with disruption of the key viral regulatory ORF E2 and a concomitant upregulation of E6 and E7. Finally, in a small percentage of cases, both *in vivo* and *in vitro*, an invasive cancer will evolve from the transformed cells (72,93–96) (Fig. 8-11). The invasive cells tend to have more overt chromosomal changes and certainly have an even

HPV-Transformed Cells Co-Transfected by Oncogene Ras

Ras

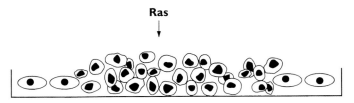

Some Cells Become Invasive

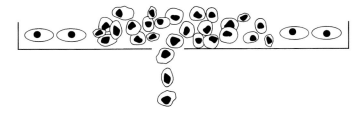

NOTE

1. Invasion can Occur Spontaneously in Immortalized Cells but is Very Rare
2. Immortalization Predisposes Cells to Effects by Other Carcinogens
3. Cytologic Appearance of Immortalized Versus Invasive Cells is Similar

Figure 8-11. *HPV infection of the cervix: invasion.* Immortalized cells, because of their persistent and uncontrolled growth, are more susceptible to other co-carcinogens, such as cigarette smoke, which can induce oncogene activation and result in *invasive* behavior. Cytologically, these cells appear similar to the immortalized cells, although nucleoli tend to be more prominent.

more dramatic shift in the cellular metabolic machinery that reflects their unique ability to invade local tissues and metastasize; this is discussed in detail below.

A key question raised by this discussion is, what is the molecular basis for the low oncogenicity of HPVs 6 and 11 and the much greater oncogenic potential of HPVs 16 and 18? The observation that the E6 and E7 ORFs alone of HPVs 16 or 18 are sufficient to cause transformation and immortalization demonstrates the importance of this part of the viral genome in the evolution of high-grade SILs and cancer. It has been demonstrated that the E6 and E7 viral products of HPV 16 but not HPV 6 can inactivate the antioncogenes p53 and

retinoblastoma gene product, respectively (57,58,60–107).

Histologic and Molecular Correlates of SILs and HPV

Let us now shift from the *in vitro* based data to the information obtained from clinical samples. Much work has been done regarding the histologic distribution of HPV DNA in cervical SILs using *in situ* hybridization (1–36). Studies have established two points: (i) HPV DNA, RNA, and proteins are most plentiful in the cells toward the surface, especially in cells that show perinuclear halos and nuclear atypia (Fig. 8-12); and (ii) the viral copy number decreases as one progresses from the low-grade SILs to high-grade SILs to invasive cancers (Fig. 8-13). In low-grade SILs the copy number varies from presumably 1 to, in many cases, over 1,000 per cell, whereas in high-grade SILs and invasive cancers the copy number is rarely over 100. In many cases, the copy number of HPV in the invasive cancers is below 10 and thus not detectable by standard *in situ* hybridization (see Fig. 8-3).

Although HPV DNA is readily detectable by *in situ* hybridization in the cells toward the surface in low-grade SILs, the distribution is often focal. Some cells with halos and nuclear atypia may be positive for HPV DNA, while their neighbors exhibiting the same cytologic

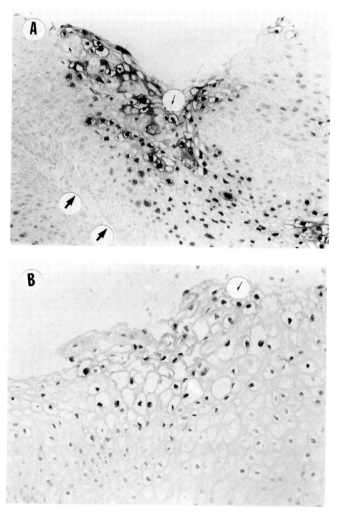

Figure 8-12. *The distribution of HPV DNA in low-grade cervical SIL.* This low-grade cervical SIL contained HPV 51. Note how the viral DNA, as detected by standard *in situ* hybridization, is most abundant toward the surface and middle zones of the lesion in the cells, which demonstrate the perinuclear halos and nuclear atypia (**A**, *small arrow*). Furthermore, viral DNA is not evident in the basal cells (*large arrows*). Similarly, note how the E4 protein of HPV detected by immunohistochemistry is most prevalent toward the superficial area of the lesion (**B**, *arrow*).

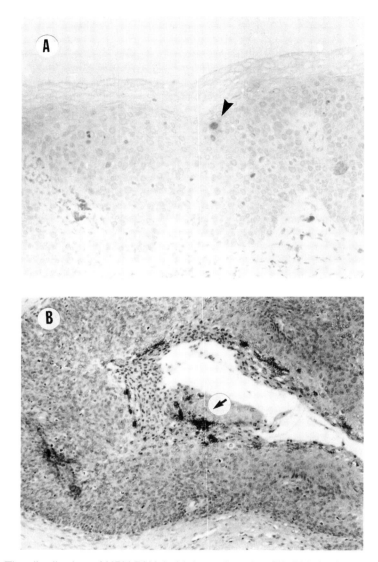

Figure 8-13. *The distribution of HPV DNA in high-grade vulva SIL.* This high-grade vulva SIL also contains HPV 16. However, note how far fewer cells have demonstrable viral DNA, as detected by standard *in situ* hybridization, when compared with low-grade cervical SILs (**A**, *arrowhead*; see Fig. 8-12). A further reflection of the lower copy number of HPV DNA in high-grade SILs is the decrease in the detection rate of viral DNA using standard *in situ* hybridization from about 90% for low-grade SILs to 70% for high-grade lesions (27). Also note that the HPV-positive cells are located toward the epithelial surface. Similarly, viral RNA is found in some of the surface cells using an ³⁵S-labeled probe that is antisense to the L1 mRNA (**B**, *arrow*).

changes may be negative (Figs. 8-12 to 8-14). Most *in situ* hybridization-based studies have claimed that HPV DNA or RNA is not detectable in the basal cells of SILs or in the directly adjacent, unremarkable epithelium. Is HPV actually absent in these areas, or is it present in copy numbers below the detection threshold of conventional *in situ* hybridization? This question as well as the issues of the synergistic viral and host molecular events that are

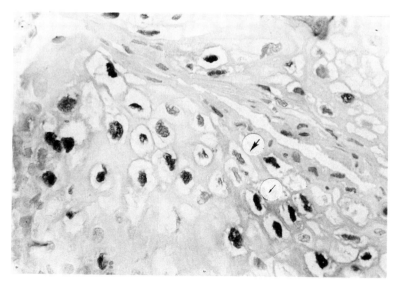

Figure 8-14. *Variable distribution of HPV DNA in cervical SIL.* This low-grade cervical SIL contains HPV 16. Viral DNA is detectable in some but not all the cells that show the cytologic changes characteristic of HPV infection (positive cell, *small arrow;* negative cell, *large arrow*).

associated with the progression from a low-grade to a high-grade SIL and then to a cancer may be addressed by the PCR *in situ* hybridization and RT *in situ* PCR methodologies.

We will begin the discussion with the SILs and then shift to the invasive cancers.

Cervical SILs

HPV 16-positive SILs and their normal-appearing adjacent epithelium were examined by both standard *in situ* hybridization and PCR *in situ* hybridization (53). These experiments also provide some insight into the utility of the hot start modification for this methodology. Figure 8-15 shows the representative results for this series of experiments in which the multiple analyses were done on the same glass slide. Note that only a few of the atypical cells in the SIL show detectable HPV 16 DNA by standard *in situ* hybridization or by PCR *in situ* hybridization if an essential reagent such as *Taq* polymerase is omitted. Figure 8-15 also shows the results of standard PCR *in situ* hybridization (not hot start) with a single primer pair.

Note the two criteria of successful PCR *in situ* hybridization: an increase in number of positive cells and a greater intensity in hybridization signal in the cells that were positive by standard *in situ* hybridization. Furthermore, the enhancement of the signal was lost if the *Taq* polymerase was omitted, if magnesium was omitted, or if irrelevant primers were substituted for the HPV 16 primers (Fig. 8-16). Although there are more positive cells after PCR *in situ* hybridization, most of the basal and parabasal cells are scored as negative. Figure 8-15 shows the results with multiple primer pairs and standard PCR *in situ* hybridization. Note that the basal and parabasal cells were positive and that the adjacent, normal-appearing epithelium was negative (insert). The observation that other cells with perinuclear halos and nuclear atypia did not appear to have detectable HPV DNA suggests that HPV DNA levels may vary widely in superficial cells having similar histologic changes and that some of these cells may indeed not contain the virus. This raises the possibility that the cytologic changes diagnostic of a SIL may, in part, be induced by host factors in response to the viral

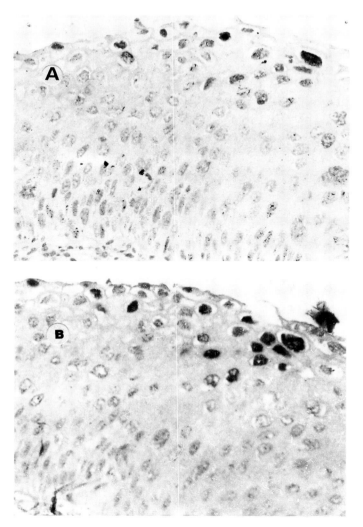

Figure 8-15. *Analysis of a cervical low-grade SIL by* in situ *hybridization after amplification by PCR.* A few superficial cells in this low-grade SIL had detectable HPV 16 DNA as demonstrated by *in situ* hybridization analysis after PCR when *Taq* polymerase was omitted from the amplifying solution (**A**). Inclusion of *Taq* polymerase and use of the oligoprimers PV1 and PV2 led to an increased hybridization signal in some superficial cells (**B**). The hybridization signal extended to the basal and parabasal cells (**C**, *arrows*) when the oligoprimers PV1 through PV7 were used; a similar signal was seen using the hot start maneuver and a single primer pair (not shown). The signal was not evident in adjacent unremarkable epithelium (*inset*).

presence. Another possible explanation is that HPV DNA was present in the cells scored as negative by PCR *in situ* hybridization but that it was removed during the sectioning process. An observation supporting this theory is that when SiHa cells were embedded in paraffin and then sectioned, about 90% were positive compared with 100% positive cells if the sample was spun down, leaving the cells intact on the glass slide. The embedded SiHa cells that were HPV negative were usually smaller than those that were HPV positive, perhaps because most of the nucleus was removed and the one copy of integrated HPV DNA was no longer present (Fig. 8-3, arrow).

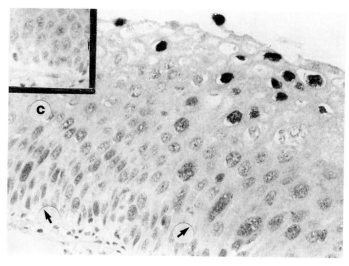

Figure 8-15. *Continued.*

You will recall that in Chapter 3 we discussed the improvement in the intensity of the hybridization signal for standard PCR *in situ* hybridization when multiple primers were used rather than a single primer pair. The strongest hybridization signal was obtained when the hot start modification was used with a single primer pair. We have noted the same results when analyzing tissue sections, as is covered later in more detail when we discuss HPV distribution patterns in vulvar and penile lesions.

We have extended the analysis of HPV infection to a comparison of the viral distribution in low-grade versus high-grade SILs using PCR *in situ* hybridization and RT *in situ* PCR. Based on these preliminary studies, the following observations have been made:

1. HPV DNA is detectable in about 90% of the cells in the middle and superficial parts of the lesion in a low-grade SIL; a similar percentage of cells of a high-grade SIL from the basal to superficial layer contain HPV DNA.
2. Expression of HPV ORFs E6 and E7 is much more limited; on average, only about 20% of the cells in a high-grade SIL contain these viral transcripts.
3. Viral nucleic acids may be detectable in the

underlying normal-appearing basal cells of a low-grade SIL.
4. The distribution of HPV DNA and RNA is highly variable in invasive squamous cell cancers. In cervical lesions, most of the malignant cells contain HPV DNA, but a smaller percentage (from 20% to 30%, as with high-grade SILs) contain E6 and E7 ORF mRNAs. However, in HPV-related squamous cell cancers of the vulva, penis, and periungual lesion, many of the malignant cells do not appear to contain either HPV DNA or HPV RNA. This mimics the viral distribution of HPV in low-grade SILs of the vulva and penis.

Points 3 and 4 are illustrated in later sections of this chapter.

Cervical Swabs

Occult infection of the cervix by HPV is presumed when the virus is detected by molecular analysis in the absence of the characteristic cytologic or histologic changes induced by HPV. Many studies have been undertaken looking for HPV in cervical swabs from women with normal Papanicolaou smears. Most investigators agree that the rate of occult infection is about

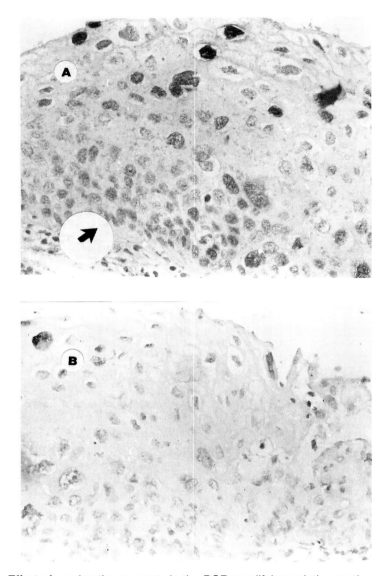

Figure 8-16. *Effect of varying the reagents in the PCR amplifying solution on the post-PCR* in situ *hybridization signal.* The weak hybridization signal evident after standard *in situ* hybridization analysis (not shown) became much stronger after PCR amplification (**A**); note the signal in the basal cells (*arrow*). The signal was lost when Mg^{2+} was omitted from the amplifying solution (**B**).

10% as determined by Southern blot or slot blot hybridization analyses (59,60,108–110). Occult infection is usually associated with low copy numbers of the virus. It is not surprising, therefore, that the rate is greater (about 30%) when determined by PCR (111). HPV DNA is typically not detectable by *in situ* hybridization in cells or tissue that lack the pathological features of HPV infection even when the virus is detected in such material by Southern blot hybridization or PCR (9,10,112,113). Again, this finding probably reflects the low copy number associated with occult infection.

Clearly, the PCR *in situ* technique may help to shed some light on the cellular distribution of HPV in occult as well as active, clinically evident infection. Preliminary studies with *in situ* PCR using consensus HPV primers, which can detect a wide variety of HPV types, have suggested the following about occult infection. (i) The endocervical cells are not involved, and (ii) the virus may be found in metaplastic or mature squamous cells that are either normal in appearance or, at most, show mild nuclear enlargement. These data again highlight two important strengths of the PCR *in situ* technology. First, one can directly correlate the viral findings with the cytologic features. Second, false positivity from contamination is not a problem, as only nuclear signal is scored as positive. We have "spiked" normal (HPV PCR negative) cervical swabs with HPV DNA and have not seen any positive cells, suggesting that the signals evident in PCR *in situ* are not the result of diffusion of amplified (HPV) DNA from the solution into the nucleus; this topic is discussed in detail in Chapter 3.

Color Plate 10 following p. 242 depicts a proposed model of HPV infection of the cervix. It is based primarily on the observations of HPV detection and morphology as demonstrated by PCR *in situ* in occult infection of the cervix and cervical SILs. In about 10% to 30% of cases, the infection is limited to relatively few squamous cells (metaplastic and the more mature intermediate and superficial cells) where the viral copy number is low. The virus apparently enters through the metaplastic squamous cell. For reasons that are still unclear, this condition may evolve into a lesion where viral DNA synthesis may increase markedly in association with the cytologic changes of perinuclear halos and nuclear atypia characteristic of a low-grade SIL. However, the virus does not appear to infect the normal basal cells in these low-grade SILs. Apparently, the lesion is overgrowing the adjacent normal epithelium; one can liken this to a clonal expansion of cells where in this case the "clonality" relates to infection by HPV. If the lesion progresses to a high-grade SIL, most cells of the lesion appear to contain virus but in numbers far below that seen in the low-grade lesions. Similarly, in cervical cancers it appears that most if not all of the malignant cells contain viral DNA but only a relatively small subpopulation are expressing viral transcripts such as the E6 and E7.

The Vulva and Penis

Cervical SILs are relatively easy to distinguish from processes that can mimic SILs on clinical examination, such as inflammatory changes, because the diagnostic histologic features are usually very well developed. More problematic are lesions on the vulva or penis. HPV is associated with the so-called venereal warts of the penis and vulva. Many lesions at these sites can mimic warts on gross examination. These include such common conditions as exaggerated skin folds, chronic candidiasis, and fibroepithelial polyps (skin tags) (39,114–134). Even when HPV DNA is detected by *in situ* hybridization in vulvar or penile lesions, often the perinuclear halos and nuclear atypia diagnostic of the infection are much less overt than in the corresponding low-grade cervical SIL (Fig. 8-17) (10,11). Thus, the histologic diagnosis of vulvar or penile warts is often more challenging and problematic than the histologic diagnosis of cervical warts, i.e., SILs. HPV-associated vulvar and penile lesions are acquired through sexual contact. Given the emotional implications of such a diagnosis, accuracy is especially important.

All vulvar and penile lesions that do demonstrate the classic histologic features of a low-grade SIL contain HPV DNA as detected by *in situ* hybridization. In over 90% of cases the HPV types are 6 or 11 (113,114). Several studies have analyzed for HPV DNA in histologically equivocal or nondiagnostic vulvar and penile tissues that were clinically suggestive of a wart. The detection rate of HPV DNA in such tissues varies from 5% to 10% by *in situ* hybridization to up to 30% by PCR (11,111). Of course, one could not directly localize the virus in the PCR-positive tissues. The pathologist is left with a dilemma. Should all equivocal tis-

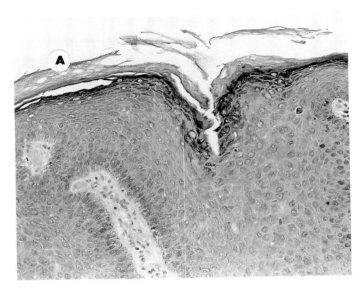

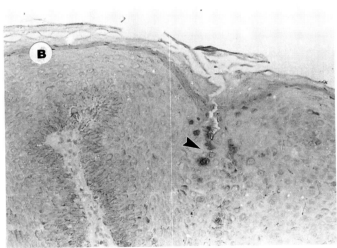

Figure 8-17. In situ *analysis of a penile lesion clinically suggestive of a low-grade SIL (condyloma).* Low-grade SILs of the vulva and penis are identifiable on histologic examination by the perinuclear halos and nuclear atypia in their granular layer (see Fig. 8-5 for the equivalent changes in the cervix). This penile tissue showed the nonspecific findings of acanthosis and parakeratosis. Furthermore, the granular layer occasionally demonstrated minimal nuclear enlargement and rare perinuclear halos (**A**). HPV 6 DNA was noted in a few cells in this area in the serial section using standard *in situ* hybridization (**B**, *arrowhead*).

sues at these sites be analyzed for HPV DNA by PCR, or is there some histological marker that may be used to distinguish the HPV-positive equivocal cases from the more common HPV-negative tissues?

PCR *in situ* hybridization has helped resolve this dilemma by allowing one to localize the virus in these equivocal tissues directly. The term *equivocal tissue* means cases where the clinical examination was sugges-

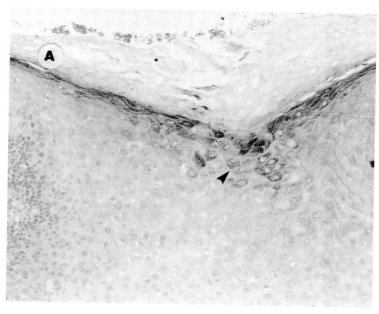

Figure 8-18. *Histologic and molecular analysis of a penile lesion.* Perinuclear halos and nuclear atypia were not evident although a thickened granular layer was noted in epithelial crevices (**A**, *arrowhead*). HPV 6 DNA was rarely detected in such cells by *in situ* analysis (**B**, *arrowhead*). An intense hybridization signal was observed in many more cells in these areas after amplification by PCR (**C**, *arrowhead*). Note the absence of a signal in the basal cells (*open arrow*).

tive of a wart but the perinuclear halos, disorganized growth pattern, and nuclear variability in the region of the granular layer were not of sufficient degree to warrant the diagnosis of a low-grade SIL on histologic examination. These analyses showed that the virus localized to specific areas in the problematic tissues that lacked perinuclear halos and nuclear atypia. The virus was found in regions where the granular layer was focally thickened, often associated with hyperkeratosis and epithelial crevices (Fig. 8-18). Interestingly, neither viral DNA nor viral RNA was detected in the basal cells using the *in situ* PCR-based techniques. Note that these results were obtained using a single primer pair and hot start PCR *in situ* hybridization (135–137). The presence of these histologic features in tissues should alert the pathologist to the possibility that HPV is present in the lesion. Alternatively, the absence of these histologic features would suggest that the le-

sion is a mimic and not HPV related (Fig. 8-19). The latter conclusion can be exceptionally important to the patient given that vulvar and penile warts are acquired through sexual contact.

Carcinoma of the Lower Genital Tract

That genital tract HPV disease is common and sexually transmitted are reasons enough to warrant a great deal of interest in the dynamics of infection by this virus. The other important reason for such interest in HPV-related disease is that this virus, as discussed above, is an essential cofactor in the development of cancer of the cervix. It is also important in the formation of cancers of the penis, vulva, periungual region of the finger, and conjunctiva. Indeed, HPV is one of the best understood and studied of the oncogenic viruses.

The association between HPV infection and the development of squamous cell neoplasms

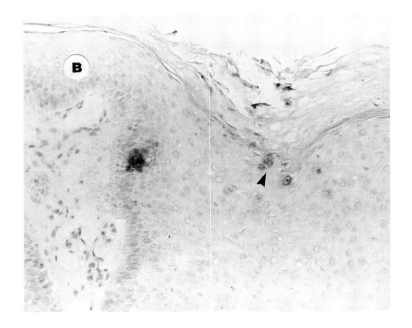

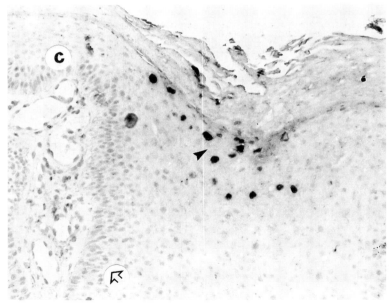

Figure 8-18. *Continued.*

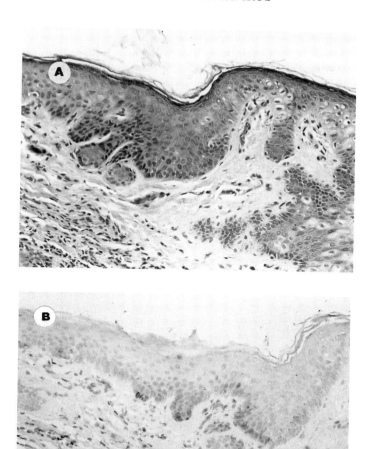

Figure 8-19. *Histologic and molecular analysis of a penile lesion.* Minimal acanthosis and a superficial perivascular infiltrate were evident; the granular layer was not focally thickened (**A**). HPV DNA was not detected in this tissue by the PCR *in situ* technique (**B**).

of the uterine cervix is based on several observations. Over 90% of squamous cell carcinomas of the cervix contain HPV DNA, usually types 16 or 18 (37,56,60). Several investigators have transfected *in vitro* these and other HPV types in normal squamous epithelium and have shown that the tissue demonstrates the histologic changes of a high-grade SIL as well as, under defined conditions, invasive and metastatic be-

havior in animal systems (37,56,60,138–142) (also see Figs. 8-9 to 8-11).

In the SILs the viral DNA exists primarily in an episomal form. The transcription pattern of the episomal form of HPV has been well characterized. The virus makes the mRNAs of the L1 and L2 capsid proteins as well as the messages and corresponding proteins of several others of its ORFs. One of the better characterized of these transcripts corresponds to the E2 ORF. The E2 message dictates the synthesis of a variety of proteins. One important function of the E2 transcript is the inhibition of the transcription of the E6 and E7 ORFs. An important event in the evolution of a high-grade SIL to an invasive cancer is the integration of the episomal viral DNA into the host genome. Although viral integration appears to occur at random in the human genome, the integration point in the viral DNA occurs selectively in the region of the E1 and E2 ORF. This integration can disrupt the E2 ORF. The concomitant loss of E2 protein can be associated with production of the E6 and E7 ORF transcripts. Both the E6 and E7 translational products are well characterized oncoproteins. E6 can bind to and inactivate the product of the antioncogene p53. E7 can inactivate the retinoblastoma gene product, which can activate a cascade of transcripts that can lead to DNA synthesis and other events necessary in oncogenesis (37,56,60,96,99).

A problem in the analysis of lower genital tract cancer is that viral integration is usually associated with a very low copy number. Although there are exceptions, such as the cell line Caski in which over 600 copies of the integrated viral genome are present, most cervical cancers contain less than 10 copies of the virus. Thus, in many cases the viral DNA cannot be detected by standard *in situ* hybridization. Similarly, although viral RNA can be detected by standard *in situ* hybridization, the copy number of the transcripts can likewise be less than 10 copies and thus escape detection by standard *in situ* hybridization.

Although most cervical carcinomas contain HPV DNA and RNA, it is not surprising based on the above discussion that the detection rate varies considerably with the detection method. While the rate of HPV detection is >90% with Southern blot hybridization or PCR, it is near 30% with *in situ* hybridization. Even when viral nucleic acids are detected in cervical cancers by *in situ* hybridization, most cancer cells appear to be HPV negative (37,38,56,60,96,99). It is unclear whether these HPV-negative carcinoma cells contain low copy numbers of the virus or indeed contain no viral DNA or RNA.

About 90% of cervical cancers are of the squamous cell type. Cervical adenocarcinomas include a morphologically diverse group of cancers that may reflect different etiologic associations, one of which is likely to be HPV infection (37,56,60). In addition to the more commonly seen mucin-producing and endometrioid variants of adenocarcinoma of the cervix, other histologic subtypes including adenoid basal carcinoma, adenoid cystic carcinoma, adenoma malignum (minimal deviation carcinoma), clear cell adenocarcinoma, villoglandular carcinoma, and small cell carcinoma can occur at this site. The use of oral contraceptives is a risk factor for villoglandular carcinoma, and diethylstilbestrol (DES) exposure is a well-documented risk factor for clear cell adenocarcinoma of the cervix. The prognosis for these tumors varies considerably from excellent for adenoid basal carcinoma and villoglandular carcinoma to poor for small cell carcinoma. Except for small cell carcinoma, which invariably contains HPV 18, only one study to date has correlated HPV detection with the specific subtype of endocervical carcinoma; Duggan et al. (143) reported that two villoglandular carcinomas and one clear cell carcinoma of the cervix were each HPV negative. We undertook a study to analyze a variety of subtypes of endocervical adenocarcinoma for the presence of HPV RNA using the RT *in situ* PCR technique.

A review of the surgical pathology files at University Hospital, Stony Brook revealed four cases of cervical adenoid basal carcinoma, one case each of adenoma malignum and villoglandular carcinoma, and three cases of cervical clear cell carcinoma as well as an *in situ* adenocarcinoma in a woman exposed to DES. Each of the tumors involved the area of the transformation zone. Positive controls included two small cell carcinomas of the cervix and two squamous cell carcinomas of the cervix, each with clear cell features. The adenoid basal carcinomas were characterized by a nested pattern of uniform basaloid cells with one or more lumina and with little or no stromal response (Fig. 8-20). Each of the four cases of adenoid basal carcinoma was accompanied by an intraepithelial or superficially invasive squamous lesion. The adenoma

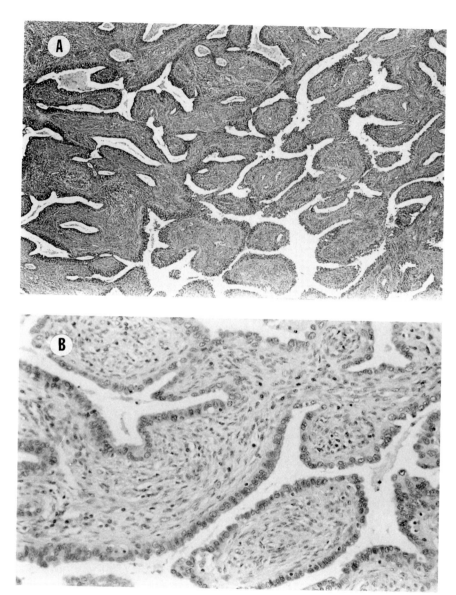

Figure 8-20. *Histologic features of different types of adenocarcinomas of the cervix.* Adenocarcinoma of the cervix consists of several subtypes. At one end of the clinical spectrum is small cell carcinoma, which has a very poor prognosis. A subtype with a good prognosis is villoglandular carcinoma, in which broad anastomosing projections invade the underlying submucosa (**A** and, at higher magnification, **B**). Another of the subtypes is adenoma malignum in which well-differentiated branching ducts invade the local tissues (**C**). Note the mitotic activity at higher magnification, which is a useful diagnostic feature of these tumors (**D**, *arrows*). These tumors have a prognosis intermediate between small cell carcinoma and villoglandular carcinoma.

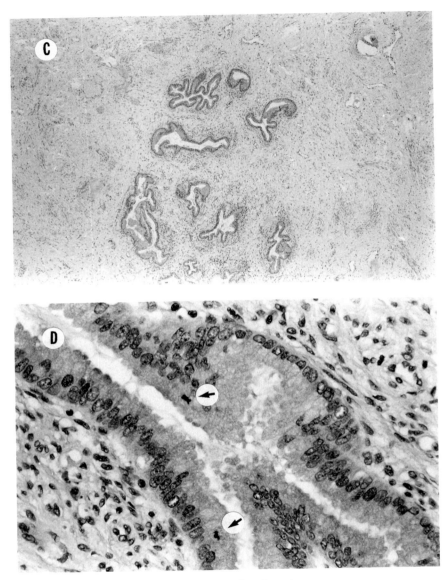

Figure 8-20. *Continued.*

malignum demonstrated deep stromal invasion by highly differentiated endocervical glands with irregular contours (Fig. 8-20). Component cells showed minimal but unequivocal cytologic atypia and readily identified mitoses. The villoglandular carcinoma was characterized by broad anastomosing papillae covered by atypical mitotically active cells (Fig. 8-20). The clear cell carcinomas grew in solid sheets and tubulocystic patterns with glycogen-rich clear cells or hobnail cells (Fig. 8-21) (143–149).

Sixteen tissues were analyzed for HPV RNA with the RT *in situ* PCR technique. The sequences of the primers used in this study are shown in Tables 8-1 and 8-2. The distribution of the cases used in this study is listed in Table 8-3. The initial analysis for HPV RNA was done with the consensus primers MO9 and

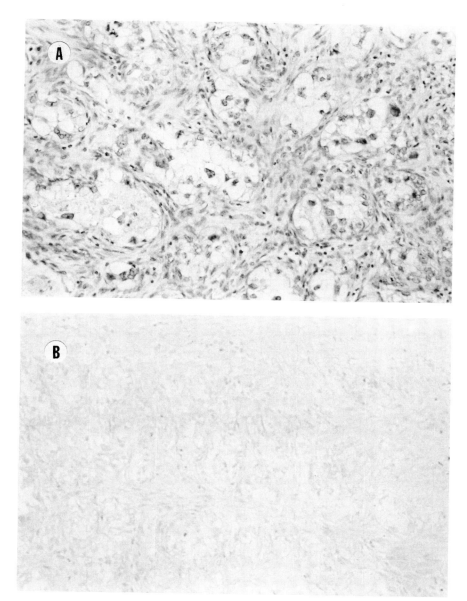

Figure 8-21. *Histologic and molecular analysis of cervical adenocarcinomas.* Another subtype of adenocarcinoma of the cervix is clear cell carcinoma, which is associated with the *in utero* exposure to DES. Note the large cells with the clear or granular cytoplasm (**A**). These tumors were uniformly negative for HPV using the RT *in situ* PCR technique (**B**). Another subtype is the adenoid basal carcinoma. Note the peripheral palisading of the tumor cells in a given nest (**C**). These tumors and the other types shown in Fig. 8-22 were each positive for HPV using the RT *in situ* PCR technique (**D**). Note that many of the tumor cells contain the E6 and E7 HPV 18 mRNAs (*large arrow*) (E7 mRNA is shown), whereas the stromal cells are HPV negative (*small arrow*).

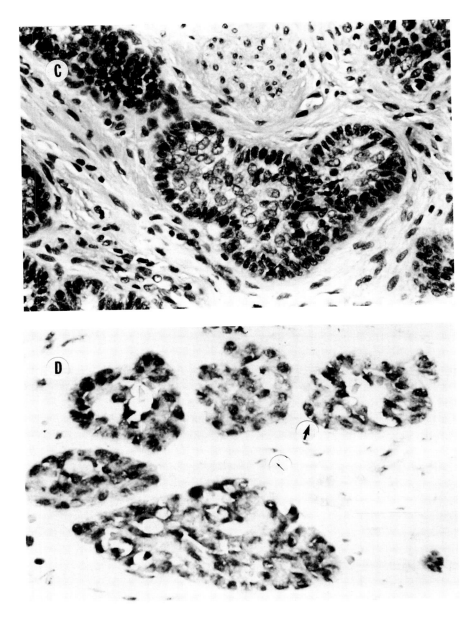

Figure 8-21. *Continued.*

MO11 (Perkin-Elmer Corporation), which can detect over 35 distinct HPV types, including most of those isolated from genital tract cancers. As is evident in Table 8-3, the two small cell carcinomas and one of the two squamous cell carcinomas were positive for HPV RNA. Each of the tissues from the adenoid basal carcinoma, adenoma malignum, and villoglandular tumor were also positive for viral transcripts (Fig. 8-21). Note that about one-half of the cells contained the E6 viral transcript in this particular tissue. In all of the cases, the average percentage of cells expressing E6 or E7 was about 25%; less than 5% of cells were expressing E2,

Table 8-1. *Oligoprimers used for amplification of HPV 16 DNA in cells in formalin-fixed tissues*

Primer	Position of first nucleotide	Sequence
PV1 (5′)	110	CAGGACCCACAGGAGCGACC
PV2 (3′)	559	TTACAGCTGGGTTTCTCTAC
PV3 (5′)	501	CCGGTCGATGTATGTCTTGT
PV4 (3′)	956	ATCCCCTGTTTTTTTTTCCA
PV5 (5′)	898	CGTACGGGATGTAATGGATG
PV6 (3′)	1,357	CCACTTCCACCACTATACTG
PV7 (5′)	1,300	AGGTAGAAGGGCGCCATGAG

which perhaps reflects the high likelihood of viral integration in the cancers with the concomitant disruption of the E2 ORF. The three clear cell carcinomas (Fig. 8-21) and the one case of an *in situ* adenocarcinoma arising in a woman exposed to DES were HPV negative, as were the two vulvar biopsies that served as negative controls. The ability to PCR amplify DNA in these cases of clear cell carcinoma was documented with the use of *bcl-2* primers. As additional negative controls, RT *in situ* PCR was performed on the tissues that contained HPV RNA using either primers specific for the hepatitis C virus or using the HPV primers but omitting the RT step. The signal was lost in the positive tissues with either of these maneuvers.

To determine the specific HPV type associated with the viral positive tissues, the adenocarcinoma cases were reanalyzed by RT *in situ* PCR using primers specific for HPV 16 and HPV 18 (Tables 8-1 and 8-2). The two small cell carcinomas were positive for HPV 18, and the one squamous cell carcinoma contained

HPV 16. Each viral-containing adenocarcinoma was positive for HPV 18 using each of the primer pairs E6 and E7–E1 and negative for HPV 16; the HPV 16 primers thus serve as an additional negative control. Viral RNA was not detected in adjacent normal squamous or glandular epithelium, although it was seen in the dysplastic squamous epithelium evident in several of the adenoid basal carcinomas.

In summary, this study demonstrated that viral RNA was detected in each of the rare endocervical adenocarcinoma variants that were analyzed, with the exception of clear cell carcinoma. All tissues that contained HPV had type 18, which is consistent with the observation that this type predominates in glandular lesions of the cervix. Viral RNA corresponding to the E6 and E7 ORFs were found in about 25% of the malignant cells, but HPV DNA was detected in over 90% of the malignant cells by PCR *in situ* hybridization. This illustrates that, even though the malignant cells appear similar to each other cytologically and all appear to contain HPV DNA, they show marked vari-

Table 8-2. *Sequences of the HPV-specific primers used in the study of adenocarcinomas*

Primer	Position of first nucleotide (reference)	Sequence
HPV 16 E6-1 (5′)	110	CAGGACCCACAGGAGCGACC
HPV 16 E6-2 (3′)	559/(26)	TTACAGCTGGGTTTCTCTAC
HPV 18 E6-1 (5′)	113	GCTTTGAGGATCCAACACGG
HPV 18 E6-2 (3′)	540/(26)	TGGTTAGTATATGTTTTACC
HPV 18 E7–E1-1 (5′)	611	TGCAAGACATTGTATTGCAT
HPV 16 E7–E1-2 (3′)	1,171/(4)	CCTCCTGCAAACTTTCGTTT
MY09 (Perkin-Elmer)	(11)	GCTCCACAAGAGGGAATACTGAT
MY11		GCACAGGGATCATAACTAATGG

Table 8-3. *Clinicopathologic features of cases analyzed in this study*

Case No.	Diagnosis	Age (years)	HPV Type
1	Adenoid basal cancer	72	18
2	Adenoid basal cancer	83	18
3	Adenoid basal cancer	NA	18
4	Adenoid basal cancer	63	18
5	Villoglandular cancer	48	18
6	Minimal deviation tumor	46	18
7	Clear cell carcinoma	22	Negative
8	Clear cell carcinoma	71	Negative
9	Clear cell carcinoma	21	Negative
10	*In situ* adenocarcinoma[a]	43	Negative
11	Squamous cell carcinoma	44	16
12	Squamous cell carcinoma	47	Negative
13	Small cell carcinoma	38	18
14	Small cell carcinoma	35	18
15	Vulva, negative for SIL	27	Negative
16	Vulva, negative for SIL	23	Negative

[a]History of DES exposure.

abilities in their expressions of viral messages. This simple but important observation is clearly evident by comparing the results from RT *in situ* PCR and PCR *in situ* hybridization. We return to this issue of differential expression in carcinoma cells below when we discuss the interaction of viral and host transcripts in the aggressiveness of cervical cancer.

HPV 18 is found in over 90% of small cell carcinomas of the cervix, which have a poor prognosis regardless of stage. The two small cell cancers included in this study were HPV 18 positive. This and other observations including the rarity of HPV 18 in SILs, its common presence in squamous cell cancers, and the more aggressive clinical behavior of cervical cancers with HPV 18 compared with those with HPV 16 has led to the hypothesis that HPV 18 has greater oncogenic potential than other HPV types (37,56,60,143–149). Villoglandular adenocarcinoma and adenoid basal carcinoma have favorable prognoses (143–149). The detection of HPV 18 in these lesions suggests that HPV type *per se* may not be an essential variable in tumor prognosis. Another study reported two cases of villoglandular carcinoma negative for HPV using filter hybridization (143). The negative result for the villoglandular adenocarcinomas may reflect the lesser sensitivity of the dot blot

assay used in that study compared with the RT PCR *in situ* test.

This study included three women with clear cell carcinoma of the cervix and one woman exposed to DES with an *in situ* adenocarcinoma; all were negative for HPV RNA. The one cervical clear cell carcinoma in another study was also HPV negative (143). The HPV negative results for the cervical clear cell carcinoma suggest that the etiological factor(s) for this tumor do not include HPV. It is not immediately evident why HPV-associated adenocarcinomas of the cervix do not apparently demonstrate the clear cell morphology. It is of interest that another histological feature of genital tract cancers found especially in vulvar cancers, extensive hyperkeratosis, is also not associated with HPV (149). About 60% of young women with clear cell carcinoma of the cervix have a history of *in utero* DES exposure. These DES-related cancers tend to be situated in the ectocervix rather than at the transformation zone, as is true for SILs and the squamous and other glandular malignancies of the cervix.

SQUAMOUS CELL CARCINOMA OF THE FINGER

Several studies have surveyed both cutaneous squamous cell and basal cell carcinomas from

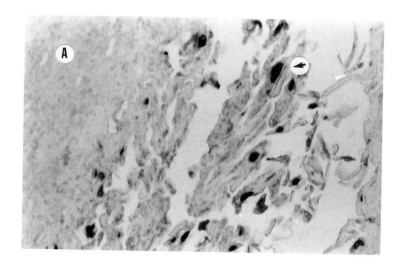

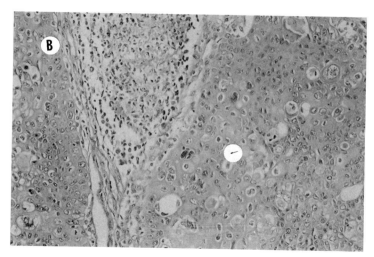

Figure 8-22. *Histologic and molecular analysis of a finger cancer and its metastases.* This periungual lesion showed areas of invasive squamous cell carcinoma as well as *in situ* carcinoma (not shown). HPV 16 DNA was detected by *in situ* hybridization (**A**, *arrow*). The tumor metastasized to a regional lymph node (**B**, *arrow* and, at higher magnification, **C**, *arrow*). The metastases also contained HPV 16 RNA as detected by RT *in situ* PCR (**D**, *arrow*).

a wide variety of sites for HPV. These studies have established that squamous cell carcinoma of the vulva and penis often contain HPV DNA and RNA (49,50,150). Most other cutaneous sites were rarely HPV positive in immunocompetent people. However, there was a notable exception to this statement. The detection rate of HPV DNA in periungual squamous cell can-

cers, either *in situ* or invasive, was almost 90% and thus equivalent to the rate in squamous cell cancers of the cervix. It has been speculated that this may represent sexual transmission from the genital tract to the periungual region.

As is true for the counterpart in the cervix, it can be difficult to detect HPV by standard *in situ* hybridization in periungual carcinomas.

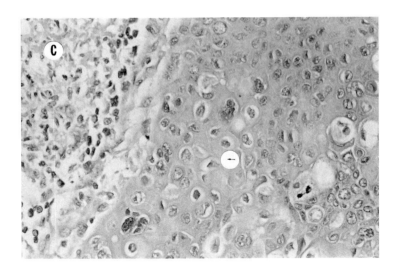

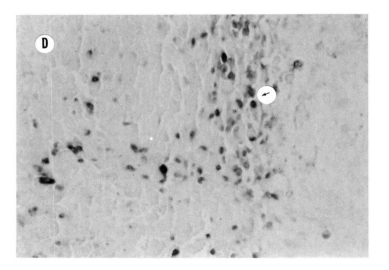

Figure 8-22. *Continued.*

Solution phase PCR showed that the lesion depicted in Fig. 8-22 contained HPV 16 DNA. Only a few cells were noted to contain viral DNA using standard *in situ* hybridization. PCR-amplified viral RNA was detected by RT *in situ* PCR in more cells (Fig. 8-22). This lesion had metastasized to a regional lymph node. Viral RNA was also detected in the carcinoma cells in the lymph nodes (Fig. 8-22).

The next lesion that is illustrated is also from the periungual region of the finger. It lacked the histologic features of a carcinoma *in situ* and is better characterized as a verruca vulgaris (Fig. 8-23). Areas of invasive cancer were seen, which is unusual for lesions that may be referred to as verrucous carcinomas. Viral DNA was not detected by standard *in situ* hybridization (Fig. 8-23). However, viral RNA was detected by RT *in situ* PCR (Fig. 8-23) and viral DNA by PCR *in situ* hybridization. Detection of oncogenic HPVs in so-called benign verruca or condyloma has been described in im-

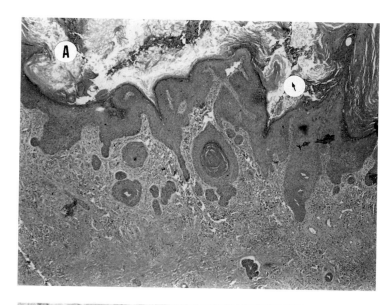

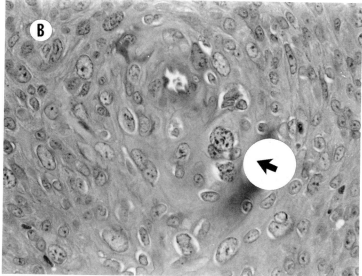

Figure 8-23. *Histologic and molecular analysis of a finger cancer.* The lesion showed extensive hyper and parakeratosis (*small arrow*) and papillary projections (**A**). These features are more typical of a benign verruca vulgaris and not carcinoma *in situ.* However, note the nests of cells invading the dermis (*large arrow*). Also, nuclear atypia is seen at higher magnification (**B**, *arrow*). HPV was not detected by standard *in situ* hybridization (**C**). However, HPV 16 RNA was detected by RT *in situ* PCR (**D**, *arrow*). Most "benign" verruca vulgaris contain HPV 2. Detection of an oncogenic HPV type, usually HPV 16, in a verruca-type lesion usually indicates that the patient is immunocompromised; this patient had AIDS.

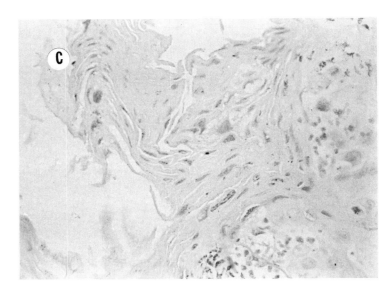

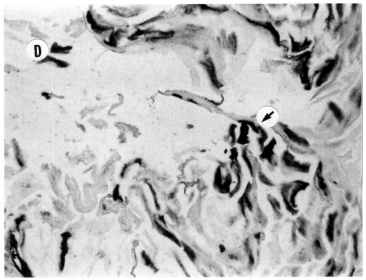

Figure 8-23. *Continued.*

munocomprised people (150). This patient indeed did have AIDS.

HPV AND HOST GENE EXPRESSION IN CERVICAL CANCERS

An exciting area in which *in situ* PCR can be of much use is in understanding the dynamics of differential expression of malignant cells. RT *in situ* PCR can compare the expression patterns of *in situ*, minimally invasive, and deeply invasive cancer cells, often in the same microscopic section, and colabeling experiments can determine if a given cell is coexpressing more than one message of interest.

As mentioned, cervical cancer is one of the best-studied tumors from the clinical and pathological standpoints. The cancer begins as a microinvasive tumor defined by less than 3 mm of invasion. In this circumstance, the cure rate with an excisional biopsy (called *cone biopsy*) is near 100%. If the tumor invades more deeply and enters the microvascular system, the prognosis decreases to 50% over 5 years (38). Is this marked worsening of prognosis due to HPV-related effects and/or host factors?

Degradation of the extracellular matrix and the endothelial cell basement membrane are necessary events in tumor invasion and metastases. Enzymes that have been implicated in the degradation of these compartments include the MMP family. Two of these enzymes, MMP-2 and MMP-9, are potent gelatinases, and their activities have been correlated with tumor cell invasion (151–160). Cancer cell invasion is the result of complex, multifactorial processes, including the transcriptional control of the genes encoding these proteinases, the activation of these degradative enzymes, and the production of their natural inhibitors TIMP-1 and TIMP-2 (151–160).

The importance of the balance in production of MMPs and TIMPs to tumor cell invasion and metastasis has been suggested by several studies. The inhibition of tumor cell invasion and metastasis in animal models has been demonstrated using *in vivo* injections of TIMP (155). The inactivation of TIMP by transfection of mouse 3T3 cells with antisense RNA converted the phenotype of these cells from noninvasive to tumorigenic and metastatic in nude mice. RNA *in situ* hybridization on archival cancer specimens correlated an increase in the number of cells expressing TIMP mRNA with less aggressive tumors (151–160).

The purpose of the first part of this study was to correlate the presence of MMP-9 and MMP-2 and TIMP-1 and TIMP-2 mRNAs, detected in serial sections using the RT *in situ* PCR technique, with prognosis in 23 cases of cervical carcinoma. PCR-amplified MMP and TIMP cDNA were restricted to the invasive cancer cells and the surrounding stromal cells. The ratios of cancer and stromal cells expressing MMP-9 and -2 to those expressing TIMP-1 and -2 were approximately one in those cancers

with a good prognosis, as is evident from the data in Table 7-2. This MMP to TIMP ratio in the cancer and stromal cells with a poor prognosis was significantly increased to 5.4 and 3.4 ($p < 0.0001$), respectively, reflecting a marked reduction in the TIMP detection rate in cancers with a poor prognosis. Note the marked increase in the MMP to TIMP ratio to over 20 in areas of vascular invasion or actual metastatic disease. In cervical cancer cell lines SiHa and HeLa, the MMP to TIMP ratio was also close to 1, and, interestingly, these cell lines are invasive but rarely metastatic in nude mice. These data suggest that the balance of MMP-9 and -2 to TIMP-1 and -2 expression is an essential factor in the aggressiveness of cervical cancer (157). Figure 8-24 shows representative data of MMP and TIMP expression in cervical cancers with a good and poor prognosis, respectively.

In the second part of the study, we addressed the question as to whether the variability in MMP and TIMP expression with clinical prognosis was also related to variations in HPV expression. We focused on two cervical cancer cell lines, HeLa and Caski. The percentages of these cells, as well as cells from archival pathology specimens from cervical carcinoma patients with good and poor prognoses, expressing MMP-9, MMP-2, TIMP-1, TIMP-2, HPV E2, HPV E6, or HPV E7 were determined to ascertain if HPV, MMP, or TIMP expression correlated with invasive behavior. The matrigel assay was used as an *in vitro* measure of the degree of invasiveness. Matrigel is composed of a filter that contains multiple pores. The filter is coated with a protein complex that contains a variety of collagens. The cell must be able to degrade the collagen, an essential event for *in vivo* invasiveness, in order to enter a pore and be counted by microscopic examination.

Transforming growth factor β1 (TGF) significantly increased the invasive behavior of the Caski cells in matrigel compared with treatment with epidermal growth factor (EGF). This TGF-induced increase in invasiveness was associated with a significant increase in the percentage of cells with MMP-9 mRNA ($p = 0.0016$) and MMP-2 mRNA ($p = 0.0042$) as determined by RT *in situ* PCR. However, there was no change

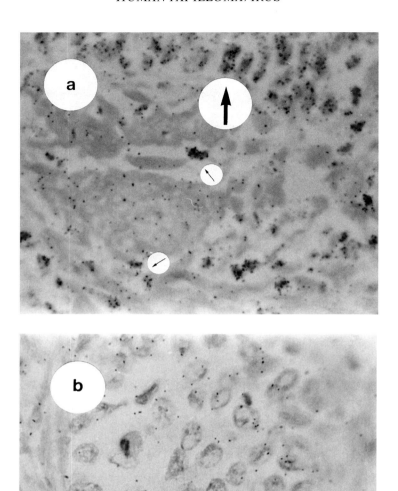

Figure 8-24. *MMP and TIMP expression in cervical cancers of good versus poor prognosis.* Cervical cancers vary greatly in their clinical prognosis. Deeply invasive cancers with microvascular invasion have a poor prognosis. Many of the cancer cells from these cancers of poor prognosis express MMP-9, as determined by RT *in situ* PCR with ³H as the reporter nucleotide (**a**, *small arrows,* stromal cells; *large arrow,* carcinoma cells). However, TIMP-2 expression is rarely evident (**b**). In comparison, microinvasive cervical cancers and rare subtypes, such as villoglandular carcinomas, have an excellent prognosis. Many of the cancer cells from these cancers of good prognosis express MMP-9 (not shown) as well as TIMP-2 (**c**, *arrow,* cancer cells; *open arrow,* stromal cells).

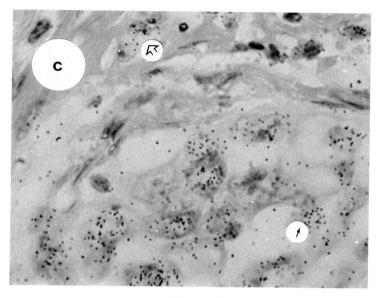

Figure 8-24. *Continued.*

MMP and TIMP expression in Caski cells

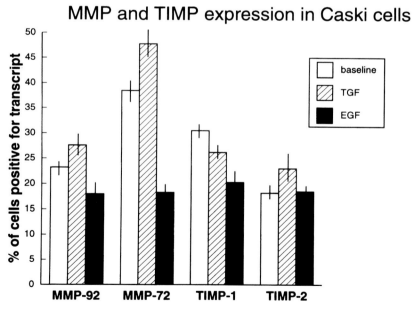

Figure 8-25. *MMP and TIMP expression in Caski cells.* TGF increases the invasiveness of Caski cells in the matrigel assay compared with treatment with EGF. Percentage of Caski cells that contain MMP-9, MMP-2, TIMP-1, or TIMP-2 mRNA as determined by RT *in situ* PCR either at baseline or after treatment with EGF or TGF. The results are those of triplicate experiments, with the vertical line representing the SEM. Note that there is a significant increase in the percentage of Caski cells that express MMP-9 or -2 after TGF treatment compared with the results after EGF treatment.

HPV transcription in Caski cells

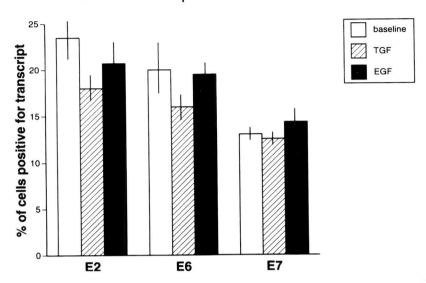

Figure 8-26. *HPV expression in Caski cells.* Percentage of Caski cells that contain either HPV E2, E6, or E7 mRNA as determined by RT *in situ* PCR either at baseline or after treatment with EGF or TGF. The results are those of triplicate experiments, with the vertical line representing the SEM. Note that there is no significant difference in HPV expression relative to changes in the invasiveness of the Caski cells.

in the percentage of cells that expressed HPV E6 or E7 (Figs. 8-25 and 8-26). Neither TGF nor EGF, which did not affect the invasive behavior of the cervical cancer-derived HeLa cells in matrigel, significantly altered the expression of MMPs or TIMPs in this cell line; HPV expression was likewise not changed. These data with the Caski and HeLa cells are further evidence that MMP expression and not HPV expression is correlated with the aggressiveness of the tumor cells. The RT *in situ* PCR technique allowed a comparison of the cells invading the matrigel with the noninvasive cells. There was a significant increase in the percentage of HeLa cells invading the matrigel expressing MMP-9 (33%) and MMP-2 (48%) compared with the noninvasive cells (11% and 12%, respectively); neither TIMP nor HPV expression was altered in the invasive versus noninvasive cells (see Color Plate 8 following p. 242 and Fig. 7-29). Increased depth of invasion and microvascular permeation in clinical samples was, as noted above, associated with

an increased percentage of cells that expressed MMP-9 and -2 and a decreased percentage that expressed TIMP-1 and -2; HPV expression was not altered.

These data suggest that the balance of MMP-9 and -2 to TIMP-1 and -2 expression, but not HPV expression, is an essential factor in the invasiveness of cervical cancer. The data from these two studies suggest a multistep process in the evolution of cervical cancer with regard to MMP-9, MMP-2 and TIMP-1, TIMP-2 expression. Expression of MMP-9, MMP-2, TIMP-1, and TIMP-2 is absent in areas of noninvasive carcinoma *in situ* directly adjacent to the invasive cervical carcinoma. Early invasion in cervical cancer probably requires activation of MMP-9 and MMP-2 expression. This is counterbalanced by an equivalent expression of TIMP-1 and TIMP-2. The controlled production of these two MMPs and two TIMPs may explain, in part, why such superficial cervical cancers, called *microinvasive carcinomas,* have a metastatic rate of less than 1% and the women have a survival rate of near 100%. The matrigel assay allows one to address directly the issue of the comparison of MMP expression in cells that are invasive versus those from the same group that are not invasive. The HeLa cells that had invaded the matrigel had a fivefold increased percentage of MMP-9 and MMP-2 expression, but the TIMP-1 and -2 expression rates were similar in the invasive versus noninvasive cells. This suggests that the process of invasion selects for cells expressing MMP-9 and MMP-2 with a concomitant increase in the MMP to TIMP ratio. The next step toward increased invasiveness requires the ability to enter microvessels. The data from the clinical samples, including direct detection of MMP and TIMP expression in tumors cells that had invaded the microvasculature, strongly suggests that, for this to occur, there must be an increased percentage of cells expressing MMP-9 and MMP-2 with very minimal expression of TIMP-1 and TIMP-2. The model that predicts that the natural selection of cancer cells expressing MMP-9 and MMP-2 and not expressing TIMP-1 and TIMP-2 is involved in the evolution of metastatic cancer is presented in Color Plate 10 following p. 242. This model would predict that cell lines that are invasive and metastatic should have greater MMP to TIMP ratios than cell lines, such as HeLa, that are invasive but not metastatic. Our preliminary data with breast cancer and squamous cancer cell lines suggest that this is indeed the case (G.J. Nuovo, *unpublished observations,* 1994).

It is very interesting that both the *in vivo* and *in vitro* data suggested that expression of HPV transcripts, specifically E6 and E7, does not appear to correlate with the invasive behavior of the cancer cells or their expression of either MMPs or TIMPs. Thus, although transfection of either E6 or E7 is an essential step in the transformation of squamous cells secondary to their ability to disrupt antioncogene activity, expression of these oncoproteins does not appear to be important in the ability of the cells to be invasive. Although one may speculate that HPV E6 and E7 transcripts, though essential for transformation and immortalization, are not needed for devel-

opment of the invasive phenotype, further studies including disruption of these viral transcripts and analysis of the expression of other HPV ORFs are needed to address this issue.

REFERENCES

1. Beckmann AM, Myerson D, Daling JR, Kiviat NB, Fenoglio CM, McDonald JM. Detection and localization of human papillomavirus DNA in human genital condylomas by *in situ* hybridization with biotinylated probes. *J Med Virol* 1983;16:265–273.
2. Collins JE, Jenkins D, McCance DJ. Detection of human papillomavirus DNA sequences by *in situ* hybridization in cervical intraepithelial neoplasia and invasive carcinoma: a retrospective study. *J Clin Pathol* 1988;41:289–295.
3. Cravador A, Herzog A, Houard S, d'Ippolito P, Carroll R, Bollen A. Selective detection of human papilloma virus DNAs by specific synthetic DNA probes. *Mol Cell Probes* 1989;3:143–158.
4. Crum CP, Symbula M, Ward BE. Topography of early HPV 16 transcription in high-grade genital precancers. *Am J Pathol* 1989;134:1183–1188.
5. Cullen AP, Reid R, Champion M, Lorincz AT. Analysis of the physical state of different human papillomavirus DNAs in intraepithelial and invasive cervical neoplasia. *J Virol* 1991;65:606–612.
6. Lorincz AT, Temple GF, Kurman RJ, Jenson AB, Lancaster WD. Oncogenic association of specific human papillomavirus types with cervical neoplasia. *J Natl Cancer Inst* 1987;79:671–677.
7. Nagai N, Nuovo GJ, Friedman D, Crum CP. Detection of papillomavirus nucleic acids in genital precancers with the *in situ* hybridization technique: a review. *Int J Gynecol Pathol* 1987;6:366–379.
8. Nuovo GJ, O'Connell M, Blanco JB, Levine RU, Silverstein SJ. Correlation of histology and human papillomavirus DNA detection in condyloma acuminatum and condyloma-like vulvar lesions. *Am J Surg Pathol* 1989;13:700–706.
9. Nuovo GJ, Friedman D. *In situ* hybridization analysis of HPV DNA segregation patterns in lesions of the female genital tract. *Gynecol Oncol* 1990;36:256–262.
10. Nuovo GJ, Blanco JS, Leipzig S, Smith D. Human papillomavirus detection in cervical lesions histologically negative for cervical intraepithelial neoplasia: correlation with Pap smear, colposcopy, and occurrence of cervical intraepithelial neoplasia. *Obstet Gynecol* 1990;75:1006–1011.
11. Nuovo GJ, Hochman H, Eliezri YD, Comite S, Lastarria D, Silvers DN. Detection of human papillomavirus DNA in penile lesions histologically negative for condylomata: analysis by *in situ* hybridization and the polymerase chain reaction. *Am J Surg Pathol* 1990;14:829–836.
12. Amortegui AJ, Meyer MP. *In situ* hybridization for the diagnosis and typing of human papillomavirus. *Clin Biochem* 1990;23:301–306.
13. Bromley SE, Darfler MM, Hammer ML, Jones-Trower A, Primus MA, Kreider JW. *In situ* hybridization to

human papillomavirus DNA in fixed tissue samples: comparison of detection methods. In Broker T, Zurhausen H, eds. *Papillomaviruses* New York:Wiley-Liss; 1990:239–259.

14. Burns J, Graham AK, Frank C, Fleming KA, Evans MF, McGee JO. Detection of low copy human papillomavirus DNA and mRNA in routine paraffin sections of the cervix by non-isotopic *in situ* hybridization. *J Clin Pathol* 1987;40:865–869.

15. Crum CP, Nagai N, Levine RU, Silverstein SJ. *In situ* hybridization analysis of human papillomavirus 16 DNA sequences in early cervical neoplasia. *Am J Pathol* 1986; 123:174–182.

16. Crum CP, Nuovo GJ, Friedman D, Silverstein SJ. A comparison of biotin and isotope labeled ribonucleic acid probes for *in situ* detection of HPV 16 ribonucleic acid in genital precancers. *Lab Invest* 1988;58:354–359.

17. Czegledy J, Gergely L, Endrodi I. Detection of human papillomavirus deoxyribonucleic acid by filter *in situ* hybridization during pregnancy. *J Med Virol* 1989;28: 250–254.

18. DelMistro A, Braunstein JD, Halwer M, Koss LG. Identification of human papillomavirus types in male urethral condylomata acuminata by *in situ* hybridization. *Hum Pathol* 1987;18:936–940.

19. Eversole LR, Laipis PJ. Oral squamous papillomas: detection of HPV DNA by *in situ* hybridization. *Oral Surg Oral Med Oral Pathol* 1988;65:545–550.

20. Farnsworth A, Laverty C, Stoler M. Human papillomavirus messenger RNA expression in adenocarcinoma *in situ* of the uterine cervix. *Int J Gynecol Pathol* 1989;8:321–330.

21. Gall AA, Saul SH, Stoler MH. *In situ* hybridization analysis of human papillomavirus in anal squamous cell carcinoma. *Mod Pathol* 1989;2:439–443.

22. Garuti G, Boselli F, Genazzani AR, Silvestri S, Ratti G. Detection and typing of human papillomavirus in histologic specimens by *in situ* hybridization with biotinylated probes. *Am J Clin Pathol* 1989;92:604–612.

23. Jacquemier J, Penault F, Durst M, et al. Detection of five different human papillomavirus types in cervical lesions by *in situ* hybridization. *Hum Pathol* 1990;21:911–917.

24. Kettler AH, Rutledge M, Tschen JA, Buffone G. Detection of human papillomavirus in nongenital Bowen's disease by *in situ* hybridization. *Arch Dermatol* 1990; 126:777–781.

25. Milde K, Loning T. Detection of papillomavirus DNA in oral papillomas and carcinomas: application of *in situ* hybridization with biotylated HPV 16 probes. *J Oral Pathol* 1986;15:292–296.

26. Ostrow RS, Manias DA, Clark BA, Okagaki T, Twiggs LB, Faras AJ. Detection of human papillomavirus DNA in invasive carcinomas of the cervix by *in situ* hybridization. *Cancer Res* 1987;47:649–653.

27. Ostrow RS, Manias DA, Clark BA, et al. The analysis of carcinomas of the vagina for human papillomavirus DNA. *Int J Gynecol Pathol* 1988;7:308–314.

28. Padayachee A, van Wyk CW. Human papillomavirus (HPV) DNA in focal epithelial hyperplasia by *in situ* hybridization. *J Oral Pathol Med* 1991;20:210–214.

29. Pilotti S, Stefanon B, dePalo G, Shah KV, Rilke F. Study of multiple human papillomavirus related lesions of the lower female genital tract by *in situ* hybridization. *Hum Pathol* 1989;20:118–123.

30. Stoler MH, Broker TR. *In situ* hybridization detection on human papillomavirus DNAs and messenger RNAs

in genital condylomata and a cervical carcinoma. *Hum Pathol* 1986;17:250–258.

31. Syrjanen S, Syrjanen K. An improved *in situ* DNA hybridization protocol for detection of human papillomavirus (HPV) DNA sequences in paraffin embedded biopsies. *J Virol Methods* 1986;14:293–304.

32. Syrjanen SM, Syrjanen KJ, Lamberg MA. Detection of human papillomavirus DNA in oral mucosal lesions using *in situ* DNA hybridization applied on paraffin sections. *Oral Surg Oral Med Oral Pathol* 1986;62.

33. Tase T, Okagaki T, Clark BA, Twiggs LB, Ostrow RS, Faras AJ. Human papillomavirus DNA in adenocarcinoma *in situ*, microinvasive adenocarcinoma of the uterine cervix, and coexisting cervical squamous intraepithelial neoplasia. *Int J Gynecol Pathol* 1989;8:8–17.

34. Vallejos H, DelMistro A, Kleinhaus S, Braunstein JD, Halwer M, Koss LG. Characterization of human papilloma virus types in condylomata acuminata in children by *in situ* hybridization. *Lab Invest* 1987;56: 611–615.

35. Walboomers JMM, Melchers WJG, Mullink H, et al. Sensitivity of *in situ* detection with biotinylated probes of human papillomavirus type 16 DNA in frozen tissue sections of squamous cell carcinoma of the cervix. *Am J Pathol* 1988;131:587–594.

36. Nuovo GJ. A comparison of slot blot, Southern blot and *in situ* hybridization analyses for human papillomavirus DNA in genital tract lesions. *Obstet Gynecol* 1989;74: 673–677.

37. Crum CP, Nuovo GJ. *Genital papillomaviruses and related neoplasms*. New York: Raven Press; 1991.

38. Nuovo GJ. *Cytopathology of the lower female genital tract: an integrated approach*. Baltimore:Williams & Wilkins;1994.

39. Slattery ML, Robison LM, Schuman KL, et al. Cigarette smoking and exposure to passive smoke are risk factors for cervical cancer. *JAMA* 1989;261:1593–1598.

40. Kessler II. Venereal factors in human cervical cancer. *Cancer* 1977;39:1912–1919.

41. LaVecchia C, Franceschi S, DeCarli A, et al. Sexual factors, venereal diseases, and the risk of intraepithelial and invasive cervical neoplasia. *Cancer* 1986;58: 935–941.

42. Oriel JD. Condylomata acuminata as a sexually transmitted disease. *Dermatol Clin* 1983;1:93–102.

43. Ostrow RS, McGlennen RC, Shaver MK, Kloster BE, Houser D, Faras AJ. A rhesus monkey model for sexual transmission of a papillomavirus isolated from a squamous cell carcinoma. *Proc Natl Acad Sci USA* 1990; 87:8170–8174.

44. Rotkin ID. A comparative review of key epidemiological studies in cervical cancer related to current searches for transmissible agents. *Cancer Res* 1973;33: 1353–1359.

45. Skegg, DCG, Corwin PA, Paul C, Doll R. Importance of the male factor in cancer of the cervix. *Lancet* 1982; ii:581–583.

46. Nuovo GJ, Smith S, Lerner J, Comite S, Eliezri Y. Human papillomavirus segregation patterns in genital and non-genital warts in children and adults. *Am J Clin Pathol* 1991;95:467–472.

47. Obalek S, Jablonska S, Favre L, Orth G. Condylomata acuminata in children: frequent association with human papillomaviruses responsible for cutaneous warts. *J Am Acad Dermatol* 1990;23:205–213.

48. Sedlacek TV, Lindheim, S, Eder C, Hasty L, Ludomirsky A, Rando, RF. Mechanism for human papillomavirus transmission at birth. *Am J Obstet Gynecol* 1989;161: 51–59.

49. Moy RL, Eliezri Y, Nuovo GJ, Bennett W, Silverstein SJ. Squamous cell carcinoma of the finger is associated with human papillomavirus type 16 DNA. *JAMA* 1989;261:2669–2673.

50. Eliezri Y, Silverstein SJ, Nuovo GJ. The occurrence of human papillomavirus DNA in cutaneous squamous and basal cell neoplasms. *Arch Dermatol* 1990;23: 836–842.

51. Nuovo GJ, Gallery F, MacConnell P, Becker J, Bloch W. An improved technique for the detection of DNA by *in situ* hybridization after PCR-amplification. *Am J Pathol* 1991;139:1239–1244.

52. Haase AT, Retzel EF, Staskus KA. Amplification and detection of lentiviral DNA inside cells. *Proc Natl Acad Sci USA* 1990;87:4971–4975.

53. Nuovo GJ, MacConnell P, Forde A, Delvenne P. Detection of human papillomavirus DNA in formalin fixed tissues by *in situ* hybridization after amplification by PCR. *Am J Pathol* 1991;139:847–854.

54. Nuovo GJ. A comparison of different methodologies (biotin based and ³⁵S based) for the detection of human papillomavirus DNA. *Lab Invest* 1989;61:471–476.

55. Walboomers JMM, Melchers WJG, Mullink H, et al. Sensitivity of *in situ* detection with biotinylated probes of human papillomavirus type 16 DNA in frozen tissue sections of squamous cell carcinoma of the cervix. *Am J Pathol* 1988;131:587–594.

56. Crum CP, Nuovo GJ. The cervix. *Diagn Surg Pathol* 1989;1557–1589.

57. Rader JS, Golub TR, Hudson JB, Patel D, Bedell MA, Laimins LA. *In vitro* differentiation of epithelial cells from cervical neoplasias resembles in vivo lesions. *Oncogene* 1990;5:571–576.

58. Rosen M, Auborn K. Duplication of the upstream regulatory sequences increases the transformation potential of human papillomavirus type 11. *J Gen Virol* 1991;19:484–487.

59. Storey A, Pim D, Murray A, Osborn K, Banks L, Crawford L. Comparison of the in vitro transforming activities of human papillomavirus types. *EMBO J* 1988;7: 1815–1820.

60. Watanabe S, Kanada T, Yoshike K. Human papillomavirus type 16 transformation of primary human embryonic fibroblasts requires expression of open reading frames E6 and E7. *J Virol* 1989;63:965–969.

60a. Colgan TJ, Percy ME, Suri M, Shier RM, Andrews DF, Lickrish GM. Human papillomavirus infection of morphologically normal cervical epithelium adjacent to squamous dysplasia and invasive carcinoma. *Hum Pathol* 1989;20:316–319.

61. deVilliers EM, Schneider A, Miklaw H, et al. Human papillomavirus infections in women with and without abnormal cervical cytology. *Lancet* 1987;i:703–706.

62. Grussendorf-Conen EI, DeVilliers EM, Gissmann L. Human papillomavirus genomes in penile smears of healthy men. *Lancet* 1986;i:1092.

63. Nuovo GJ, Cottral S. Occult infection of the uterine cervix by human papillomavirus in postmenopausal women. *Am J Obstet Gynecol* 1989;160:340–344.

64. Nuovo GJ, Nuovo MA, Cottral S, Gordon S, Silverstein SJ, Crum CP. Histological correlates of clinically occult human papillomavirus infection of the uterine cervix. *Am J Surg Pathol* 1988;12:198–204.

65. Bauer HM, Ting Y, Greer CE, et al. Genital human papillomavirus infection in female university students as determined by a PCR-based method. *JAMA* 1991;265: 472–477.

66. Crum CP, Fu Y, Kurman RJ, Okagaki T, Twiggs LB, Silverberg SG. Practical approach to cervical human papillomavirus-related intraepithelial lesions. *Int J Gynecol Oncol* 1989;8:388–399.

67. Nuovo GJ, Darfler MM, Impraim CC, Bromley SE. Occurrence of multiple types of human papillomavirus in genital tract lesions: analysis by *in situ* hybridization and the polymerase chain reaction. *Am J Pathol* 1991;58: 518–523.

68. Barrasso R, DeBrux J, Croissant O, Orth G. High prevalance of papillomavirus associated penile intraepithelial neoplasia in sexual partners of women with cervical intraepithelial neoplasia. *N Engl J Med* 1987; 317:916–923.

69. Boon ME, Schneider A, Hogewoning CJA, van der Kwast TH, Bolhuis P, Kok LP. Penile studies and heterosexual partners: peniscopy, cytology, histology and immunocytochemistry. *Cancer* 1988;61:1652–1659.

70. DelMistro A, Braunstein JD, Halwer M, Koss LG. Identification of human papillomavirus types in male urethral condylomata acuminata by *in situ* hybridization. *Hum Pathol* 1987;18:936–940.

71. Levine RA, Crum CP, Herman E, Silvers D, Ferenczy A. Cervical papillomavirus infection and intraepithelial neoplasia: a study of male sexual partners. *Obstet Gynecol* 1984;64:16–20.

72. Roman A, Fife K. Human papillomavirus DNA associated with foreskins of normal newborns. *J Infect Dis* 1986;153:855–860.

73. Schneider A, Kirchmayr R, deVilliers EM, Gissmann L. Subclinical human papillomavirus infections in male sexual partners of female carriers. *J Urol* 1988;140: 1431–1434.

74. Schultz RE, Skelton HG. Value of acetic acid screening for flat genital condylomata in men. *J Urol* 1988; 139:777–779.

75. Zderic SA, Carpiniello VL, Malloy TR, Rando RF. Urological applications of human papillomavirus typing using deoxyribonucleic acid probes for the diagnosis and treatment of genital condyloma. *J Urol* 1989;141: 63–65.

76. Buscema J, Naghashfar Z, Sowada E, Daniel R, Woodruff JD. The predominance of human papillomavirus type 16 in vulvar neoplasia. *Obstet Gynecol* 1988;71:601–605.

77. Crum CP, Burkett BJ. Papillomavirus and vulvovaginal neoplasia. *J Reprod Med* 1989;34:566–571.

78. McKay M. Subsets of vulvodynia. *J Reprod Med* 1988;33:695–698.

79. Park JS, Jones RW, McLean MR, Currie JL, Woodruff JD, Shah KV. Possible etiologic heterogeneity of vulvar intraepithelial neoplasia. *Cancer* 1991;67:1599–1607.

80. Pilotti S, Stefanon B, dePalo G, Shah KV, Rilke F. Study of multiple human papillomavirus related lesions of the lower female genital tract by *in situ* hybridization. *Hum Pathol* 1989;20:118–123.

81. Reid R, Greenberg M, Jenson AB, et al. Sexually transmitted papillomaviral infections. I. The anatomic distribution and pathologic grade of neoplastic lesions as-

sociated with different viral types. *Am J Obstet Gynecol* 1987;156:212–222.

82. Schneider A, Sawada E, Gissmann L, Shah K. Human papillomaviruses in women with a history of abnormal Papanicolaou smears and in their male partners. *Obstet Gynecol* 1987;69:554–561.

83. Sfameni SF, Ostor AG, Chanen W, Fortune DW. The association between vulvar condylomata acuminata, cervical wart virus infection and cervical intraepithelial neoplasia. *Aust NZ J Obstet Gynaecol* 1986;26:149–150.

84. Waliknshaw SA, Cordiner JW, Clements JB, MacNab JCM. Prognosis of women with human papillomavirus DNA in normal tissue distal to invasive cervical and vulvar cancer. *Lancet* 1987;i:563.

85. Carpiniello V, Sedlacek TV, Cunnane M, Schlecker B, Malloy T, Wein AJ. Magnified penile surface scanning in diagnosis of penile condyloma. *Urology* 1986;28:190–192.

86. Carpiniello VL, Zderic SA, Malloy TR, Sedlacek T. Carbon dioxide laser therapy of subclinical condyloma found by magnified penile surface scanning. *Urology* 1987;29:608–610.

87. Crum CP, Fu Y, Kurman RJ, Okagaki T, Twiggs LB, Silverberg SG. Practical approach to cervical human papillomavirus-related intraepithelial lesions. *Int J Gynecol Oncol* 1989;8:388–399.

88. Nuovo GJ. Comparison of Bouin's solution and buffered formalin fixation on the detection rate by *in situ* hybridization of human papillomavirus DNA in genital tract lesions. *J Histotech* 1991;14:13–18.

89. Nuovo GJ. Human papillomavirus DNA in genital tract lesions histologically negative for condylomata: analysis by *in situ*, Southern blot hybridization and the polymerase chain reaction. *Am J Surg Pathol* 1990;14:643–651.

90. Nuovo GJ, Gallery F, MacConnell P. Analysis of the distribution pattern of PCR-amplified HPV 6 DNA in vulvar warts by *in situ* hybridization. *Mod Pathol* 1992;5:444–448.

91. Nuovo GJ, Becker J, MacConnell P, Margiotta M, Comite S, Hochman H. Histological distribution of PCR-amplified HPV 6 and 11 DNA in penile lesions. *Am J Surg Pathol* 1992;16:269–275.

92. Barbosa MS, Edmonds C, Fisher C. The region of the HPV E7 oncoprotein homologous to adenovirus E1a and SV40 large T antigen contains separate domains for Rb binding and casein kinase II phosphorylation. *EMBO J* 1990;9:153–160.

93. Chen S, Mounts P. Transforming activity of E5a protein of human papillomavirus type 6 in NIH 3T3 and C127 cells. *J Virol* 1990;64:3226–3233.

94. Cook T, Morgenstern JP, Crawford L, Banks L. Continued expression of HPV 16 E7 protein is required for maintenance of the transformed phenotype of cells cotransformed by HPV 16 plus EJ-ras. *EMBO J* 1989;8:513–519.

95. Crook T, Greenfild I, Howard J, Stanley M. Alterations in growth properties of human papilloma virus type 16 immortalised human cervical keratinocyte cell line correlate with amplification and overexpression of c-myc oncogene. *Oncogene* 1990;5:619–622.

96. Dyson N, Howley PM, Munger K, Harlow E. The human papilloma virus-16 E7 oncoprotein is able to bind to the retinoblastoma gene product. *Science* 1989;243:934–936.

97. Bedell MA, Jones KH, Grossman SR, Laimins L. Identification of human papillomavirus type 18 transforming genes in immortalized and primary cells. *J Virol* 1989;63:1247–1255.

98. Cerni C, Bineruy B, Schiller JT, Lowy DR, Meneguzzi G, Cuzin F. Successive steps in the process of immortalization identified by transfer of separate bovine papillomavirus genes into rat fibroblasts. *Proc Natl Acad Sci USA* 1989;86:3266–3270.

99. Gage JR, Meyers C, Wettstein FO. The E7 proteins of the nononcogenic human papillomavirus type 6b (HPV-6b) and the oncogenic HPV-16 differ in retinoblastoma protein binding and other properties. *J Virol* 1990;64:723–730.

100. Hurlin PJ, Kaur P, Smith PP, Perez-Reyes N, Blanton RA, McDougall JK. Progression of human papillomavirus type 18-immortalized human keratinocytes to a malignant phenotype. *Proc Natl Acad Sci USA* 1991;88:570–574.

101. Iwasaka T, Yokoyama M, Hayashi Y, Sugimori H. Combined herpes simplex virus type 2 and human papillomavirus type 16 or 18 deoxyribonucleic acid leads to oncogenic transformation. *Am J Obstet Gynecol* 1988;159:1251–1255.

102. Kanada T, Furuno A, Yoshike K. Human papillomavirus type 16 open reading frame E7 encodes a transforming gene for rat 3Y1 cells. *J Virol* 1988;62:610–613.

103. Le J, Defendi V. A viral–cellular junction fragment from a human papillomavirus type 16-positive tumor is competent in transformation of NIH 3T3 cells. *J Virol* 1988;62:4420–4426.

104. Matlashewski G, Osborn K, Banks L, Stanley M, Crawford L. Transformation of primary human fibroblast cells with human papillomavirus type 16 DNA and EJ-ras. *Int J Cancer* 1988;42:232–238.

105. O'Banion MK, Reichmann ME, Sundberg JP. Cloning and characterization of a papillomavirus associated with papillomas and carcinomas in the European harvest mouse (Micromys minutus). *J Virol* 1988;62:226–233.

106. Pecoraro G, Lee M, Morgan D, Defendi V. Evolution of in vitro transformation and tumorigenesis of HPV 16 and HPV 18 immortalized primary cervical epithelial cells. *Am J Pathol* 1991;138:1–8.

107. Pirisi L, Yasumoto S, Feller M, Doniger J, DiPaolo JA. Transformation of human fibroblasts and keratinocytes with human papillomavirus type 16 DNA. *J Virol* 1987;61:1061–1066.

108. Yasumoto S, Doniger J, DiPaolo JA. Differential early viral gene expression in two stages of human papillomavirus type 16 DNA-induced malignant transformation. *Mol Cell Biol* 1987;7:2165–2172.

109. Cernie C, Patocka K, Meneguzzi G. Immortalization of primary rat embryo cells by human papillomavirus type 11 DNA is enhanced upon cotransfer of ras. *Virology* 1990;177:427–436.

110. Woodworth CD, Doniger J, DiPaolo JA. Immortalization of human foreskin keratinocytes by various human papillomavirus DNAs corresponds to their association with cervical carcinoma. *J Virol* 1989;63:159–164.

111. Amortegui AJ, Meyer MP. *In situ* hybridization for the diagnosis and typing of human papillomavirus. *Clin Biochem* 1990;23:301–306.

112. Byrne MA, Wickenden C, Coleman DV. Prevalence of human papillomavirus types in the cervices of women

before and after laser ablation. *Br J Obstet Gynaecol* 1988;95:201–202.

113. Dinh TV, Powell LC, Hannigan EV, Yang HL, Wirt DP, Yandell RB. Simultaneously occurring condylomata acuminata, carcinoma *in situ* and verrucous carcinoma of the vulva and carcinoma *in situ* of the cervix in a young woman. *J Reprod Med* 1988;33:510–513.

114. Fey SJ, Hansen K, Frandsen K, Vetner M, Gissmann L, Larsen PM. The type of human papillomavirus present in cervical infections can be determined by the occurrence of specific marker proteins. *Cell Biol Int Rep* 1986;10:905–913.

115. Garuti G, Boselli F, Genazzani AR, Silvestri S, Ratti G. Detection and typing of human papillomavirus in histologic specimens by *in situ* hybridization with biotinylated probes. *Am J Clin Pathol* 1989;92:604–612.

116. Griffin NR, Bevan IS, Lewis FA, Young LS. Demonstration of multiple HPV types in normal cervix and in cervical squamous cell carcinoma using the polymerase chain reaction on paraffin wax embedded material. *J Clin Pathol* 1990;45:52–56.

117. Kadish AS, Burk RD, Kress Y, Calderin S, Romney SL. Human papillomavirus of different types in precancerous lesions of the uterine cervix: histologic, immunocytochemical and ultrastructural studies. *Hum Pathol* 1986;17:384–392.

118. Villa LL, Franco ELL. Epidemiologic correlates of cervical neoplasia and risk of human papillomavirus infection in asymptomatic women in Brazil. *J Natl Cancer Inst* 1989;81:337–340.

119. Woodworth CD, Notario V, DiPaolo JA. Transforming growth factors beta 1 and 2 transcriptionally regulate human papillomavirus (HPV) type 16 early gene expression in HPV–immortalized human genital epithelial cells. *J Virol* 1990;64:4767–4775.

120. Takami Y, Kondoh G, Saito J, et al. Cloning and characterization of human papillomavirus type 52 from cervical carcinoma in Indonesia. *Int J Cancer* 1991;48:516–522.

121. Woodworth CD, Waggoner S, Barnes W, Stoler MH, DiPaolo JA. Human cervical and foreskin epithelial cells immortalized by human papillomavirus DNAs exhibit dysplastic differentiation in vivo. *Cancer Res* 1990;50:3709–3715.

122. Popescu NC, DiPaolo JA. Integration of human papillomavirus 16 DNA and genomic rearrangements in immortalized human keratinocyte lines. *Cancer Res* 1990;50:1316–1323.

123. Gall AA, Saul SH, Stoler MH. *In situ* hybridization analysis of human papillomavirus in anal squamous cell carcinoma. *Mod Pathol* 1989;2:439–443.

124. Liang XM, Wieczorek RL, Koss LG. *In situ* hybridization with human papillomavirus using biotinylated DNA probes on archival cervical smears. *J Histochem Cytochem* 1991;39:771–775.

125. Syrjanen SM, Syryjanen K, Lamberg MA. Detection of human papillomavirus DNA in oral mucosal lesions using *in situ* DNA hybridization applied on paraffin sections. *Oral Surg Oral Med Oral Pathol* 1986;62:660–667.

126. van der Brule AJC, Cromme FV, Snijders PJF, et al. Nonradioactive RNA *in situ* hybridization detection of human papillomavirus 16 E7 transcripts in squamous cell carcinomas of the uterine cervix using confocal laser scan microscopy. *Am J Pathol* 1991;139:1037–1045.

127. Syrjanen S, Saastamoinen J, Chang F, Ji H, Syrjanen K. Colposcopy, punch biopsy, *in situ* DNA hybridization, and the polymerase chain reaction in searching for genital human papillomavirus infections in women with normal pap smears. *J Med Virol* 1990;31:259–266.

128. Abdelatif OMA, Chandler FW, Pantazis CG, McGuire BS. Enhanced expression of c-myc and H-ras oncogenes in Letterer-Siwe disease. *Arch Pathol Lab Med* 1991;114:1254–1260.

129. Benz CC, Scott GK, Santos GF, Smith HS. Expression of c-myc, c-Ha-ras1, and c-erbB-2 proto-oncogenes in normal and malignant human breast epithelial cells. *J Natl Cancer Inst* 1989;81:1704–1709.

130. Crook T, Almond N, Murray A, Stanley M, Crawford L. Constitutive expression of c-myc oncogene confers hormone independence and enhanced growth-factor responsiveness on cells transformed by human papillomavirus type 16. *Proc Natl Acad Sci USA* 1989;86:5713–5717.

131. DiPaolo JA, Woodworth CD, Popescu NC, Notario V, Doniger J. Induction of human cervical squamous cell carcinoma by sequential transfection with human papillomavirus 16 DNA and viral Harvey ras. *Oncogene* 1989;4:395–399.

132. Farr A, Wang H, Kasher MS, Roman A. Relative enhancer activity and transforming potential of authentic human papillomavirus type 6 genomes from benign and malignant lesions. *J Gen Virol* 1991;72:519–526.

133. Ishibashi T, Matsushima S, Tsunokawa Y. Human papillomavirus DNA in squamous cell carcinoma of the upper aerodigestive tract. *Arch Otolaryngol Head Neck Surg* 1990;116:294–298.

134. Liotta LA, Steeg PS, Stetler-Stevenson WG. Cancer metastasis and angiogenesis: an imbalance of positive and negative regulation. *Cell* 1991;64:327–336.

135. Sato H, Kida Y, Mai M, et al. Expression of genes encoding type IV collagen-degrading metalloproteinases and tissue inhibitors of metalloproteinases in various human tumor cells. *Cell* 1992;66:302–326.

136. Syrjanen K, Mantyjarvi R, Vayrynen M, et al. Human papillomavirus (HPV) infections involved in the neoplastic process of the uterine cervix as established by prospective followup of 513 women for two years. *Eur J Gynaecol Oncol* 1987;8:5–14.

137. ElAwady MK, Kaplan JB, O'Brien SJ, Burk RD. Molecular analysis of integrated human papillomavirus 16 sequences in the cervical cancer line SiHa. *Virology* 1987;159:389–398.

138. Lehn H, Villa LL, Marziona F, Hilgarth M, Hillemans HG, Sauer G. Physical state and biological activity of human papillomavirus genomes in precancerous lesions of the female genital tract. *J Gen Virol* 1988;69:187–196.

139. McCance DJ, Kopan R, Fuchs E, Laimins LA. Human papillomavirus type 16 alters human epithelial cell differentiation in vitro. *Proc Natl Acad Sci USA* 1988;85:7169–7173.

140. Meanwell CA, Cox MF, Blackledge G, Maitland NJ. HPV 16 DNA in normal and malignant cervical epithelium: implications for the aetiology and behaviour of cervical neoplasia. *Lancet* 1987;i:703–707.

141. Sastre-Garau X, Schneider-Maunoury S, Couturier J, Orth G. Human papillomavirus type 16 DNA is integrated into chromosome region 12q14–q15 in a cell line

derived from a vulvar intraepithelial neoplasia. *Cancer Genet Cytogenet* 1990;44:243–251.

142. Schneider-Maunoury S, Croissant O, Orth G. Integration of human papillomavirus type 16 DNA sequences: a possible early event in the progression of genital tumors. *J Virol* 1987;61:3295–3298.

143. Duggan MA, Benoit JL, McGregor SE, Nation JG, Inoue M, Stuart GCE: The human papillomavirus status of 114 endocervical adenocarcinoma cases by dot blot hybridization. *Hum Pathol* 1993;24:121.

144. Harding U, Teglbjaerg CS, Visfeldt J, Bock JEE: Human papillomavirus types 16 and 18 in adenocarcinoma of the uterine cervix. *Gynecol Oncol* 1992;46:313.

145. Jones MW, Silverberg SG, Kurman RJ: Well-differentiated villoglandular adenocarcinoma of the uterine cervix: a clinicopathological study of 24 cases. *Int J Gynaecol Pathol* 1993;12:1.

146. Stoler MH, Mills SE, Gersell DJ, Walker AN: Small cell neuroendocrine carcinoma of the cervix. A human papillomavirus type 18 associated cancer. *Am J Surg Pathol* 1991;15:28.

147. Ferry JA, Scully RE: Adenoid cystic carcinoma and adenoid basal carcinoma of the uterine cervix. A study of 28 cases. *Am J Surg Pathol* 1988;12:134.

148. Barnes W, Delgado G, Kurman RJ, et al. Possible prognostic significance of human papillomavirus type in cervical cancer. *Gynecol Oncol* 1988;29:267.

149. Nuovo GJ, Delvenne P, MacConnell P, Neto C, Chalas E, Mann W: Correlation of histology and detection of human papillomavirus DNA in vulvar cancers. *Gynecol Oncol* 1991;43:275.

150. Bradshaw BR, Nuovo GJ, DiCostanzo D, Cohen SR. Human papillomavirus type 16 associated perianal carcinoma *in situ* and condylomata acuminata in a homosexual male. *Arch Dermatol* 1992;128:949-952.

151. Reich R, Thompson E, Iwamoto Y, et al. Effects of inhibitors of plasminogen activator, serine proteinases, and collagenase IV on the invasion of basement membrane by metastatic cells. *Cancer Res* 1988;48:3307–3312.

152. Mignatti P, Robbins E, Rifkin DB: Tumor invasion through the human amniotic membrane: requirement for a protease cascade. *Cell* 1986;47:487–498.

153. Liotta LA, Steeg PS, Stetler-Stevenson WG: Cancer metastasis and angiogenesis: an imbalance of positive and negative regulation. *Cell* 1991;64:327–336.

154. McDonnell S, Matrisian LM: Stromelysin in tumor progression and metastasis. *Cancer Metastasis Rev* 1990;9:305–319.

155. Khokha R, Waterhouse P, Yagel S, et al. Antisense RNA-induced reduction in murine TIMP levels confers oncogenicity on Swiss 3T3 cells. *Science* 1989;243:947–950.

156. Polette M, Clavel C, Birembaut P, DeClerck YA: Localization by *in situ* hybridization of mRNAs encoding stromelysin 3 and tissue inhibitors of metalloproteases TIMP-1 and TIMP-2 in human head and neck cancers. *Pathol Res Pract* 1993;189:1052–1057.

157. Nuovo GJ, MacConnell P, French DL: Correlation of the *in situ* detection of PCR-amplified metalloprotease cDNAs and their inhibitors with prognosis in cervical carcinoma. *Cancer Res* 1995;55:267–275.

158. Riklund KE, Makiya RA, Sundstrom BE, Thornell L, Stigbrand TI: Experimental radioimmunotherapy of HeLa tumours in nude mice with ^{131}I-labeled monoclonal antibodies. *Anticancer Res* 1992;10:379–384.

159. Agarwal C, Hembree JR, Rorke EA, Eckert RL: Transforming growth factor beta1 regulation of metalloprotease production in cultured human cervical epithelial cells. *Cancer Res* 1994;54:943–949.

160. Bernhard EJ, Gruber SB, Muschel RJ: Direct evidence linking the expression of MMP-9 to the transformed phenotype in transformed rat cells. *Proc Natl Acad Sci USA* 1993;91:1993–1998.

9

Applications of PCR *in situ* Hybridization: Human Immunodeficiency Virus-1

The proliferation of research directed at understanding the pathogenesis of AIDS and developing treatments for the disease has been one of the major driving forces for the development of *in situ* PCR. No disease of this generation has caused as much emotional, physical, and financial distress as AIDS, and the causative agent of AIDS is a retrovirus designated HIV-1 (1–12). Members of this family are RNA viruses that have the ability, once they enter a cell, to synthesize DNA complementary to their RNA (called cDNA) using the enzyme reverse transcriptase. Once the cDNA is made, it often integrates into the chromosome of the host cell. The virus may remain quiescent in this form for long periods of time, even years (13–15). Thus, cells can be latently infected with one or a few copies of integrated HIV-1 DNA and otherwise appear normal, both cytologically and functionally. Standard *in situ* hybridization would not be able to detect HIV–1 in this latent form. Solution phase PCR could, of course, detect the proviral DNA, but could not localize the target to the specific infected cell and, importantly, could not give us a reliable measure of the percentage of a given cell type infected.

A critical distinction in HIV-1 pathogenesis is latent versus activated or productive infection. In latent infection, either no or rare incomplete viral mRNAs are being made. Under these conditions the cell will not be killed, and its function may be minimally altered, if at all. The viral transcripts that may be produced in latent infection are usually few and do not include some of the multiply spliced messages associated with widespread disruption of the cellular machinery that presages cell death. Cells that are latently infected by HIV-1 are "walking time bombs," for eventually the virus may become activated and begin to synthesize a variety of full-length and multiply spliced transcripts, which may lead to the production of infectious virions. Some of these transcripts involve late gene expression from the nucleocapsid (*gag*), envelope (*env*), and RNA polymerase regions (*pol*) that are needed for the production of intact, infectious particles, whereas others involve the early gene regions, which help modulate viral nucleic acid production, including active versus latent infection (*tat* and *rev* genes). Thus, activation can be associated with the production of infectious viral particles, which can then reach other cells, and cell death (Fig. 9-1). If the cell actively infected by HIV-1 does not immediately die, it is certain that there will be a marked interference with its normal functioning. Intensive research has focused on agents, such as interleukin-1 and NK-B, that may induce productive HIV-1 RNA synthesis in latently infected cells (1,13,16). This process is obviously very important and is the essential step in the evolution of asymptomatic HIV-1 infection to clinically evident disease and ultimately to the person's demise.

The PCR *in situ* hybridization analysis in combination with RT *in situ* PCR can easily provide some very important information about

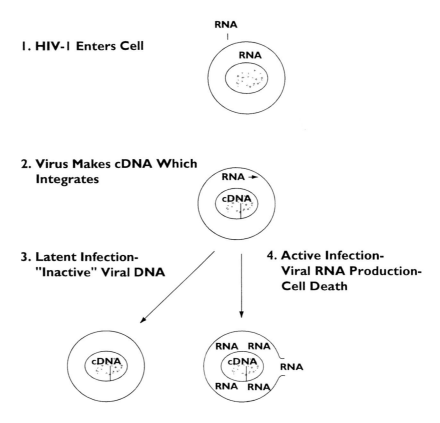

Figure 9-1. *Possible consequences of HIV-1 infection.* After HIV-1 RNA enters a cell, it can synthesize the corresponding cDNA using the enzyme reverse transcriptase. The cDNA can integrate into the host genome. It can remain in this latent state with no or minimal viral RNA production for years with no evident deleterious effect on the cell. However, if viral RNA synthesis is activated, one consequence may be the production of a relatively high copy number of a variety of cell transcripts, the production of infectious viral particles, and cell death.

HIV-1 infection and the evolution of AIDS. These tests can show

1. The specific cell type(s) infected
2. The percentage of a specific cell type infected
3. The percentage of latently infected cells and the percentage containing the multiply spliced transcripts associated with productive lethal infection

The discussion of the above points in this chapter will show how the *in situ* PCR analyses provide us with a wealth of information about HIV-1 pathogenesis.

With regard to the specific cell type(s) infected, it is well documented that HIV-1 attacks a subpopulation of T lymphocytes called *helper cells* (1,13,17–20). These cells have a specific receptor called *CD4,* which is the usual port of entry of the virus. However, because many other sites, including the brain, kidney, bone marrow, skeletal muscle, cervix, testes, and heart, can be involved in AIDS, it has long been postulated that HIV-1 may be able to enter cells via other receptors (19,21–62). One group was able to show that the astrocyte receptor galactosylceramide is a portal of entry for the AIDS virus (19). *In situ* PCR, in combination with routine histological analysis or colabeling experiments, has provided a wealth of data demonstrating cell types that lack the CD4 receptor and that can be infected by HIV-1, which are discussed in detail later in this chapter.

Early detection of HIV-1 infection has become an important issue, especially now that several different classes of antiretroviral drugs are available. The current methods of detection rely on the host's ability to develop antibodies against the AIDS virus. Although these tests—the ELISA and Western blot analyses—have good specificity (especially the Western blot analysis), it is well documented that it may take months or even years after the initial infection by the virus for them to become positive. Obviously, a prolonged period of uncertainty may be an eternity for someone who fears having been exposed to the virus. Studies have shown that, given its extreme sensitivity, PCR positivity may precede seroconversion (13,14,30–32). The PCR has also been very helpful in the analysis of children borne to women with AIDS. These children will usually be seropositive for about 1 year due to circulating maternal antibodies. It has been shown that PCR analysis is a good predictor in such children of those who will remain seropositive and develop AIDS versus those children who will become seronegative and not develop the disease (31). Considering these accomplishments and potential benefits, one may ask why PCR analysis has not played a large role in the diagnosis of infection by HIV-1? One issue has been the contamination problem. Although much progress has been made in reducing the risk of contamination, especially "crossover" contamination, the extreme sensitivity of PCR makes contamination a possibility that, even when a very rare event, may be unacceptably high for a disease such as HIV-1. An incorrect positive result (false positive) can have extreme emotional and medical–legal implications. While the potential for cross-contamination continues to hinder the use of solution phase PCR, it simply does not occur during *in situ* PCR, as discussed in detail in Chapter 3. It is possible that *in situ* PCR will play an important role in the initial diagnosis of HIV-1 infection and in monitoring the progress of the disease, especially in response to antiretroviral therapy.

IDENTIFICATION OF HIV-1 DNA AND HIV-1 RNA IN INFECTED CELL LINES

Lymphocyte Cell Lines

Many lymphocyte cell lines infected by HIV-1 are available for research purposes. We have used the CR10 cell line and normal pooled lymphocytes infected *in vitro* by the virus in order to study HIV-1 nucleic acids by standard *in situ* hybridization and PCR *in situ*. The cells were fixed overnight in 10% buffered formalin and either embedded in paraffin or washed and then placed directly on a silane-coated glass slide. Several 4 μm sections or cell suspension samples could then be placed on each glass slide for analysis. When a digoxigenin-labeled DNA probe made from the internal SK19 fragment corresponding to the *gag* region of the viral genome was used, HIV-1 DNA was not detectable, as would be expected given the low copy number of the provirus in the infected cells (Fig. 9-2). We next amplified HIV-1 DNA using the corresponding primers SK38 and SK39. After hot start PCR amplification, *in situ* analysis was done under the conditions described above; indeed, the compared *in situ* and PCR *in situ* hybridization analyses were done on the same glass slide. HIV-1 DNA was now detectable in about 90% of the CR10 cells from the paraffin-embedded block and in about one-third of the infected pooled lymphocytes (Fig. 9-2). This comparative analysis shows that of the cells infected by the virus, the DNA was apparently present in one to a few copies per cell integrated into the host genome. Two other important points need to be highlighted: (i) the negative cells in the paraffin-embedded section may well have contained HIV-1 DNA that was removed as the cell block was sectioned, cutting cells into parts; and (ii) the DNA was amplified under the hot start conditions using a single primer pair that dictated the synthesis of a small (115 base pair) fragment. Good results

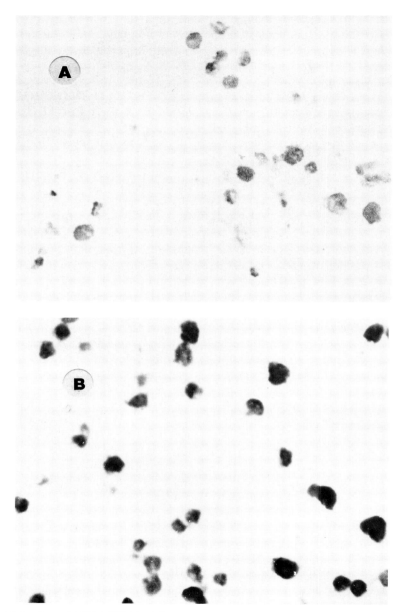

Figure 9-2. *Detection of HIV-1 DNA in CR10 cells by PCR* in situ *hybridization.* HIV-1 DNA was not detected in an infected CR10 line by standard *in situ* hybridization analysis (**A**). HIV-1 DNA was detected in most of the cells, however, by *in situ* hybridization analysis after PCR amplification (**B**). The hybridization signal was lost when the DNA polymerase was omitted from the amplifying solution (**C**). About 10% of the cells that contained HIV-1 DNA were producing abundant transcripts, as detected with a panel of ^{35}S-labeled probes and a serial section to that shown in B (**D**, *arrows*) (the probe is from ONCOR and detects transcripts in all viral regions except the *gag* ORF).

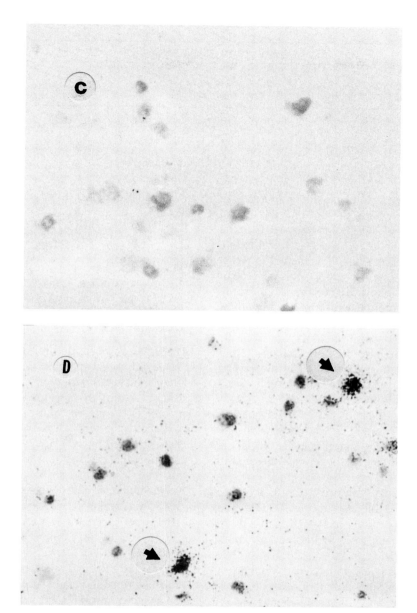

Figure 9-2. *Continued.*

with the small fragment reinforces the concept that the degree of target-specific amplification and not the size of the final amplified product is the key factor in successful PCR *in situ* hybridization. Recall that several groups have theorized that the size of the final product had to be >900 base pairs for successful PCR *in situ* (33). However, their tests were done under standard conditions where the competing nonspecific pathways decreased the amount of target-specific amplified DNA (34).

We next attempted to distinguish infected cells that contain presumably only the integrated viral DNA (latent infection) from those in which active HIV-1 RNA synthesis is occurring. To this end, the CR10 cells were analyzed with

Table 9-1. *Latent versus activated infection by HIV-1 in quiescent versus activated lymphocytes*

Sample	% of cells HIV-1 DNA+/RNA+	Localization of signal
Mock infected	0/0	—
Quiescent lymphocytes	10/8	Cytoplasm
Activated lymphocytes	34/31	Nucleus

Data were obtained by counting 100 to 210 cells; experiments were done twice.

a pool of ^{35}S probes that cover most of the transcribing region of HIV-1 (ONCOR, Gaithersburg, MD). The results are shown in Fig. 9-2. Note that whereas about 90% of the cells had detectable HIV-1 DNA, only about 10% of the cells had detectable HIV-1 RNA. It is possible that a higher percentage of cells were expressing viral RNA that was not detected because of low copy number or due to their containing transcripts in regions excluded in the pool of ^{35}S-labeled RNAs employed in this study. These possibilities cannot be ruled out; however, the intensity of the hybridization signal noted in cells with detectable HIV-1 RNA suggests a basic difference at the molecular level between these cells and those negative for RNA synthesis. RT *in situ* PCR for HIV-1 RNA has yielded similar data (G.J. Nuovo, *unpublished observations,* 1993), suggesting that only about one in every nine cells is actively infected in this cell line.

Pooled normal lymphocytes infected with HIV-1 were obtained by adding 100,000 cpm (by isotopic RT assay) of IV-1-IIIB to 5 ml of PHA-P stimulated peripheral blood mononuclear cells (PBMC) at 2×10^6 cells/ml. The PHA-P activates the lymphocytes, which leads to their proliferation and production of a variety of cytokines and differential phenotypic expression. T-cell activation, as routinely occurs with any stimulus of the immune system such as with an infection, likely predisposes the cell to HIV-1 infection. To test this, we studied quiescent, nonactivated lymphocytes versus those stimulated by PHA-P. These experiments were done in collaboration with Drs. Michael Bukrinsky and Helena Schmidtmayerova of the Picower Institute. The lymphocytes were exposed to HIV-1 and the percentage of cells that were latently versus actively infected were determined by PCR *in situ* hybridization and RT *in situ* PCR analyses, respectively. The results are provided in Table 9-1. Several observations were made:

1. Activation of the lymphocytes is associated with a higher rate of infection of the cells by HIV-1.
2. Lymphocyte activation is apparently needed to induce nuclear localization of the HIV-1 DNA (Fig. 9-3 and Color Plate 11 following p. 242).

The latter observation highlights a simple but powerful utility of *in situ* PCR: the ability to localize a signal to a specific cellular compartment. Although the actual mechanism whereby HIV-1 migrates from the cytoplasmic membrane to the nucleus is not well known, the data provided by PCR *in situ* hybridization demonstrate that cellular activation is essential in this regard.

Another lymphocyte cell line that was studied for HIV-1 was supplied by Dr. Kenneth Wieder of Beth Israel Medical Center in Boston. This was an especially interesting cell line as it was derived from a mouse. HIV-1 is exceptionally trophic for humans, and other animals, including related primates, cannot successfully be infected by the virus. Of course, neither can mice. However, Dr. Wieder was able to generate some CD4 mutant lymphocyte cell lines from a mouse that it appeared were capable of sustaining a long-term HIV-1 infection. This, and the transgenic mouse that could be generated from the construct, would be a valuable tool in the study of HIV-1, especially in possible antiretroviral drugs as it would, in affect, provide an animal model to study the disease process. However, documentation of long-term infection could not reliably be done by solution phase PCR, as it is possible that a

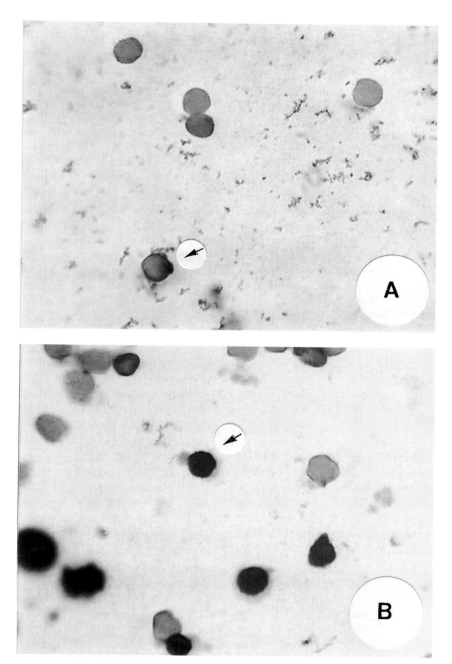

Figure 9-3. *Nuclear versus cytoplasmic localization of HIV-1 DNA as determined by PCR* in situ *hybridization: quiescent versus activated CD4 lymphocytes.* **A:** These cells are quiescent lymphocytes that were infected with HIV-1. A signal was noted in about 10% of these lymphocytes and it localized to the cell membrane and the thin rim of cytoplasm characteristic of these cells. **B:** In comparison, T-helper cells activated by PHA and then infected with HIV-1 show a threefold increase of infected cells and the signal localizes to the nucleus. This observation, readily made with PCR *in situ* hyridization, implies that proviral transport from the surface CD4 receptor to the nucleus is dependent on cellular activation.

signal may represent virus nonspecifically bound to the cell membrane. Here is another example where *in situ* PCR can readily and unequivocally determine if the cells indeed are infected by the virus. Recall that if one adds microgram amounts of labeled HIV-1 DNA to the amplifying solution and does *in situ* PCR with cells known to be viral negative, then no nuclear signal is seen (discussed in detail in Chapter 3).

We performed PCR *in situ* hybridization using the mouse cells that possessed the mutant CD4 molecule, which apparently allowed for HIV-1 infection. The data follows:

Sample	Detection rate of HIV-1 DNA (%)	Detection rate of HIV-1 RNA (%)
Mouse cell line, normal CD4	6	3
Mutant mouse CD4	29	26
Mutant mouse CD4 (sham)	0	0
Human cell line	27	ND
Human cell line (sham)	0	0

These data clearly demonstrate that HIV-1 can infect the mouse cells that contain the CD4 mutant at an efficiency similar to the human cell lines. Viral infection is active with a similar percentage of cells containing viral DNA and RNA. Surprisingly, a small but definite and reproducible number of the mouse cells with the normal CD4 (the line was leukemia derived) did show viral DNA that localized to their nuclei. This raises the intriguing question of whether HIV-1 can infect cells of other species but other factors prevent the development of an AIDS-type syndrome.

Macrophage Cell Lines

The genetic variability of HIV-1 is extraordinary. Any given person infected by this virus will actually have many different "quasispecies" or strains of the virus at a given time. This can be compared with the human papillomavirus (HPV), described in a previous chapter, where there is minimal genomic variability of a given HPV type. Indeed, it has been demonstrated that the HPV 16 that infects someone in the United States, for example, will in many cases have the exact same genomic sequence as an HPV that infects someone in Germany. One ramification of the marked genetic variability of HIV-1 is that some strains are more efficient at infecting T-helper lymphocytes, whereas other strains have a greater affinity for infecting the other major target of this virus—macrophages. The importance of the distinction between the so-called macrophage-tropic strains and lymphocytic-tropic strains of HIV-1 was demonstrated by Ho et al. (61). In their study of heterosexual transmission of HIV-1 they showed that, whereas lymphocytic-tropic strains predominate in the male donor, macrophage-tropic strains predominate in the female recipient early in her disease course. Possible explanations for this observation are discussed below when we analyze the *in situ* distribution of PCR-amplified HIV-1 DNA and cDNA in the genital tract.

In collaboration with Drs. Michael Bukrinsky and Helena Schmidtmayerova of the Picower Institute, I studied the infection rates and differential localization of HIV-1 in macrophages infected with a variety of viral strains. The LAV and NDK strains are lymphocytic tropic, whereas the ADA strain is macrophage tropic. One difference between these strains was evident on routine hematoxylin and eosin stain; 36% of the ADA-infected cells at day 9 of infection showed multinucleated forms (this is the so-called syncytial response) compared with only 7% to 8% for the lymphocytic-tropic LAV and NDK strains. As expected, only rare cells were positive for HIV-1 DNA using standard *in situ* hybridization. The detection rates increased over 40-fold when PCR *in situ* hybridization was performed. There were also some interesting differences in the localization of the signal between these different strains, as evident from the data at day 9 of infection:

HIV-1 strain	% of cells HIV-1 DNA+ (nuclear signal)	% of cells HIV-1 DNA+ (cytoplasmic signal)
LAV	22	5
NDK	43	5
ADA	32	0
Control	0	0

Representative photographs are shown in Fig. 9-4. Note that the cytoplasmic signal in the LAV infected cells localizes to the cytoplasmic membrane, suggesting the virus was actually associated with the membrane. This may represent a failed attempt to actually enter the cell or, perhaps, viral entry but retarded migration from the cytoplasm to the nucleus. It is clear that the lymphocytic-tropic strains are as effective as the ADA strain in the initial infection of the macrophages. The enhanced ability of the ADA strain for a long term productive infection must relate to other factors including, perhaps, migration to the nuclei; the ADA strain provirus was never detected in the cytoplasm in this study. Another interesting difference between the macrophage and lymphocytic-tropic strains was the ratio of latent to activated infection. Using RT *in situ* PCR and primers that detect spliced transcripts that are present in activated infection (as compared to primers that detect the intact viral RNA genome which could be present in quiescent infection), 32% of the cells infected by the ADA strain contained these spliced HIV-1 transcripts, demonstrating that infection in all cells which contained the virus was activated. In contrast, about 50% of the LAV infected cells did not contain these spliced viral transcripts. These data again demonstrate the simple but useful information provided by PCR *in situ* hybridization and RT *in situ* PCR in understanding the important topic of the molecular basis for the variable infection rates of lymphocytes and macrophages of different HIV-1 strains.

Another area where *in situ* PCR might provide some key insights is the effect of zidovu-dine (AZT) on the dynamics of HIV-1 infection. We analyzed the effect of AZT on the percentage of macrophages affected by the different strains of the virus. The results were:

	% of cells HIV-1 DNA+	
Strain	NO AZT	AZT
NDK	15	2
LAV	11	5
ADA	13	2

Note that, although the percentage of infected cells dropped considerably after AZT treatment, some HIV-1–infected cells persist. One explanation is that the high sensitivity of *in situ* PCR detects the low percentage of cells that "escape" AZT blockage, either by resistance or by the low probability that a given virus may not be exposed to HIV-1 prior to making its cDNA.

The final series of experiments in the macrophages addressed the question of cellular activation and HIV-1 detection. Macrophage activation can be measured by a variety of means, including cytokine expression and increased uptake of labeled nucleotides. *In situ* PCR was done for HIV-1 DNA after the macrophages were exposed to ^{3}H-labeled nucleotides for several days. Colocalization of HIV-1 and macrophage activation could be done by detecting the digoxigenin dUTP (HIV-1–labeled probe) and ^{3}H (activated macrophages). Colocalization of two different targets, in my experience, is best performed using a colorimetric and radioactive isotope. The radioactive isotope should be developed first, followed by xylene and ethanol washes to remove residual emulsion, which may interfere with detection of the digoxigenin (or biotin). The results of experiments with the macrophages were as follows:

	^{3}H positive cells
HIV-1–positive	47%
HIV-1 negative	1%

Clearly, over 97% of the macrophages that were infected by HIV-1 were activated, as determined by detection of ^{3}H nucleotide incor-

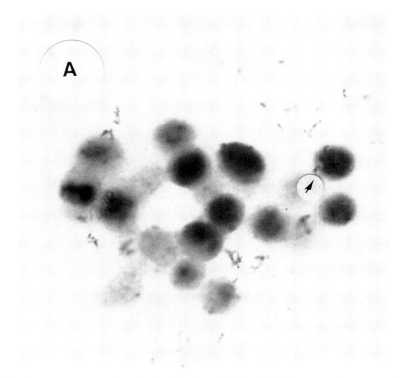

Figure 9-4. *Nuclear versus cytoplasmic localization of HIV-1 DNA in macrophages as determined by PCR* in situ *hybridization: macrophage-tropic versus lymphocyte-trophic strains.* HIV-1 DNA localized to the nucleus of macrophages infected with the macrophage-tropic HIV-1 strain ADA; cell membrane signal was rarely evident (**A**, *arrow*). Viral DNA localized to the nucleus (**B**, *large arrow*) in macrophages infected with the lymphocyte-tropic strain LAV; however, cell membrane staining was also readily evident (*small arrow*). This observation, readily made with PCR *in situ* hybridization, suggests that the efficiency of proviral transport from the cell surface to the nucleus may be one factor that differentiates macrophage from lymphocyte tropic strains.

poration. It should be added that it is very doubtful that HIV-1 could incorporate enough ^{3}H to produce a signal, given the small size of the viral genome relative to the human DNA (see related discussion in Chapter 6). The utility of colocalization of two separate targets will be especially useful in the analysis of the contributions of HIV-1 and cytokine expression to AIDS dementia, which are discussed later in this chapter.

IDENTIFICATION OF HIV-1 DNA IN PERIPHERAL BLOOD LEUKOCYTES

T-helper (CD4) cells are plentiful in the circulating blood. Thus, identification of HIV-1 DNA and RNA in PBMC might seem to be the logical basis of a diagnostic test for infection by the virus and for testing to monitor the effectiveness of anti-HIV therapy.

Thus far, we have analyzed PBMC from about 70 patients with AIDS or pre-AIDS (seropositive for the virus without any AIDS-defining illness). Standard *in situ* analysis did not detect HIV-1 DNA in any peripheral leukocytes. However, in all but one of the cases of HIV-1 infection the proviral DNA was detected by *in situ* PCR. The data from these experiments are separated according to patients with pre-AIDS and those with AIDS and listed in Table 9-2. Note that the percentage of CD4 cells in the peripheral blood that is infected by HIV-1 in the asymptomatic group ranged from 1% to 10%. This is much higher than originally

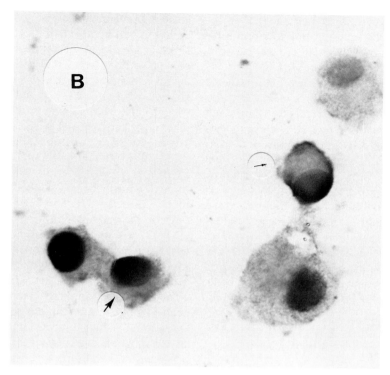

Figure 9-4. *Continued.*

Table 9-2. *Detection of PCR-amplified HIV-1 nucleic acids in PBMC from patients with asymptomatic and advanced-stage AIDS*

Case no.	Total peripheral blood CD4 count	PBMC		CD4+	
		% CD4+	%HIV-1 DNA+	%HIV-1 DNA+	%HIV-1 RNA+
Asymptomatic					
1	426	19.5	1.5	7.7	1.2
2	859	12.5	0.5	4.0	0
3	327	16.5	0.3	1.8	0.6
4	630	NA	0.7	NA	NA
5	560	20.1	0.2	1.0	0.2
6	400	17.3	2.0	11.0	0.8
Advanced stage					
1	40	1.7	1.1	64.7	30.2
2	32	4.1	1.7	41.4	42.2
3	38	3.8	2.5	65.7	79.8
4	18	1.2	0.6	50.0	41.6

NA, not available

estimated. However, this percentage (HIV-1–infected CD4 cells/total peripheral circulating CD4 cells) was often over 50% in patients with end-stage AIDS. This high rate of infection addresses a central dilemma regarding the cause of AIDS. Due to the low estimates of HIV-1 detection in PBMC made several years ago, some people questioned whether HIV-1 was the actual cause of the AIDS disease. The data from the study of PBMCs suggest that infection and destruction of T-helper cells by HIV-1 is a slow but inexorable process that continues until so few (about 1%) T-helper cells are left that the patient eventually succumbs to some other infection or to a malignancy. We will return to this important concept in the discussion of the tissue that is the major site of HIV-1 infection in the asymptomatic person—the lymph node.

SPECIFICITY OF THE HIV-1 SIGNAL IN THE PBMC

The need for carefully monitored controls for PCR *in situ* hybridization and RT *in situ* PCR cannot be overstated. An important negative control for the experiments described above was to use PBMCs from subjects who are HIV-1 negative. Over 20,000 cells from such individuals have been analyzed without obtaining a signal. Another negative control used for studies of viral infected cells is sham-infected cells, as recorded above. This control was used for the HIV studies with no signal noted after the PCR *in situ* hybridization. The signal in the infected pooled lymphocytes was eliminated by overnight DNase digestion but not by RNase digestion (Fig. 9-5). Another way to address the specificity of the *in situ* PCR technique for studies using PBMCs is to make use of the fact that most infected PBMCs will be CD4-positive T-helper cells. By using an immunohistochemical assay for CD4 and other leukocyte phenotypic markers in combination with *in situ* PCR, the infected cells can be colabeled. The chromogen used to detect the amplified DNA–antidigoxigenin dUTP antibody complex was new fuchsin (DAKO, Carpinteria, CA). New fuchsin yields a moderately in-

tense red precipitate that is preferable in colabeling experiments when two different color schemes are used to detect the targets to chromogens such as NBT/BCIP, which yields precipitates that are so intense that it is difficult to see any other colored precipitate. NBT/BCIP is acceptable for colabeling experiments if the other reporter nucleotide is ^{3}H, as the dark black silver grains are not obscured by the blue NBT/BCIP-induced precipitate. After *in situ* PCR, the PBMC sample was dehydrated through graded ethanols and the slides were air dried. The cells were then incubated overnight with a mouse CD4 monoclonal antibody (DAKO) at a dilution of 1:10. The PBMC samples were next incubated for 30 minutes with biotinylated rabbit antimouse antibody (Zymed Laboratories, San Francisco, CA). The primary and secondary antibody complexes were detected using streptavidin–horseradish peroxidase with a 3,3-diaminobenzidine/H_2O_2 solution as the substrate. The cells were treated with a 1% osmium solution for 15 to 30 seconds to intensify the staining, which is manifest as a dark brown rim on the CD4-positive cells. The counterstain was a 1% hematoxylin solution used for 5 minutes. This colabeling experiment demonstrated that almost all of the HIV-1–positive cells were CD4 positive as well (65) (see Color Plate 12 following p. 242). In such colabeling experiments, I have found it preferable to perform the *in situ* PCR reaction first and then to do the immunohistochemical stain.

DETECTION OF HIV-1 INFECTION

In the Lymph Nodes

Of all the anatomic sites that HIV-1 can infect, the most dramatic histologic changes early in the disease process are to be found in the lymph nodes. The systemic lymph adenopathy that characterizes the early, asymptomatic stage of HIV-1 infection is marked by an intense follicular hyperplasia (Fig. 9-6). The germinal centers, which comprise the central region of the follicles, may be expanded to three to five times normal size. The predominant cell in the nor-

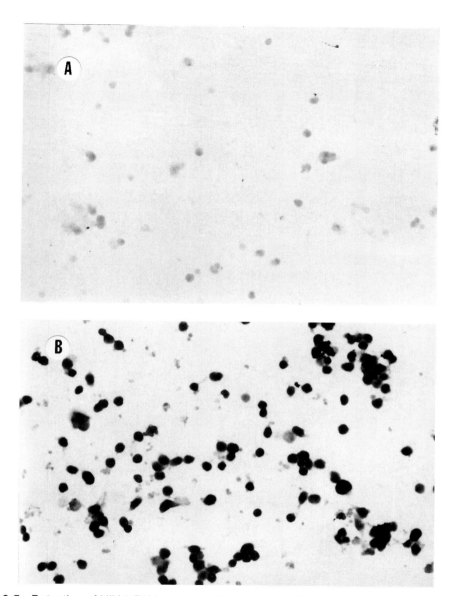

Figure 9-5. *Detection of HIV-1 DNA in infected lymphocytes.* HIV-1 DNA was not detected in lymphocytes infected by HIV-1 when standard *in situ* hybridization was used (**A**). Viral DNA was detectable when *in situ* hybridization was preceded by PCR (**B**). The hybridization signal was lost when the cells were pretreated in DNase (**C**) but persisted when the cells were digested in RNase (**D**).

mal and expanded germinal centers is the dendritic cell. This cell, which contains surface epitopes that react with the antibody against CD21, is the antigen-presenting cell. Thus, it is one of the first cell types to encounter a foreign antigen, which it subsequently "presents" to the CD4 cells and other cells, including the B-cell progenitor immunoblasts, that are also located in the germinal center. As will be discussed later, the CD21 dendritic cell in the lymph node has functional counterparts at other sites, such as the Langerhans cell in the skin and mucosa of the cervix and anus, which also serve as portals of entry for the virus, and, possibly, the as-

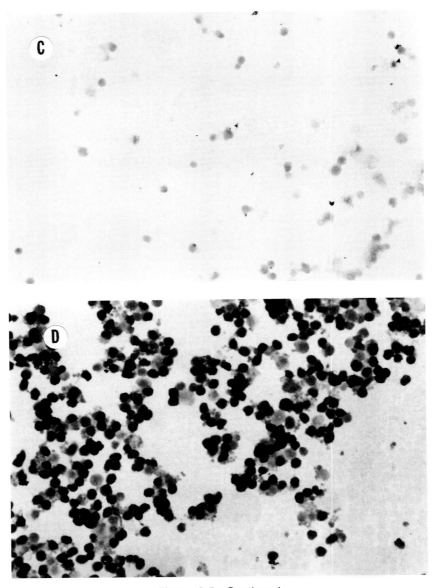

Figure 9-5. *Continued.*

trocytes in the central nervous system (CNS) may have an antigen-presenting function for the resident macrophages. The germinal center in the lymph node is surrounded by a relatively thin mantle zone in which B cells and some CD4 cells are located. This mantle zone is often disrupted in people with the lymphadenopathy that is characteristic of early asymptomatic HIV-1 infection. The lymph node has three other zones, including the parafollic-

ular area, the medullary zone, and the sinus histiocytes. Of these, only the parafollicular zone typically shows changes in pre-AIDS, often being substantially increased in size (Fig. 9-6). This zone is also rich in CD4 cells.

As the disease progresses, certain histologic changes are invariably noted in the lymph nodes. Specifically, in the patient with advanced-stage AIDS, the nodes will have undergone marked atrophy. The follicles are no

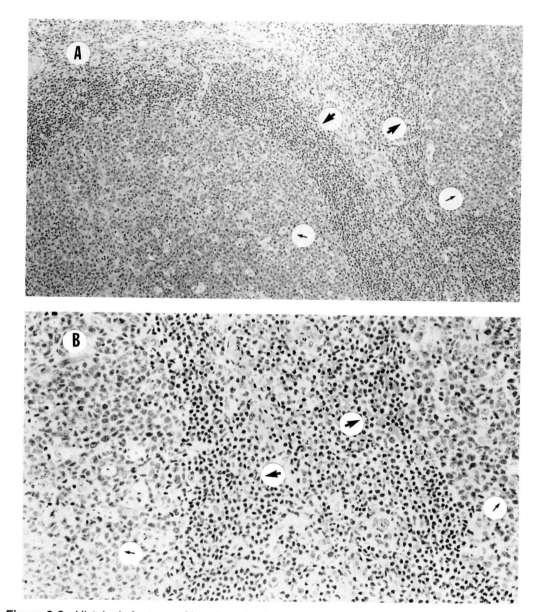

Figure 9-6. *Histologic features of lymph nodes from HIV-1–seropositive patients who are asymptomatic.* The lymph node, which was about three times the normal size, showed marked expansion of the germinal centers on histologic examination (**A**, *small arrows*). Note the surrounding partly disrupted mantle zone and parafollicular zones (A, *large arrows,* and at higher magnification in **B**). Many of the cells in the germinal center are CD21-positive dendritic cells (**C**), whereas the CD4 cells are most plentiful in the parafollicular area (The large and small *arrows* in B and C correspond to those in A.)

longer evident. Rather, one finds a scattering of small and large lymphocytes, histiocytes, and plasma cells. The plasma cell is rarely a predominant cell type in the lymph nodes of patients with asymptomatic HIV-1 infection.

In advanced-stage AIDS, CD21-positive cells are usually not found, but, if present, only rare dendritic cells will be located (Fig. 9-7). Clearly, their scarcity reflects destruction during the evolution of the infection by HIV-1. Similarly,

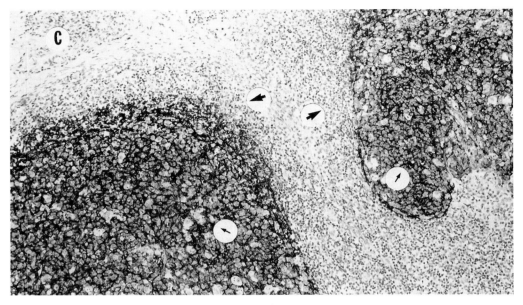

Figure 9-6. *Continued.*

there are few CD4 cells in the lymph nodes of a patient with advanced-stage AIDS, where the CD4 count will be less than 50, which, again, reflects the destruction of these cells during the disease process.

The *in situ* localization of HIV-1 RNA in lymphocytes both in lymph nodes and in peripheral blood has been documented by several groups (61–73). Studies using standard *in situ* hybridization to detect HIV-1 in lymph nodes have shown that viral RNA is routinely detectable, mostly in the dendritic cells found in the germinal center, in patients with AIDS in which follicular hyperplasia is evident. The detection of the viral RNA by standard *in situ* hybridization analyses in these studies suggests that the virus is actively proliferating, as, you will recall, it is difficult to detect latent infection due to the low copy number of the proviral DNA. Lymphocytes that contain viral RNA are not commonly found in patients with advanced-stage AIDS when tested with *in situ* hybridization. The failure to detect this RNA corresponds with the marked depletion of the CD4 T-helper cells and dendritic cells that characterizes advanced-stage AIDS. Few studies report on the detection of HIV-1 DNA in lymph

nodes; Shapshank et al. (49) noted a detection rate of the provirus with standard *in situ* hybridization of about 1%.

The *in situ* detection of PCR-amplified HIV-1 DNA in PBMCs and lymph nodes has been documented by three laboratories at the time this chapter was written (61–73). Each of these groups has independently reported that from 1% to 10% of PBMCs contain HIV-1 DNA, even early in the disease. Furthermore, each has reported that even in the asymptomatic HIV-1 infection as many as 30% of the CD4 lymphocytes in the lymph node can be latently infected by the virus. Recall that the rate estimated by standard *in situ* hybridization is about 1%. As noted above, a central problem in dealing with AIDS is that the detection rate of HIV-1, especially in early-stage asymptomatic infection, has been extremely low using methodologies other than PCR *in situ*. This difficulty with early detection of HIV-1 infection led to uncertainty and concern that the virus may not be the cause of AIDS. PCR *in situ* hybridization was required to demonstrate that a much higher rate of CD4 lymphocytes are infected by the virus even before the patient shows any symptoms.

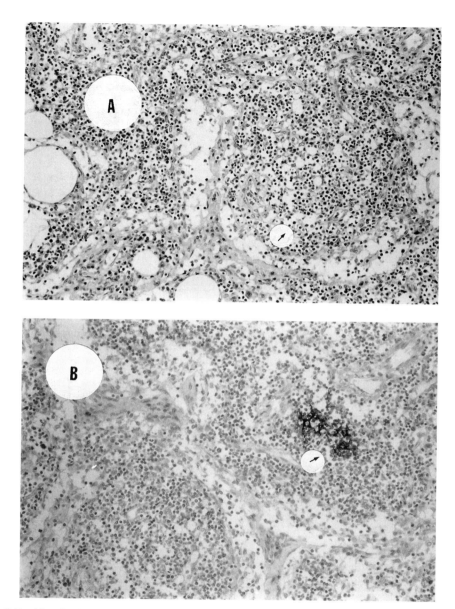

Figure 9-7. *Histologic features of lymph nodes from a patient who died of AIDS.* The lymph node, which was about one-half the normal size, showed loss of the germinal centers and parafollicular zones (**A**). The marked atrophic pattern consists of scattered small and large lymphocytes, macrophages, and plasma cells. Rare CD4 cells are scattered throughout the node (not shown) and either no or only a few CD 21-positive dendritic cells will be detected (**B**). (*Arrows* mark residual germinal center.)

We undertook a study to compare the detection rates of HIV-1 DNA and HIV-1 RNA in cells in the lymph nodes of persons with asymptomatic HIV-1 infection and with late-stage AIDS. The viral distribution was initially de-termined in the lymph nodes of six people with asymptomatic infection and then compared with the distribution in the nodes of six people who died of advanced-stage AIDS. Included in this study were six control lymph nodes from peo-

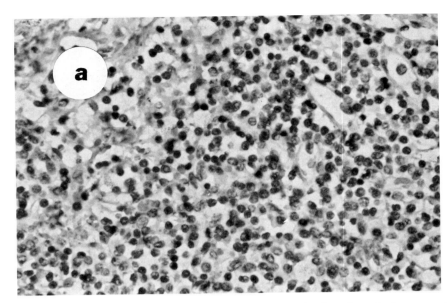

Figure 9-8. *Molecular and immunohistochemical analyses of a lymph node from a patient with advanced AIDS.* The lymph node from this patient, who died of AIDS, showed no CD21-positive dendritic cells, scattered CD4-positive lymphocytes, and many macrophages secondary to infection by *Mycobacterium avium-intracellulare.* **a** shows the routine H&E stain. PCR-amplified HIV-1 DNA (**b**) was detected in scattered lymphocytes and in macrophages. The proportion of cells that contained HIV-1 DNA was similar to the proportion in the serial section that contained HIV-1 RNA as detected by RT *in situ* PCR (**c**). Furthermore, the percentage of HIV-1–infected cells was similar to the percentage of CD4 cells in the lymph node, suggesting, at end-stage AIDS, that basically all remaining CD4 T lymphocytes are actively infected by the virus. (*Arrows* mark viral-positive cells.)

ple who had no risk factors for HIV-1 infection (74).

The 18 lymph nodes were analyzed for HIV-1 DNA using standard *in situ* hybridization. Occasional positive cells that localized to the germinal centers were noted in one of the six lymph nodes from patients with asymptomatic HIV-1 infection. None of the six tissues from patients with advanced-stage AIDS had detectable virus using standard *in situ* hybridization. HIV-1 was not detected in any of the six controls. However, PCR-amplified HIV-1 DNA was detected *in situ* in each of the 12 lymph nodes from the HIV-1–infected patients and in none of the six controls. The specificity of the signal was demonstrated by its absence with the omission of *Taq* polymerase or with the use of irrelevant (HPV-specific) primers. Furthermore, the pattern of distribution of the PCR-amplified HIV-1 DNA was equivalent with two different primer pairs and corresponding probes

(i.e., the SK38 and SK39 primers and the SK19 probe, as well as the SK145 and SK431 primers and the SK102 probe) used in this study. The use of serial tissue sections, which are 4μm apart, provides an opportunity for positive controls by permitting comparative tests on the same cells in adjacent sections. When examined by PCR *in situ* hybridization, the number of cells with detectable provirus increased by at least 100-fold in the one tissue that was positive by standard *in situ* hybridization. This increased sensitivity again highlights the importance of using PCR amplification for the provirus. Recall that the SK19 oligoprobe does not detect the viral message as it is in the sense direction.

As noted, the virus was found to localize to the germinal centers and to the parafollicular zones in lymph nodes from patients with asymptomatic HIV-1 infection. Immunohistochemical analysis of the serial sections showed

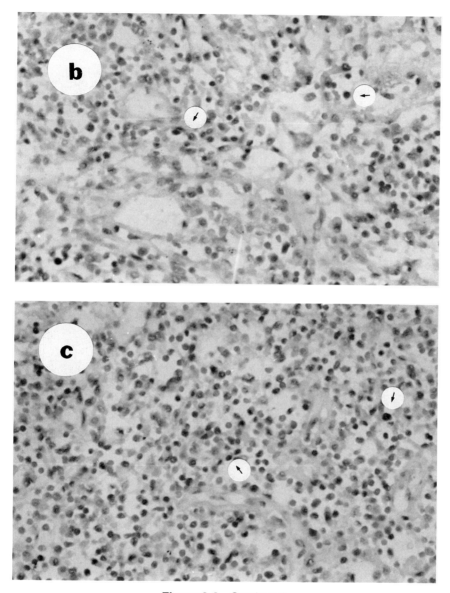

Figure 9-8. *Continued.*

that the HIV-1–positive cells corresponded to the areas where the CD21-positive dendritic cells and CD4-positive lymphocytes were most numerous (see Color Plate 13 following p. 242). The PCR-amplified viral DNA was not detected in the medullary zone, where CD4-positive cells are rarely seen, and viral DNA was rarely noted in sinusoidal histiocytes. Lymph nodes from patients with advanced-stage AIDS demon-strated, in general, fewer HIV-1–positive cells, reflecting the marked depletion of lymphocytes and dendritic cells. The positive cells found in patients with advanced-stage AIDS were dispersed throughout the lymph node, although they tended to be more frequent toward the capsular sinus (Fig. 9-8). This was the same pattern seen with the immunohistochemical stain for CD4. Each of the six lymph nodes from the

Table 9-3. *Viral and CD4 findings in lymph nodes in HIV-1–infected patients*

Case no.	% of small lymphocytes positive for CD4[a]	Ratio of HIV-1 DNA+ cells to CD4+ cells in identical area of serial section	Ratio of HIV-1 RNA+ cells to HIV-1 DNA+ cells in identical area of serial section
Asymptomatic			
1	32	0.4	0.8
2	24	0.2	0.2
3	22	0.8	0.5
4	20	0.05	0.0
5	30	0.5	0.05
6	25	0.2	0.3
Advanced stage			
1	1	1.0	1.0
2	1	1.0	1.0
3	9	1.0	1.1
4	8	1.0	1.1
5	5	1.2	1.2
6	8	1.0	1.0

[a]The CD4+ cells localized to the parafollicular areas in the lymph nodes from asymptomatic patients and toward the capsular area in the lymph nodes from the patients who died of AIDS. Because the colabeling of PCR-amplified HIV-1 nucleic acids and CD4 led to a decrease in the number of CD4+ cells, these analyses were done using the identical regions in serial sections of the regions where the CD4+ cells were most plentiful. The numbers are based on counting 100 to 350 cells in each serial section (74).

patients who died of AIDS had many plasma cells that did not show HIV-1 DNA by PCR *in situ* hybridization. These plasma cells served as an internal negative control.

To quantify the proportion of CD21-positive and CD4-positive cells that were infected by HIV-1, the subjacent (i.e., serial) sections were incubated with monoclonal antibodies to CD21 and CD4 and compared with the next serial section analyzed by PCR *in situ* hybridization. These separate analyses were required for quantification of the number of target-infected cells because, although HIV-1 DNA-positive cells could be colabeled with antibodies to CD4 or CD21, it was noted that there was a significant decrease in the number of antigen-positive cells after cycling and hybridization. The CD4 analyses were done by comparing the number of CD4-positive cells with the number of HIV-1 DNA- and HIV-1 RNA-positive cells using identical regions in serial sections of areas where the CD4-positive cells were most plentiful. Similarly, the dendritic cell analyses were done by comparing the number of CD21-positive cells in a germinal center with the HIV-1 DNA- and HIV-1 RNA-positive cells in serial sections of the same germinal center.

The results of these experiments are listed in Tables 9-3 and 9-4. The percentage of CD4-positive cells present in the lymph nodes from patients with asymptomatic HIV-1 infection ranged from 20% to 32% of the small parafollicular lymphocytes, which was slightly less than the percentage found in the non-HIV-1–infected controls. In marked contrast, the proportion of CD4-positive small lymphocytes in the lymph nodes of the people with advanced-stage AIDS was only 1% to 9% in parallel with the loss of CD4-positive cells in their blood (Table 9-3). Furthermore, CD21-positive dendritic cells were not detected in four of the six lymph nodes from people who died of AIDS while the other two patients had only rare dendritic cells. This finding is in contrast to the predominance of this cell type in the lymph nodes from the asymptomatic patients (Table 9-4). It is also evident that the proportion of HIV-1 DNA-positive/CD4-positive cells was close to 100% in all people with advanced-stage AIDS (Table 9-3). In contrast, this proportion ranged from 5% to 80% (mean 35%) in patients with asymptomatic infection.

PCR-amplified viral RNA (cDNA) was detected in serial sections using RT *in situ* PCR (Fig. 9-8). These results are also compiled in

Table 9-4. *Viral and CD21 findings in lymph nodes in patients with asymptomatic HIV-1 infection*[a]

Case no.	% of cells in the germinal center positive for CD21	Ratio of HIV-1 DNA+ cells to CD21+ cells in identical area of serial section	Ratio of HIV-1 RNA+ cells to HIV-1 DNA+ cells in identical area of serial section
1	45	0.2	0.5
2	25	0.1	1.0
3	33	0.5	0.4
4	5	0.0	0.0
5	20	0.3	0.0
6	25	0.1	0.3

[a]CD21+ dendritic cells were not seen in four of six lymph nodes in patients with advanced-stage AIDS, and only rare CD21+ cells were seen in the other two nodes. The CD21+ cells are found in the germinal centers. Because the colabeling of PCR-amplified HIV-1 nucleic acids and CD21 led to a decrease in the number of CD21+ cells, these analyses were done using the identical regions of the germinal centers in serial sections. The numbers are based on counting 100 to 350 cells in each serial section (74).

Tables 9-3 and 9-4. To demonstrate the integrity of the RNA in the lymph nodes, RT *in situ* PCR was done using primers for CD3 mRNA (kindly provided by Dr. D. Volkmann, SUNY at Stony Brook). The distribution and number of CD3-positive cells were consistent with the distribution of the T cells in the lymph nodes. Virtually all of the cells with HIV-1 DNA also had viral RNA in each of the lymph nodes from patients with advanced-stage AIDS. This result differed markedly from the findings in the lymph nodes of patients with asymptomatic infection where the ratio of HIV-1 RNA-positive to HIV-1 DNA-positive cells in the parafollicular zone ranged from 0 to 0.8, with a mean of 0.3. The SK38 and SK39 primers cannot distinguish between genomic HIV-1 RNA and spliced transcripts (see Color Plate 14 following p. 242). A primer pair that either does not amplify or poorly amplifies a target in genomic viral RNA due to its large size of 3,500 base pairs and robustly amplifies 250 base pairs after splicing in the *rev* and *tat* exons (kindly provided by Dr. Roger Pomerantz) produced an intense signal after RT *in situ* PCR in most of the cells that showed a signal using the other primer pairs. Plasma cells, common in the advanced-stage nodes, were uniformly HIV-1 RNA negative. Macrophages were common only in the lymph nodes of patients with advanced AIDS, and their rate of HIV-1 DNA positivity ranged from 5% to 15%; the virus in the infected macrophages was actively replicating as the de-

tection rate of HIV-1 RNA in these cells was also 5% to 15%.

In summary, there were two primary findings in this study. First, the percentage of HIV-1–infected CD4 cells in the lymph nodes (and peripheral blood) of patients with advanced disease was about 100%, whereas this rate was much lower (from 5% to 80% in lymph nodes and 1% to 5% in blood) in the asymptomatic HIV-1–infected patients. Second, in the advanced stage of AIDS the infection is marked by the ubiquitous presence of genomic and multiply spliced viral transcripts, suggesting actively replicating virus. In marked contrast, in asymptomatic patients the infection is primarily latent, as typically a relatively small percentage of the HIV-1 DNA positive cells have viral transcripts.

Although the 5% to 80% (mean 30%) of infected CD4 cells may seem low compared with the rate for patients with end-stage AIDS, this is 30% of the total CD4 pool of the body, which resides primarily in the lymph nodes. There are about 60 billion CD4 cells in the body. Thus, about 20 billion CD4 cells, on average, are infected in the person with pre-AIDS. Of these about 1:20 are actively infected, corresponding to about 1 billion cells. This is an enormous viral load. Early in the disease process, the body is capable of replacing these 1 billion CD4 cells that are being destroyed by the virus, presumably on a daily basis. At end stage, only about 2 billion CD4 cells remain, and basically all are actively infected. These numbers certainly are consistent with the notion that HIV-1 infection is the primary agent in the pathogenesis of AIDS.

This study provided confirmation that the dendritic cells are a major target of HIV-1 infection in asymptomatic HIV-1 infection, as noted by several groups (61–73). The virtual absence of CD21 cells in lymph nodes from patients with CD4 counts less than 50 and the paucity of CD4 cells in these nodes explains why the total number of HIV-1–positive cells is lower in these nodes relative to patients with asymptomatic HIV-1 infection, as noted in this study. These observations are consistent with those of Pantaleo et al. (68,73). Our finding that a greater percentage of CD4 cells are infected in the lymph nodes relative to the blood in asymptomatic HIV-1 infection is also consistent with the findings of others (68,73). However, our results as well as those reported by others (61–74) using PCR *in situ* hybridization suggest that in advanced AIDS most of the circulating CD4 PBMCs are HIV-1 positive, as is true in the lymph nodes. These results are in contrast to findings in other studies in which PCR *in situ*–based techniques were not employed where much smaller percentages of HIV-1–infected PBMC were noted.

The observations in this study in conjunction with other studies using PCR *in situ* hybridization suggest a model for the evolution of HIV-1 infection (Fig. 9-9). In asymptomatic HIV-1 infection an average of about 30% of the CD4 cells in the lymph nodes are HIV-1 DNA positive. These HIV-1–infected T-helper cells are concentrated around the germinal centers, where the viral-infected CD21 follicular dendritic cell predominates. Typically, most of the infected cells, including the lymphocytes and follicular dendritic cells, do not have detectable viral RNA. It is not clear whether the cells that contain provirus alone or contain provirus and rare transcripts are dysfunctional, although it is feasible that latently infected cells are still able to function normally. Regardless, at this stage of HIV-1 infection most CD4 lymphocytes do not contain HIV-1 DNA or RNA and, despite large-scale latent infection, the person does not show any symptoms.

As noted above, many of the dendritic cells in the nodes are also infected by HIV-1. Studies based on standard HIV-1 RNA *in situ* hybridization have suggested that the virus is trapped on the cell membranes of the dendritic cells. Using PCR *in situ* hybridization we were able to show that the dendritic cells contained HIV-1 DNA in their nucleus, demonstrating that the virus has entered the cells.

A key concept is that disease progression is secondary to activation of viral transcription, spread of the infection to the other CD4 cells, and a concomitant loss of CD21 and CD4 cells. At the end stage, virtually all CD4 PBMCs and lymphocytes in lymph nodes are actively infected by the virus and are presumably dysfunctional. This model suggests that a key parameter for therapeutic interventions against HIV-1 infection is the ratio of HIV-1 DNA-positive to HIV-1 RNA-positive target cells. One may speculate that the marked variability in the proportion of HIV-1-positive to CD4 lymphocytes and HIV-1 RNA-positive to HIV-1 DNA-positive cells in the lymph nodes of asymptomatic patients may be predictive of the subsequent clinical course. This suggestion should be addressed by prospective studies. We are in the process of performing such studies. Such analyses are best done using lymph node biopsies given the small number of HIV-1 RNA-positive PBMCs early in the disease and will likely require the *in situ* PCR-based technologies given the markedly increased detection rate compared with standard *in situ* hybridization.

Although there is massive, primarily latent infection of the CD4 and CD21 cells in the lymph node by HIV-1 early in the disease process, it is reasonable to speculate that the dramatic histological changes may reflect the presence of another virus. A prime suspect would be Epstein-Barr virus (EBV), given its strong tropism for B lymphocytes and its association with several diseases in people with AIDS, notably lymphoma. We analyzed six lymph nodes from people with asymptomatic HIV-1 infection for EBV as well as an additional 15 lymph nodes from additional people at various stages of HIV-1 disease. Analysis of these additional 15 lymph nodes for HIV-1 DNA and

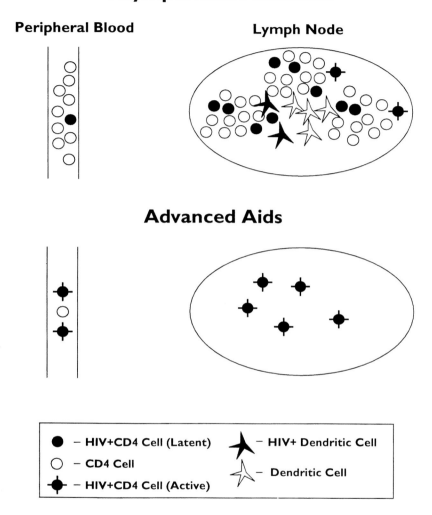

Figure 9-9. *Proposed model for the natural progression of HIV-1 infection.* The key elements of this model include latent infection of many CD4-positive lymphocytes and dendritic cells in the lymph nodes and relatively few CD4-positive PBMCs during the asymptomatic phase of the disease. It should be stressed that the proportions of HIV-1–infected CD4-positive lymphocytes and the ratio of latent to active infection appear to be highly variable while the patient is asymptomatic. Disease progression is marked by activation of viral RNA synthesis and destruction of the dendritic cells and the CD4-positive lymphocytes. Thus, at the end stage of AIDS, many of the few remaining CD4-positive lymphocytes are actively infected both in the lymph node and in the peripheral blood.

RNA yielded data similar to those presented in Tables 9-3 and 9-4. EBV DNA was detectable in each of these lymph nodes by PCR *in situ* hybridization; the percentage of infected cells detected was much greater than with standard *in situ* hybridization. The EBV-infected cells localized to the mantle zone, where B cells are plentiful; the B cells colabeled with the phenotypic marker L26 (Fig. 9-10). PCR-amplified EBV DNA was noted, on average, in about 20%

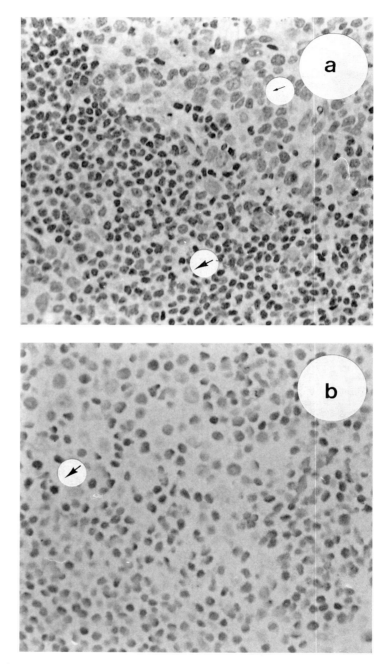

Figure 9-10. *Histologic and molecular analyses of a hyperplastic lymph node in an asymptomatic person seropositive for HIV-1.* **a:** The lymph node was grossly enlarged and showed expanded germinal centers (*small arrow*) and mantle zones (*large arrow*) as well as enlarged parafollicular zones. **b:** EBV DNA was detected in a few cells from this region using standard *in situ* hybridization (*arrow*). **c:** Many more EBV-positive cells were evident after PCR *in situ* hybridization after analysis of the serial section on the same glass slide. **d:** PCR-amplified HIV-1 DNA was also detected in this area.

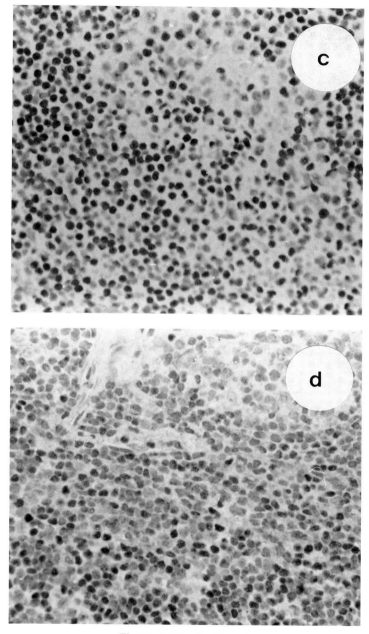

Figure 9-10. *Continued.*

of the L26-containing cells. Thus, the dramatic lymphadenopathy characteristic of early HIV-1 infection reflects the synergistic involvement by HIV-1 and EBV that are infecting different target cells that are in close proximity.

As noted above, EBV has been associated with AIDS lymphoma. We used PCR *in situ* hybridization to study the distribution of HIV-1 and EBV DNA in AIDS lymphomas (J. Becker and G.J. Nuovo, *unpublished observations,*

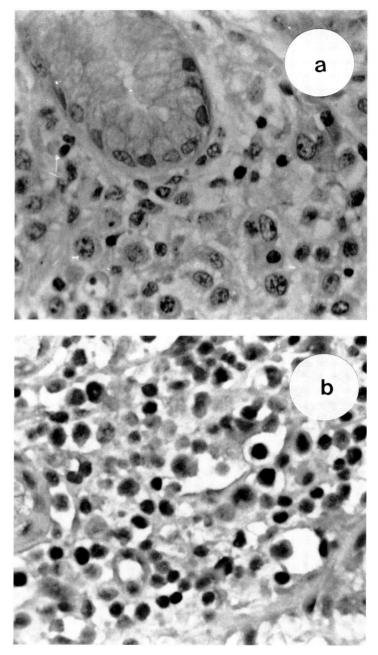

Figure 9-11. *Histologic and molecular analyses of an AIDS-related lymphoma.* This immunoblastic lymphoma was detected in the submandibular gland. Rare benign lymphocytes are admixed with the malignant lymphocytes (**a**). EBV DNA was detected in many of the malignant cells when PCR *in situ* hybridization was performed (**b**). Only rare nonmalignant lymphoid cells contained PCR-amplified HIV-1 DNA (**c**, *arrow*).

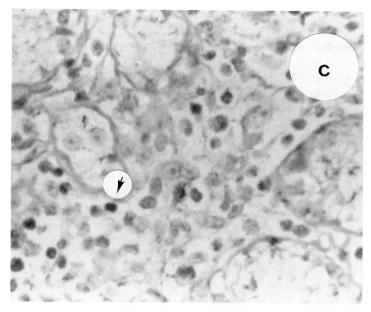

Figure 9-11. *Continued.*

1996). Amplified EBV DNA was detected in five of eight AIDS non-Hodgkin's lymphomas, but in only three of these tissues did the viral DNA localize to the malignant cells. HIV-1 DNA was detected in four of these lymphomas and localized to non-neoplastic lymphocytes; the proviral DNA was not detected directly in lymphoma cells (Fig. 9-11). It is concluded that, although many cells in hyperplastic lymph nodes from people with early HIV-1 infection contain HIV-1 and EBV DNA, HIV-1 is absent and EBV is variably present in the malignant cells of AIDS-related lymphoma. This is in marked contrast to HPV, which is invariably found in cervical cancers as discussed in Chapter 8. This suggests that, although infection by EBV and HIV-1 and the concomitant lymphoid hyperplasia may predispose to lymphoma, the viruses are not required for maintenance of the malignant phenotype.

In Skeletal Muscle in Patients with Myopathy

The association of muscle disease and HIV-1 infection is well documented (75–84). Myopathy can occur early in the course of the dis-

ease and may be the first manifestation. The course of muscle disease in patients with AIDS is commonly a subacute progression of proximal weakness with elevation of creatinine kinase, although a rhabdomyolytic episode may be the presenting feature. Several morphologic categories of primary HIV-associated myopathy have been described. These include polymyositis characterized by inflammatory cell infiltrates and myocyte necrosis, necrotizing myopathy without inflammatory infiltrates, and myopathy with nemaline rods. In addition to primary HIV-1–associated muscle disease, secondary involvement of muscle by other pathogens and drug toxicity, notably AZT, has been reported.

It is not known if primary HIV-associated myopathy is a direct consequence of HIV-1 infection of muscle tissue. As was true in the lymph nodes and PBMCs, a major impediment to understanding HIV-1–induced skeletal muscle disease is that the viral DNA and, at times, RNA may be difficult to localize directly by *in situ* hybridization.

The question of HIV-1 localization in the skeletal muscle was examined by our group. Thirteen skeletal muscle biopsies were includ-

Table 9-5. *Clinical and pathological findings in the HIV-1–infected patients included in one study*[a]

Case no.	Age (years)/ sex	Clinical features	HIV-1 serostatus at biopsy	AZT treatment	CPK value	Pathology (necrosis/ inflammation)	HIV-1 DNA/RNA
1a	41/M	Increasing weakness	Positive	Stopped 6 weeks prior to biopsy	Elevated	+/+	+/+
1b	36/M	Subacute progressive proximal weakness	Unknown; positive 5 years later (see 1a)	No	1,000	+/+	+/+
2	30/M	Progressive muscle weakness, myalgia	Positive	Not known	500	+/Mild	–/–
3	36/M	Progressive muscle weakness	Positive	Yes	390	+/+	+/+
4	29/F	Fever?, vasculitis	Positive	Unknown	Unknown	+/Mild	–/–
5	30/M	Acute weakness, myalgia	Positive	No	6,000	+/Mild	+/–
6	38/M	1-year progressive proximal weakness	Unknown (positive 1 year later)	No	2,000	+/+	–/–

[a]Analysis by PCR *in situ* hybridization and RT *in situ* PCR, respectively (86).

ed in this study. Seven of these tissues were from patients diagnosed as HIV-1 positive either at the time of biopsy (five cases) or subsequent to the biopsy (two cases). Although there is no serological evidence to support or refute that the latter two patients had HIV-1 infection at the time of biopsy, it was decided to include these patients in the category of "HIV-1 positive" given that the infection was documented by serological testing subsequently. The other six biopsy specimens were controls from patients with no evidence of HIV-1 infection. Clinical and pathological information concerning these patients is provided in Table 9-5 (see also ref. 86).

Of the seven muscle biopsies from patients with HIV-1 infection, five had pathological findings consistent with polymyositis. The other two patients also showed muscle fiber necrosis, but the degree of inflammation was deemed not substantial enough for a diagnosis of myositis (Table 9-5). The control tissues showed myositis associated with rheumatoid arthritis, polymyositis, inclusion body myositis, and unremarkable muscle. These 13 tissues were analyzed for sequences homologous to HIV-1

DNA using *in situ* hybridization with and without prior PCR amplification. Serial sections were studied using the probes SK19, and probe SK102, respectively, which each correspond to the *gag* region. A hybridization signal was evident in only one of the seven muscle biopsies from the patients with HIV-1 infection using standard *in situ* hybridization; only rare positive cells were noted in that given case (Fig. 9-12). When *in situ* hybridization was preceded by PCR amplification with the appropriate oligomers (SK38/SK39 and SK145/SK431 for SK19 and SK102, respectively), the detection rate increased to four of seven for the patients with HIV-1 infection. Furthermore, the number of cells with detectable viral DNA in the positive case increased by about 100-fold (Fig. 9-12). This increase in detection rate is equivalent to the increase observed in the lymph node study and again underscores the importance of using the PCR *in situ* hybridization technique to ascertain the histologic distribution of the virus in tissues and organs.

Reflecting the sensitivity of the technique, features defining successful PCR *in situ* hybridization that are evident in Fig. 9-12 include

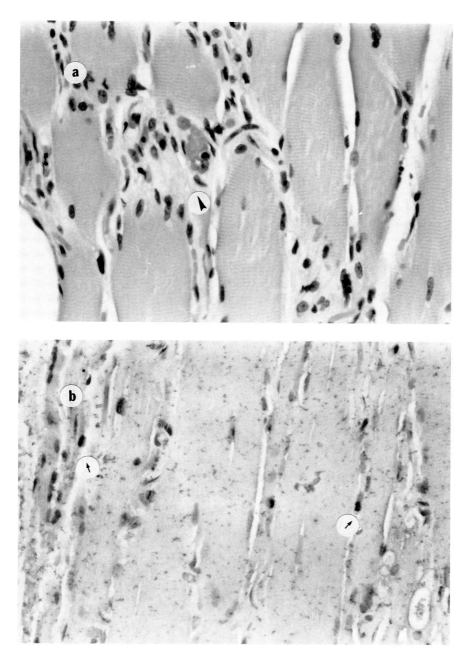

Figure 9-12. *Detection of HIV-1 DNA in skeletal muscle biopsy material from a patient with AIDS.* This tissue showed areas of myocyte necrosis and inflammation (**a**, *arrowhead*). Rare HIV-1 DNA-positive cells were detected in these areas by standard *in situ* hybridization (**b**, *arrows*). The number of cells with detectable provirus increased markedly when the *in situ* assay was preceded by PCR amplification as seen in the serial section (**c**, *arrows*).

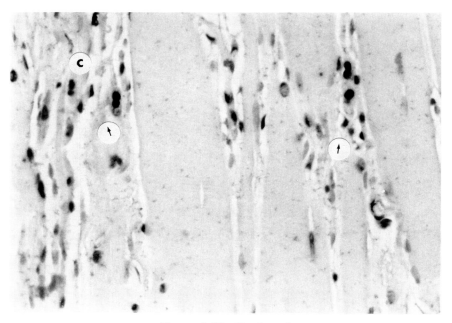

Figure 9-12. *Continued.*

(i) an increase in the number of positive cells after PCR *in situ* hybridization compared with the results for *in situ* hybridization in a serial section and (ii) increased intensity after PCR amplification in some of the cells that were positive by standard *in situ* hybridization. The PCR-enhanced hybridization signal was not evident when the tissue was DNased prior to PCR if the *Taq* polymerase was omitted or if irrelevant primers specific for HPV type 18 (which does not infect muscle tissue) were employed, again underscoring the need for the negative controls when interpreting test results. It cannot be overstated that the negative controls should be routine in the PCR *in situ* assay as they provide additional information concerning the specificity of the signal. PCR-amplified HIV-1 DNA was not detected in any of the six control cases. This is a critical negative control because tissues can differ markedly in their background (nonspecific) signal, especially when using internal oligoprobes (G.J. Nuovo, *unpublished observations,* 1993; discussed in detail in Chapter 4).

The HIV-1 DNA-positive cells often localized to areas of myocyte necrosis (Fig. 9-12).

Many of the viral-infected cells had round to oval nuclei and ample cytoplasm suggestive of macrophages. Other nuclei were elongated and located subjacent to the sarcolemmal membrane and, thus, were cytologically suggestive of myocytes. Perhaps the most powerful aspect of PCR *in situ* hybridization, unlike solution phase PCR, is that the target can be directly localized to a specific cell type. Still, it is often useful to confirm further the identity of the positive cells using double labeling with immunohistochemistry. This double labeling was done with the skeletal muscle biopsies after PCR *in situ* hybridization by using antibodies that react against epitopes for LCA (specific for lymphocytes and macrophages) and Mac387 (specific for macrophages). There was little loss of the immunologic signal for these two antigens after PCR *in situ* amplification of the viral DNA in contrast with the CD4 and CD21, which, as noted above, were not as reliably detected after the PCR *in situ* hybridization step. Although the immunohistochemistry was attempted first, it was noted that the PCR signal was diminished in such cases and that the chromogen that marks the antigen–antibody complex became less intense after the PCR cycling. These colabeling experiments demonstrated that many of the HIV-1–infected cells were macrophages and that some of the viral-infected cells that did not colabel with either LCA or Mac387 had the elongate nuclei and subsarcolemmal localization of myocyte nuclei (86).

To ascertain whether the infection was latent or active with viral transcription, the positive tissues were analyzed for HIV-1 RNA with RT *in situ* PCR and the downstream primers SK39 and SK431, respectively. These results were equivalent to the results for the detection of HIV-1 DNA: four of the seven cases were positive, and none of the controls showed a signal. The number and distribution of HIV-1 RNA-positive cells from the viral positive biopsies were equivalent with that of PCR-amplified HIV-1 DNA (Fig. 9-13). This 1:1 ratio of HIV-1 DNA/HIV-1 RNA implies an activated infection. The specificity of the signal using RT *in situ* PCR was demonstrated by its loss with the omission of the RT step, the use of the HPV 18-specific primers (Fig. 9-13), the absence of a signal in any of the viral negative controls, and its persistence with the use of the internal oligoprobe in the absence of the direct incorporation of digoxigenin dUTP, i.e., RT PCR *in situ* hybridization (9,11). The controls in this study serve to illustrate that the DNase/no RT and DNase/irrelevant primer RT are critical negative controls that must be done for every tissue when performing direct incorporation RT *in situ* PCR. The primer pair that dictates a product of about 3,500 base pairs in genomic viral RNA and 250 base pairs after multiple splicing (kindly provided by Dr. Roger Pomerantz, as noted above) but does not or only poorly amplifies genomic length RNA produced a signal after RT *in situ* PCR in most of the cells that showed a signal using the other primer pairs. This implies that the infection was "wild type," i.e., with the production of multiply spliced transcripts and, presumably, infectious particles. Cells positive for p24 were identified in two of the four viral-positive tissues, but in far fewer cells than had detectable viral DNA or transcripts. This observation is certainly true for HIV-1 infection in a wide variety of tissues

and is reminiscent of the poor detection rate of HPV proteins by immunohistochemistry in high-grade SILs and cancers when compared with localization of the viral-associated nucleic acids.

In summary, this study based on PCR *in situ* hybridization showed that HIV-1 DNA and RNA could be detected in the muscle biopsies of patients with myopathy (85). This does not prove that HIV-1 is the cause of myopathy in these patients. The HIV-1–positive macrophages could be "innocent bystanders" that simply were "captured" in the skeletal muscle at the time of biopsy. However, certain observations suggest that HIV-1 may indeed have a causative role in AIDS myopathy. First, the macrophages that were viral positive were much more common in the areas of muscle fiber necrosis. Macrophages in adjoining fascicles where there was no myocyte necrosis were usually HIV-1 negative. If HIV-1–positive macrophages in the muscle tissues simply reflected viral-infected "transients," one would anticipate that they would be as common in regions of normal muscle fibers. Second, the observation that occasional myocyte nuclei were HIV-1 positive also supports a direct role for the virus in AIDS myopathy. These observations illustrate the ability to ascertain and evaluate the geographic distribution of the target of interest using PCR *in situ* hybridization. Cells can be seen that *do not* have the target (even one copy of the target) of interest, which is information that, in the case of HIV-1 and other viral infections, is often as useful as knowing which cells do contain the target of interest.

An intriguing result in this study was that muscle biopsy material from one patient was positive for HIV-1 prior to documentation of seroconversion. This suggests that infection by HIV-1 of certain tissues besides the lymph nodes and CD4 PBMCs may be an early event and may precede clinically evident disease. CNS involvement was also found to be an early manifestation of HIV-1 infection in some cases, as is discussed below.

The absence of HIV-1 nucleic acids in three of the cases suggests that either the virus was present but not detected due to sampling or that

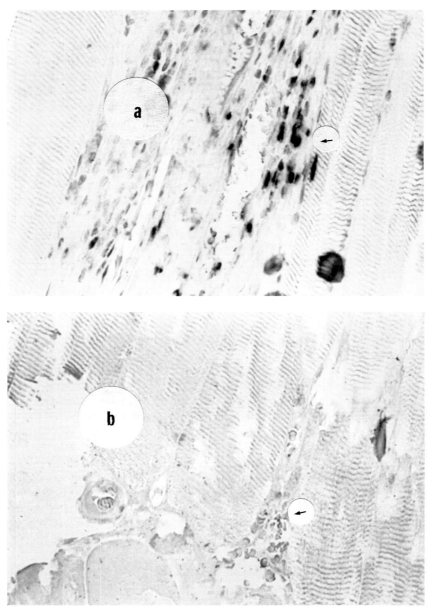

Figure 9-13. *Detection of activated viral infection in skeletal muscle tissue of a patient with AIDS.* HIV-1 DNA was detected by PCR *in situ* hybridization in this biopsy (not shown). In this same muscle biopsy, HIV-1 RNA was detected in areas of myocyte necrosis and inflammation by the RT *in situ* PCR technique (**a**, *arrow*). The RNA-derived signal was eliminated when the RT step was omitted or when the RT and PCR steps were done with HPV-specific nonsense primers (**b**).

HIV-1 may play a role in some but not all cases of HIV-1 myopathy. Further studies are needed to determine whether the virus can be routinely detected in the skeletal muscle of HIV-1–infected patients without myopathy and, if so, if the infection is active or in a latent form. Specifically, it would be interesting to see how often HIV-1 is detected in the skeletal muscle from patients who die of AIDS, and an extensive study would be possible as the size of the tissue in autopsy material is not a limiting factor for the analyses. Our preliminary data in this regard are that viral DNA is rarely detected in the skeletal muscle of people who die of AIDS and who have muscle-specific symptoms.

Leon-Monzon et al. (86) have recently reported the inability to culture HIV-1 from myotubules of patients with AIDS myopathy. Whether this reflects that the culturing technique is less sensitive than the *in situ* PCR requires further study. It is interesting in this regard that the ability of HIV-1–related retroviruses SAIDS D and the human foamy retrovirus to infect myocyte tissue cultures and skeletal muscle in a transgenic mouse model, respectively, have been reported (83,84), suggesting that HIV-1 may be able to infect myocytes directly, presumably those that are regenerating and are mitotically active.

In the Central Nervous System

The presence of HIV-1 in skeletal muscle tissues, in lymph nodes, and in PBMCs provides very important information about the nature of some of the clinical manifestations of AIDS. From a clinical standpoint, perhaps the CNS is the most critical site to study. Clinically overt dysfunction of the CNS is found in the majority of patients with AIDS, especially in the later stages of their disease (87–98). The symptoms are often profound and among the most severe suffered by patients with AIDS. Several observations including the neurotropism of the retroviral family, to which HIV-1 belongs, and detection of the virus or its antigens in cerebrospinal fluid (CSF) prior to neurological symptomatology suggest that early CNS infection is common. The clinical manifestations of AIDS dementia suggests a diffuse CNS process in that most of the different regions of the brain and spinal cord may show clinical evidence of dysfunction, although cerebral involvement predominates based on clinical findings that include memory loss and difficulty in a variety of cognitive functions. The histological changes that may be seen in AIDS dementia include neuronal loss, myelin loss, and the char-

acteristic microglial nodules. Multinucleated macrophage cells are sometimes seen, although these may not be evident even in sections of the CNS from patients who have clear-cut neurological symptomatology.

In the attempt to understand the clinical presentation of AIDS CNS disease and the histological changes observed, it is important to discover which specific cells are susceptible to HIV-1 infection in the CNS. *In vivo* and *in vitro* studies have suggested that all the cell components of the CNS—neurons, astrocytes, macrophages/microglial cells, and oligodendroglial cells—can be infected by the virus (87–98). The molecular mechanism for CNS damage induced by HIV-1 is also unclear at this time. Several nonexclusive hypotheses include gp120 neuronal toxicity, immunologic-mediated damage due to common epitopes such as gp41 and an astrocyte cell surface antigen, and the production of cytokines such as tumor necrosis factor (TNF) by microglial cells and/or astrocytes that hinders neuronal function and can cause oligodendroglial cell death and, thus, demyelinization (Fig. 9-14).

Although several investigators have detected HIV-1 in the CNS using standard *in situ* hybridization, the number of infected cells seemed too low relative to the patient's neurologic status to explain the profound clinical dysfunction. It is clear that PCR *in situ* hybridization may be able to offer important insights into the CNS disease that is commonly found in patients with AIDS. Our group undertook a study with the purpose to use the *in situ* PCR-amplification techniques for viral DNA and RNA with the colabeling of the cell phenotype to identify the cells in the CNS that are infected by HIV-1. In addition, the initial part of the study would explore the extent and cell localization of the cytokines TNF and interleukin-1 (IL-1), as these have each been implicated in AIDS dementia. Subsequently, expression of the cytokines macrophage inflammatory protein-α (MIP-1α) and -β (MIP-1β) as well as inducible nitric oxide synthetase (iNOS) were also studied. The colabeling experiments were done with antibodies against leukocyte common antigen (LCA; lymphocytes and macrophages, 1:40), Mac 387 (macrophages, 1:500), GFAP (astro-

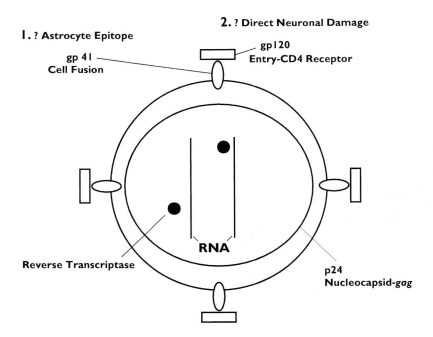

1. ? Astrocyte Epitope

gp 41
Cell Fusion

2. ? Direct Neuronal Damage

gp120
Entry-CD4 Receptor

RNA

Reverse Transcriptase

p24
Nucleocapsid-*gag*

3. Direct infection of Neurons and Astrocytes

4. Viral Induced Cytokine Production (eg, TNF)

Figure 9-14. *Potential causes for AIDS dementia.* Possible explanations for the dementia that is common in patients with AIDS is presented. These hypotheses include direct neuronal damage by gp120, cross-reactivity between HIV-1 and astrocyte antigens, direct viral infection, and upregulation of cytokine production by the virus.

cytes, 1:400), neuron-specific enolase (neurons, 1:30) monoclonal antibody (DAKO), biotin-labeled RCA-1 (microglial cells/macrophages, 1:6,000) (Sigma Chemicals), or rabbit anti-galactose cerebroside (oligodendroglial cells, 1:100) (Sigma) (dilutions in parentheses), which covers the entire range of cell types that can be found in the CNS. It was demonstrated that the antigenicities of these epitopes were either not affected or, at most, minimally decreased by the protease digestion and heating from the PCR cycling and hybridization steps.

Initially a total of 21 CNS tissues were studied. Tissue samples were taken from the cerebrum, cerebellum, brain stem, and spinal cord from seven patients with AIDS (14 tissue samples; one to three blocks per patient) and seven patients without evidence of HIV-1 infection (seven tissue samples). Several of the patients

had severe dementia that correlated with widespread CNS histologic changes, including marked neuronal loss evident on routine histological staining, demyelinization, and the microglial nodules and multinucleated giant cells diagnostic of HIV-1 encephalitis. Other cases showed either minimal or "nonspecific" CNS changes in patients who did not have any overt clinical evidence of AIDS dementia. The tissues were analyzed for sequences homologous to HIV-1 DNA using standard *in situ* hybridization with and without prior PCR amplification. Serial sections were studied using probes SK19 and SK102, respectively. The results can be summarized as follows:

1. HIV-1 DNA was detected by standard *in situ* hybridization in less than one-half of the tissues of patients with AIDS; the pos-

itive tissues were from patients with AIDS dementia.

2. HIV-1 DNA was detected by PCR *in situ* hybridization in over 90% of the tissues of people with AIDS. In the cases that were positive by standard *in situ* hybridization, up to 100 times more cells were found to contain the provirus when analyzed by PCR *in situ* hybridization (Fig. 9-15).

3. p24 protein was detected in less than one-half of the tissues from AIDS patients, and only rare positive cells were detected.

As with the studies of other tissues, analysis of adjacent serial sections demonstrated a similar distribution of the PCR-amplified signal using the SK19 and the SK102 probes with their respective primers. I recommend using these two sets of HIV-1 primer pairs, as they are both readily available from commercial sources and a similar distribution of the PCR-amplified HIV-1 DNA with each set provides further evidence of the specificity of the results. The PCR-enhanced hybridization signal was not evident when the tissue was DNased prior to PCR or when the *Taq* polymerase was omitted (Fig. 9-15).

The histologic localization of the PCR-amplified signal in the tissue samples from these patients provided a dramatic and interesting result in that there was a marked disparity in the location and number of cells positive for PCR-amplified HIV-1 DNA. The tissue samples from people with minimal or no CNS-specific symptoms, where neuronal or myelin loss was not seen or was minimal, showed rare small, round to oval viral positive cells that localized in and around the perivascular spaces (Fig. 9-16). In addition to HIV-1 DNA-positive cells in these areas, many other positive cells most evident in the gray matter were seen in the tissues from the people with AIDS dementia. Although provirus was most readily identified in the tissues from the people with AIDS dementia in areas of demyelinization, microglial nodules, and/or neuronal loss, it was also evident in areas where these pathological features were not evident. Therefore, it appeared that in patients with CNS disease, the number of positive cells

correlated with the clinical disease state (see Table 9-6). This correlation has also been reported in the spinal cord (24).

The next goal was to determine the phenotype of the HIV-1–infected cells. Immunohistochemistry was done after PCR *in situ* hybridization using antibodies that react against epitopes for RCA-1, LCA, and Mac387 (for microglial/macrophage cells), GFAP (for astrocytes), neuron-specific enolase (for neurons), and galactocerebroside (for oligodendroglial cells). These colabeling experiments demonstrated that the perivascular HIV-1–positive cells were microglia and that in patients with AIDS dementia many of the infected cells were neurons, astrocytes, and microglia (see Color Plate 15 following p. 242). The demonstration that some of the infected cells were astrocytes, microglia, or neurons was best made based on determination of the phenotype by combined *in situ* PCR and immunohistochemistry. In addition, the cytologic features of the infected cells also assisted in the identification of the specific cell type. For example, the cells that colabeled with the astrocyte marker GFAP usually had long, thin, branching cellular processes that are characteristic of astrocytes. Also, many of the neuron-specific enolase-positive cells that were also infected by HIV-1 contained large halos around the nucleus as well as nucleoli that are found in neurons. Similarly, the RCA-1–positive, HIV-1–positive cells showed, at times, the elongate, thinned nuclei of microglia. The helpful recognition of the cytological features of these cells in this case illustrates the value of a knowledge of histology and tissue structure for interpreting the results. Clearly, someone trained in histopathology or surgical pathology is well suited to make these interpretations. Those investigators who do not have a strong background in the histologic analysis of tissue would do well to consult with a person trained in this area when interpreting the PCR *in situ* hybridization results. This author certainly found it helpful to consult with Dr. Alex Braun, a neuropathologist, when interpreting the CNS results to identify the specific cell types that were viral positive.

To ascertain whether the infection was latent or active with viral transcription, the positive tis-

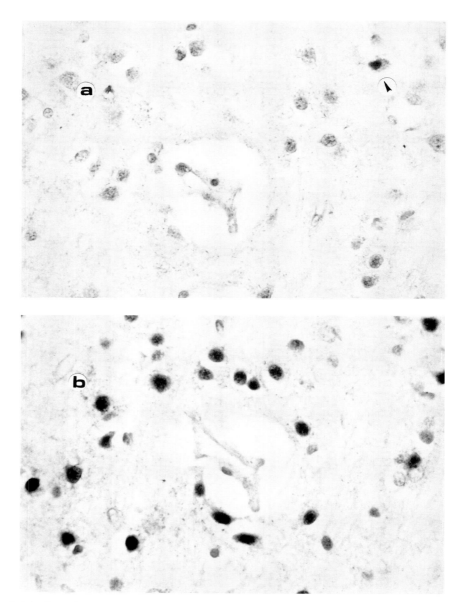

Figure 9-15. *Correlation of the detection of PCR-amplified HIV-1 DNA in the CNS with the clinical disease state.* HIV-1 DNA was detected in a few cells (**a**, *arrowhead*) with standard *in situ* hybridization in this tissue from patient 1, who was severely demented. Many more positive cells were detected in the serial section done on the same slide when the *in situ* analysis was preceded by PCR (**b**). The signal was eliminated by omission of the *Taq* polymerase, use of HPV-specific irrelevant primers, or prior digestion in DNase (**c**).

sues were analyzed for HIV-1 RNA with RT *in situ* PCR and the downstream primers SK39 and SK431, respectively (Tables 9-6 and 9-7). The number and distribution of HIV-1 RNA-positive cells from patients with AIDS dementia were equivalent with the results for PCR-amplified HIV-1 DNA (Fig. 9-17). The specificity of the signal with RT *in situ* PCR was again demonstrated by its loss with the omission of the RT step (Fig. 9-17), the use of HPV 18-specific

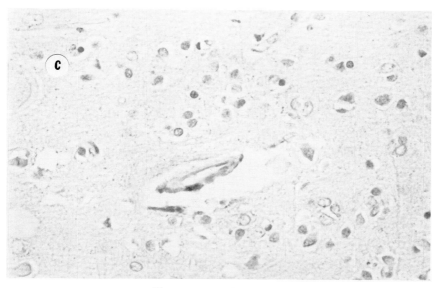

Figure 9-15. *Continued.*

primers, and its persistence with the use of the internal oligoprobe in the absence of the direct incorporation of digoxigenin dUTP (RT PCR *in situ* hybridization). Note that viral RNA was not detectable in the rare HIV-1 DNA-positive cells in the tissues from the patients without AIDS dementia, which is consistent with latent infection (Table 9-6). Interestingly, there were areas in the tissues from patients with AIDS dementia where rare HIV-1 DNA-positive cells were seen that were HIV-1 RNA negative, especially in the region of the midbrain and cerebellum, where CNS symptoms are rare in AIDS dementia (Table 9-7). This suggests that, in patients with AIDS dementia, latent CNS infection may coexist with areas of activated infection. The SK38/39 and SK145/431 primer pairs cannot distinguish between genomic HIV-1 RNA and spliced transcripts. This primer pair, which either does not amplify or poorly amplifies a target in genomic viral RNA due to its large size of 3,500 base pairs and robustly amplifies 250 base pairs after splicing in the *rev* and *tat* exons, produced an intense signal after RT *in situ* PCR in most of the cells that showed a signal using the other primer pairs. Cells positive for p24 were identified in tissues from patients 1 to 3, but in far fewer cells that had detectable viral DNA or

transcripts (Table 9-6), as was noted in the skeletal muscle biopsy study.

TNF and IL-1β have each been implicated in HIV-1 CNS pathogenesis. Tissues from the seven AIDS patients were analyzed for the corresponding mRNAs using RT *in situ* PCR. Amplified IL-1 cDNA was not identified. However, many cells with detectable amplified TNF cDNA were identified in the cases of AIDS dementia only and were found exclusively in those areas where there were many viral infected cells (Table 9-6). By analyzing subjacent serial sections for HIV-1 RNA and TNF RNA it was found that the positive cells were similar in number and had an equivalent distribution pattern. Astrocytes and microglial cells positive for TNF were identified, and neurons were invariably negative (Fig. 9-16). We have extended this study and demonstrated that other cytokines, notably nitrous oxide synthetase, and MIP-α and -β mRNAs are increased in the tissues of patients with AIDS dementia in the region of activated viral infection (Table 9-7).

In summary, HIV-1 DNA was detected in this study by PCR *in situ* hybridization in the CNS from each patient who had AIDS, even when there was minimal clinical or pathological evidence of neurological disease (98). However,

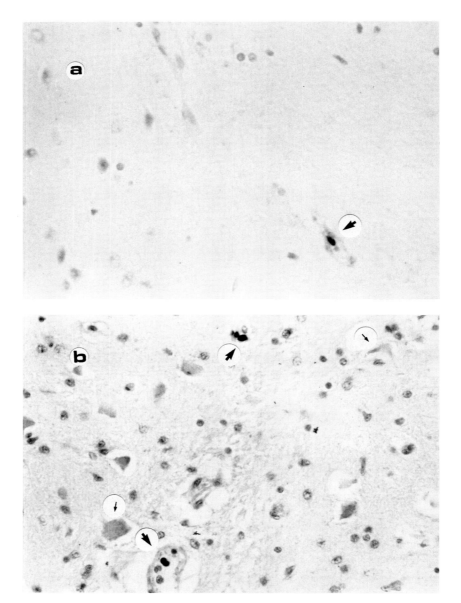

Figure 9-16. *Correlation of the detection of PCR-amplified HIV-1 DNA in the CNS with the clinical disease state.* This tissue is from a patient who died of AIDS but who had minimal CNS-related symptoms. HIV-1 DNA was detectable only after amplification in rare perivascular cells or intravascular monocytes (**a** and **b**, *large arrows*). Note the negative neurons in b (*small arrows*).

in most cases viral DNA was detectable only when the *in situ* hybridization was preceded by PCR, and, in those cases where the provirus was demonstrated by standard *in situ* hybridization, the number of positive cells was dramatically increased after amplification. The data derived from

AIDS patients who do not have CNS-specific symptoms suggested latent infection by HIV-1. Specifically, few HIV-1 DNA-positive cells were identified, and these cells were negative for viral RNA. The cells localized within or adjacent to perivascular spaces and were shown by colabel-

Table 9-6. *Correlation of detection of amplified HIV-1 DNA, RNA, TNF-α RNA, and p24 protein with the cell type in the CNS of patients with AIDS[a]*

	Microglia/macrophages	Astrocytes	Neurons
Case 1—AIDS dementia			
HIV DNA	23/202 (11%)	8/198 (1%)	28/189 (15%)[b]
HIV RNA	13/202 (6%)	6/192 (3%)	30/177 (17%)
TNF-α	7/199 (4%)	10/204 (5%)	0/182
p24	3/167 (2%)	0/202	2/192 (1%)
Case 2—AIDS dementia			
HIV DNA	6/160 (4%)	6/192 (3%)	5/174 (3%)
HIV RNA	5/148 (3%)	5/198 (3%)	6/184 (3%)
TNF-α	3/140 (2%)	6/188 (3%)	0/169
p24	1/167 (<1%)	0/202	1/192 (<1%)
Case 3—AIDS dementia			
HIV DNA	5/172 (3%)	4/189 (2%)	5/179 (3%)
HIV RNA	4/157 (2%)	5/170 (3%)	3/180 (2%)
TNF-α	3/136 (2%)	3/189 (1%)	0/159
p24	1/165 (<1%)	0/200	0/187
Cases 4–7—no CNS symptoms			
HIV DNA	8/558 (1%)	0/480	0/477
HIV RNA	0	0	0[c]

[a]Cell type was determined by colabeling with GFAP, neuron-specific enolase, and RCA-1 (see Fig. 9-2) as well as by specific cytologic features of the cells. These numbers were generated by counting the cells in multiple serial sections of the tissue from a given case.

[b]The most variability in the number of infected cells was in case 1, where the range of infected neurons was from 5% to 30% in different areas of the same tissue.

[c]For cases 4 to 7, neither TNF-α nor p24 was detected (98).

ing experiments to be mononuclear or microglial cells, which is consistent with the observations of others (87–97). One may speculate that this represents asymptomatic infection with entry of the virus from the peripheral blood to the CNS via monocytes (Fig. 9-18).

The results from the people with AIDS dementia suggest that the infection by HIV-1 was activated. The ratio of HIV-1 DNA/HIV-1 RNA detection in these tissues was about 1. Furthermore, the detection of HIV-1 RNA with the primers that correspond to the *gag* region and the exons from the *tat* and *rev* regions is the pattern seen in wild-type infection, suggesting the presence of multiply spliced and full-length genom-

ic transcripts. Another difference between the viral results in the patients with minimal CNS disease and dementia was the range of cell types infected by the virus. In patients with minimal CNS disease, only rare microglia cells appeared to be infected by the virus. Alternatively, in patients with dementia, microglia and macrophages were infected as well as astrocytes and neurons. Some infected cells appeared cytologically to be oligodendroglial cells, although we could not prove this phenotype with the colabeling experiments. Nonetheless, it was clear that the other cell types were the most commonly infected.

Another enigmatic issue that was partly addressed is the molecular mechanism for CNS

Table 9-7. *Detection of HIV-1 DNA and RNA and cellular RNA by in situ PCR in AIDS patients*

	HIV-1 DNA	HIV-1 RNA	iNOS RNA	TNF RNA	MIP-1α RNA	MIP-1β RNA
No CNS symptoms	3/5	1/5	0/5	0/5	0/5	0/5
AIDS dementia						
Cerebrum	8/8	8/8	7/8	8/8	7/8	7/8
Noncerebrum	4/4	2/4	1/3	1/2	2/3	1/3

Number of positive tissues/total tissues tested

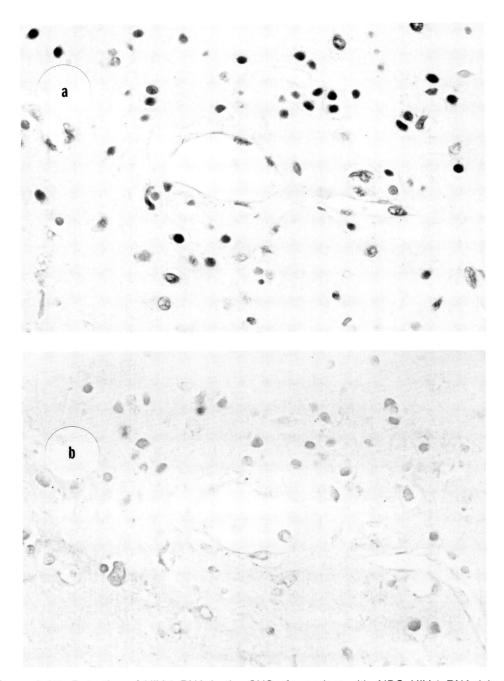

Figure 9-17. *Detection of HIV-1 RNA in the CNS of a patient with AIDS.* HIV-1 RNA (**a**) was detected by RT *in situ* PCR in a similar distribution to the amplified HIV-1 DNA in patients with AIDS dementia in the areas from the cerebrum. The signal was lost when the RT step was omitted (**b**). TNF mRNA was also detected by RT *in situ* PCR (**c**). The positive cells had the cytologic features of astrocytes and microglia/macrophages (*small arrows*); the neurons were negative for TNF (*large arrow*).

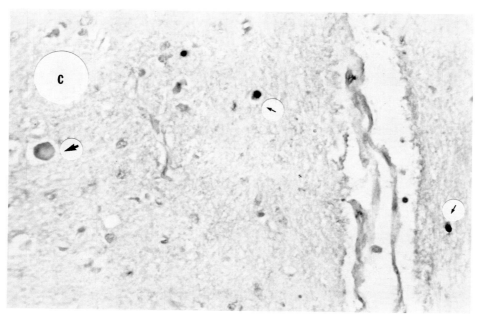

Figure 9-17. *Continued.*

damage induced by HIV-1. A variety of hypotheses including gp120 neuronal toxicity, immunologic-mediated damage, and the production of cytokines such as TNF have been proposed (87–98). The study did not address the issue of immune-mediated damage or HIV-1 antigen-induced toxicity. However, it was observed that when there was clinically evident CNS dysfunction many neurons were directly infected, and expression of TNF, iNOS, MIP-1α and MIP-1β was readily demonstrated in microglial cells, astrocytes, and in some neurons. Direct neuronal infection could partly explain the clinical and pathological features of HIV-1–induced CNS damage. Furthermore, the detection of TNF, which can hinder neuronal function, cause increased viral production in infected glial cells, and cause oligodendroglial cell death, supports a role for this cytokine in the pathogenesis of CNS dysfunction in AIDS. Expression of iNOS, MIP-1α, and MIP-1β clearly could enhance local tissue damage, increase viral transcription, and, in combination with the direct viral infection of the neurons, ultimately lead to the devastating symptoms characteristic of AIDS dementia (see Color Plate 16 following p. 242).

One important issue not addressed by these data is which cells are expressing the cytokines—the HIV-1–infected cells or their HIV-1–negative neighbors? Although analyses of serial sections clearly demonstrated that expression of the different cytokines was in the same areas as where HIV-1–infected cells were most plentiful, such analyses do not allow us to answer this important question. To address this issue, colocalizing RT *in situ* PCR was done. First, HIV-1 RNA was amplified using the rTth-based RT *in situ* PCR protocol (discussed in detail in Chapter 7) with digoxigenin as the reporter molecule. This was followed by a separate RT *in situ* PCR assay for a cytokine, using ³H as the reporter system. A representative photograph of these data is presented in Color Plate 16 following p. 242. It is evident that the HIV-1–infected cells were not expressing cytokines; rather, it was the neighboring HIV-1–negative cells. Quantitative analyses showed that five times as many HIV-1–negative cells were expressing a cytokine as HIV-1–infected cells. This suggests an "amplification" mechanism for neuronal damage in AIDS dementia, where neuronal damage results from direct viral infection and the effects of cytokines produced by neighboring, viral negative

Asymptomatic Infection

1. HIV-1 Enters Through Infected mononuclear cells
2. Rare Perivascular Microglia Cells are Latently Infected

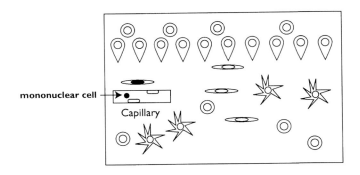

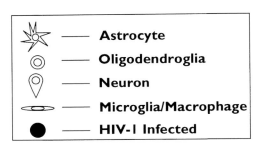

Figure 9-18. *Model for HIV-1–induced CNS disease: asymptomatic disease.* It is speculated that HIV-1 enters the CNS early in the disease process. The virus gains entry through infected lymphocytes and macrophages where it can be transmitted to perivascular microglia cells. The rare infected cells appear to be scattered throughout the CNS. The disease is presumably latent, as viral RNA is usually not detected with RT *in situ* PCR.

cells. A model that emphasizes the common early asymptomatic infection as well as the importance of viral activation and cytokine production is presented in Figs. 9-18 and 9-19.

It is hoped that these colabeling experiments will help to elucidate the early cellular response to HIV-1 infection in lymph nodes in general and lymphocytes in particular. Such data may help us understand which factors are important to viral activation. Preliminary data in this regard have demonstrated expression of interferon-γ and in-

terleukin-4 in response to challenge with HIV-1–derived antigens, done as part of a study to develop a vaccine effective against HIV-1 (Fig. 9-20).

In the Genital Tract

It has been documented that heterosexual transmission of HIV-1 is the primary mode of spread of the virus on a worldwide basis. With the added observation that homosexual contact

AIDS Dementia

1. **Active Viral RNA Production**
2. **Virus Infects Astrocytes and Neurons**
3. **Expression of TNF, NOS, MIP∂ and MIPß by surrounding viral negative cells**

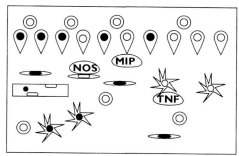

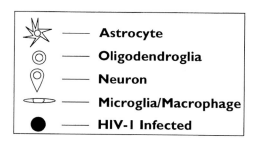

Figure 9-19. *Model for HIV-1–induced CNS disease: AIDS dementia.* For reasons that are not clear, certain foci of latent infection in the CNS may become activated. In patients with AIDS dementia, the infection is activated in the CNS based on the ready detection of viral RNA. Furthermore, many more cells are infected by the virus, including astrocytes and neurons. Viral activation is also correlated with production of TNF iNOS and MIP mRNA by astrocytes and microglia/macrophages, which can damage neighboring neurons.

between an infected man and his partner often leads to infection by HIV-1 in the viral-negative man, it becomes apparent that transmission through sexual intercourse is the major route for viral transmission. Despite the certainty about this mode of transmission, the specific cell types that the virus infects in the male and female genital tracts have, until recently, not been well characterized. As for the other sites mentioned above, a major problem in identifying the cell types infected with the virus in the male and female genital tracts is that the viral nucleic acid copy number is often below the detection threshold for standard *in situ* hybridization, and the viral-associated proteins are usually below the immunohistochemical threshold. The last section of this chapter discusses the histologic distributions of PCR-amplified HIV-1 DNA and RNA in the genital tract tissues of men and women.

The Cervix

One of the epidemiologic observations to be explained in the study of the distribution of HIV-1 in the genital tract is that women are

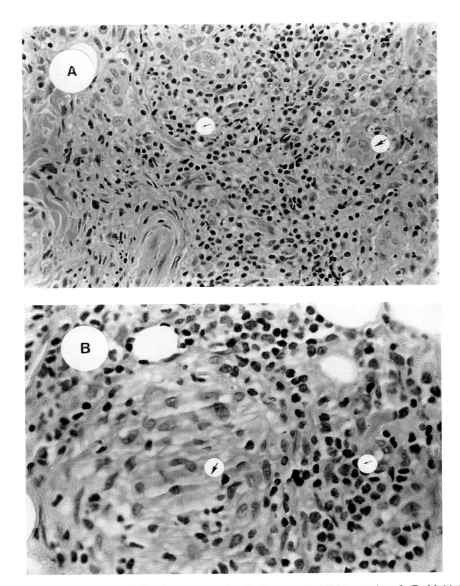

Figure 9-20. *Cytokine upregulation in response to challenge with HIV-1 vaccine.* **A, B:** Multiple granulomas were noted in response to repeated challenges with HIV-1–specific vaccine. The clusters of epithelioid histocytes (*large arrows*) and lymphocytes (*small arrows*), which form the granuloma, are evident. HIV-1 DNA was detected in scattered lymphocytes by PCR *in situ* hybridization (not shown). **C, D:** Some of the lymphocytes in the region of the granulomas were shown to express IL-4 (C) and interferon-γ (D). (Arrows in C and D correspond to those in A and B.)

about ten times more likely to acquire AIDS through heterosexual contact than are men (66,99–102). That is, a woman who has unprotected intercourse with a man with HIV-1 infection is ten times more likely to become infected than a man who has unprotected inter-

course with a woman who is infected by the virus. Another interesting observation about the heterosexual transmission of HIV-1 is that macrophage-tropic strains predominate in the woman recipient, even though lymphocytic-tropic strains usually predominate in the man

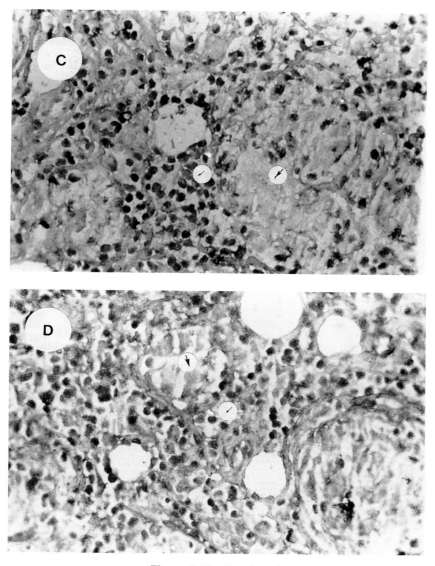

Figure 9-20. *Continued.*

who was the donor. We analyzed the distributions of PCR-amplified HIV-1 DNA and cDNA in cervical biopsy tissues from 31 women (66). These were obtained from lesions discovered at colposcopic examination that had been prompted by a previous abnormal Papanicolaou smear. Of these 31 women, 21 had AIDS and 10 were HIV-1–negative controls. The histological diagnoses for these tissues were 12 low-grade SIL, 3 high-grade SIL, and 16 nonspecific inflammation and/or squamous meta-

plasia. We also studied eight cervical tissues from children who had acquired HIV-1 infection *in utero*. These eight tissues showed no microscopic abnormalities.

The tissues were analyzed for sequences homologous to HIV-1 DNA by *in situ* hybridization after PCR amplification. Amplified viral DNA was detected in each of the 21 tissues from the HIV-1–seropositive adult women (see Color Plate 17 following p. 242). No histologic feature, such as degree of inflammation, type

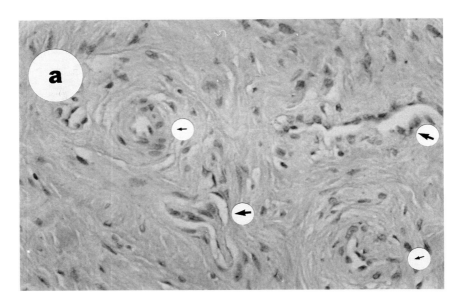

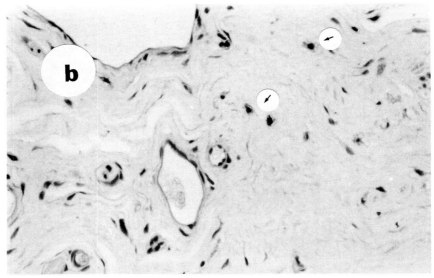

Figure 9-21. *Molecular and immunohistochemical analyses of a cervical tissue from an adult woman with AIDS.* **a:** Typical arrangement of the microvessels in the cervical submucosa: thick-walled arterioles (*small arrows*) and thin-walled venules and lymphatics (*large arrows*). **b:** Epitopes against the macrophage marker Mac387 also localized to the region around the microvessels (*arrow*). PCR-amplified HIV-1 DNA (not shown), TNF cDNA and HIV-1 RNA (**c**, *arrows*) localized to the same area.

of inflammatory cell, or presence of SIL, seemed to distinguish the HIV-1–positive tissues from the HIV-1–negative cases. There was a dramatic and specific geographic distribution of the PCR-amplified HIV-1 DNA. Specifically, the PCR product localized to two areas:

(i) the cells in the endocervical aspect of the transformation zone at the interface of the endocervical glands and submucosa and (ii) the cells in the deep submucosa around microvessels (Fig. 9-21). For comparison, recall that PCR-amplified HPV DNA localized in the

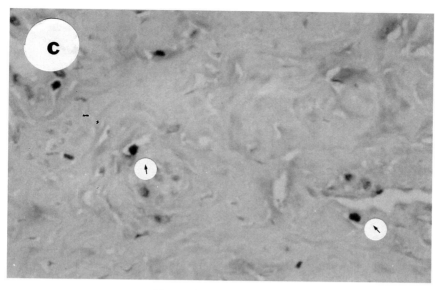

Figure 9-21. *Continued.*

cervix to the squamous component of the transformation zone. HPV is not detected in the glandular cells or the cells in the submucosa of the transformation zone (see Chapter 8). When PCR *in situ* hybridization was done on serial sections on the same glass slide without the *Taq* DNA polymerase or with the enzyme but with irrelevant (HPV-specific) primers, a hybridization signal was not evident in the positive cases. Amplified HIV-1 DNA was not detected in any of the ten controls. Of the eight cervical tissues from children who acquired HIV-1 *in utero*, only one had detectable PCR-amplified viral DNA. Some of the positive cells in this case were intravascular, although others were in the stroma.

The histological distribution of viral DNA was compared with the distribution of PCR-amplified HIV-1 cDNA in serial sections. Viral cDNA was noted in the 21 seropositive cases and the distribution was identical to that with the amplified HIV-1 DNA (see Color Plate 17 following p. 242). The number of cells infected by HIV-1 in a given tissue section ranged from about 20 to about 1,000. The cDNA-based signal was eliminated when the RT step was omitted, or when nonsense primers were substituted for the RT and PCR steps. HIV-1–amplified nucleic acids were not evident in the normal, metaplastic, or dysplastic squamous epithelium. Amplified HIV-1 cDNA was not detected in the ten controls and was present in the tissue from one of eight seropositive children, which was also positive for HIV-1 PCR-amplified DNA.

The cells positive for HIV-1–amplified nucleic acids rarely had the cytologic features of lymphocytes. This was unexpected considering the large number of lymphocytes that are typically present in the transformation zone of the cervix. However, this is consistent with the observation that macrophage-tropic strains predominate in the women who acquire HIV-1 through heterosexual transmission. More often the viral-infected cells were large with oval- to spindle-shaped nuclei, inconspicuous, finely dispersed chromatin, and a minimal to moderate amount of cytoplasm. These features suggest that they may have been macrophages. HIV-1 DNA and RNA were rarely detected in some cells above the basement membrane of the glandular epithelium as well as in occasional endothelial cells. The rare HIV-1–positive cells that were located in the mucosal lining of the endocervix may have been epithelial cells or, more

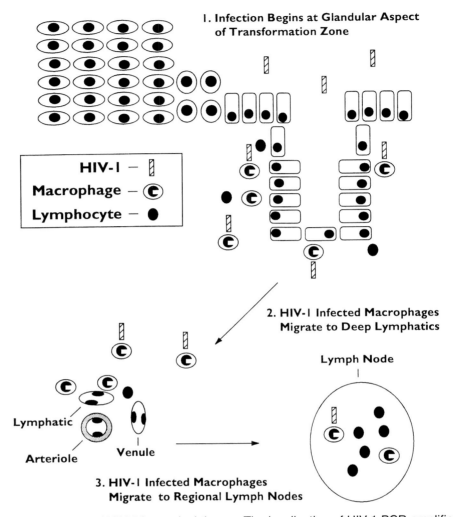

Figure 9-22. *Distribution of HIV-1 in cervical tissues.* The localization of HIV-1 PCR-amplified nucleic acids to the endocervical aspect of the transformation zone and around the deep microvessels is depicted as a proposed model for the systemic spread of HIV-1 infection via the cervical macrophages.

likely, Langerhans cells, which are antigen-presenting macrophages. We were not able to identify the phenotypes of these cells using S100 antibody, which stains Langerhans cells, because these cells were rarely seen.

To determine if HIV-1 nucleic acids routinely localized to sites other than the cervix in seropositive adults, we analyzed three other tissues (vulva, endometrium, and esophagus) available from the 21 AIDS-positive women included in this study. PCR-amplified viral nucleic acids were not identified at these sites.

The next issue addressed was determining the phenotypes of the HIV-1–infected cells. As noted above, most of the infected cells had cytologic features suggestive of macrophages. Furthermore, it was clear that the epithelial cells were routinely negative for HIV-1. The specific cell type infected by the virus was examined with sections directly adjacent to those analyzed by PCR *in situ* hybridization. Because most of the infected cells were about 10 to 20 μm in size, each would be present in several of the 3 to 4 μM serial sections. The antibodies used were for LCA which reacts with epitopes on both macrophages and lymphocytes; Mac387, which reacts with epitopes on macrophages; CD4, which is present in both T-helper cells and macrophages; and p24, an HIV-1–associated core protein. Epitopes cross-re-active to the LCA and Mac387 antibodies had a distribution similar to that of the amplified viral nucleic acids. Specifically, the antigens that complexed with these antibodies localized primarily to the mucosal–submucosal interface and to the deeper stroma around the vessels (see Color Plate 17 following p. 242). Note in Fig. 9-21 that the microvessels are arranged in groups that consist of the thick-walled arterioles, thin-walled larger venules, and thin-walled smaller lymphatics. A direct comparison of the phenotypic markers to cells positive for PCR-amplified HIV-1 nucleic acids showed that many of the HIV-1–positive cells colabeled with LCA and about one-half of these LCA-positive cells colabeled with Mac387 and CD4. As noted above, LCA stains both lymphocytes and macrophages.

To distinguish between the lymphocytes and the macrophages and to determine if the macrophages were activated, serial sections were assayed for TNF-α mRNA using RT *in situ* PCR. TNF may be found in "activated" macrophages but would not be expected to be present in lymphocytes. Amplified TNF cDNA was detected in most of the HIV-1 DNA- and cDNA-positive cells, demonstrating (Fig. 9-20), with the LCA data as well as the Mac387 results, that many of these viral-infected cells were indeed activated macrophages. It should be emphasized that LCA- and Mac387-positive cells are much more common in the endocervical aspect of the transformation zone. This no doubt reflects that this part of the cervix, where the squamous cells meet the columnar cells, is the site where most sexually transmitted pathogens and other foreign antigens enter the female genital tract. For example, HPV localizes almost exclusively to the squamous cells here, whereas *Chlamydia* and *Neisseria gonorrhea* attack the endocervical glands. Also, recall that the endocervical glands present a thin, one-cell barrier in contrast with the much

thicker squamous part toward the vagina. The observation that scattered viral-infected macrophages were also found about the deep lymphatics suggests that there may be migratory macrophages that move to the regional lymph nodes where they could present any foreign antigens to the wide variety of cell types found at these sites. This is reminiscent of the much more extensively studied migratory macrophage population in the upper airways of the lung.

The detection rates of PCR amplified HIV-1 DNA and cDNA were next compared with the rates for standard *in situ* hybridization and p24 detection using immunohistochemistry. There was sufficient tissue available to do comparative studies on 10 of the 21 HIV-1–positive cases. Epitopes reactive against p24 were detected in seven of these ten tissues. The histologic distribution was the same as for the amplified nucleic acids. However, the number of positive cells in the cases with detectable p24 decreased by 10- to 100-fold when compared with the amplified HIV-1 nucleic acids. The detection rate for HIV-1 nucleic acids using the SK19 probe, which could detect both viral DNA and RNA under the reaction conditions, three of ten if the tissues were first DNased and four of ten if the tissues were not digested in DNase. The positive cases were ones in which many cells (>100) had detectable HIV-1 DNA and cDNA after amplification. The primer pair, which dictates a product of about 3,500 base pairs in genomic viral RNA and 250 base pairs after splicing (kindly provided by Dr. Roger Pomerantz), produced a signal after RT PCR *in situ* in most of the cells that had a signal using the SK38 and SK39 primers.

The observations made in this study suggest that HIV-1, when exposed to the cervix, enters through the endocervical aspect of the transformation zone and infects primarily the tissue macrophages. Alternatively, the viral nucleic acids detected in the cervix may represent hematogenous spread and not direct infection from sexual contact. Although the distinction between these two possibilities could not be made in this study, certain facts suggest that infection of the cervix by direct sexual contact is a tenable hypothesis. First, HIV-1 DNA and cDNA were detected in 21 of 21 cervical biopsy specimens from the women with AIDS. We did not detect HIV-1 DNA or RNA at other sites in these women, although few such tissues were available. In a larger study, Shibata and Klatt (102) detected HIV-1 DNA by PCR in only 3 of 55 (5%) of nonlymphoid, noncervical tissues (1 of 2 cervices was positive). Second, HIV-1 nucleic acids were detected in the cervices of only one of eight children who acquired AIDS *in utero*. This last result must be tempered by the realization that the cervices of children are quite different both histologically and immunologically from adults. Third, the virus was readily detected in the macrophages at the endocervical aspect of the transformation zone of the cervix but not in the squamous aspect. If the virus reaches the cervix by hematogenous spread, why is it evident only in the macrophages in the deep stroma and endocervical–stromal interface and not in the directly adjoining squamous component? It is speculated that HIV-1, having entered at the cervix, may be transported via the infected macrophages that migrate to the regional lymph nodes or directly into the circulation through venules where systemic infection could then occur. This proposed model of HIV-1 spread is presented in Fig. 9-22. To test this model, we are attempting to obtain tissue from the cervices of women who acquired AIDS through transfusions and who have no other risk factors for the disease. The goal would be to determine whether HIV-1–infected macrophages are absent in these cervices, as would be predicted by this model.

The theory that the ubiquitous macrophages present in the endocervical aspect of the transformation zone are the target cell for HIV-1 infection in the cervix could explain why a woman is so susceptible to HIV-1 infection through unprotected heterosexual contact with an infected man. Clearly, the target cell would be directly exposed to the HIV-1 virions that have been routinely detected in the semen of infected men. This theory could also explain why unprotected homosexual contact between an infected male and noninfected male is such a strong risk fac-

tor for acquiring HIV-1 disease. The rectal–anal junction is similar to the transformation zone of the cervix in that there are many macrophages present that may be inadvertently recruited to carry the virus to the regional lymph nodes and then to the systemic circulation. As noted above, that the macrophage is the primary target in the female genital tract would also explain why macrophage-tropic strains dominate early in the disease of women who acquire the virus through homosexual transmission. Although speculative, it is interesting to theorize that the macrophage-tropic strains would have stronger tropism for the CD21 cell in the germinal center of the lymph node, which would be the initial primary target of the virus. Massive CD21 infection could then serve as the nidus for infection of the adjoining CD4 cells, beginning the process of their inexorable loss, which is the ultimate factor responsible for much of the pathogenesis of AIDS.

In the Male Genital Tract

It seems apparent that the microenvironment of the female genital tract provides a portal of entry for the HIV-1 virus. The results of the experiments describing the mechanism of viral entry in the cervix lead to questions about the histologic correlates in the male genital tract. Although there has been little information available in this important area due to the limitations of detecting the viral nucleic acids and proteins by standard *in situ* hybridization and immunohistochemistry, the following observations based on epidemiologic and molecular studies have been made.

1. As noted above, men are about one in ten as likely to acquire AIDS through unprotected heterosexual contact with infected women compared with the risk to women having unprotected intercourse with men who are HIV-1–positive.

2. Infectious HIV-1 virions can be detected in about 50% of the semen samples from men with early-stage AIDS.

3. Initial studies stated that PCR-amplified HIV-1 DNA can be detected in over 90%

of the cell-free fraction and inflammatory cell fraction of semen but very rarely in the spermatids in semen. Subsequent analysis showed that HIV-1 DNA was readily detected in the spermatid fraction of semen after inactivation of an inhibitor to the PCR reaction.

4. HIV-1 DNA–RNA or proteins are found infrequently *in situ* in the testes and prostatic tissue of men with AIDS and appear to localize to inflammatory cells (103–108). The several studies that have attempted to localize the virus directly in tissue sections from the male genital tract are based on detection of viral-related antigens by immunohistochemistry in patients with advanced-stage AIDS. They have produced conflicting results, with one report stating that the viral protein could be found in 57% of testes, localizing to the germ cells, while another study reported a detection rate of 39%, with the viral proteins being present in lymphocytes and macrophages (103–108).

5. In over 90% of men with AIDS, there is marked testicular atrophy with near to complete arrest of spermatogenesis. Although the prostate may show nonspecific inflammation, the most dramatic histologic changes in the genital tract of males with AIDS are to be found in the testes.

We undertook a study to ascertain the histological distribution of PCR-amplified HIV-1 DNA and RNA in the male genital tract, including the penis, epididymus, prostate, seminal vesicles, and testes (108). Genital tract tissues from 14 men were available for study. Of the 14 patients, 11 had AIDS and 3 were controls. Thirty-six tissues from these 11 men were analyzed for sequences homologous to HIV-1. There were 11 tissue samples from the testes, 11 samples from the prostate, 8 from the epididymus, 3 from the seminal vesicles, and 3 from the penis. All tissues were obtained from autopsy material, and the advanced-stage AIDS of these patients was reflected in the low CD4 counts (<50) in the tissues. However, one case was unique in that the man died immediately after learning he was seropositive for HIV-1. This patient had no symptoms attributable to immunosuppression at the time of his demise. Each of the ten testicular tissues from AIDS patients showed either retarded maturation or arrest of spermatogenesis. Only four cases demonstrated evidence of spermatid production, while the other cases contained either only spermatogonia or, more commonly, spermatogonia and spermatocytes with the Sertoli cells. Alternatively, the testicular tissue from the one HIV-1–positive, AIDS-negative man was histologically normal (Fig. 9-23).

The 36 biopsy specimens were analyzed for sequences homologous to HIV-1 DNA by standard *in situ* hybridization. The provirus was detected in only 2 of the 36 tissues, and these were testes tissues from HIV-1–positive men in whom spermatid production was evident. Serial sections of these tissues were then analyzed for HIV-1 DNA by *in situ* hybridization after PCR amplification. Amplified viral DNA was detected in each of the 11 testicular tissues (Fig. 9-24), in 3 of the 11 prostatic tissues (Fig. 9-25), in 1 of the 8 epididymal tissues, and in none of the tissues from the seminal vesicles or the penises of the men with HIV-1 infection (Table 9-7). The distribution of the PCR-amplified viral DNA was equivalent when serial sections were compared using the SK38 and SK39 primers with the SK19 probe and the SK145 and SK431 primers and the SK102 probe.

The histologic distribution of the PCR-amplified HIV-1 DNA was equivalent for the 11 testicular tissues. Specifically, the virus was found in the spermatogonia, spermatocytes, and in the spermatids when they were present (Fig. 9-24). The virus was not detected in the Sertoli cells, Leydig cells, or endothelial cells, which served as internal negative controls. The number of viral positive cells in the testes was inversely related to the degree of spermatogenesis maturation arrest. That is, in the testes where spermatid production was still evident, hundreds of viral-positive cells were noted, often numbering 5 to 20 in a given seminiferous tubule (Fig. 9-24). The positive cells often clustered, suggesting that they represented infec-

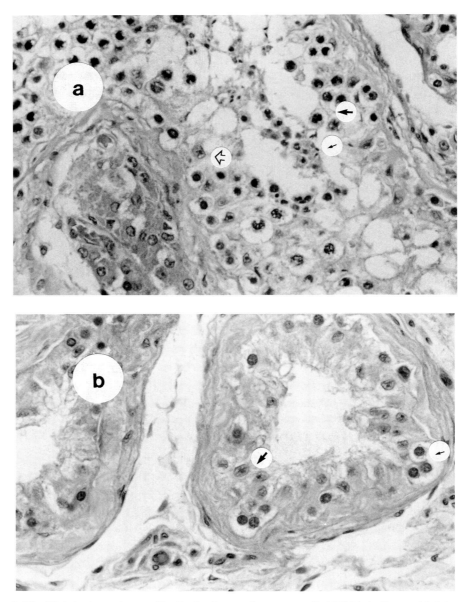

Figure 9-23. *Histologic analyses of testicular tissues from men with HIV-1 infection.* **a:** Histology of the testes from a 37-year-old man with HIV infection, pre-AIDS. Note the active spermatid production (*small arrow,* spermatid; *large arrow,* spermatogonia and spermatocytes; *open arrow,* Sertoli cells). **b:** The other testes is from a 44-year-old man; only rare spermatogonia (*small arrow*) are seen among the Sertoli cells (*large arrow*). The arrest of spermatogenesis depicted in b is typical of men with advanced-stage AIDS.

tion of a common progenitor cell. Conversely, in the testes in which Sertoli cells and rare spermatogonia were evident in the tubules, only rare viral-positive cells were seen (Fig. 9-24). PCR-amplified viral DNA was noted in occasional stromal cells that cytologically appeared to be

macrophages, and analysis of serial sections showed that these cells did label with LCA and Mac387.

Four of the prostatic tissues showed moderate to severe inflammation as indicated by the presence of many macrophages and lympho-

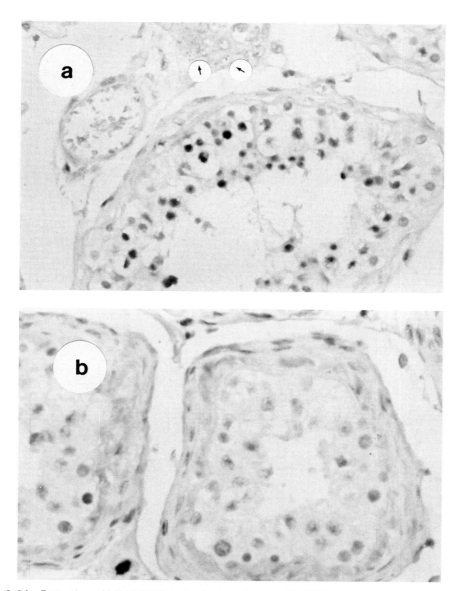

Figure 9-24. *Detection of HIV-1 DNA in the testes of men with AIDS: correlation with spermatogenesis.* **a:** HIV-1 DNA was detected by PCR *in situ* hybridization in many of the spermatogonia and their progeny in the testes of a man with active spermatid production. Note the negative interstitial cells (*small arrows*). The signal was lost when the tissues were pretreated in DNase, when the *Taq* polymerase was omitted, when nonsense primers were used, or, in this tissue, when standard *in situ* hybridization was done (not shown). **b:** Testes from a man with little spermatogenesis where only rare HIV-1–positive spermatogonia were evident.

cytes on histologic examination and substantiated by analysis with LCA and Mac387. Three of these tissues were positive for PCR-amplified HIV-1 DNA. Most of the viral-infected cells were in the lumen and were macrophages, as determined by their cytologic appearance and by labeling with Mac387 (Fig. 9-25). It should be stressed that only 1% to 5% of the macrophages and lymphocytes in these tissues were HIV-1–positive. Furthermore, the epithelial tissue samples from the prostate and epididymus were invariably negative.

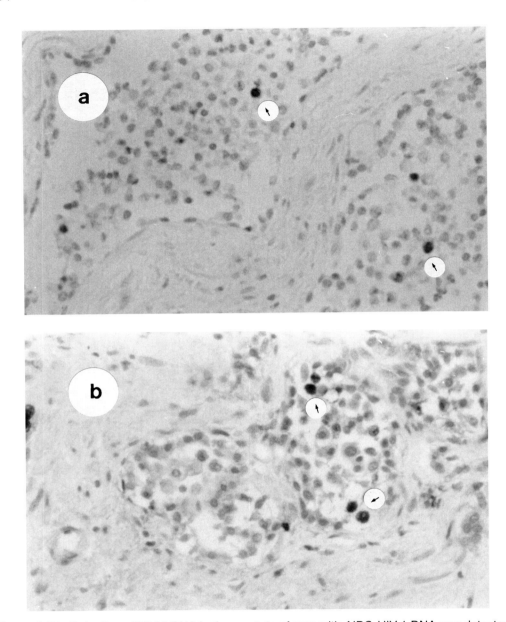

Figure 9-25. *Detection of HIV-1 DNA in the prostate of men with AIDS.* HIV-1 DNA was detected in the rare cells in the prostate from about 30% of men with AIDS by PCR *in situ* hybridization. **a:** The infected cells were present in the interstitium and the glandular lumen and had the cytological appearance of macrophages (*arrows*). **b:** These cells did label with the macrophage marker Mac387 when the serial section was analyzed by immunohistochemistry (*arrows*). Infection of the prostatic epithelium by HIV-1 was not evident.

The histologic distribution of viral DNA was compared with the distribution of PCR-amplified HIV-1 cDNA in serial sections. Viral cDNA was noted in each of the 15 HIV-1 DNA-positive cases, and the distribution was identical to the amplified HIV-1 DNA (Fig. 9-26). The cell types that most commonly contained viral RNA were the spermatogonia, spermatocytes, and, when present, the spermatids. The viral transcription appeared to be activated based

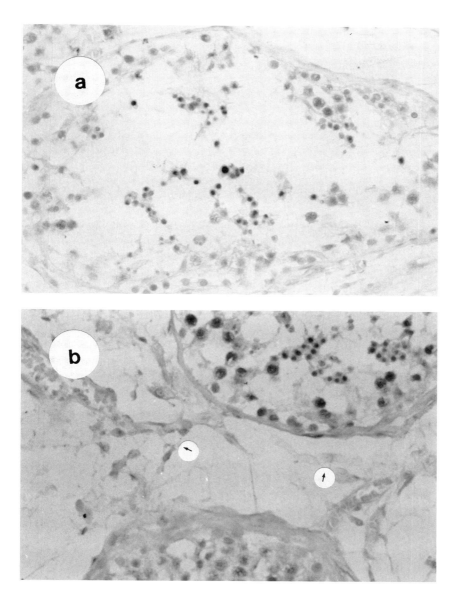

Figure 9-26. *Detection of HIV-1 RNA in the testes of men with AIDS: correlation with spermatogenesis.* HIV-1 DNA (**a**) and cDNA (**b**) were detected by PCR *in situ* hybridization and RT *in situ* PCR, respectively, in many of the spermatogonia and their progeny in the testes of the men with AIDS who still had active spermatogenesis. Far fewer viral-infected cells were detected in the testes of men with marked retardation of sperm production. In the positive control (no DNase) for RT *in situ* PCR (**c**), note the positive interstitial cells whose signal reflects DNA repair and mispriming (*arrow;* these cells are negative in b, as indicated by the *small arrows* in b). The negative control (**d**) shows the absence of signal with DNase and the omission of the RT step; it is essential that the negative and positive controls be done on the same tissue section as the RT *in situ* PCR test reaction.

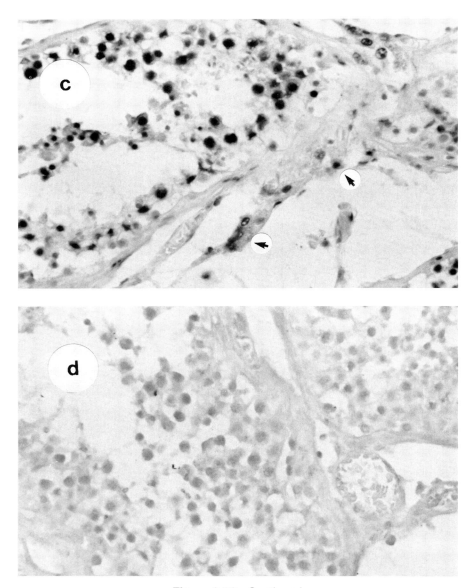

Figure 9-26. *Continued.*

on positive results using the primer pairs described above that were used to detect HIV-1 transcripts after splicing in the *rev* and *tat* exons.

Based on the findings in this study, one may speculate that direct HIV-1 infection of the spermatogonia and their progeny may retard their maturation as well as lead to their death. Further study, including *in vitro* infection of spermagonia-type cell lines, is needed to address this issue. However, this certainly could explain, in part, the marked atrophy and inhibition of spermatogenesis typical of HIV-1 infection. Although lymphocytes and macrophages are noted in the testes of patients with AIDS, their number does not seem sufficient to explain the histologic changes.

Another implication of this study relates to the route of transmission of the virus through

Table 9-8. *Detection of HIV-1 in the testes and prostate*

	HIV-1 DNA (ISH)	HIV-1 DNA (PCR ISH)	HIV-1 RNA RT *in situ* PCR
HIV-1 infected: men[a]			
Testes	3/12	11/12	11/12
Prostate	1/11	3/11[b]	2/11
HIV-1 infected: children			
Testes	0/3	0/3	0/3
No HIV-1 infection: men			
Testes	0/3	0/3	0/3
Prostate	0/3	0/3	0/3

ISH, standard *in situ* hybridization.
[a]11/12 men had AIDS.
[b]Rare HIV-1–infected macrophages and lymphocytes were seen. PCR-amplified viral nucleic acids were not detected in epithelia from the prostate, seminal vesicles, epididymus, or penis (108).

heterosexual contact. One may speculate that viral infection of the spermatogonia leads to the release of infectious virions due to the concomitant destruction of the cells prior to spermatid maturation. This may serve as the primary viral source in the ejaculated material that enters the cervix during unprotected intercourse. This hypothesis needs further study by *in vitro* experiments and correlation of viral burden in the semen in relation to the testes. The ability of HIV-1 to infect spermatogonia and their progeny has been suggested by immunologic studies that have described HLA-DR binding ligands on these cells that could initiate CD4-positive type effects, including viral entry (106,107), as well as in studies by Bagasra et al. (*personal communication,* 1993) using PCR *in situ* hybridization. The skin of the male genital tract lacks the target cells that can be infected by HIV-1. The penile urethra also presents a transformation zone–type histology that is much smaller and less active than the corresponding zone in the cervix. This may explain why the male is at a lower risk for acquiring AIDS through heterosexual contact. The primary target in the male genital tract, the spermatogonia, is presumably infected by hematogenous spread. However, the anorectal junction in the male presents a large and active transformation zone, which may relate to the high risk of transmission of HIV-1–infection from man to man through unprotected anal intercourse.

ACKNOWLEDGMENTS

This chapter is dedicated to the memories of Mr. Freddie Bulsara and Dr. John J. Fenoglio.

REFERENCES

1. Greene W. The molecular biology of human immunodeficiency virus type 1 infection. *N Engl J Med* 1991;324:301–307.
2. Genesca J, Wang RYH, Alter HJ, Shih JWK. Clinical correlation and genetic polymorphism of the immunodeficiency virus proviral DNA obtained after polymerase chain reaction amplification. *J Infect Dis* 1990; 162:1025–1030.
3. Broder S, Gallo RC. A pathogenic retrovirus (HTLV-III) linked to AIDS. *N Engl J Med* 1984;311:1292–1297.
4. Selik RM, Starcher ET, Curran JW. Opportunistic diseases reported in AIDS patients: frequencies, associations and trends. *AIDS* 1987;1:175–182.
5. Curran JW, Jaffe HW, Hardy AM, et al. Epidemiology of HIV infection and AIDS in the United States. *Science* 1988;239:610–616.
6. Selik RM, Haverkos HW, Curran JW. Acquired immune deficiency syndrome (AIDS) trends in the United States. *Am J Med* 1984;76:493–500.
7. Fauci AS. The immune deficiency virus: infectivity and mechanisms of pathogenicity. *Science* 1988;239: 617–622.
8. Baccheti P, Moss AR. Incubation period of AIDS in San Francisco. *Nature* 1989;338:251–253.
9. Fahey JL, Prince H, Weaver M. Quantitative changes in T helper or T suppresser/cytotoxic lymphocyte subsets that distinguishes acquired immune deficiency syndrome from other immune subset disorders. *Am J Med* 1984; 76:95–100.
10. Ziegler JL, Drew WL, Miner RC. Outbreak of Burkitt's-like lymphoma in homosexual men. *Lancet* 1982;2: 631–633.
11. Levine AM, Gill PS, Meyer PR. Retrovirus and malignant lymphomas in homosexual men. *JAMA* 1985;254: 1921–1925.

12. Knowles DM. Malignant lymphomas occurring in association with acquired immunodeficiency syndrome. *Lab Med* 1986;17:674–678.

13. Sninsky JJ, Kwok S. Detection of human immunodeficiency viruses by the polymerase chain reaction. *Arch Pathol Lab Med* 1990;114:259–262.

14. Ou CY, Kwok S, Mitchell SW, et al. DNA amplification for direct detection of HIV-1 in DNA of peripheral blood mononuclear cells. *Science* 1988;239: 295–297.

15. Besansky NJ, Butera ST, Sinha S, Folks TM. Unintegrated human immunodeficiency virus type 1 DNA in chronically infected cell lines is not correlated with surface CD4 expression. *J Virol* 1991;65:2695–2698.

16. Pomerantz RJ, Trono D, Feinberg MB, Baltimore D. Cells nonproductively infected with HIV-1 exhibit an aberrant pattern of viral RNA expression: a molecular model for latency. *Cell* 1990;61:1271–1276.

17. Orloff GM, Orloff SL, Kennedy MS, Maddon PJ, McDougal JS. The CD4 receptor does not internalize with HIV, and CD4-related signal transduction events are not required for entry. *J Immunol* 1991;146: 2578–2587.

18. Lusso P, DeMaria A, Malnati M, et al. Induction of CD4 and susceptibility to HIV-1 infection in human CD8+ T lymphocytes by human herpesvirus 6. *Nature* 1991;349: 533–535.

19. Harouse JM, Bhat S, Spitalnik SL, et al. Inhibition of entry of HIV-1 in neural cell lines by antibodies against galactosyl ceramide. *Science* 1991;253:320–322.

20. Clerici M, Berzofsky JA, Shearer GM, Tacket CO. Exposure to human immunodeficiency virus type 1-specific T helper cell responses before detection of infection by the polymerase chain reaction and serum antibodies. *J Infect Dis* 1991;164:178–182.

21. Nast CC. HIV-associated nephropathy: a unique combined glomerular, tubular, and interstitial lesion. *Mod Pathol* 1988;1:87–96.

22. Cohen AH, Sun NC, Shapshak P, Imagawa DT. Demonstration of human immunodeficiency virus in renal epithelium in HIV-associated nephropathy. *Mod Pathol* 1989;2:125–128.

23. D'Agati V, Suh JI, Carbone L, Cheng JT, Appel G. Pathology of HIV-associated nephropathy: a detailed morphologic and comparative study. *Kidney Int* 1989;35: 1358–1370.

24. Eilbott DJ, Peress N, Burger H, et al. Human immunodeficiency virus type 1 in spinal cords of acquired immunodeficiency syndrome patients with myelopathy: expression and replication in macrophages. *Proc Natl Acad Sci USA* 1989;86:3337–3341.

25. Major EO, Amemiya K, Elder G, Houff SA. Glial cells of the human developing brain and B cells of the immune system share a common DNA binding factor for recognition of the regulatory sequences of the human polyomavirus, *J Clin Virol* 1990;27:461–471.

26. Shaw GM, Harper ME, Hahn BH, et al. HTLV-III infection in brains of children and adults with AIDS encephalopathy. *Science* 1985;227:177–181.

27. Steinberg HN, Crumpacker CS, Chatis PA. In vitro suppression of normal human bone marrow progenitor cells by human immunodeficiency virus. *J Virol* 1991;65: 1765–1769.

28. Weiser B, Peress N, LaNeve D, Eilbott DJ, Seidman R, Burger H. Human immunodeficiency virus type 1 expression in the central nervous system correlates directly with extent of disease. *Proc Natl Acad Sci USA* 1990; 87:3997–4001.

29. Hair LS, Nuovo GJ, Powers JM, Sisti MB, Britton CB, Miller JR. Progressive multifocal leukoencephalopathy in patients with human immunodeficiency virus. *Hum Pathol* 1992;23:663–667.

30. Chadwick EG, Yogev R, Kwok S, Sninsky JJ, Kellogg DE, Wolinsky SM. Enzymatic amplification of the human immunodeficiency virus in peripheral blood mononuclear cells from pediatric patients. *J Infect Dis* 1989;160:954–959.

31. Escaich S, Wallon M, Baginski I, et al. Comparison of HIV detection by virus isolation in lymphocyte cultures and molecular amplification of HIV DNA and RNA by PCR in offspring of seropositive mothers. *J AIDS* 1991; 4:130–135.

32. Horsburgh CR, Ou C, Jason J, et al. Concordance of polymerase chain reaction with human immunodeficiency virus antibody detection. *J Infect Dis* 1990; 162:542–545.

33. Haase AT, Retzel EF, Staskus KA. Amplification and detection of lentiviral DNA inside cells. *Proc Natl Acad Sci USA* 1990;87:4971–4975.

34. Nuovo GJ, MacConnell P, Forde A, Delvenne P. Detection of human papillomavirus DNA in formalin fixed tissues by *in situ* hybridization after amplification by PCR. *Am J Pathol* 1991;139:847–854.

35. Aksamit AJ, Sever JL, Major EO. Progressive multifocal leukoencephalopathy: JC virus detection by *in situ* hybridization compared with immunohistochemistry. *Neurology* 1986;36:499–504.

36. Besansky NJ, Butera ST, Sinha S, Folks TM. Unintegrated human immunodeficiency virus type 1 DNA in chronically infected cell lines is not correlated with surface CD4 expression. *J Virol* 1991;65:2695–2698.

37. Clayton F, Klein EB, Kotler DP. Correlation of *in situ* hybridization with histology and viral culture in patients with acquired immunodeficiency syndrome with cytomegalovirus. *Arch Pathol Lab Med* 1989;113: 1124–1126.

38. Davis BR, Schwartz DH, Marx JC, et al. Absent or rare human immunodeficiency virus infection of bone marrow stem/progenitor cells in vivo. *J Virol* 1991;65: 1985–1990.

39. Dickover RE, Donovan RM, Goldstein E, Dandekar S, Bush CE, Carlson JR. Quantitation of human immunodeficiency virus DNA by using the polymerase chain reaction. *J Clin Microbiol* 1990;28:2130–2133.

40. Drysdale CM, Pavlakis GN. Rapid activation and subsequent downregulation of the human immunodeficiency virus type 1 promoter in the presence of Tat: possible mechanisms contributing to latency. *J Virol* 1991;65: 3044–3051.

41. Garcia-Blanco M, Cullen BR. Molecular basis of latency in pathogenic human viruses. *Science* 1991;254: 815–819.

42. Harper ME, Marselle LM, Gallo RC, Wong-Staal F. Detection of lymphocytes expressing human T-lymphotropic virus type III in lymph nodes and peripheral blood from infected individuals by *in situ* hybridization. *Proc Natl Acad Sci USA* 1986;83:772–776.

43. Henry MJ, Stanley MW, Cruikshank S, Carson L. Association of human immunodeficiency virus-induced immunosuppression with human papillomavirus infec-

tion and cervical intraepithelial neoplasia. *Am J Obstet Gynecol* 1989;160:352–353.

44. Kalter DC, Greenhouse JJ, Orenstein JM, Schnittman SM, Gendelman HE, Meltzer MS. Epidermal Langerhans cells are not principal reservoirs of virus in HIV disease. *J Immunol* 1991;146:3396–3404.

45. Lewis DE, Minshall M, Wray NP, Paddock SW, Smith LC, Crane MM. Confocal microscopic detection of human immunodeficiency virus RNA-producing cells. *J Infect Dis* 1990;162:1373–1378.

46. Matorras R, Ariceta JM, Rementeria A, et al. Human immunodeficiency virus-induced immunosuppression: a risk factor for human papillomavirus infection. *Am J Obstet Gynecol* 1991;164:42–44.

47. Nakamine H, Okano M, Taguchi Y, et al. Hematological features of Epstein-Barr virus–induced human B-lymphoproliferation in mice with severe combined immunodeficiency. *Lab Invest* 1991;65:389–398.

48. Provencher D, Valme B, Averette HE, et al. HIV status and positive Papanicolaou screening: identification of a high risk population. *Gynecol Oncol* 1988;31:184–188.

49. Shapshak P, Sun NCJ, Resnick L, et al. The detection of HIV by *in situ* hybridization. *Mod Pathol* 1990;3:146–152.

50. Shibata S, Brynes RK, Nathwani B, Kwok S, Sninsky J, Arnheim N. Human immunodeficiency viral DNA is readily found in lymph node biopsies from seropositive individuals. *Am J Pathol* 1989;135:697–702.

51. Yoffe B, Petrie BL, Noonan CA, Hollinger FB. In vivo and in vitro ultrastructural alterations induced by human immunodeficiency virus in human lymphoid cells. *Lab Invest* 1989;61:303–309.

52. Wiley CA, Schrier RD, Nelson JA. Cellular localization of human immunodeficiency virus infection within brains of AIDS patients. *Proc Natl Acad Sci USA* 1986;83:7089–7093.

53. Reka S, Kotler DP. An inflammatory bowel disease associated with HIV infection. *Gastroenterology* 1990;98:A472.

54. Chaisson RE, Hopewell PC. Mycobacteria and AIDS mortality. *Am Rev Respir Dis* 1989;139:1–3.

55. Reka S, Kotler DP. An inflammatory bowel disease associated with HIV infection. *Gastroenterology* 1990;98:A472.

56. Levine AM, Gill PS, Muggia F. Malignancies in the acquired immunodeficiency syndrome. *Curr Probl Cancer* 1987;11:209–255.

57. Cotton P. AIDS giving rise to cardiac problems. *JAMA* 1990;263:2149.

58. Anderson DW, Virmani R. Emerging patterns of heart disease in human immunodeficiency virus infection. *Hum Pathol* 1990;21:253–259.

59. Coldiron BM, Bergstresser PR. Prevalence and clinical spectrum of skin disease in patients infected with the immunodeficiency virus. *Arch Dermatol* 1989;125:357–361.

60. Britton CB, Miller JB. Neurologic complications in acquired immunodeficiency syndrome. *Neurol Clin* 1984;2:315–339.

61. Ho DD, Pomerantz RJ, Kaplan JC. Pathogenesis of infection with human immunodeficiency virus. *N Engl J Med* 1987;321:278–286.

62. Bagasra O, Hauptman SP, Lischer HW, Sachs M, Pomerantz RJ. Detection of human immunodeficiency virus type 1 provirus in mononuclear cells by *in situ* poly-merase chain reaction. *New Engl J Med* 1992,326:1385–1391.

63. Burke AP, Benson W, Ribas JL. Postmortem localization of HIV-1 RNA by *in situ* hybridization in lymphoid tissues of intravenous drug addicts who died unexpectedly. *Am J Pathol* 1993;142:1701–1713.

64. Harper ME, Marselle LM, Gallo RC, Wong-Staal F. Detection of lymphocytes expressing human T-lymphotropic virus type III in lymph nodes and peripheral blood from infected individuals by *in situ* hybridization. *Proc Natl Acad Sci USA* 1986;83:772–776.

65. Nuovo GJ, Margiotta M, MacConnell P, Becker J. Rapid *in situ* detection of PCR-amplified HIV-1 DNA. *Diagn Mol Pathol* 1992;1:98–102.

66. Nuovo GJ, Forde A, MacConnell P, Fahrenwald R. *In situ* detection of PCR-amplified HIV-1 nucleic acids and tumor necrosis factor cDNA in cervical tissues. *Am J Pathol* 1993;143:40–48.

67. Patterson BK, Till M, Otto P, et al. Detection of HIV-1 DNA and messenger RNA in individual cells by PCR-driven *in situ* hybridization and flow cytometry. *Science* 1993;260:976–979.

68. Pantaleo G, Graziosi C, Demarest JF, et al. HIV infection is active and progressive in lymphoid tissue during the clinically latent stage of the disease. *Nature* 1993;362:355–358.

69. Fox CH, Tenner-Racz K, Racz P, Firpo A, Pizzo PA, Fauci AS. Lymphoid germinal centers are reservoirs of human immunodeficiency virus type 1 RNA. *J Infect Dis* 1991;164:1051–1057.

69a. Embretson J, Zupancic M, Ribas JL, Racz P, Tenner-Racz T, Haase AT. Massive covert infection of helper T lymphocytes and macrophages by HIV during the incubation period of AIDS. *Nature* 1993;362:359–362.

70. Hsia K, Spector SA. Human immunodeficiency virus DNA is present in a high percentage of CD4+ lymphocytes of seropositive individuals. *J Infect Dis* 1991;164:470–475.

71. Embretson J, Zupancic M, Beneke J, Ribas JL, Burke A, Haase AT. Analysis of human immunodeficiency virus infected tissues by amplification and *in situ* hybridization reveals latent and permissive infections at single cell resolution. *Proc Natl Acad Sci USA* 1993;90:357–361.

72. Spiegel H, Herbst H, Niedobitek G, Foss HD, Stein H. Follicular dendritic cells are a major reservoir for human immunodeficiency virus type 1 in lymphoid tissue facilitating infection of CD4+ T helper cells. *Am J Pathol* 1992;140:15–22.

73. Pantaleo G, Graziosi C, Fauci AS. The immunopathogenesis of human immunodeficiency virus infection. *N Engl J Med* 1993;328:327–335.

74. Nuovo GJ, Becker J, Margiotta M, Burke M, Fuhrer J, Steigbigel R. *In situ* detection of PCR-amplified HIV-1 nucleic acids in lymph nodes and peripheral blood in asymptomatic infection and advanced-stage AIDS. *J AIDS* 1994;7:916–923.

75. Simpson DM, Bender AN. Human immunodeficiency virus associated myopathy: analysis of 11 patients. *Ann Neurol* 1988;24:79.

76. Dalakas MC, Pezeshkpour GH. Neuromuscular diseases associated with human immunodeficiency virus infection. *Ann Neurol* 1988;23:38.

77. Wrzolek MA, Sher JH, Kozlowski PB, Rao C. Skeletal muscle pathology in AIDS: an autopsy study. *Muscle Nerve* 1990;13:508.

78. Lange DJ, Britton CB, Younger DS, Hays AP. The neuro-muscular manifestations of human immunodeficiency virus infections. *Arch Neurol* 1988;45:1084.

78a. Hantai D, Fournier JG, Vazeux R, Collin H, Baudrimont M, Fardeau M. Skeletal muscle involvement in human immunodeficiency virus infection. *Acta Neuropathol* 1991;81:496.

79. Ilia I, Nath A, Dalakas M. Immunocytochemical and virological characteristics of HIV-associated inflammatory myopathies: similarities with seronegative polymyositis. *Ann Neurol* 1991;29:474.

80. Mhiri C, Baudrimont M, Bonne G, et al. Zidovudine myopathy: a distinctive disorder associated with mitochondrial dysfunction. *Ann Neurol* 1991;29:606.

81. Arnaudo E, Dalakas M, Shanske S, Morales CT, Di-Mauro S, Schon EA. Depletion of muscle mitochondrial DNA in AIDS patients with zidovudine-induced myopathy. *Lancet* 1991;337:508.

82. Chad DA, Smith TW, Blumenfeld A, Fairchild PG, De-Girolami U. Human immunodeficiency virus associated myopathy: immunohistochemical identification of an HIV-antigen (gp 41) in muscle macrophages. *Ann Neurol* 1990;28:579.

83. Dalakas MC, London WT, Gravell M, Sever JL. Polymyositis in an immunodeficiency disease in monkeys induced by a type D retrovirus. *Neurology* 1986;36: 569.

84. Bothe K, Aguzzi A, Lassmann H, Rethwilm A, Horak I. Progressive encephalopathy and myopathy in transgenic mice expressing human foamy virus genes. *Science* 1991;253:555.

85. Seidman R, Peress N, Nuovo GJ. *In situ* detection of PCR-amplified HIV-1 nucleic acids in skeletal muscle in patients with myopathy. *Mod Pathol* 1994;7:369–375.

86. Leon-Monzon M, Lamperth L, Dalakas MC. Search for HIV proviral DNA and amplified sequences in the muscle biopsies of patients with HIV polymyositis. *Muscle Nerve* 1993;16:408–413.

87. Price RW, Brew B, Sidti J, Rosenblum M, Scheck, AC, Cleary P. The brain in AIDS: central nervous system HIV-1 infection and AIDS dementia complex. *Science* 1988;239:586–592.

88. Grant I, Atkinson JH, Hesselink JR. Evidence for early central nervous system involvement in acquired immunodeficiency syndrome and other human immunodeficiency virus infections. *Ann Intern Med* 1987; 107:828–836.

89. Weiser B, Peress N, LaNeve D, Eilbott DJ, Seidman R, Burger H. Human immunodeficiency virus type 1 expression in the central nervous system correlates directly with extent of disease. *Proc Natl Acad Sci USA* 1990; 87:3997–4001.

90. Wiley CA, Schrier RD, Nelson JA, Lampert PW, Oldstone MBA. Cellular localization of human immunodeficiency virus infection within the brains of acquired immune deficiency syndrome patients. *Proc Natl Acad Sci USA* 1986;83:7089–7093.

91. Tornatore C, Nath A, Amemiya K, Major EO. Persistent human immunodeficiency virus type 1 infection in human fetal glial cells reactivated by T-cell factor(s) or by the cytokines tumor necrosis factor alpha and interleukin-1 beta. *J Virol* 1990;65:6094–6100.

92. Watkins B, Dorn H, Kelley H, et al. Specific tropism of HIV-1 for microglial cells in primary human brain cultures. *Science* 1990;249:549–553.

93. Cvetkovich TA, Lazar E, Blumberg BM, et al. Human immunodeficiency virus type 1 infection of neural xenografts. *Proc Natl Acad Sci USA* 1992;89:5162–5166.

94. Lipton SA: HIV-1 related neurotoxicity. *Brain Pathol* 1991;1:193–199.

95. Yamada M, Zurbriggen A, Oldstone M, Fujinami R. Common immunologic determinant between human immunodeficiency virus type 1 gp41 and astrocytes. *J Virol* 1991;65:1370–1376.

96. Seshamma P, Bagasra O, Oakes J, Pomerantz RJ: Quantitative RT PCR for HIV-1 RNA specific species. *J Virol Methods* 1992;40:331–346.

97. Budka H. Human immunodeficiency virus (HIV) envelope and core proteins in CNS tissues of patients with AIDS and progressive encephalopathy. *Acta Neuropathol* 1990;79:611–619.

98. Nuovo GJ, Gallery F, MacConnell P, Braun A. *In situ* detection of PCR-amplified HIV-1 nucleic acids and tumor necrosis factor RNA in the central nervous system. *Am J Pathol* 1994;148:659–666.

99. Voeller B, Anderson DJ. Vaginal pH and HIV transmission. *JAMA* 1992;267:1917–1919.

100. Vande Perre P, DeClercq A, Cogniaux-Leclerc J, Nzaramba D, Butzler JP, Sprecher-Goldberger S. Detection of HIV p17 antigen in lymphocytes but not epithelial cells from cervicovaginal secretions of women seropositive for HIV: implications for heterosexual transmission of the virus. *Genitourin Med* 1988;64:30–37.

101. Pomerantz RJ, de la Monte SM, Donegan SP, et al: Human immunodeficiency virus (HIV) infection of the uterine cervix. *Ann Intern Med* 1988;108:321–327.

102. Shibata D, Klatt EC. Analysis of human immunodeficiency virus and cytomegalovirus infection by the polymerase chain reaction in the acquired immunodeficiency syndrome. *Arch Pathol Lab Med* 1989;113:1239–1244.

103. Mermim JH, Holodniy M, Katzenstein DA, Merigan TC: Detection of human immunodeficiency virus DNA and RNA in semen by the polymerase chain reaction. *J Infect Dis* 1991;164:769–772.

104. Pudney J, Anderson D. Orchitis and human immunodeficiency type 1 infected cells in reproductive tissues from men with the acquired immunodeficiency syndrome. *Am J Pathol* 1991;139:149–159.

105. DaSilva M, Shevchuk MM, Cronin WJ, et al. Detection of HIV-1 related protein in testes and prostates of patients with AIDS. *Am J Clin Pathol* 1990;93: 196–201.

106. Krieger JN, Coombs RW, Collier AC. Recovery of human immunodeficiency type 1 from semen: minimal impact of stage of infection and current antiviral chemotherapy. *J Infect Dis* 1991;163:386–388.

107. Ashida RA, Scofield SL. Lymphocyte major incompatibility complex-coded class II structures may act as sperm receptors. *Proc Natl Acad Sci USA* 1987;84:3395–3399.

108. Nuovo GJ, Becker J, Simsir A, Margiotta M, Shevchuck M. *In situ* localization of PCR-amplified HIV-1 nucleic acids in the male genital tract. *Am J Pathol* 1994;144: 142–148.

10

Instrumentation for *in situ* PCR

John G. Atwood

In the past, much *in situ* PCR has been performed by very labor-intensive and skill-intensive techniques. Most techniques have been developed by the scientists who have pioneered this new field in their own laboratories. Typically they have used available laboratory apparati and materials to address the special needs of containing the PCR reagent in contact with the specimen to be amplified and of controlling evaporation during thermal cycling.

The author's technique described in Chapter 6 is one of several in the literature that require fastening of a coverslip to the slide with an adhesive (e.g., nail polish) or building a covered reagent well around the sample using a plastic element. Usually, an overlay of oil is used to inhibit evaporation of the reagent during cycling.

Although these published techniques for performing *in situ* PCR do work well when carefully performed, they are less than ideal and inadequate for the future development of the field. Generally, they do not successfully address issues of large sample throughput, easy and reliable assembly reactions, and rapid thermal cycling at accurately controlled reaction temperatures. Their reagents are seldom designed for portability of robust protocols from one laboratory to another. These attributes of *in situ* PCR are necessary if it is to fulfill its great promise as a broadly useful method in biotechnology.

REQUIREMENTS UNIQUE TO *IN SITU* PCR

Several key differences between *in situ* PCR and PCR in solution present difficult challenges to the developer of optimized equipment for this field. These include relatively large surface area occupied by typical tissue samples, need to prevent evaporation of reagent spread in a thin layer over such samples, and sheer bulk of the glass slides to which the samples to be amplified are typically attached.

In situ PCR typically requires careful optimization of the fixation and protease permeabilization steps. Other than those steps, however, there are actually only a few special requirements for conducting *in situ* PCR compared with solution phase PCR. Per-cycle step efficiencies of *in situ* PCR tend to be rather low, probably due to the environment of cross-linked protein and DNA. However, because even single copy genes are in rather high concentration in the cells' nuclei, only rather modest amounts of amplification are required for detection. Generally, 25 thermal cycles or even fewer suffice. Protocols generally resemble those conducted in 500-μl plastic reaction tubes, requiring typically 1 minute for denaturation and 2 to 3 minutes for primer annealing and extension. Typical *in situ* amplifications thus require about 100 minutes. Many protocols specify higher levels of polymerase than are employed in solution phase PCR. This may reflect the reduced ability of *Taq* DNA polymerase to diffuse into the highly cross-linked environment as well as possible absorptive effects on glass slides.

Surface-to-Volume Ratio

Consider 50 μl of *in situ* PCR reagent spread in a layer 250 μm thick under a 14-mm^2 coverslip. It touches a total of 400 mm^2 of silanized glass, fixed cells or tissue, and coverslip. Its surface-to-volume ratio is 400 mm^2/50 mm^3, or 8 mm^{-1}. The same reagent volume in a 200-μl reaction tube would touch about 60 mm^2 of polypropylene and a smaller area of air, for a wetted surface-to-volume ratio about 1.2 mm^{-1}. The additional surface area exposes the *in situ* reagent to much greater loss of polymerase enzyme to the surfaces by adsorption and to much greater risk of enzyme inhibition by contaminants eluted from the surfaces.

The specific activity of *Taq* polymerase is so high that a typical 50-μl PCR containing 1.25 units of the enzyme has only about 5 $\times$ 10^{-14} mols of enzyme. If this reagent were contained under the *in situ* coverslip described above, and if only one-one thousandth of the wetted areas contained sites that could adsorb a monolayer of enzyme molecules, they would be sufficient to remove *all* the enzyme from solution.

For this reason, materials that can be used in containing *in situ* PCR reagents on a slide are much more sharply limited to those that are free of even slight harmful effects that would be tolerable for PCRs in solution. Also, reagents optimized for *in situ* PCR must be designed to give greater protection of the reaction from loss of enzyme activity. Many investigators compensate for adsorptive effects by substantially increasing the concentration of *Taq* DNA polymerase in the PCR mixture. Often, adding a comparatively high concentration (1 mg/ml) of an inert protein such as bovine serum albumin appears to serve the same purpose.

The Containment Challenge

Unless the *in situ* reagent is contained against the slide by a gas-tight seal to prevent evaporation, it will generally be necessary to rely on either an oil overlay with its attendant inconvenience or a humidity-controlled environment over the slides. Since the time required for the dew point in the controlled environment to follow the cycle temperatures are quite long

for a large volume, this approach is appropriate only for very slow cycles.

On the first heating of a room-temperature reagent to 95°C, about 40% of the air dissolved in the reagent comes out, forming bubbles with volumes of about 1% of the reagent, unless the containment system puts the reagent under pressure or the reagent is previously degassed. If the containment is rigid, the pressure within it at 95°C will rise by almost one atmosphere. This makes it unfeasible to attempt to contain a sealed, pressure-tight cover on a slide by adhesives alone, since the forces tending to lift it off become very large, while the adhesion where the boundary of the containment crosses tissue sections on the glass may be poor.

Slides as Bulky Sample Holders

Ninety-six PCRs in 200-μl tubes occupy the area of one microtiter plate. Ninety-six 25 $\times$ 75 mm microscope slides close-packed in a single horizontal layer occupy an area of about 2 square feet. In systems that depend on oil overlay, slides must be horizontal during cycling. Containment systems that are freed from the horizontal cycling requirement will be needed in the future.

Some researchers have placed samples to be amplified on tiny slivers of glass, small enough to be placed inside conventional PCR reaction tubes. But to depart from the standard slide format cuts the technique apart from centuries of development of histology techniques and apparatus.

Although bulky, slides are not inherently bad from the thermal point of view. Glass is roughly four times as good a conductor of heat as polyprolene. Thus, if a 1-mm-thick slide is brought into the same good thermal contact with a metal cycling block as the PCR reaction tube in a conventional thermal cycler, the *in situ* cycling speed can be roughly the same as for a plastic tube with a much thinner wall. The thermal mass of tissue sample itself is negligible, but the mass of any antievaporation cover may increase the thermal response time.

INSTRUMENTATION

Until now the most commonly employed instrumentation for thermal cycling of slides has been the top surfaces of cycler blocks intended for reaction in tubes. Recently, the same equipment with flat blocks without tube wells was used.

Typically, these cyclers, as well as the containment systems used with them, require that the slide be horizontal during cycling. Since most present-day cycles designed for use with tubes have rather small areas, only a few (typically three) slides at a time can be cycled. Furthermore, cycles designed for microcentrifuge tubes typically control the temperature in wells in a metal block that completely surrounds the reaction mixture in the tube, minimizing its loss of heat to the ambient environment. When slides are placed on top of a thermal cycler block, there is a considerable heat loss upward to ambient. Even with good thermal coupling from block to slide, the vertical temperature gradient through the slide caused by this heat flow can cause a difference between actual sample temperature and programmed block temperature of several degrees at 95°C and less at lower block temperatures. If the thermal coupling between block and slide is variable, as when aluminum foil boats are used, the difference can be much larger, more than 5°C and variable.

One problem with such systems with upward heat loss is that it is difficult for the user to measure the actual temperature achieved at the sample. It requires a special slide with a hair-thin thermocouple bonded to the glass under the containment system used on actual samples so that the actual vertical temperature gradient is simulated.

To cycle larger numbers of slides at one time, convection ovens have been adapted. Generally, the slides are placed in oil-filled plastic bags disposed on trays. Cycling is typically very slow. In one published protocol using an oven, the time for one cycle was 19 minutes (1). Uniformity of temperature is reported to be within ±1°C. With ovens, the ability to perform physical hot starts is apparently lost.

Almost all systems until recently do not address the containment issue, leaving the user to the laborious manual assembly of reactions under glued down coverslips, and so forth.

A Complete *in situ* PCR System

To make *in situ* PCR broadly useful and easy to perform, a complete system from sample prepartion to PCR product detection is needed that meets all the unique requirements.

A complete system for *in situ* PCR is described here that addresses the need to reduce the labor intensity and skill required to assemble each reaction. It employs an engineered system for thermal cycling ten slides with up to three specimens per slide with speed and accuracy comparable with those achieved with PCR in solution in 500-μl reaction tubes. It uses no adhesives or oil to control evaporation. It easily permits one to use thermal hot starts.

Reagent Containment System

The new system uses a purely mechanical approach for containing the reagent over the tissue specimen on a microscope slide. A concave rubber diaphragm is clamped over the specimen by a thin, stainless steel clip. The space between the diaphragm and the slide contains about 25 μl of reagent. The rim of the steel clip compresses the edge of the rubber diaphragm against the slide with considerable force, making a water- and gas-tight seal. The force is supplied by two stainless steel parts attached to the ends of the clamp that extend over the edges of the slide and are made to slide under and grip the bottom edges of the slide.

Figure 10-1 shows a microscope slide with three serial tissue sections. Above it are two rubber diaphragms and two steel clamps. Those on the right are oriented as they would be on the side. Those on the left are upside down to show the cavity in the clamp into which the rubber diaphragm is placed. Figure 10-2 shows the rubber diaphragm (it is made of transparent

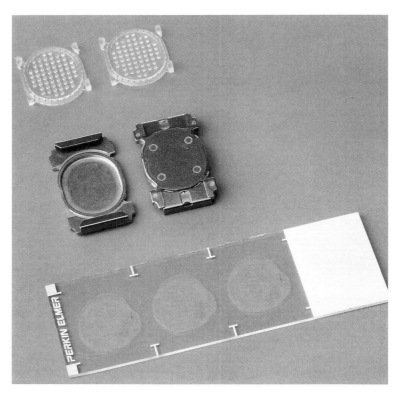

Figure 10-1. *Components of slide containment system.* Three deparaffinized tissue sections are shown mounted on a silane-treated slide. On the right, a silicone diaphragm and the mounting clip are shown in the orientation in which they would be mounted over the specimen. On the left, both the silicone diaphragm and clip are shown inverted.

silicone rubber) being placed in the cavity of the steel clamp.

Figure 10-3 shows the two clamps and diaphragms applied to the slide. The view is from the underside of the slide, showing how the sliding grips reach over the edges of the slide to compress the rubber diaphragms on the top of the slide tightly against the glass. The reagent is trapped between the diaphragm and the slide. The working area is an oval about 14 × 17 mm in size.

A special assembly tool is used to make the assemblies quickly and easily (Fig. 10-4). The slide with sample specimens can be seen placed on the platen in the center of the tool. A steel clamp and diaphragm are visible mounted on the vertical swinging arm.

As shown in Fig. 10-5, a droplet of about 30 μl of reagent is pipetted onto the slide over one of the samples. The arm is then swung down to a horizontal position over the reagent droplet. The arm automatically engages a hook-like cam. The user then turns the knob, rotating the cam. This pulls the arm down against the slide with a pre-engineered force (Fig.10-6). The cam is rotated by the user's right hand.

As the diaphragm moves down on the reagent droplet, the liquid spreads uniformly out toward the edges of the diaphragm, expelling all the air ahead of it. Since the volume in the droplet is a few microliters larger than will fit in the concavity between the diaphragm and the slide, a small amount of reagent is expelled as the diaphragm's edge

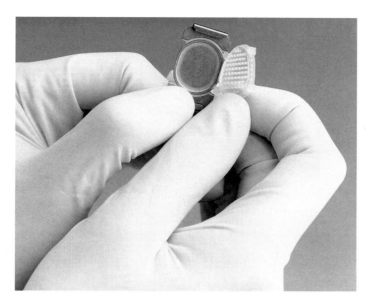

Figure 10-2. *Assembly of diaphragm into clip.* The male portion of the diaphragm (the bottom of the diaphragm on the left side of Fig. 10-1) slips into and is held by the complementary-shaped cavity of the clip.

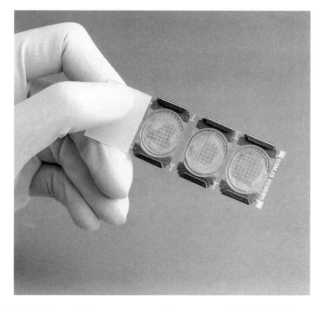

Figure 10-3. *Assembled slide containment system.* Once assembled, liquid is trapped over the specimens and cannot be lost. The dark color that appears in the center is due to the presence of an inert dye, which confirms that no bubbles are present over the specimen.

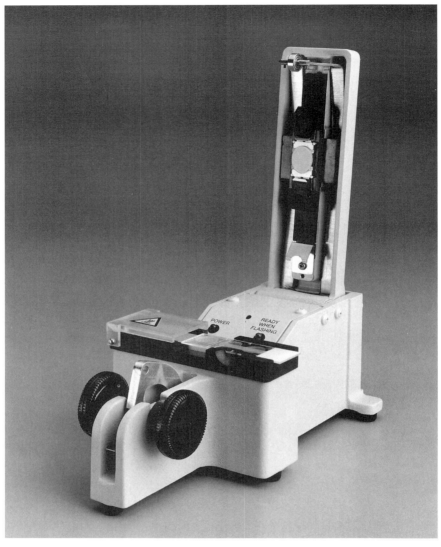

Figure 10-4. *Assembly tool.* The slide with sample specimens is placed on the platen in the center of the tool. This platen is heated for hot starts. The assembled silicone diaphragm and clamp are held in the middle portion of the handle of the tool shown in the vertical position. Magnets hold the clamp and keep the arms of the clamp open.

seals against the slide. No air bubbles remain inside the cavity. Air bubbles are to be avoided because they create a localized dry spot on the specimen that may fail to amplify. Generally, an inert, easily visualized dye is added to the PCR mixture so that any air bubbles trapped under the containment system can be detected.

Further force compresses the sealing edge of the diaphragm and puts the trapped reagent under pressure. The sliding steel grips are now in a position to be pushed under the edge of the slide. The user pinches together two sliding handles on the top of the arm, which push the grips under the slide. In Fig. 10-6, this action is being performed by the user's left hand.

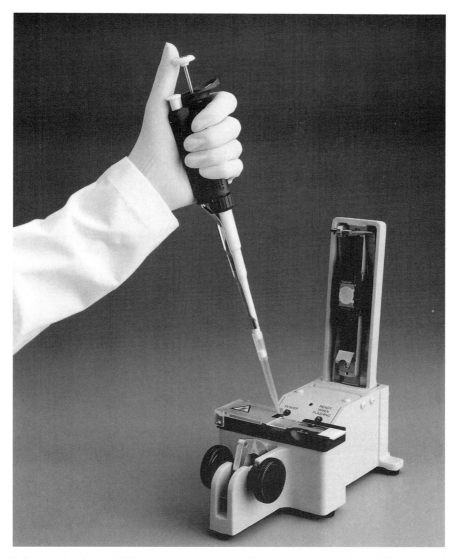

Figure 10-5. *Application of PCR mixture to samples.* Approximately 30 μl of PCR mixture is applied to the slide, which is heated in the case of hot start PCR. The PCR mixture heats quickly.

Now, by rotating the cam back to its original position, the user releases the arm and returns it to the original upright position. The slide can be removed, or it can be moved to a new position and another reaction can be assembled. Up to three reactions can be assembled on each slide. Each assembly takes about 30 seconds.

The assembled slide can now be placed in a specially designed *in situ* thermal cycler, shown in Fig. 10-7. Its sample block has 10 vertical slots, each of which can hold one slide with any number of clamps and diaphragms in almost any position. The left side of each slot is especially flat and has grooves at the top and bottom to accommodate the grips so that the entire central region of each slide can be pressed firmly into contact with the flat surface.

Twenty small springs, one at each end of each slot, are opened by a single cam lever to permit placing slides in the slots (Fig. 10-8).

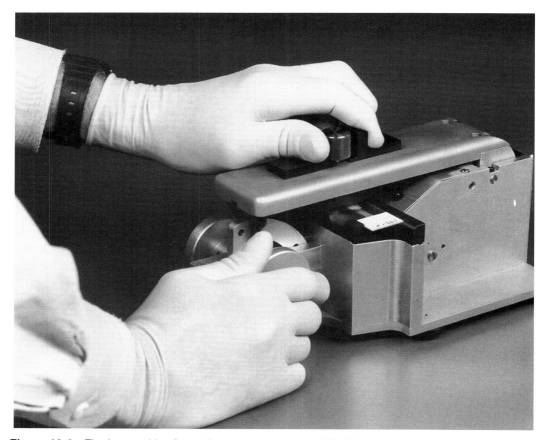

Figure 10-6. *Final assembly of containment system upon slide.* The vertical arm is dropped, and the user rotates a knob to pull the arm down against the slide. Pinching the two sliding handles on top of the arm completes the mounting of the clip and diaphragm onto the slide. The sample is now mounted with the PCR mixture under pressure and without bubbles.

When the cam lever is moved to the closed position, the springs push and hold each slide against the left wall of its slot. The block cover (shown open in Fig. 10-8) can now be closed, and cycling can begin.

Because the containment system completely traps the reagent with no air inside, the slides can be handled in any position and cycled on edge, permitting ten slides to be cycled in a space that would hold at most three if horizontal cycling were required. In addition, each slide is entirely embedded in the block. It is heated and cooled from both sides. Little heat is lost upward, so there is little vertical gradient, and excellent temperature accuracy and uniformity are achieved (Fig. 10-9).

Response times during cycling are shown in Fig. 10-10. The sample temperature lags the block temperature by about 18 seconds in this prototype unit.

Hot Starts

As previously discussed (Chapter 3), hot starts are often critically important to the success of an *in situ* amplification. In some cases, chemical reagents such as single-stranded binding proteins can substitute for physical hot start methods. In the case of solution phase PCR, physical hot starts can be fully automated with the use of wax beads (available under the name of Ampliwax). This type of physical hot start is unsuitable for *in situ* amplification of samples on slides.

However, physical *in situ* hot starts can be easily implemented due to the unique property of, with *in situ* PCR, the DNA in the sample being immobilized on the slide. This means that a complete PCR mixture with all the reactants except DNA can be assembled prior to addition of the PCR mixture on the (heated) slide without fear of nonspecific priming. In theory, this should not prevent the possible formation of one type of nonspecific product, primer oligomers. In practice, it appears that primer oligomerization rarely causes problems with *in situ* PCR due to the limited number of thermal cycles generally performed. In the rare case that primer oligomer-

ization does cause problems, the reaction mixture can be kept warm before applying it to the *in situ* specimen.

Actual thermal hot starts can be easily implemented in this system. The metal platen on which the slide is placed in the assembly tool has a heater and temperature sensor attached to it. It is thermostatted at a fixed, user-determined temperature, typically about 80°C.

When a slide is placed on the platen it rises rapidly toward the thermostatted temperature. Since all the double-stranded DNA, both genomic and template, is on the slide, the complete reagent including polymerase enzyme can be mixed before assembly. Studies show that when a room temperature reagent is pipetted onto the slide, the part that touches the slide immediately rises in temperature to the average between the slide temperature and the reagent temperature. If the reagent temperature is a bit

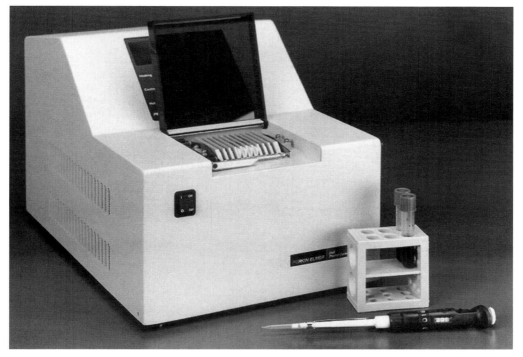

Figure 10-7. *Prototype of* in situ *thermal cycler.* The sample block has ten slots, each of which can hold one slide with up to three containment vessels over the slide.

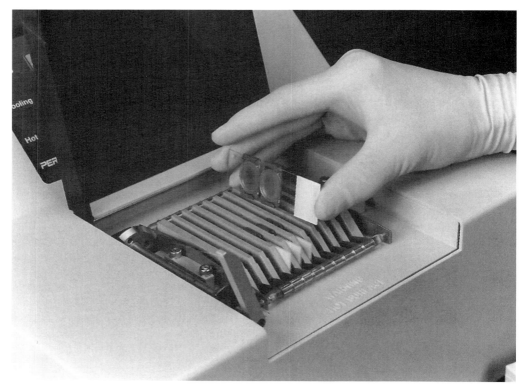

Figure 10-8. *Mounting of assembled slides in the* in situ *thermal cycler.* Each slot can accept a single slide. The top of the diaphragm faces the right, and the bottom of the clips is on the left. After loading up to ten slides, a mounting lever is engaged to seat each slide firmly against the block.

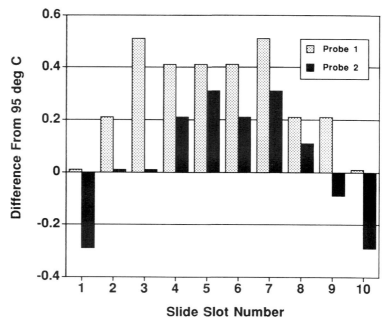

Figure 10-9. *Measured steady-state thermal uniformity of a ten-slot* in situ *block at 95°C before and after calibration of the thermal cycler.* Measurements were made with a calibrated miniature platinum resistance thermometer chip bonded to a microscope slide.

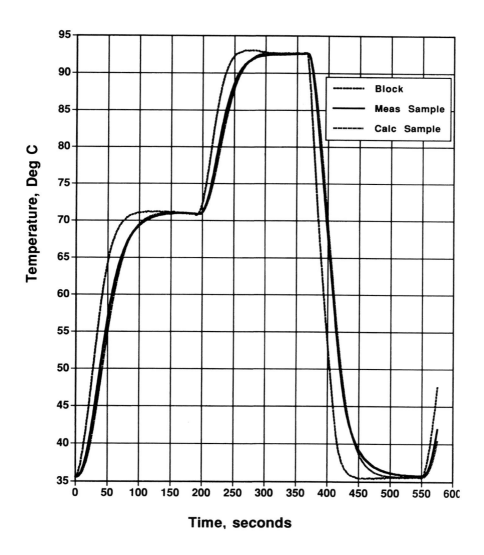

Figure 10-10. *Measured temperature profiles on a slide in the block of the* in situ *thermal cycle.* Temperature cycle was 2 minutes at 72°C, 2 minutes at 94°C, and 2 minutes at 35°C. Sample and block temperatures were measured with an uncalibrated, fine-wire thermocouple bonded to a slide. Calculated sample temperature was computed from the measured block temperature assuming a pure exponential thermal line constant of 17.8 seconds.

above room temperature, there will never be any contact between reagent and sample DNA at temperatures low enough to cause mispriming.

If the cycler is set in a hold at, say, 80°C during preparation of slides, each reaction can be placed in an open slot and will not cool to a mispriming temperature. Cycling with a true hot start can begin when the last slide has been placed in the cycler. An example of DNA target-specific direct incorporation of the reporter mol-

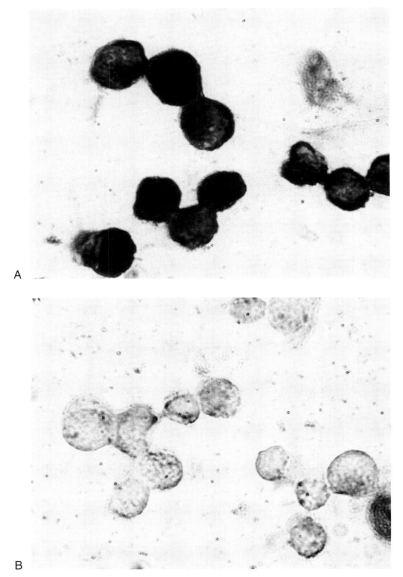

A

B

Figure 10-11. *Results of amplification of HLA-DRB target sequence in JW-5 cells.* The cells were formalin fixed, treated with pepsin, and thermal cycled on the *in situ* DNA thermal cycler prototype in the presence of digoxigenin-dUTP. Direct detection of total amplified sequences was accomplished with antidigoxigenin–alkaline phosphatase conjugate and NBT/BCP reagent (Boehringer Mannheim). **A:** Amplification with DRB-specific primers. Nucleic are intensely stained. **B:** Amplification with mismatched primers. The amplification was conducted with human papillomavirus (HPV)-specific primers. JW-5 cells are HPV negative, and only a very weak nuclear signal was observed. **C:** Amplification without primers. Only a very weak nuclear signal is observed, much the same as with amplification with HPV-specific primers. **D:** Amplification without *Taq* DNA polymerase. No signal observed.

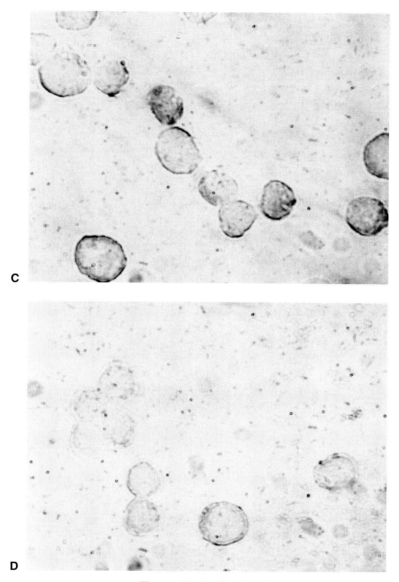

C

D

Figure 10-11. *Continued.*

ecule using hot start *in situ* PCR is provided in Fig. 10-11. Many examples of RT *in situ* PCR in tissue sections using the Perkin-Elmer *in situ* 1000 thermal cycler are provided in this book (Fig. 10-12; see also Figs. 7.25, 7.26, 7.30, and 7.31).

REFERENCE

1. Staskus KA, Couch L, Bitterman P, et al. *In situ* amplification of visna virus DNA in tissue sections reveals a reservoir of latently infected cells. *Microbiol Pathogenesis* 1991;39:67–76.

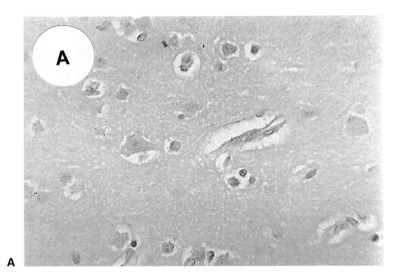

A

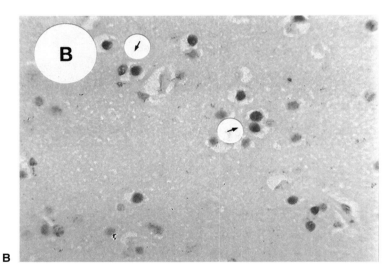

B

Figure 10-12. *Detection of PCR-amplified HIV-1 DNA using the Perkin-Elmer* in situ *PCR cycler.* HIV-1 DNA was not detected by *in situ* hybridization in this brain tissue of a patient with AIDS dementia (**A**). The viral DNA was detected in many cells after PCR *in situ* hybridization (**B**, *arrow*).

Appendix: Glossary of Terms and Reagents for Molecular Biological Analyses

This appendix provides the reader with a glossary of commonly used terms and a listing of reagents that can be used for filter hybridization, *in situ* hybridization, PCR, RT *in situ* PCR, and PCR *in situ* hybridization. It is important to stress that this listing does not imply that these products are the ones I recommend to the exclusion of others. However, for the most part, I have tried these products with good results. I would like to thank Mr. Bernie Janossen (Boehringer Mannheim), John Atwood (Perkin-Elmer), Dr. Norman Kelker (Enzo), and Barbara Keech (ONCOR) for contributing to the list of reagents.

Glossary of Terms

A

adenovirus   DNA virus that causes typical "smudge" nuclei and is associated with large copy numbers, easily detectable by standard *in situ* hybridization.

alkaline phosphatase   Enzyme ultimately responsible for production of signal by being linked to molecule that attaches to reporter nucleotide, e.g., streptavidin to biotin.

alu probe/sequence   Common repetitive DNA sequence in mammalian cells that comprises about 5% of the total genome. Thus, the *alu* sequence is present as hundreds of copies in a given cell and can be used as a positive control for *in situ* hybridization.

Ampliwax   A hardened wax at room temperature that can be used to separate amplification solution from *Taq* polymerase. At 55°C, it melts and allows mixing, permitting hot start PCR.

annealing   The binding of one DNA strand to another via base pair matching.

B

background   In general, any nonspecific signal. For *in situ* hybridization, this involves nonspecific sticking of the probe to cellular proteins or, less commonly, DNA, from too low stringent washing (see below). For *in situ* PCR, background also includes primer-independent DNA synthesis and mispriming-based DNA synthesis.

base pair matching   The complexing of A and T (two hydrogen bonds) or G and C (three hydrogen bonds) during hybridization.

biotin   Common reporter nucleotide that binds to streptavidin–alkaline phosphatase conjugate.

bovine serum albumin   Protein commonly used with *in situ* hybridization and immunohistochemistry to block nonspecific adsorption of the detection reagent (usually alkaline phosphatase conjugate) to the tissue and thus reduce background. It can also raise the effective concentration of *Taq* polymerase during *in situ* PCR by blocking adsorption to the glass slide and tissue.

C

Caski cells   A human cervical cancer cell line that contains about 600 copies of HPV 16 DNA.

chemical hot start   Inhibition of mispriming and primer oligomerization by using molecules that can complex to primers and thus require high homology for persistence of binding of primer to DNA (e.g., single-stranded binding protein of *Escherichia coli*). Another mechanism of chemical hot start is the degradation of dUTP-containing DNA made at temperatures <55°C by uracil *N*-glycosylase.

chromatin   The complex of DNA and proteins in the nucleus.

chromogen   Molecule(s) that, typically, are precipitated by alkaline phosphatase and thus produce a signal, e.g., NBT/BCIP.

copy number   The number of target molecules per a given cell. The detection threshold for *in situ* hybridization is 10 copies per cell.

counterstain   A stain used to visualize tissue better, it must not mask the signal. A common example is nuclear fast red (light pink) versus the chromogen NBT/BCIP (blue).

cross-hybridization   The hybridization of a DNA strand with a similar but not identical DNA strand.

cytomegalovirus   A DNA virus that infects (primarily) endothelial cells and macrophages. It causes a large nuclear inclusion and multiple small cytoplasmic inclusions.

D

denature   The separation of a hybridized double-stranded DNA complex due to disruption of their hydrogen bonds.

dideoxynucleotide   A nucleotide that lacks the 3' OH group and, thus, will terminate DNA synthesis.

digoxigenin   Common reporter nucleotide that binds to antidigoxigen–alkaline phosphatase conjugate. Unlike biotin, it does not occur in mammalian cells and is less likely to produce background.

DNA repair   See **primer-independent signal.**

DNase digestion   Elimination of genomic-based DNA synthesis by overnight DNase digestion after optimal protease digestion.

E

endonuclease   A DNase that disrupts the phosphodiester bond between two nucleotides internal to the terminal 5' and 3' ends. Endonucleases are often highly specific for a 6 to 10 base pair region.

eosin   Common stain used in pathology. It stains proteins pink/red.

Epstein-Barr virus   A DNA virus that infects B lymphocytes and squamous cells. It is found in hairy leukoplakia, infectious mononucleosis, and commonly in the lymphomas of AIDS patients. Does not produce diagnostic cytopathic effects and thus requires *in situ* or PCR *in situ* hybridization for direct detection.

ethidium   A carcinogen that intercalates into DNA. It can be used to detect DNA by its ability to react with ultraviolet light and produce an intense fluorescence.

EZ RT *in situ* PCR   Detection of RNA *in situ* using the enzyme rTth, which is capable of synthesizing cDNA and amplifying it in the same reaction mixture inside the cell.

F

filter hybridization   Detection of DNA after direct transfer to filter (slot blot) or after electrophoretic separation and transfer to a filter (Southern blot). Detection of RNA, usually after electrophoretic separation, is called Northern blot.

formalin   A commonly used fixative that cross-links nucleic acids and proteins.

formamide   A chemical that can disrupt hydrogen bonds. It is commonly used to reduce background.

G

glutaraldehyde   A cross-linking fixative commonly used in electron microscopy.

H

HeLa cells   A cervical cancer cell line that contains 20 copies of HPV 18 per cell.

hematoxylin   Common stain used in pathology. It stains nucleic acids blue.

herpes simplex virus   DNA virus that infects squamous cells and causes multinucleation and chromatin clearing.

homology   The percentage of base pairs that match (A–T and G–C) when two antiparallel DNA strands attempt to hybridize.

hot start   Withholding one of the key reagents for DNA amplification, such as the *Taq* polymerase or the magnesium until the temperature of the block reaches at least 55°C. This will reduce mispriming and primer oligomerization.

hybridization   The binding of two DNA strands via base pair matching.

hydrogen bond   The chemical attraction that is the major force responsible for hybridization of two DNA strands or RNA with cDNA.

I

immortalization   Persistent cell growth in tissue culture.

inadequate protease digestion: DNA   Inability to generate a hybridization signal using a probe known to correspond to an abundant target in the tissue. It is assumed that other variables, such as correct fixative, denaturation, and so forth, are adequate. This is an unusual cause of a lack of a signal with *in situ* hybridization or PCR *in situ* hybridization.

inadequate protease digestion: RNA   Inability to generate intense primer-independent and primer-dependent signals with *in situ* PCR with an enhancement of the signal after DNase digestion. This is the most common cause of a lack of signal with RT *in situ* PCR.

in situ **hybridization**   Detection of a DNA or RNA target in an intact cell; it requires ten copies per cell to be able to visualize the signal.

in situ **PCR**   Direct incorporation of the labeled nucleotide in the PCR product as it is formed inside the cell.

J

JC virus   A DNA virus that is the cause of progressive multifocal leukoencephalopathy. This is a condition seen in AIDS patients that is associated with oligodendroglial cells and is evident as enlarged, smudged nuclei.

L

leukocyte   A white blood cell; includes neutrophils, lymphocytes, and macrophages.

ligation   The attachment of two DNA strands by a phosphodiester bond via the enzyme DNA ligase.

low stringency   Conditions of either hybridization or, more commonly, the posthybridization wash that do not require a high degree of homology for two hybridized strands to remain attached.

lymphocyte   A leukocyte associated with chronic inflammation; it has a round, dark nucleus and minimal cytoplasm.

M

macrophage   A leukocyte associated with chronic inflammation. It has a large, folded (kidney bean shaped) nucleus and ample cytoplasm that often has vacuoles.

measles   An RNA virus that infects epithelium and leukocytes, producing multinucleated cells.

melting temperature   The temperature under defined reactions conditions (including salt and formamide concentration) at which one-half of a hybridized DNA complex remains hybridized and the other one-half denatured.

mispriming   DNA synthesis during PCR or *in situ* PCR based on annealing of the primer to nontarget DNA, e.g., an HIV-1 primer and human DNA. This can be blocked by the hot start maneuver.

N

new fuschin   A chromogen that can be used with hematoxylin and eosin as the counterstain.

nick translation   Synthesis of a DNA probe from controlled DNase digestion and DNA polymerase activity.

Northern blot hybridization   See **filter hybridization**.

NBT/BCIP   The two chemicals that, when acted upon by alkaline phosphatase, produce an intense blue precipitate.

nuclear fast red   A counterstain to be used with NBT/BCIP (see **NBT/BCIP**). It stains intact DNA and RNA a pale pink. Loss of this pink staining implies protease overdigestion (see **overdigestion**).

nucleotide   The building block of DNA and RNA, it consists of a ribose sugar, a 5' triphosphate, and a 1' base (A,C,G,T or, for RNA, U).

nuclear matrix   A complex, three-dimensional array of proteins, DNA, and RNA. Unmasking of the proteins with a protease is needed to detect or amplify a target of interest.

nuclear membrane   A bilayer protein–lipid structure. It probably serves as part of the migration "barrier" with *in situ* PCR, presupposing optimal protease digestion.

O

oligomerization   DNA synthesis during PCR based on annealing of one primer to another primer. This can be blocked by the hot start maneuver.

oligoprobe   A small (20–40mer) probe that can be used to detect the PCR product.

organosilane   See **silane**.

overdigestion Destruction of the basic skeleton of the cell by too much protease digestion. In the initial stages, the nuclear membrane (see **nuclear membrane**) is destroyed, and DNA targets migrate to the cytoplasm. At the end stage, the signal is lost and the cytoplasmic membrane is no longer clearly evident. Loss of DNA in the nucleus from overdigestion results in the loss of the pink color with the counterstain nuclear fast red (see **nuclear fast red**).

P

paraformaldehyde A cross-linking fixative.

paraffin A wax used to embed formalin-fixed tissue. It is removed by xylene.

parvovirus A DNA virus that selectively infects nucleated red blood cells, causing a large intranuclear inclusion.

PCR *in situ* hybridization Detection of amplified DNA inside an intact cell by using a labeled probe.

pepsin A protease commonly used in molecular diagnostics. It is less likely than proteinase K to cause overdigestion.

picric acid A fixative sometimes used in pathology, causing a yellow color in the tissue. It causes extensive degradation of the DNA and, thus, is not compatible with PCR or *in situ* PCR.

plasmid A self-replicating circular DNA molecule used to clone an insert after ligation.

primer A short (20–40) base pair sequence of DNA used either to amplify a specific DNA target in PCR or to initiate cDNA synthesis from RNA by reverse transcriptase. Primers are typically unlabeled.

primer-independent signal Direct incorporation of a labeled nucleotide during *in situ* PCR in the absence of primers. It results from repair of gaps in the double-stranded DNA complex caused by the "dry" heating of the cells. It is also apparent in solution phase PCR under the following conditions: heated DNA that is treated with a cross-linking fixative in the presence of a protein and intact protein–DNA cross-links.

probe A labeled DNA or RNA sequence used to detect a specific target. There usu-

ally is 100% homology between the target and probe.

R

ramping The change of one temperature to another by the thermal cycler.

random priming The synthesis of a DNA probe via many hexanucleotides that bind to homologous regions after denaturation.

respiratory syncytial virus An RNA virus that causes multinucleation usually of alveolar lining cells.

reverse transcriptase Synthesizes cDNA from an RNA molecule.

rTth A DNA polymerase that can synthesize cDNA using the same reagent conditions as for PCR amplification.

S

sensitivity The ability to detect a DNA or RNA sequence when present in a given cell or tissue sample.

serial section A paraffin-embedded tissue section slice that is 4 μM away from the adjacent section.

SiHa cells A cervical cancer cell line that contains one copy of HPV 16 per cell.

silane An adhesive that, when used to treat glass, greatly improves tissue adherence during *in situ* PCR.

slot blot hybridization See **filter hybridization**.

Southern blot hybridization See **filter hybridization**.

Stoffel fragment of DNA polymerase A DNA polymerase that lacks the exonuclease activity of *Taq*. It can be used to study the effects of the exonuclease activity of *Taq* on the DNA repair-based signal.

stringency The conditions of, typically, the post-hybridization wash that determine the degree of homology needed for persistent binding of the probe to the target and non-target sequences. Stringency is increased by raising the temperature, by using formamide, or by reducing the salt concentration.

T

***Taq* polymerase** The thermal stable enzyme that can synthesize DNA during PCR.

target   A DNA or RNA sequence one is attempting to detect by use of a specific primer or probe.

terminal transferase   An enzyme used to label an oligoprobe.

Tm   See **melting temperature.**

trypsin   A commonly used protease.

U

Uracil *N*-glycosylase   An enzyme that degrades DNA that contains dUTP. Can be used for chemical hot start in PCR as it is inactivated by temperatures above 55°C.

W

Western blot analysis   Detection of a protein after electrophoretic separation and transfer to a filter.

X

xylene   A chemical used to remove paraffin from tissue after it is placed on a glass slide. It also removes the mineral oil overlay that is used with the aluminum boat method of *in situ* PCR.

Boehringer Mannheim Corporation, 9115 Hague Road, PO Box 50414, Indianapolis, Indiana 46250-0414

Genius™ System

The Genius™ System, developed by Boehringer Mannheim, allows specific labeling and detection of biomolecules. The steroid hapten digoxigenin, covalently bound to nucleotides, nucleic acids, proteins or carbohydrates, is recognized by digoxigenin antibodies that are labeled with fluorescent dyes or enzymes.

The process for use of digoxigenin-labeled RNA, DNA, and oligonucleotides is claimed in European Patent No. 0 324 474 and corresponding patent rights in other countries. The price of the products include a prepaid royalty in consideration for which royalty the purchaser hereby acquires a non-exclusive license to use the appropriate product in the above-mentioned process in their own internal research. Licenses for uses other than internal research are subject to a separate agreement. Please address a corresponding request to International Product Management, Biochemical Reagents, Sandhofer Str. 116, 68298 Mannheim, Germany.

Support Material for Nonradioactive Alternatives

Genius™ System User's Guide for Filter Hybridization*	101 023	1 book
This guide contains the definitive protocols and technical tips for using the Genius™ System in blotting applications.		
Genius™ System Bibliography	101 087	1 book
This bibliography features the most current list of published papers in which the Genius™ System was used. It is updated regularly and is arranged by technique for ease of use.		
Genius™ System Video*	101 089	1 video
Nonradioactive *In Situ* Hybridization Application Manual		
This manual provides complete *in situ* hybridization protocols (e.g., PRINS) for using the Genius™System on whole chromosomes, fixed sections, and cultured cells.	101 091	1 book

*Supplied free of charge with a Genius™kit purchase.

Genius™ Labeling and Detection Kits

DNA Labeling and Detection Kit, Nonradioactive (Genius™ 1)	1093 657	1 kit (25 labeling and 50 detection [100 cm²] reactions)
25 labeling reactions (10 ng to 3 μg DNA per reaction). Typically, 125 ng of labeled DNA is enough to detect homologous DNA on a 100 cm² nitrocellulose filter. Labeled probes can detect as little as 0.1 pg DNA. A labeled DNA probe can detect a single copy gene on a Southern blot of 1 μg human placental DNA. When control DNA is labeled and used as a hybridization probe on Southern or dot blots, it can detect 0.1 pg homologous DNA after 12-hour incubation (1 pg after 1-hour incubation). No hybridization occurs to a control containing 100 ng heterologous DNA. This kit uses the random primed labeling technique to prepare DNA hybridization probes with a nonradioactive label (digoxigenin-11-dUTP). Labeled DNA is detected with an enzyme-labeled antibody to digoxigenin.		
DNA Labeling Kit, Nonradioactive (Genius™ 2)	1175 033	1 kit (40 reactions)
For random primed labeling of DNA with the nonradioactive label digoxigenin-dUTP.		
Labeled probes can detect as little as 0.1 pg of homologous DNA. A labeled DNA probe can detect a single copy gene on a Southern blot of 1 μg human placental DNA. When control DNA is labeled and used as a hybridization probe on Southern or dot blots, it can detect 0.1 pg homologous DNA after 12-hour incubation (1 pg after 1-hour incubation). No hybridization occurs to a control containing 100 ng of heterologous DNA. This kit uses the random primed labeling technique to prepare DNA hybridization probes with the non-radioactive label, digoxigenin-11-dUTP. For colorimetric detection of probes made with this kit, use the Genius™ 3 Nucleic Acid Detection Kit (Cat. No. 1175 041) or the Genius™ 7 Luminescent Detection Kit (Cat No. 1363 514).		
Nucleic Acid Detection Kit, Nonradioactive (Genius™ 3)	1175 041	1 kit (40 blots, 100 cm²)

For detection of digoxigenin-labeled DNA or RNA by enzyme immunoassay.

The kit can detect a digoxigenin-labeled DNA probe hybridized to 0.1 pg homologous DNA in a Southern blot. The kit can also detect a digoxigenin-labeled RNA probe hybridized to 0.1 pg homologous DNA (Southern blot) or RNA (Northern blot). When labeled control DNA (vial 1) is used as hybridization probe on a Southern or dot blot, the kit can detect 0.1 pg homologous DNA after 12-hour incubation (1 pg after 1-hour incubation). The kit gives no color reaction when 100 ng of heterologous DNA is probed with the labeled control DNA. When digoxigenin-labeled RNA is used as hybridization probe on a Northern or dot blot, the kit can detect 0.1 pg homologous RNA after 12-hour incubation (1 pg after 1-hour incubation). This kit detects digoxigenin-labeled nucleic acid (either DNA or RNA prepared with the Genius™ 2 or 4 Nonradioactive Labeling Kits) with an enzyme-labeled antibody to digoxigenin.

RNA Labeling Kit, Nonradioactive (Genius™ 4)	1175 025	1 kit (2 × 10 reactions)

For *in vitro* labeling of RNA with the nonradioactive label digoxigenin-UTP.

Labeled RNA probes can detect as little as 0.1 pg homologous DNA. Digoxigenin-labeled Neo RNA, transcribed from the pSPT19-Neo template with SP6 RNA polymerase, can detect 0.3 pg homologous (pSPT19-Neo) DNA or 0.3 pg homologous (Neo) RNA on a dot blot after 12-hour color development (1 pg after 1-hour color development). No hybridization occurs to controls containing 100 ng heterologous DNA or RNA. For detection of probes made with this kit, use the Genius™ 3 Nucleic Acid Detection Kit (Cat. No. 1175 041) or the Genius™7 Luminescent Detection Kit (Cat. No. 1363 514).

Oligonucleotide 3′-End Labeling Kit, Nonradioactive (Genius™ 5)	1362 372	1 kit (25 reactions)

For the preparation of nonradioactively labeled oligonucleotide probes.

The kit contains enough reagents to label 25 different oligonucleotides, each 14 to 100 nucleotides long. Each reaction can label up to 100 pmol of an oligonucleotide (equivalent to 1 μg of a 30-mer). Oligonucleotide probes prepared with the Oligonucleotide 3′-End Labeling Kit, Nonradioactive may be used for *in situ* hybridization experiments and blotting applications.

Oligonucleotide Tailing Kit (Genius™ 6)	1417 231	1 kit (25 tailing reactions)

For nonradioactive 3′-tailing of oligonucleotides.

The kit contains all of the reagents needed to perform 25 tailing reactions (100 pmol of oligonucleotide per reaction). The digoxigenin Oligonucleotide Tailing Kit is a nonradioactive system used to place an oligonucleotide tail on the 3′-end of hybridization probes using DIG-dUTP and dATP. Following hybridization, the digoxigenin-labeled probes may be detected with an anti-DIG enzyme conjugate. Dig-tailed probes can be used in any standard hybridization procedure (e.g., Southern blots, Northern blots, *in situ* hybridizations, DNA footprinting).

Luminescent Detection Kit (Genius™ 7)	1363 514	1 kit (50 blots 100 cm^2)

For chemiluminescent detection of digoxigenin-labeled DNA or RNA by enzyme immunoassay on 50 blots, each 100 cm^2. The kit can detect 0.03 pg of homologous DNA in a dot blot after a 30-minute exposure to x-ray film. This kit detects digoxigenin-labeled nucleic acids (either DNA or RNA) with an alkaline phosphatase-conjugated antibody to digoxigenin and the chemiluminescent substrate Lumigen PPD. This kit should be used only for filter hybridization experiments.

Oligonucleotide 5′-End Labeling Set, Nonradioactive (Genius™ 8)	1480 863	1 set (10 reactions)

For the preparation of 5′-digoxigenin–labeled sequencing primers, PCR primers, and hybridization probes using an automatic DNA synthesizer.

Oligonucleotides are reacted with the phosphoramidite in a final synthesis step according to the solid phase phosphoramidite method to create a 5′-terminal activated amino group. The oligonucleotide is then released from the solid support, and, after cleavage of the protecting groups, the digoxigenin moiety is introduced at the 5′-end. Note: The bottle with the phosphoramidite directly fits to the appropriate position of the automatic DNA synthesizers from Applied Biosystems, Eppendorf, and Pharmacia.

Nonradioactive Nucleic Acid Labeling Reagents

AMCA-6-dUTP	1534 386	25 nmol
(Amino-4-methyl-coumarin-6-2′-deoxyuridine-5′-triphosphate)		(25 μl)

1 mM aqueous tetralithium salt solution.

AMCA-6-dUTP is used for nonradioactive labeling of DNA. The modified nucleoside is a substrate for *E. coli* DNA polymerase I (holoenzyme and Klenow fragment), T4 and T7 DNA polymerase, *Taq* DNA polymerase, and reverse transcriptases (AMV and M-MuLV). Amino-coumarin–labeled probes used in direct *in situ* hybridizations give a bright blue fluorescent signal.

Biotin-16-dUTP, solution   1427 598   25 nmol (25 μl)

Tetralithium salt, 1 mM, in H$_2$O. 2′-Deoxyuridine-5′-triphosphate, coupled to biotin via a 16-atom spacer arm.

Biotin-16-dUTP, an analogue of dTTP, may be incorporated into DNA by standard enzymatic techniques (e.g., random primed labeling, nick translation) to produce a non-radioactive hybridization probe. Biotinylated DNA may be detected with an avidin or streptavidin conjugate.

Biotin-16-ddUTP, solution   1093 070   50 nmol (50 μl)

Tetralithium salt, 1 mM aqueous solution. 2′,3′-dideoxyuridine-5′-triphosphate, coupled to biotin via a 16-atom spacer arm.

Oligonucleotides can be enzymatically labeled at the 3′ end with a single biotin-16–ddUTP molecule to produce nonradioactive probes. Biotin-16-ddUTP–labeled probes can be used in standard DNA hybridization techniques (e.g., colony and plaque screening, *in situ* hybridization, screening gene libraries) and can be detected with avidin or streptavidin conjugates.

Dig-DNA labeling mixture (10×)	1277 065	50μl
For random primed labeling of DNA with digoxigenin-dUTP, alkali-labile.		(25 reactions)

Solution containing 1 mM dATP, 1 mM dCTP, 1 mM dGTP, 0.65 mM dTTP, 0.35 mM dig-dUTP; pH 6.5.

The labeling mixture may be used for random primed labeling of DNA with digoxigenin-dUTP (dig-dUTP). The mixture contains enough nucleotides for 25 standard DNA labeling reactions (10 ng to 3 μg DNA each).

Dig-RNA labeling mixture (10×)	1277 073	40 μl
For transcriptional labeling of RNA with digoxigenin-UTP.		(20 reactions)

Solution containing 10 mM ATP, 10 mM CTP, 10 mM GTP, 6.5 mM UTP, 3.5 mM dig-UTP; pH 6.5.

The labeling mixture may be used for transcriptional labeling of RNA with digoxigenin-UTP (dig-UTP). The mixture contains enough nucleotides to label 20 RNA samples (up to 10 μg RNA each) with SP6, T7, or T3 RNA polymerase.

Digoxigenin-3-O-methylcarbonyl-ε-amino-caproic acid N-hydroxysuccinimide ester   1333 054   5 mg

(Digoxigenin-NHS-ester)

Powder.

Digoxigenin-NHS-ester may be covalently coupled to amino groups of proteins or oligonucleotides. Digoxigenin-labeled proteins may be easily detected with the Digoxigenin Detection Kit. Labeled oligonucleotides can be detected using the Genius™ 3 Kit, the Genius™ 7 Kit, or Lumi-Phos‑ 530.

Digoxigenin-16-dATP, solution	1558 714	2.5 nmol
		(25 μl)

Tetralithium salt, 1 mM, in H$_2$O. 2′-Deoxyadenosine-5′-triphosphate coupled to digoxigenin via a 16-atom spacer arm.

Digoxigenin-16-dATP, an analogue of dATP, may be used as a substrate for T7 DNA polymerase for internal digoxigenin labeling of DNA fragments. The modified nucleotide is a poor substrate for *Taq* DNA polymerase. Digoxigenin-labeled DNA may be detected with an antibody–enzyme conjugate, such as antidigoxigenin–alkaline phosphatase.

| **Digoxigenin-11-ddUTP, solution** | 1363 905 | 25 nmol (25 ml) |

Lithium salt, 1 mM, in aqueous solution. 2′,3′-Dideoxyuridine-5′-triphosphate, coupled to digoxigenin via an 11-atom spacer arm.

Digoxigenin-11-ddUTP, an analogue of ddTTP, may be used, with terminal transferase, to add a nonradioactive label to the 3′-end of a DNA probe. Digoxigenin-labeled DNA may be detected with the Genius™ 3 Nonradioactive Nucleic Acid Detection Kit or the Genius™ 7 Luminescent Detection Kit.

| **Digoxigenin-11-dUTP, alkali-labile, solution** | 1573 152 | 25 nmol (25 µl) |
| | 1573 179 | 125 nmol (125 µl) |

Tetralithium salt, 1 mM, in H$_2$O. 2′-Deoxyuridine-5′-triphosphate, coupled to digoxigenin via an 11-atom spacer arm.

Digoxigenin-11-dUTP, an analogue of dTTP, may be incorporated into DNA by standard enzymatic techniques (e.g., random primed labeling, nick translation) to produce a nonradioactive hybridization probe. Digoxigenin-labeled DNA may be detected with an antibody–enzyme conjugate, antidigoxigenin–alkaline phosphatase. Application: The alkali-labile form is more suitable than the alkali-stable form for probe labeling when stripping and reprobing (especially when multiple reprobing) of blots is intended. The alkali-labile form is sensitive to treatment with NaOH and cannot be used when alkali probe denaturation is required.

| **Digoxigenin-11-dUTP, alkali-stable, solution** | 1093 088 | 25 nmol (25 µl) |
| | 1558 706 | 125 nmol (125 µl) |

Tetralithium salt, 1 mM, in H$_2$O. 2′-Deoxyuridine-5′-triphosphate, coupled to digoxigenin via an 11-atom spacer arm.

Digoxigenin-11-dUTP, an analogue of dTTP, may be incorporated into DNA by standard enzymatic techniques (e.g., random primed labeling, nick translation) to produce a nonradioactive hybridization probe. Digoxigenin-labeled DNA may be detected with an antibody–enzyme conjugate, such as antidigoxigenin–alkaline phosphatase.

| **Digoxigenin-11-UTP, solution** | 1209 256 | 250 nmol (25 µl) |

10 mM tetralithium salt solution, in H$_2$O. Uridine-5′-triphosphate coupled to digoxigenin via an 11-atom spacer arm.

Digoxigenin-11-UTP, an analog of UTP, may be incorporated into RNA by standard enzymatic techniques (e.g., in vitro transcription with SP6, T3 or T7 RNA polymerase) to produce a nonradioactive hybridization probe. Digoxigenin-labeled RNA may be detected with an antibody-enzyme conjugate such as anti-digoxigenin-alkaline phosphatase.

| **Fluorescein-15-dATP, solution** | 1498 142 | 25 nmol (25 µl) |

1 mM aqueous tetralithium salt solution. 2′-Deoxyadenosine-5′-triphosphate coupled to fluorescein via a 15-atom spacer arm.

Fluorescein-15-dATP is incorporated into DNA by DNA polymerases and reverse transcriptases for nonradioactive labeling of DNA. Fluorescein-labeled DNA may be used as a nonradioactive *in situ* hybridization probe and is detectable by fluorescence microscopy or with an antifluorescein antibody conjugate. Fluorescein-15-dATP can also be used to label DNA for nonradioactive DNA sequencing according to Ansorge, W. et al. (1992) Methods Mol. Cell. Biol. 3, in press.

Fluorescein-12-ddUTP, solution   1427 849   25 nmoles
(25 µl)

1 mM aqueous tetralithium salt solution. 2′,3′-dideoxyuridine-5′-triphosphate coupled to fluorescein via a 12-atom spacer arm.

Oligonucleotides can be enzymatically labeled at the 3′-end with a single fluorescein-12-ddUTP molecule to produce nonradioactive probes. Fluorescein-labeled DNA may be detected directly with fluorescein microscopy or indirectly with an antibody to fluorescein conjugated to alkaline phosphatase.

Fluorescein-12-dUTP solution   1427 857   250 nmol
(25 µl)

1 mM aqueous lithium salt solution. 2′-Deoxyuridine-5′-triphosphate coupled to fluorescein via a 12-atom spacer arm.

Fluorescein-12-dUTP, an analogue of dTTP, is incorporated into DNA by DNA polymerases, reverse transcriptases, or terminal transferase. Fluorescein-labeled DNA may be used as a nonradioactive *in situ* hybridization probe and is detectable by fluorescence microscopy or with an antifluorescein antibody conjugate.

High Prime Biotin DNA Labeling Mix   1585 649   100 µl
(25 reactions)

For nonradioactive labeling of DNA using random oligonucleotide primers and biotin-16-dUTP.

5× concentrated aqueous solution in 50% glycerol containing 12-mer random primers; a nucleotide mixture with biotin-16-dUTP, Klenow enzyme, and reaction buffer.

Biotin-labeled DNA probes can be used in Southern and Northern blot hybridizations, colony or plaque screenings, *in situ* hybridizations, and as capture probes in streptavidin-coated microtiter plate immunoassays. Biotin-labeled DNA probes can be detected with streptavidin–POD or –AP conjugates and color or chemiluminescent substrates.

High Prime Digoxigenin DNA Labeling Mix   1585 606   160 µl
(40 reactions)

For nonradioactive labeling of DNA using random oligonucleotide primers and digoxigenin-11-dUTP.

5× concentrated aqueous solution in 50% glycerol containing 12-mer random primers; a nucleotide mixture with digoxigenin-11-dUTP, Klenow enzyme, and reaction buffer.

Digoxigenin-labeled DNA probes can be used in Southern and Northern blot hybridizations and colony or plaque screenings and *in situ* hybridizations. Digoxigenin-labeled DNA probes can be detected with the Genius™ 3 Nucleic Acid Detection Kit or the Genius™ 7 Luminescent Detection Kit.

High Prime Fluorescein DNA Labeling Mix   1585 622   100 µl
(25 reactions)

For nonradioactive labeling of DNA using random oligonucleotide primers and fluorescein-12-dUTP.

5× concentrated aqueous solution in 50% glycerol containing 12-mer random primers; a nucleotide mixture with fluorescein-12-dUTP, Klenow enzyme, and reaction buffer.

Fluorescein-labeled DNA probes can be used in Southern and Northern blot hybridizations and colony or plaque screenings. They can be detected with an antifluorescein antibody conjugate and a color or luminescent substrate.

PCR DIG Labeling Mix*   1585 550   50 reactions

Two vials: each vial contains the lithium salt solutions in water (10× concentrated) of dATP, dCTP, dGTP, each at a concentration of 2 mM; TTP (1.9 mM); and digoxigenin-dUTP (0.1 mM); pH 7.0.

This ready-to-use solution can be added directly to polymerase chain reactions. The dig-labeled nucleotide will be incorporated by both *Taq* and Tth DNA polymerases into the PCR product allowing sensitive detection of amplification products.

*This product is sold under licensing arrangements with Roche Molecular Systems and The Perkin-Elmer Corporation. Purchase of this product is accompanied by a license to use it in the Polymerase Chain Reaction (PCR) process in conjunction with an Authorized Thermal Cycler.

Rhodamine-6-dUTP	1534 378	25 nmol (25 µl)

(Tetramethyl-rhodamine-6-2'-deoxyuridine-5'-triphosphate)

1 mM aqueous tetralithium salt solution.

Rhodamine-6-dUTP is used for nonradioactive labeling of DNA. The modified nucleoside is a substrate for *E. coli* DNA polymerase I (holoenzyme and Klenow fragment), T4 and T7 DNA polymerase, *Taq* DNA polymerase, and reverse transcriptases (AMV and M-MuLV). Rhodamine-labeled probes used in direct *in situ* hybridizations give a red fluorescent signal.

Antibodies for Nonradioactive Detection

Antidigoxigenin Fab fragment	unlabeled	1214 667	1 mg
Form: Solution (alkaline phosphatase conjugate) and lyophilized,	alkaline	1093 274	150 U
stabilized (all others). **Type:** Affinity purified polyclonal, Fab fragments.	phosphatase		
Host species: Sheep. **Specificity:** Antidigoxigenin reacts with the cardiac			
glycoside digoxigenin. The antibody shows <1% cross-reactivity with other	AMCA	1533 878	200 mg
steroids. The Fab fragments prepared by proteolytic digestion of the			
purified antibody retain the antigen-binding sites of the native molecule.	fluorescein	1207 741	200 ug
Contaminants: Essentially free of nonspecific antibodies.			
Stability: Stable at +4°C. Store the AMCA, fluorescein, and rhodamine	peroxidase	1207 733	150 U
conjugates protected from light. **Note:** The AMCA conjugate fluoresces			
bright blue, the fluorescein conjugate gives a yellow fluorescent signal, and	rhodamine	1207 750	200 ug
the rhodamine conjugate fluoresces red. **Application:** To detect digoxigenin-			
labeled compounds, e.g., in a nonradioactive DNA or RNA hybridization			
assay or in a glycoprotein assay. A Fab preparation eliminates nonspecific			
adsorption to cellular Fc receptors.			

Antidigoxigenin	1333 062	100 µg

Form: Lyophilized, stabilized. **Type:** Monoclonal. **Host species:** Mouse. **Clone:** 1.71.256. **Subclass:** IgG₁k. **Characterization and specificity:** Antibody, subclass IgG₁, binds to free or immobilized digoxigenin. **Application:** For nonradioactive assay of digoxigenin-conjugated macromolecules (e.g., proteins, nucleic acids) on nitrocellulose membranes, microtiter plates, and tissue sections.

Antidigoxigenin	1333 089	200 µg

Form: Lyophilized, stabilized. **Type:** Affinity purified polyclonal. **Host species:** Sheep. **Specificity:** Reacts with free or immobilized digoxigenin. **Application:** For nonradioactive assay of digoxigenin-conjugated macromolecules (e.g., proteins, nucleic acids) on nitrocellulose membranes, microtiter plates, and tissue sections.

Nonradioactive Hybridization and Detection Reagents

Blocking reagent for nucleic acid hybridization	1096 176	50 g

Form: Powder. **Typical analysis:** Tested for performance in a nonradioactive DNA hybridization assay. **Suggested working concentration:** 3% (w/v). Treatment of a nitrocellulose or nylon filter containing "blotted" DNA with blocking reagent will minimize the nonspecific binding of detecting antibody in a nonradioactive DNA hybridization assay.

BM blue, precipitating (POD substrate)	1442 066	100 ml

Form: Ready-to-use solution. The preparation is a chromogenic substrate for horseradish peroxidase (POD) designed for precipitating enzyme immunoassays. It can also be used for immunoblots and other techniques.

BM purple, precipitating (AP substrate)	1442 074	100 ml

Form: Ready-to-use solution. The preparation is a chromogenic substrate for alkaline phosphate (AP) designed for precipitating enzyme immunoassays. It can also be used for immunoblots and other techniques.

5-Bromo-4-chloro-3-indolyl-phosphate (BCIP, X-phosphate)	1383 221	3 ml (150 mg)

Form: Toluidine salt solution, 50 mg/ml, in dimethylformamide. X-phosphate is a substrate for phosphatases (particularly alkaline phosphatase), which cleave it to form an insoluble blue dye. X-phosphate is particularly useful in immunohistochemical studies to localize a phosphatase-conjugated antibody.

Digoxigenin 3′-end labeled control oligonucleotide	1585 754	125 pmol (50 µl)

Form: Aqueous solution containing 125 pmol of an oligonucleotide (30-mer) with the following sequence: 5′-pTTG GGT AAC GCC AGG GTT TTC CCA GTC ACG-DIG-3′. The oligonucleotide is homologous to the *lacZ* region of the pUC and M13 plasmids. **Concentration:** 2.5 nmol/ml. **Application:** As a control hybridization probe in blots and for estimating the yield of digoxigenin-labeled oligonucleotide probes.

Digoxigenin-labeled control DNA (pBR328)	1585 738	250 ng (50 µl)

Form: Aqueous solution of linearized pBR328 DNA (1 µg of template DNA and approx. 250 ng of digoxigenin-labeled DNA). **Application:** As a control hybridization probe in blots and for estimating the yield of digoxigenin-labeled DNA probes.

Digoxigenin-labeled control RNA	1585 746	5 µg (50 µl)

Form: Aqueous solution containing approx. 5 µg of digoxigenin-labeled antisense neopA-RNA. **Stability:** Stable for at least 12 months when stored at −20°C. **Application:** As a control hybridization probe in blots and for estimating the yield of digoxigenin-labeled RNA probes.

Lumigen® PPD	1357 328	1 ml (100× conc.)

Chemiluminescent substrate for alkaline phosphatase, for use with the Genius™ Nonradioactive Nucleic Acid Labeling and Detection System.

Form: Solution, containing 4-methoxy-4-(3-phosphatephenyl)-spiro-(1,2-dioxetane-3,2′-adamantane), disodium salt; 10 mg/ml (23.5 mM). **Note:** Lumigen PPD, a chemiluminescent substrate for alkaline phosphatase, emits light as it is enzymatically cleaved. The light released is directly proportional to the amount of alkaline phosphatase (or alkaline phosphatase-conjugated antibody) present and will produce a signal on a piece of x-ray film. When used with the Genius™System on a Southern blot, Lumigen PPD produces enough light in 15 to 30 minutes to visualize a single copy gene.

Lumi-Phos® 530	1413 155	40 ml
	1275 470	100 ml
	1413 163	200 ml

Chemiluminescent substrate for alkaline phosphatase, for use with the Genius™ Nonradioactive Nucleic Acid Detection System.

Form: Solution, containing 4-methoxy-4-(3-phosphatephenyl)-spiro-(1,2-dioxetane-3,2′-adamantane), disodium salt, 0.33 mM; 2-amino-2-methyl-1-propanol (pH 9.6), 750 mM; $MgCl_2$, 0.88 mM; cetyltrimethylammonium bromide, 1.13 mM; fluorescein surfactant, 0.035 mM. **Note:** Lumi-Phos 530, a chemiluminescent substrate for alkaline phosphatase, emits light as it is enzymatically cleaved. The light released is directly proportional to the amount of alkaline phosphatase (or alkaline phosphatase-conjugated antibody) present and will produce a signal on a piece of x-ray film. When used with the Genius™System to assay a Southern blot, Lumi-Phos 530 produces enough light in 15 to 30 minutes to visualize a single copy gene.

Multi-Color DNA Detection Set[4]	14650341	3 × 50 tablets

Provides three colorimetric alkaline phosphatase substrates in tablet form and allows discrete nucleic acid sequences to be detected with differently colored hybridization signals on the same blot.

The set includes

1. 50 alkaline phosphatase substrate tablets (green). Each tablet contains 2 mg of naphthol-AS-GR-phosphate and 3.5 mg of Fast Blue B.

2. 50 alkaline phosphatase substrate tablets (red). Each tablet contains 2 mg of naphthol-AS-phosphate and 1 mg of Fast Red TR.

3. 50 alkaline phosphatase substrate tablets (blue). Each tablet contains 2 mg of naphthol-AS-phosphate and 3.5 mg of Fast Blue B.

Quality control: Using labeled control DNA (e.g., pBR328), 0.3 pg of homologous DNA diluted with 50 ng of heterologous DNA is detected on a dot blot with the Multi-Color DNA Detection Set after 2 hours of color development. Under identical conditions, 50 ng of heterologous DNA is not detected when probed with labeled control DNA (e.g., pBR328).
Applications: For detection of multiple target sequences on the same blot or specimen. Useful applications include genomic Southern blots of lower eukaryotes, plasmid mapping, Northern blots comparing the abundance of different mRNAs, and colony and plaque hybridizations.

Labeling and Hybridization

	Cat. No.	Size
PRINS Reaction Sets		
Dig PRINS Reaction Set	1695 932	1 set (40 reactions, 5 controls)
Rhodamine PRINS Reaction Set	1768 514	1 set (40 reactions, 5 controls)
PRINS Oligunucleotide Primers		
Human Chromosome 1 specific	1695 959	100 ml (20 reactions)
Human Chromosome 1 + 16 specific	1768 549	100 ml (20 reactions)
Human Chromosome 3 specific	1695 967	100 ml (20 reactions)
Human Chromosome 7 specific	1695 975	100 ml (20 reactions)
Human Chromosome 8 specific	1695 983	100 ml (20 reactions)
Human Chromosome 9 (SAT) specific	1768 565	100 ml (20 reactions)
Human Chromosome 10 specific	1768 522	100 ml (20 reactions)
Human Chromosome 11 specific	1695 991	100 ml (20 reactions)
Human Chromosome 12 specific	1696 009	100 ml (20 reactions)
Human Chromosome 14 + 22 specific	1768 557	100 ml (20 reactions)
Human Chromosome 17 specific	1696 017	100 ml (20 reactions)
Human Chromosome 18 specific	1696 025	100 ml (20 reactions)
Human Chromosome X specific	1696 033	100 ml (20 reactions)
Human Chromosome Y specific	1696 041	100 ml (20 reactions)
All Human Chromosome specific	1699 172	100 ml (20 reactions)
Human Telomere Specific	1699 199	100 ml (20 reactions)
DNA probes, human chromosomes		
1 specific, digoxigenin-labeled	1558 765	1 mg (50 ml)
1 specific, fluorescein-labeled	1558 684	1 mg (50 ml)
1 + 5 + 19 specific, digoxigenin-labeled	1690 507	1 mg (50 ml)
1 + 5 + 19 specific, fluorescein-labeled	1690 647	1 mg (50 ml)
2 specific, digoxigenin-labeled	1666 479	1 mg (50 ml)
2 specific, fluorescein-labeled	1666 380	1 mg (50 ml)
3 specific, digoxigenin-labeled	1690 515	1 mg (50 ml)
4 specific, digoxigenin-labeled	1690 523	1 mg (50 ml)
6 specific, digoxigenin-labeled	1690 531	1 mg (50 ml)
7 specific, digoxigenin-labeled	1690 639	1 mg (50 ml)
7 specific, fluorescein-labeled	1694 375	1 mg (50 ml)
8 specific, digoxigenin-labeled	1666 487	1 mg (50 ml)
8 specific, fluorescein-labeled	1666 398	1 mg (50 ml)
9 specific, digoxigenin-labeled	1690 540	1 mg (50 ml)
10 specific, digoxigenin-labeled	1690 558	1 mg (50 ml)
10 specific, fluorescein-labeled	1690 655	1 mg (50 ml)
11 specific, digoxigenin-labeled	1690 566	1 mg (50 ml)
11 specific, fluorescein-labeled	1690 663	1 mg (50 ml)
12 specific, digoxigenin-labeled	1690 574	1 mg (50 ml)
12 specific, fluorescein-labeled	1690 671	1 mg (50 ml)
13 + 21 specific, digoxigenin-labeled	1690 582	1 mg (50 ml)

14 + 22 specific, digoxigenin-labeled	1666 495	1 mg (50 ml)
14 + 22 specific, fluorescein-labeled	1666 401	1 mg (50 ml)
15 specific, digoxigenin-labeled	1690 604	1 mg (50 ml)
16 specific, digoxigenin-labeled	1699 091	1 mg (50 ml)
17 specific, digoxigenin-labeled	1666 452	1 mg (50 ml)
17 specific, fluorescein-labeled	1666 371	1 mg (50 ml)
18 specific, digoxigenin-labeled	1666 509	1 mg (50 ml)
18 specific, fluorescein-labeled	1666 428	1 mg (50 ml)
20 specific, digoxigenin-labeled	1666 517	1 mg (50 ml)
20 specific, fluorescein-labeled	1666 436	1 mg (50 ml)
22 specific, digoxigenin-labeled	1690 612	1 mg (50 ml)
X specific, digoxigenin-labeled	1666 525	1 mg (50 ml)
X specific, fluorescein-labeled	1666 444	1 mg (50 ml)
Y specific, digoxigenin-labeled	1558 196	1 mg (50 ml)
Y specific, fluorescein-labeled	1558 692	1 mg (50 ml)
Specific for all human chromosomes, digoxigenin-labeled	1558 757	1 mg (50 ml)
Specific for all human chromosomes, fluorescein-labeled	1558 676	1 mg (50 ml)

Enzo Diagnostics, 60 Executive Boulevard, Farmingdale, New York 11735
Telephone (516)755-5500

Hybridization/Detection Reagents

Nonradioactive Labeling of Nucleic Acids—Modified Nucleotides

Enzo's proprietary labeling systems have been formatted for a wide variety of research needs. Each labeling kit contains all the necessary reagents and a detailed protocol for the preparation of labeled probes. Detection of these probes after hybridization requires the use of visualization reagents such as DETEK® Signal Generating Sysems. For those scientists who wish to adapt the *BioProbe*® technology to their own specific needs, Enzo offers proprietary biotin as well as digoxigenin, fluorescent modified nucleotides.

BioProbe® Nick Translation DNA Labeling Systems

Cat. No.	Product
	Nick Translation Labeling Kits
42710-11	Nick Translation Kit with Bio-11-dUTP, 25 x 1 μg reactions
42710-12	Nick Translation Kit with Bio-16-dUTP, 25 x 1 μg reactions
42710-13	Nick Translation Kit with Bio-11-dCTP, 25 x 1 μg reactions
42710-14	Nick Translation Kit with Bio-7-dATP, 25 x 1 μg reactions
42710-15	Nick Translation Kit with Digoxigenin-11-dUTP, 25 x 1 μg reactions
42710-16	Nick Translation Kit with Fluorescein-12-dUTP, 25 x 1 μg reactions
	Nick Translation Deoxynucleotide Packs
Cat. No.	Product
42711	Bio-11-dUTP for Nick Translation, 25 reactions
42712	Bio-16-dUTP for Nick Translation, 25 reactions
42713	Bio-11-dCTP for Nick Translation, 25 reactions
42714	Bio-7-dATP for Nick Translation, 25 reactions
42715	Digoxigenin-11-dUTP for Nick Translation, 25 reactions
42716	Fluorescein-12-dUTP for Nick Translation, 25 reactions
	Nick Translation Reagent Pack
Cat. No.	Product
42710	Reagent Pack for Nick Translation, 25 reactions

BioProbe® Random Primed DNA Labeling Systems

Random Primed Labeling Kits

Cat. No.	Product
42720-21	Random Primed Labeling Kit with Bio-11-dUTP, 25 x 1 µg reactions
42720-22	Random Primed Labeling Kit with Bio-16-dUTP, 25 x 1 µg reactions
42720-23	Random Primed Labeling Kit with Bio-11-dCTP, 25 x 1 µg reactions
42720-24	Random Primed Labeling Kit with Bio-7-dATP, 25 x 1 µg reactions
42720-25	Random Primed Labeling Kit with Digoxigenin-11-dUTP, 25 x 1 µg reactions
42720-26	Random Primed Labeling Kit with Fluorescein-12-dUTP, 25 x 1 µg reactions

Random Primed Deoxynucleotide Packs

Cat. No.	Product
42721	Bio-11-dUTP for Random Primed Labeling, 25 reactions
42722	Bio-16-dUTP for Random Primed Labeling, 25 reactions
42723	Bio-11-dCTP for Random Primed Labeling, 25 reactions
42724	Bio-7-dATP for Random Primed Labeling, 25 reactions
42725	Digoxigenin-11-dUTP for Random Primed Labeling, 25 reactions
42726	Fluorescein-12-dUTP for Random Primed Labeling, 25 reactions

Random Primed Labeling Reagent Pack

Cat. No.	Product
42720	Reagent Pack for Random Primed Labeling, 25 reactions

BioProbe® 3′-Oligonucleotide Labeling Systems

3′-Oligo Labeling Kits

Cat. No.	Product
42730-31	3′-Oligo Labeling Kit with Bio-16-ddUTP, 25 x 100 picomoles reactions
42730-32	3′-Oligo Labeling Kit with Digoxigenin-11-ddUTP, 25 x 100 picomoles reactions
42730-33	3′-Oligo Labeling Kit with Fluorescein-12-ddUTP, 25 x 100 picomoles reactions

3′-Oligo Dideoxynucleotide Packs

Cat. No.	Product
42731	Bio-16-ddUTP for 3′-Oligo Labeling
42732	Digoxigenin-11-ddUTP for 3′-Oligo Labeling, 25 reactions
42733	Fluorescein-12-ddUTP for 3′-Oligo Labeling, 25 reactions

3′-Oligo Tailing Kits

Cat. No.	Product
42730-41	3′-Oligo Tailing Kit with Bio-11-dUTP, 25 x 100 picomoles reactions
42730-42	3′-Oligo Tailing Kit with Bio-16-dUTP, 25 x 100 picomoles reactions
42730-43	3′-Oligo Tailing Kit with Bio-11-dCTP, 25 x 100 picomoles reactions
42730-44	3′-Oligo Tailing Kit with Bio-7-dATP, 25 x 100 picomoles reactions
42730-45	3′-Oligo Tailing Kit with Digoxigenin-11-dUTP, 25 x 100 picomoles reactions
42730-46	3′-Oligo Tailing Kit with Fluorescein-12-dUTP, 25 x 100 picomoles reactions

3′-Oligo Deoxynucleotide Packs

Cat. No.	Product
42741	Bio-11-dUTP for 3′-Oligo Tailing, 25 reactions
42742	Bio-16-dUTP for 3′-Oligo Tailing, 25 reactions
42743	Bio-11-dCTP for 3′-Oligo Tailing, 25 reactions

42744	Bio-7-dATP for 3'-Oligo Tailing, 25 reactions
42745	Digoxigenin-11-dUTP for 3'-Oligo Tailing, 25 reactions
42746	Fluorescein-12-dUTP for 3'-Oligo Tailing, 25 reactions

OligoBridge™ Labeling Kits

Cat. No.	Product
42730-36	OligoBridge™ Labeling Kit, 25 x 100 picomoles reactions

OligoBridge™ Nucleotide Pack

Cat. No.	Product
42736	Nucleotide Pack for OligoBridge™ Labeling, 25 reactions

Oligo Labeling Reagent Pack

Cat. No.	Product
42730	Reagent Pack for Oligonucleotide Labeling, 25 reactions

BioProbe® RNA Transcript Labeling Systems

RNA Labeling Kits

Cat. No.	Product
42750-51	RNA Labeling Kit with Bio-11-UTP, 20 x 1 µg reactions
42750-52	RNA Labeling Kit with Bio-16-UTP, 20 x 1 µg reactions
42750-53	RNA Labeling Kit with Bio-11-CTP, 20 x 1 µg reactions
42750-54	RNA Labeling Kit with Bio-17-ATP, 20 x 1 µg reactions
42750-55	RNA Labeling Kit with Digoxigenin-11-UTP, 20 x 1 µg reactions
42750-56	RNA Labeling Kit with Fluorescein-12-UTP, 20 x 1 µg reactions

RNA Ribonucleotide Packs

Cat. No.	Product
42751	Bio-11-UTP for RNA Labeling, 20 reactions
42752	Bio-16-UTP for RNA Labeling, 20 reactions
42753	Bio-11-CTP for RNA Labeling, 20 reactions
42754	Bio-17-ATP for RNA Labeling, 20 reactions
42755	Digoxigenin-11-UTP for RNA Labeling, 20 reactions
42756	Fluorescein-12-UTP for RNA Labeling, 20 reactions

RNA Labeling Reagent Pack

Cat. No.	Product
42750	Reagent Pack for RNA Labeling, 20 reactions

Modified Deoxynucleotides

Cat. No.	Product
42806	Bio-11-dUTP, 1.0 mM
42811	Bio-16-dUTP, 1.0 mM
42816	Bio-11-dCTP, 1.0 mM
42812	Bio-AP3-dCTP, 0.3 mM
42819	Bio-7-dATP, 1.0 mM
42821	Digoxigenin-11-dUTP, alkali labile, 1.0 mM
42822	Digoxigenin-11-dUTP, alkali stable, 1.0 mM
42831	Fluorescein-12-dUTP, 1.0 mM
42841	Rhodamine-dUTP, 1.0 mM

42851   Coumarin-dUTP, 1.0 mM

Modified Dideoxynucleotides

Cat. No.	Product
42813	Bio-16-ddUTP, 1.0 mM
42823	Digoxigenin-11-ddUTP, 1.0 mM
42833	Fluorescein-12-ddUTP, 1.0 mM

Modified Ribonucleotides

Cat. No.	Product
42815	Bio-11-UTP, 10 mM
42814	Bio-16-UTP, 10 mM
42818	Bio-11-CTP, 10 mM
42817	Bio-17-ATP, 10 mM
42824	Digoxigenin-11-UTP, 10 mM
42834	Fluorescein-12-UTP, 10 mM

Membrane Hybridization and Detection

Enzo's *MaxSense*™ Membrane Hybridization and Detection Systems offer the scientist all the reagents required for nonradioactive Southern, Northern or dot blot analyses. The many labeling opportunities provided by Enzo are complemented with a complete line of products for specific, problem-free, maximum sensitivity membrane hybridization and detection of biotin- digoxigenin- and flurorescein-labeled nucleic acid probes.

MaxSense™ Membrane Hybridization Systems

Cat. No.	Product
45500	*MaxSense*™ *BioProbe*® Membrane Hybridization System *(for DNA & RNA Probes)*, 10 blots 10 × 10 cm each
45600	*MaxSense*™ *OligoProbe*™ Membrane Hybridization System *(for Oligonucleotide Probes)*, 10 blots 10 × 10 cm each

MaxSense™ Detection Systems

Cat. No.	Product
45401	*BioDETEK*® HP Hrp Membrane Detection System, 1000 cm^2
45402	*BioDETEK*® Alk Membrane Detection System, 1000 cm^2
45403	*DigDETEK*® HP Hrp Membrane Detection System, 1000 cm^2
45404	*DigDETEK*® AP Membrane Detection System, 1000 cm^2
45405	*FluorDETEK*® Hrp Membrane Detection System, 1000 cm^2
45406	*FluorDETEK*® AP Membrane Detection System, 1000 cm^2

MaxSense™ BioProbe® Hybridization and Detection System Kits for DNA and RNA Probes

Cat. No.	Product
	Horseradish Peroxidase Detection Systems
45501	*BioDETEK*® HP Hrp Complete *BioProbe*® Membrane System, 10 blots 10 x 10 cm each
45503	*DigDETEK*® HP Hrp Complete *BioProbe*® Membrane System, 10 blots 10 x 10 cm each
45505	*FluorDETEK*® Hrp Complete *BioProbe*® Membrane System, 10 blots 10 x 10 cm each
	Alkaline Phosphatase Detection Systems
45502	*BioDETEK*® Alk Complete *BioProbe*® Membrane System, 10 blots 10 x 10 cm each
45504	*DigDETEK*® AP Complete *BioProbe*® Membrane System, 10 blots 10 x 10 cm each
45506	*FluorDETEK*®AP Complete *BioProbe*® Membrane System, 10 blots 10 x 10 cm each

MaxSense™ OligoProbe™ Hybridization and Detection System Kits for Oligonucleotide Probes

Cat. No.	Product
	Horseradish Peroxidase Detection System
45601	*BioDETEK*® HP Hrp Complete *OligoProbe*™ Membrane System, 10 blots 10 x 10 cm each
45603	*DigDETEK*® HP Hrp Complete *OligoProbe*™ Membrane System, 10 blots 10 x 10 cm each
45605	*FluorDETEK*® Hrp Complete *OligoProbe*™ Membrane System, 10 blots 10 x 10 cm each
	Alkaline Phosphatase Detection System
45602	*BioDETEK*® Alk Complete *OligoProbe*™ Membrane System, 10 blots 10 x 10 cm each
45604	*DigDETEK*® AP Complete *OligoProbe*™ Membrane System, 10 blots 10 x 10 cm each
45606	*FluorDETEK*® AP Complete *OligoProbe*™ Membrane System, 10 blots 10 x 10 cm each

MaxSense™ Hybridization and Detection System Accessories

Cat. No.	Product
45701	Hybridization Membrane *(roll)*, 30 cm x 3 m
45702	Hybridization Membrane *(pre-cut sheets)*, 10 sheets, 15 cm x 10 cm
45703	Blocking Solution *(ready-to-use)*, 100 ml
45704	Liquid Blocking Reagent *(concentrated)*, 100 ml
45705	*MaxSense*™ *BioProbe*® Hybridization Buffer, 150 ml
45706	*MaxSense*™ *OligoProbe*™ Hybridization Buffer, 150 ml

Dot Blot System

Cat. No.	Product
46305	Dot Blot Hybridization and Detection Assay Kit, 100 tests
46305/C	Dot Blot Control DNA Pack
46307	Dot Blot CMV Control DNA Pack
46308	Dot Blot HBV Control DNA Pack

In Situ Hybridization Assay Systems

Enzo's *PathoGene*® DNA Probe Assays and Apop*DETEK*®Cell Death Assays are comprised of two parts, a Probe Pack or Labeling Pack and a Detection System of choice, thus allowing for either colorimetric or fluorescence detection of in situ hybridization. Each of the systems is complete with all the necessay ready-to-use reagents and complete easy-to-follow protocols. Enzo's *PathoGene*® HPV and *BioPap*® HPV kits have been formatted for *in situ* hybridization reactions and contain all the necessary reagents, including probe, buffers and detection reagents.

Detection Assays

Cat. No.	Product
	SimplySensitive™ Detection Systems
32830	Hrp - AEC System for *in situ* Detection, 20 slides
32840	Hrp - DAB System for *in situ* Detection, 20 slides
32850	Fl-SA System for *in situ* Detection, 20 slides
32860	Alk Phos - INT/BCIP System for *in situ* Detection, 20 slides
32870	Alk Phos - NBT/BCIP System for *in situ* Detection, 20 slides
	UltraSensitive™ Enhanced Detection Systems
32300	Enhanced Hrp - AEC System for *in situ* Detection, 30 slides
32400	Enhanced Hrp - DAB System for *in situ* Detection, 30 slides
32500	Enhanced Fl -SA System for *in situ* Detection, 30 slides

32600   Enhanced Alk Phos - INT/BCIP System for *in situ* Detection, 30 slides
32700   Enhanced Alk Phos - NBT/BCIP System for *in situ* Detection, 30 slides

PathoGene® DNA Probe Assays

Cat. No.   **Product**

SimplySensitive™ - Horseradish Peroxidase - AEC Detection

32801-30   *PathoGene®* Assay for Adenovirus/Hrp - AEC, 20 slides
32802-30   *PathoGene®* Assay for Cytomegalovirus/Hrp - AEC, 20 slides
32803-30   *PathoGene®* Assay for Epstein-Barr Virus/Hrp - AEC, 20 slides
32804-30   *PathoGene®* Assay for Hepatitis B Virus/Hrp - AEC, 20 slides
32805-30   *PathoGene®* Assay for Herpes Simplex Virus/Hrp - AEC, 20 slides
32806-30   *PathoGene®* Assay for *Chlamydia trachomatis*/Hrp - AEC, 20 slides

SimplySensitive™ - Horseradish Peroxidase - DAB Detection

32801-40   *PathoGene®* Assay for Adenovirus/Hrp - DAB, 20 slides
32802-40   *PathoGene®* Assay for Cytomegalovirus/Hrp - DAB, 20 slides
32803-40   *PathoGene®* Assay for Epstein-Barr Virus/Hrp - DAB, 20 slides
32804-40   *PathoGene®* Assay for Hepatitis B Virus/Hrp - DAB, 20 slides
32805-40   *PathoGene®* Assay for Herpes Simplex Virus/Hrp - DAB, 20 slides
32806-40   *PathoGene®* Assay for *Chlamydia trachomatis*/Hrp - DAB, 20 slides

SimplySensitive™ - Fluorescent Streptavidin Detection

32801-50   *PathoGene®* Assay for Adenovirus/Fl-SA, 20 slides
32802-50   *PathoGene®* Assay for Cytomegalovirus/Fl-SA, 20 slides
32803-50   *PathoGene®* Assay for Epstein-Barr Virus/Fl-SA, 20 slides
32804-50   *PathoGene®* Assay for Hepatitis B Virus/Fl-SA, 20 slides
32805-50   *PathoGene®* Assay for Herpes Simplex Virus/Fl-SA, 20 slides
32806-50   *PathoGene®* Assay for *Chlamydia trachomatis*/Fl-SA, 20 slides

SimplySensitive™ - Alkaline Phosphatase - INT/BCIP Detection

32801-60   *PathoGene®* Assay for Adenovirus/Alk Phos - NBT/BCIP, 20 slides
32802-60   *PathoGene®* Assay for Cytomegalovirus/Alk Phos - NBT/BCIP, 20 slides
32803-60   *PathoGene®* Assay for Epstein-Barr Virus/Alk Phos - NBT/BCIP, 20 slides
32804-60   *PathoGene®* Assay for Hepatitis B Virus/Alk Phos - NBT/BCIP, 20 slides
32805-60   *PathoGene®* Assay for Herpes Simplex Virus/Alk Phos - NBT/BCIP, 20 slides
32806-60   *PathoGene®* Assay for *Chlamydia trachomatis*/Alk Phos - NBT/BCIP, 20 slides

SimplySensitive™ - Alkaline Phosphatase - NBT/BCIP Detection

32801-70   *PathoGene®* Assay for Adenovirus/Alk Phos - NBT/BCIP, 20 slides
32802-70   *PathoGene®* Assay for Cytomegalovirus/Alk Phos - NBT/BCIP, 20 slides
32803-70   *PathoGene®* Assay for Epstein-Barr Virus/Alk Phos - NBT/BCIP, 20 slides
32804-70   *PathoGene®* Assay for Hepatitis B Virus/Alk Phos - NBT/BCIP, 20 slides
32805-70   *PathoGene®* Assay for Herpes Simplex Virus/Alk Phos - NBT/BCIP, 20 slides
32806-70   *PathoGene®* Assay for *Chlamydia trachomatis*/Alk Phos - NBT/BCIP, 20 slides

UltraSensitive™ Enhanced - Horseradish Peroxidase - AEC Detection

32801-33   *PathoGene®* Assay for Adenovirus/Enhanced Hrp - AEC, 20 slides
32802-33   *PathoGene®* Assay for Cytomegalovirus/Enhanced Hrp - AEC, 20 slides
32803-33   *PathoGene®* Assay for Epstein-Barr Virus/Enhanced Hrp - AEC, 20 slides
32804-33   *PathoGene®* Assay for Hepatitis B Virus/Enhanced Hrp - AEC, 20 slides
32805-33   *PathoGene®* Assay for Herpes Simplex Virus/Enhanced Hrp - AEC, 20 slides
32806-33   *PathoGene®* Assay for *Chlamydia trachomatis*/Enhanced Hrp - AEC, 20 slides

UltraSensitive™ Enhanced - Horseradish Peroxidase - DAB Detection

32801-44   *PathoGene®* Assay for Adenovirus/Enhanced Hrp - DAB, 20 slides
32802-44   *PathoGene®* Assay for Cytomegalovirus/Enhanced Hrp - DAB, 20 slides

32803-44	*PathoGene*® Assay for Epstein-Barr Virus/Enhanced Hrp - DAB, 20 slides
32804-44	*PathoGene*® Assay for Hepatitis B Virus/Enhanced Hrp - DAB, 20 slides
32805-44	*PathoGene*® Assay for Herpes Simplex Virus/Enhanced Hrp - DAB, 20 slides
32806-44	*PathoGene*® Assay for *Chlamydia trachomatis*/Enhanced Hrp - DAB, 20 slides

UltraSensitive™ Enhanced - Fluorescent Streptavidin Detection

32801-55	*PathoGene*® Assay for Adenovirus/Enhanced Fl -SA, 20 slides
32802-55	*PathoGene*® Assay for Cytomegalovirus/Enhanced Fl -SA, 20 slides
32803-55	*PathoGene*® Assay for Epstein-Barr Virus/Enhanced Fl -SA, 20 slides
32804-55	*PathoGene*® Assay for Hepatitis B Virus/Enhanced Fl -SA, 20 slides
32805-55	*PathoGene*® Assay for Herpes Simplex Virus/Enhanced Fl -SA, 20 slides
32806-55	*PathoGene*® Assay for *Chlamydia trachomatis*/Enhanced Fl -SA, 20 slides

UltraSensitive™ Enhanced - Alkaline Phosphatase - INT/BCIP Detection

32801-66	*PathoGene*® Assay for Adenovirus/Enhanced Alk Phos - INT/BCIP, 20 slides
32802-66	*PathoGene*® Assay for Cytomegalovirus/Enhanced Alk Phos - INT/BCIP, 20 slides
32803-66	*PathoGene*® Assay for Epstein-Barr Virus/Enhanced Alk Phos - INT/BCIP, 20 slides
32804-66	*PathoGene*® Assay for Hepatitis B Virus/Enhanced Alk Phos - INT/BCIP, 20 slides
32805-66	*PathoGene*® Assay for Herpes Simplex Virus/Enhanced Alk Phos - INT/BCIP, 20 slides
32806-66	*PathoGene*® Assay for *Chlamydia trachomatis*/Enhanced Alk Phos - INT/BCIP, 20 slides

Ultrasensitive™ Enhanced - Alkaline Phosphatase - NBT/BCIP Detection

32801-77	*PathoGene*® Assay for Adenovirus/Enhanced Alk Phos - NBT/BCIP, 20 slides
32802-77	*PathoGene*® Assay for Cytomegalovirus/Enhanced Alk Phos - NBT/BCIP, 20 slides
32803-77	*PathoGene*® Assay for Epstein-Barr Virus/Enhanced Alk Phos - NBT/BCIP, 20 slides
32804-77	*PathoGene*® Assay for Hepatitis B Virus/Enhanced Alk Phos - NBT/BCIP, 20 slides
32805-77	*PathoGene*® Assay for Herpes Simplex Virus/Enhanced Alk Phos - NBT/BCIP, 20 slides
32806-77	*PathoGene*® Assay for *Chlamydia trachomatis*/Enhanced Alk Phos - NBT/BCIP, 20 slides

PathoGene® Tissue Preparation Kit and Control Slides

Cat. No.	Product
32800	*PathoGene*® Tissue Preparation Kit, 20 specimens
31871	Adenovirus Control Slide
31872	Cytomegalovirus Control Slide
31873	Epstein-Barr Control Slide
31875	Herpes Simplex Virus Control Slide
31876	*Chlamydia trachomatis* Control Slide
31877	HPV 16 Probe Control Slide

ApopDETEK® *In Situ* Cell Death Assay Systems

Cat. No.	Product
32930	*ApopDETEK*® *in situ* Cell Death Assay/Hrp - AEC, 20 slides
32940	*ApopDETEK*® *in situ* Cell Death Assay/Hrp - DAB, 20 slides
32950	*ApopDETEK*® *in situ* Cell Death Assay/Fl -SA, 20 slides
32960	*ApopDETEK*® *in situ* Cell Death Assay/Alk Phos - INT/BCIP, 20 slides
32970	*ApopDETEK*® *in situ* Cell Death Assay/Alk Phos - NBT/BCIP, 20 slides

Human Papillomavirus Identification Systems

Cat. No.	Product
32881	*BioPap*® Human Papillomavirus *in situ* Screening Assay for Cervical Smears, 20 tests
32892	*BioPap*® Human Papillomavirus *in situ* Typing Assay for Cervical Specimens *(Types 6/11, 16/18 and 31/33/51),* 10 tests
32883	*BioPap*® Human Papillomavirus *in situ* Typing Assay Cervical Specimen Transport Kit, 10 specimens
32879	*PathoGene*® Human Papillomavirus *in situ* Screening Assay for Tissue Sections, 20 tests
32895	*PathoGene*® Human Papillomavirus *in situ* Typing Assay for Tissue Sections *(Types 6/11, 16/18 and 31/33/51),* 10 tests

| 32877 | *PathoGene®* Hrp-AEC Human Papillomavirus *in situ* Typing Assay for Tissue Sections *(Types 6/11, 16/18 and 31/33/51),* 20 tests |
| 32874 | *PathoGene®* Hrp-DAB Human Papillomavirus *in situ* Typing Assay for Tissue Sections *(Types 6/11, 16/18 and 31/33/51),* 20 tests |

In Situ Hybridization Accessories

Cat. No.	Product

Specimen Slides

31802/20	Pretreated slides/single well, 20 slides
31802/100	Pretreated slides/single well, 100 slides
31803/20	Pretreated slides/double well, 20 slides
31803/100	Pretreated slides/double well, 100 slides

Heating Blocks and Surface Thermometer

31500	Heating Block for use with 110V, 50/60 Hz
31508	Heating Block for use with 220V, 50 Hz
31580	Surface Thermometer

Biological Reagents and Buffers

33801	Proteinase K, 2×5 mg
33802	Enzo Wash Buffer Salts, 3×1L packets
33803	Enzo *SignaSure®* Wash Buffer, 3×1L packets
33804	Dilution Buffer for Horseradish Peroxidase-linked Detection Reagents, 100 ml
33805	Dilution Buffer for Alkaline Phosphatase-linked Detection Reagents, 100 ml
33806	Dilution Buffer for Fluorescence-linked Streptavidin, 100 ml
33807	Dilution Buffer for Double Antibody Enhancement Procedures, 100 ml
33808	*In situ* Hybridization Buffer *(1.25 × concentrate),* 10 ml
33809	*In situ* Hybridization Wash Reagent, 30 ml

Bioprobe® Labeled Probes

Enzo offers biotin-labeled probes for those researchers who wish to design their own hybridization procedures. These concentrated probes can be used for hybridization in an *in situ* format or for hybridization to nucleic acids immobilized on a solid matrix for Southern blot, Northern blot or dot blot analysis.

Cat. No.	Product

Infectious Agents

40834	Adenovirus, 2 µg
40835	Cytomegalovirus, 2 µg
40836	Epstein-Barr Virus, 2 µg
40837	Hepatitis B Virus, 2 µg
40838	Herpes Simplex Virus, 2 µg
40839	*Chlamydia trachomatis,* 2 µg
40842	Hepatitis A Virus, 2 µg
40843	*Mycoplasma pneumonia,* 2 µg
40845	SV40, 2 µg
40846	*Campylobacter jejuni,* 2 µg
40847	JC Virus, 2 µg
40848	BK Virus, 2 µg

Oncogenes

| 40717 | c-*Myc,* 2 µg |
| 40718 | N-*Myc,* 2 µg |

Hybridization Controls

| 40840 | Lambda, 2 µg |
| 40849 | Blur 8 (human *alu* repeat), 2 µg |

DETEK® Signal Generating Systems

Enzo offers a wide variety of systems for the detection labeled nucleic acids, proteins and antibodies. Detection systems are available for biotin, digoxigenin, fluorescein haptens. The systems are based on recognition of biotin by streptavidin or anti-biotin antibodies, of digoxigenin by anti-digoxigenin conjugate and of fluorescein by anti-fluorescein conjugate.

Cat. No.	Product
	Fluorescent Biotin Detection
43818	DETEK® 1-f *(Double Antibody Fluorescence Detection)*, 200 slides
43821	DETEK® FS *(Fluorescent Streptavidin Detection)*, 100 slides
	DETEK® **Colorimetric Signal Generating Systems**
43820	DETEK® Hrp Kit *(Hrp - AEC Detection)*, 500ml working soln or 40 membranes
43830	DigDETEK® Hrp Kit *(Hrp - AEC Detection)*, 500ml working soln or 40 membranes
43840	FluorDETEK® Hrp Kit *(Hrp - AEC Detection)*, 500ml working soln or 40 membranes
43822	DETEK® Alk Kit *(Alk Phos- NBT/BCIP Detection)*, 500ml working soln or 40 membranes
43832	DigDETEK® AP Kit *(Alk Phos- NBT/BCIP Detection)*, 500ml working soln or 40 membranes
43842	FluorDETEK® AP Kit *(Alk Phos- NBT/BCIP Detection)*, 500ml working soln or 40 membranes
	Anti-Biotin Antibody Reagents
43823	DETEK® Enhancer Kit *(Double Antibody Enhanced Detection)*, 30 slides
43861	Rabbit anti-Biotin Antibody Concentrate, 400ml working soln
	Colorimetric Signal Generating Reagents
43825	AEC Substrate Kit, 300ml working soln
43826	DAB Substrate Kit, 300ml working soln
43827	NBT/BCIP Substrate Kit, 400ml working soln
43828	INT/BCIP Substrate Kit, 400ml working soln

Microplate Hybridization Assays

The Enzo Microplate Hybridization Assay System is an easy-to-use, rapid and nonradioactive kit for detecting DNA in a microtiter well. The assay procedure, based on a two probe hybridization method can be carried out either directly, if there is sufficinet target DNA present, or following DNA amplification procedures.

Cat. No.	Product
46330	HIV 1 Microplate Hybridization Assay, 96 test kit
46340	MTB Microplate Hybridization Assay, 96 test kit
46350	HBV *(core antigen sequences)* Microplate Hybridization Assay, 96 test kit
46360	HIV 2 Microplate Hybridization Assay, 96 test kit
46380	HBV *(surface antigen sequences)* Microplate Hybridization Assay, 96 test kit
46353	Enhanced Microplate Hybridization Assay for Hepatitis B, 96 test kit
46354	Enhanced Microplate Hybridization Assay for Hepatitis B Serum Titration Standards, 4 runs
46331	Oligonucleotide Pair SK38/SK39, 2 x 5 nmol
46341	Oligonucleotide Pair MTB10/MTB11, 2 x 5 nmol
46351	Oligonucleotide Pair HB01/HB02, 2 x 5 nmol
46355	Oligonucleotide Pair HB07/HB08, 2 x 5 nmol
46361	Oligonucleotide Pair VB306/VB310, 2 x 5 nmol
46381	Oligonucleotide Pair HB011/HB014, 2 x 5 nmol
46382	Oligonucleotide Pair HB012/HB013, 2 x 5 nmol

Oncor Corporation, 209 Perry Parkway, Gaithersburg, Maryland 20877

Pre-Mixed Hybridization Solutions

Description	Catalog No.	Quantity
Hybrisol®[VI]	S1370-30	$10 \times 750 \, \mu l$

(65% Formamide, 2×SSC, dextran sulfate, and other blocking reagents)
For nonisotopic *in situ* detection of chromosome-specific probes.

Description	Catalog No.	Quantity
Hybrisol®[VII]	S1390-10	$10 \times 750 \, \mu l$

(50% Formamide, 2×SSC, dextran sulfate, and other blocking reagents)
For nonisotopic *in situ* detection of chromosome-specific probes.

Description	Catalog No.	Quantity
Hybrisol®[VIII]	S1372-10	$10 \times 750 \, \mu l$

(78% Formamide, 2.4×SSC, dextran sulfate, and other blocking reagents)
For nonisotopic *in situ* detection of chromosome-specific probes.

Description	Catalog No.	Quantity
Hybridization Mix I	S1319	$10 \times 180 \, \mu l$

(55% Formamide, 2.2×SSC, 1 mM DTT, and other blocking reagents)
For isotopic *in situ* detection with RNA probes.

Description	Catalog No.	Quantity
Hybridization Mix II	S1320	$10 \times 180 \, \mu l$

(55% Formamide, 2.2×SSC, 1 mM DTT, 11% dextran sulfate, and other blocking reagents)
For isotopic *in situ* detection with DNA probes.

Other Hybridization Reagents and Accessories

Description	Catalog No.	Quantity
Formamide	S4117	500 ml

Triple-distilled and packaged under nitrogen to ensure high performance in isotopic or nonisotopic hybridization procedures.

Description	Catalog No.	Quantity
Dextran sulfate, powder	S4010	100 g
Dextran sulfate, 50% solution	S4030	100 ml/500 ml bottle
Dextran Sulfate, 50% solution	S4031	200 ml/1000 ml bottle

Dextran sulfate (MW > 500,000) is supplied in either powder or 50% solution form (autoclaved). The 50% solution is packaged in a convenient oversized bottle with enough room to add all other ingredients for a final concentration of 10% dextran sulfate.

Description	Catalog No.	Quantity
Silanized slides	S1308	100 slides and 1 oz. box of coverslips

Silanized slides are acid washed, ethanol dried, and then treated with 3-aminopropyltriethoxysilane. Slides are then washed in deionized water, air dried, and packaged into a reusable slide box. Qualified for paraffin-embedded or fresh frozen tissues and cytospins.

Labeling Kits

Description	Catalog No.	Quantity
Probe Labeling Kit	S4089-KIT	Labels 20 µg DNA

Complete reagent set and protocol for preparing biotin, digoxigenin, or isotopically labeled probes. The kit utilizes the nick translation technique, which relies on the concerted action of DNase I and *E. coli* DNA polymerase I.

Large Fragment Probe Labeling Kit	S4099-KIT	Labels 20 µg DNA

Efficiently labels cosmids and YACs with either biotin or digoxigenin for nonisotopic *in situ* hybridization. Reagent con-centrations are optimized for fragments larger than 30 kb, and probe sizes of 300 to 600 base pairs are routinely achieved for maximum *in situ* signal strength.

Perkin-Elmer Corporation, Applied Biosystems Division, 850 Lincoln Center Drive, Foster City, CA 94404
Telephone: (415)570-6667; For more information call 1-800-345-5224. For PCR technical support call 1-800-762-4001.

In Situ **PCR**

As your research uncovers new challenges, PCR technology must advance to meet your needs. Since, 1987, Perkin-Elmer has been delivering PCR solutions to laboratories worldwide. New standards in PCR performance are being established as the needs of amplifying RNA and DNA targets, within a cell or a population of cell types becomes of interest. The power of PCR amplification to amplify DNA and RNA targets starting from a single copy of target has been demonstrated in solution. How-ever, it is not possible to identify after solution PCR which cells within the multiple cell population contain the target sequence of interest. The major technological breakthrough of *in situ* PCR is the localization of amplified sequences within the cell.

GeneAmp® *In situ* **PCR System 1000**

Another milestone in PCR Technology

Description

The GeneAmp *in situ* PCR System 1000 offers a complete solution to your needs of performing PCR *in situ* within a cell. The technology offers a major revolution in the art of performing the technique. Perkin-Elmer offers an integrated instru-ment design, uniquely engineered vertical block, novel consumables, oil and adhesive free operation, optimized reagents and controls, unsurpassed cycle time reproducibility and high performance PCR protocols. The GeneAmp *In situ* PCR System 1000 with our high quality GeneAmp *In situ* PCR Core Kit (PE No. N808-0197), can be quickly and reliably used for a variety of applications, some of which are listed below:

• Identification of cells with latent viral infections
• Unique gene alterations associated with neoplastic disorders
• Gene rearrangements
• Chromosomal translocation
• Gene expression in specific cell types
• Monitor progression of diseases of effect of therapy

Because of the demands for *in situ* PCR technology, the innovative engineering and advanced system design of the GeneAmp *In situ* PCR System 1000 introduces new standards of precision, accuracy, efficiency, reproducibility, and conve-nience. The GeneAmp *In situ* PCR System 1000 offers the following advantages:

Unique sample block
Sample temperature display
High throughput 10 slides, 30 samples
Oil and adhesive free operation
Novel containment system

Ability to do the hot start technique
Optimized reagents and protocols

Unique Sample Block Design for unmatched temperature uniformity

The only vertical block that offers the capacity of 10 slides and throughput of 30 samples. The new design of the DNA thermal cycler sample block provides advanced uniform heating and cooling throughout the entire sample block. The glass slides are entirely embedded in the aluminum block and heated and cooled to ensure excellent temperature accuracy. The block is engineered to optimize the thermal contact between the slots and glass slides.

The special block design along with enhanced specifications improves uniformity cycle to cycle and slide to slide to ensure the highest reproducibility of results. This offers guaranteed optimal performance in every sample and every run.

Advanced software with Sample temperature display

The GeneAmp® *In situ* PCR System 1000 has advanced software with calculated sample temperature displays. It eliminates the need of any external temperature probes and provides temperature precision of actual cycling parameters. Temperature can be set in 0.1°C increments. There are 99 user files, 4 preprogrammed files and 93 user storage files.

Novel Reagent Containment System

To make *in situ* PCR broadly useful and easy to perform, Perkin-Elmer introduces specially engineered consumables as part of the GeneAmp *In situ* PCR System 1000 to optimize the *in situ* PCR process and to ensure highest temperature and amplification uniformity of your samples. Their patent pending design eliminates the need of oil overlays and creates a tight seal preventing samples from drying.

The consumables comprise of AmpliCovers™ discs and Clips that are clamped over the microscopic slides containing the sample. The AmpliCover disc is a concave silicone rubber diaphragm that holds the reagents over the sample to be amplified and is PCR compatible. The Clips are made of stainless steel and slide over the AmpliCover discs with a considerable force, making a pressure-tight seal. The AmpliCover disc and Clip together provide an environment that is favorable for *in situ* PCR and offers a unique solution to the use of nail-polish and other adhesives. This significantly reduces handling time. The size of the AmpliCovers discs and Clips allows assembly of up to three samples on each microscopic slide, giving a throughput of 30 samples per run. The Assembly Tool described below is used for quick and easy assembly of the AmpliCovers discs and Clips.

Assembly Tool

Our advanced engineering of the Assembly Tool allows quick and easy assembly of your samples prior to cycling, as well as provides the ability to do physical hot starts. Hot starts are often critical to the success of an *in situ* PCR amplification. In the case of solution PCR, physical hot starts can be easily done using AmpliWax™ PCR Gems, an approach that is not feasible for *in situ* PCR amplification.

Thermal hot start can be implemented using our Assembly Tool. The tool has a heater and a temperature sensor. The slide is placed on a metal platen. The platen is thermostated at a pre-fixed temperature of 80°C. When the slide is placed on the platen, the temperature rapidly rises to 80°C. The complete reagent mixture including the enzyme is then placed over the sample. Since all the DNA is inside the cell, the chances of cooling to a mispriming temperature is minimized.

The vertical swinging arm of the assembly tool has a magnet that holds the Clip and the AmpliCover discs and is swung down over the reagent and clamped onto the microscopic slide. The reagent is spread uniformly over the sample and ready for PCR amplification. The process is simple.

In situ PCR Glass Slides

Perkin-Elmer provides silane-coated glass slides that are quality controlled and tested for *in situ* PCR amplification. The slides are routinely checked for their thermal tolerance and heat transferability.

Optimized protocols

The GeneAmp® *In situ* PCR System 1000 is backed by Perkin-Elmer PCR performance guarantee. Using the GeneAmp® *In situ* PCR System 1000 with the GeneAmp® *In situ* PCR Core and the protocols included in the package inserts, *in situ* PCR amplification of a single coy gene (HLADRB) can be achieved.

Components

- GeneAmp® *In situ* PCR System 1000 (Part Nos. N804-0001, N804-0002, N804-0003).
  A thermal cycler that is designed for doing *in situ* PCR and offers high throughput and uniform performance

- AmpliCovers (Part No. N804-0500) and Clips (Part No. N804-0501).
  Each set contains 50 AmpliCovers and 10 Clips respectively

- Assembly Tool (Part No. N804-0100).
  A tool to place the AmpliCovers and Clips on the glass slides

- *In situ* PCR Glass Slides (Part No. N804-0502).
  Each set contains 50 glass slides that have been pretested for *in situ* PCR

- GeneAmp *In situ* PCR Core Kit (Part No. N808-0197).
  A 100 reaction kit that has a formulation of AmpliTaq® DNA Polymerase, buffer, dNTPs for *In situ* PCR amplifications.

- GeneAmp *In situ* PCR cell Control Kit (Part No. N808-0198).
  Contains 10 silane coated glass slides each with 3 samples per slide of K-562 human leukemia cells prefixed with buffered formalin and ready for amplifications. Also included are a set of HLA DRB and Lambda Primer sets that serve as positive and negative controls respectively.

- Use Manual

GeneAmp® In situ **PCR Core Kit**	**PE No.**	**Qty**
The first kit for *in situ* PCR optimized for a wide range of samples	N808-0197	1 Kit

Description

The GeneAmp *In situ* PCR Core Kit provides all the basic reagents needed for PCR amplification *in vivo* utilizing the GeneAmp PCR process. This Kit is optimized for use with the controls in our GeneAmp *In situ* PCR cell Control Kit C (PE No. N808-0198) on our GeneAmp® *In situ* PCR system 1000, and is an integral part of the first complete system enabling efficient, reproducible and convenient *In situ* PCR, with cells or tissue samples of your choice.

The GeneAmp PCR process within cells and tissues is performed after fixation of the sample with standard fixatives. It is important to preserve the morphology of the tissue for accurate result interpretation. Unlike solution phase PCR, the amplification reagents do not have easy access to the target. A protease treatment may be required to allow the penetration of PCR reagents within the cells or desired tissue sample. The amplification is performed using this Kit with tailored primers on a sample of choice.

The GeneAmp *In situ* PCR Core Kit includes GeneAmp10X *In situ* PCR Buffer and a separate mM MgCl₂ Solution set of all four nucleotides designed for use with your own primers and samples. It also includes AmpliTaq® DNA Polymerase, *IS,* a magnesium ion-dependent enzyme, that is the key to the GeneAmp PCR process *in vivo.* The reagents have been optimized for use on a GeneAmp *In situ* PCR System 1000.

Components

- AmpliTaq® DNA Polymerase, *IS* (20 Units/μL)

- GeneAmp® dNTPs
  Set of four, consists of dATP, dTTP, dGTP, and dCTP, each vial containing 320 μL of a 10 mM solution of the specified deoxynucleoside triphosphate

- GeneAmp® 10X *In situ* PCR Buffer mL consisting of 500 mM KCl and 100 mM Tris-HCl, pH 8.3

- MGCl₂ Solution, 1.5 mL, 25 mM

- Package insert with *In situ* PCR protocols

PCR Performance Guarantee

The performance of the GeneAmp *In situ* PCR Core Kit is guaranteed for PCR amplification when it is used with a GeneAmp *In situ* PCR System 1000 and with protocols included in the package inserts . *In situ* PCR amplification of a single copy gene HLA DRB can be achieved.

Related Products

GeneAmp® *In situ* PCR Cell Control Kit C (PE No. N808-0198), GeneAmp® *In situ* PCR System 1000 (PE Nos. N804-0001, N804-0002, N804-0003), Assembly Tool (PE No. N804-0100), AmpliCovers (PE No. N804-0500), Clips (PE No. N804-0501), *In situ* PCR glass slides (PE No. N804-0502).

GeneAmp® *In situ* **PCR Control Kit C**	**PE No.**	**Qty**
The only *In situ* PCR control kit optimized for guaranteed PCR performance	N808-0198	1 Kit

Description

GeneAmp® *In situ* Cell PCR Control Kit C is the first and only commercially available kit that consists of a cell sample that has been pretreated and optimized for PCR amplification using our GeneAmp® *In situ* PCR Core Kit (PE No. N808-0197) on our GeneAmp® *In situ* PCR System 1000 (see Chapter 10). The kit comprises of 10 silane-coated glass slides with 3 spots per slide of K-562 human leukemia cells that have been fixed in buffered formalin.

K-562 is a continuous cell line of chronic myelogenous leukemia of a 53-year-old female. The cell population has been characterized as highly undifferentiated terminal blast cells of the granulocytic series. These blast cells are multipotential, hematopoietic malignant cells that spontaneously differentiate into progenitors of erythrocytic, granulocytic, and monocytic series.

Also included are HLA DRB and Lambda Primer sets that serve as positive and negative controls, respectively. These synthetic oligonucleotide primers are HPLC-purified and checked for base composition.

Components

- *In situ* PCR Cell Control Slides
  10 silanized glass slides with spots each of K-562 cells prefixed for 4 hrs in 10% buffered formalin
- HLA DRB Primer GH46 (Positive Control Primer #1)
  Sequence: 5′-CCGGATCCTTCGTGTCCCCACAGCACG-3′
- HLA DRB Primer AB60 (Positive Control Primer #2)
  Sequence: 5′-CCGAATTCCGCTGCACTGTGAAGCTCTC-3′
- Lambda Control Primer #1 (Negative Control Primer #1)
  Sequence: 5′-GATGAGTTCGTGTCCGTACAACTGG-3′
- Lambda Control Primer #2 (Negative Control Primer #2)
  Sequence: 5′-GGTTATCGAAATCAGCCACAGCGCC-3′

These products are designed and intended for research use only, and not for medical or diagnostic use.

Related Products

GeneAmp® *In situ* PCR Kit (PE No. N808-0197), GeneAmp® *In situ* PCR System 1000 (PE Nos. N804-0001, N804-0002, N804-0003), Assembly Tool (PE No. N804-0100), AmpliCovers (PE No. N804-0500), Clips (PE No. N804-0501).

Subject Index

Subject Index

ISBN 0-397-58749-X

9 780397 587490